Amy Chaudhury MD

MULTIPLE SCLEROSIS

MULTIPLE SCLEROSIS

Clinical and pathogenetic basis

EDITED BY

Cedric S. Raine,

Henry F. McFarland

and

Wallace W. Tourtellotte

CHAPMAN & HALL MEDICAL

London · Weinheim · New York · Tokyo · Melbourne · Madras

Published by Chapman & Hall, 2–6 Boundary Row, London SE1 8HN

Chapman & Hall, 2–6 Boundary Row, London SE1 8HN, UK

Chapman & Hall GmbH, Pappelallee 3, 69469 Weinheim, Germany

Chapman & Hall USA, 115 Fifth Avenue, New York, NY 10003, USA

Chapman & Hall Japan, ITP-Japan, Kyowa Building, 3F, 2-2–1 Hirakawacho, Chiyoda-ku, Tokyo 102, Japan

Chapman & Hall Australia, 102 Dodds Street, South Melbourne, Victoria 3205, Australia

Chapman & Hall India, R. Seshadri, 32 Second Main Road, CIT East, Madras 600 035, India

First edition 1997

© 1997 Chapman & Hall

Typeset in 10/12 Sabon by Genesis Typesetting, Rochester, Kent
Printed at The University Press, Cambridge

ISBN 0 412 30890 8

A catalogue record for this book is available from the British Library

Library of Congress Catalog Card Number: 96–85631

CONTENTS

CONTRIBUTORS

ROBERT W. BAUMHEFNER, MD
Neurology Service,
West Los Angeles VA Medical Center,
11301 Wilshire Blvd,
Los Angeles, CA 90073,
USA

GEORGE S. BENSON, MD
Department of Surgery,
Division of Urology,
University of Texas Medical School,
6431 Fannin, Suite 6.018,
Houston, TX 77030,
USA

MOHAMED BIDAIR, MD
Division of Urology,
University of California, San Diego,
UCSD Medical Center (8897),
200 West Arbor Drive,
San Diego, CA 92103–8897,
USA

CELIA BROSNAN, PhD
Department of Pathology,
Albert Einstein College of Medicine,
1300 Morris Park Avenue,
The Bronx, NY 10461,
USA

DIANE L. COOKFAIR, MD
Department of Neurology,
State University of New York at Buffalo,
Buffalo General Hospital,
100 Goodrich Street,
Buffalo, NY 14203,
USA

MARGARET M. ESIRI, DM, FRCPath
Department of Neuropathology,
Radcliffe Infirmary,
Oxford, OX2 6HE
UK

DEREK GAY, MD
Department of Biomedical Science,
Anglia Polytechnic University,
Cambridge CB1 1PT
UK

DONALD E. GOODKIN, MD
The UCSF/MT Zion Multiple Sclerosis Center,
1600 Divisadero Street,
San Francisco, CA 94115
USA

MICHAEL KATZ, MD
March of Dimes Birth Defects Foundation,
National Office,
1275 Mamaroneck Avenue,
White Plains, NY 10605
USA

JOHN F. KURTZKE, MD
Department of Neurology, Georgetown University
   School of Medicine;
Neuroepidemiology Section, Neurology Service,
Veterans Affairs Medical Center, Washington, DC;
c/o 7509 Salem Road,
Falls Church,
VA 22043–3240,
USA

GREG LEMKE, PhD
Molecular Neurobiology Laboratory,
The Salk Institute,
PO Box 85800,
San Diego, CA 92186,
USA

ROLAND MARTIN, MD
Neurologische Universitätsklinik,
Hoppe-Seyler-Str. 3,
D-72076 Tübingen,
Germany

HENRY F. McFARLAND, MD
Neuroimmunology Branch,
National Institute of Neurological Disorders and
    Stroke,
Building 10, Room 5B–16,
10 Center DR MSC 1400,
Bethesda, MD 20892–1400,
USA

DALE E. McFARLIN, MD
Neuroimmunology Branch, NINDS,
National Institutes of Health,
Bethesda MD 20892,
USA

VOLKER TER MEULEN, MD
Institut für Virologie und Immunbiologie,
Universität Würzburg,
Versbacher-Str.-7,
D-97078 Würzburg,
Germany

DAVID H. MILLER, MD, FRCP
Institute of Neurology,
National Hospital for Neurology and Neurosurgery,
Queen Square,
London WC1N 3BG,
UK

GALEN W. MITCHELL, MD
Department of Neurology,
The University of Alabama at Birmingham,
Birmingham Veterans Medical Center,
Suite 1052, Tinsley Harrison Tower,
Birmingham, AL 35294–0007
USA

MARC R. NUWER, MD, PhD
UCLA Department of Neurology,
Reed Neurological Research Center,
710 Westwood Plaza,
Los Angeles, CA 90024–6987
USA

C. LOWELL PARSONS, MD
Division of Urology,
University of California, San Diego,
UCSD Medical Center (8897),
200 West Arbor Drive,
San Diego, CA 92103–8897
USA

MICHAEL K. RACKE, MD
Department of Neurology,
Washington University,
660 South Euclid Avenue,
St Louis, MO 63110
USA

STEPHEN M. RAO, PhD
Department of Neurology,
Medical College of Wisconsin,
9200 West Wisconsin Avenue,
Milwaukee, WI 53226
USA

CEDRIC S. RAINE, PhD, DSc, FRCPath
Department of Pathology (Neuropathology),
Albert Einstein College of Medicine,
1300 Morris Park Avenue,
The Bronx, NY 10461, USA

RICHARD A. RUDICK, MD
Department of Neurology,
The Mellen Center U10,
Cleveland Clinic Foundation,
9500 Euclid Avenue,
Cleveland, OH 44195,
USA

E. MICHAEL SEDGWICK, MD, FRCP
Clinical Neurological Sciences,
University of Southampton,
General Hospital,
Tremona Road,
Southampton, SO16 6YD,
UK

KRZYSZTOF SELMAJ, MD, PhD
Department of Neurology,
Medical Academy of Lodz,
22 Kopcinskiego Street,
Lodz,
Poland 90–153

RANDALL T. SCHAPIRO, MD
The Fairview MS Center,
701 25th Avenue South, Suite 200,
Minneapolis, MN 55454
USA

WILLIAM A. SIBLEY, MD
Department of Neurology,
University of Arizona College of Medicine,
Health Sciences Center,
1501 N. Campbell Avenue, Room 7329,
Tucson, AZ 85724–5023,
USA

WALLACE W. TOURTELLOTTE, MD, PhD
Neurology Service (127),
West Los Angeles VA Medical Center,
11301 Wilshire Blvd,
Los Angeles, CA 90073,
USA

HAYRETTIN TUMANI, MD
Klinik und Poliklinik für Neurologie,
Georg-August-Universität,
Robert Koch Str.-40,
D-37075 Göttingen,
Germany

BRIAN G. WEINSHENKER, MD
Mayo Clinic,
Department of Neurology,
200 First Street, SW,
Rochester, MN 55905,
USA

JOHN N. WHITAKER, MD
Department of Neurology,
The University of Alabama at Birmingham,
Birmingham Veterans Medical Center,
625 South 19th Street,
Birmingham, AL 35294–0007,
USA

SHIRLEY H. WRAY, MD, PhD, FRCP
Unit for Neurovisual Visual Disorders,
Department of Neurology,
Massachusetts General Hospital,
15 Parkman Street – ACC 837,
Boston, MA 02114,
USA

PREFACE

Fully cognizant of the challenge and somewhat intimidated by the rapidity of developments in the field, it was with no small degree of trepidation that the Editors undertook the task of compiling for the clinician, the investigator and the student, a state-of-the-art text on multiple sclerosis. Further, we recognized that thousands of publications about multiple sclerosis already existed and that to have a single volume that delivers facts, controversy and practical aspects comprehensively might give a timely push to the momentum to eradicate multiple sclerosis and to ease the disease in the afflicted. Attempts to define multiple sclerosis fully have never met with everyone's approval since, like the canvas of the master painter, details always need to be added or changed. Multiple sclerosis is a serious condition to the patient and the family who have to live with it, an awesome task to the clinician who confronts it, and a formidable challenge to the investigator who chooses to research it. With evidence implicating an immunologic basis for lesion pathogenesis and the myelin sheath as the primary target, there has been in recent years a heavy bias towards a break in self-tolerance and autoimmunity as major mechanisms. This and other immunologic anomalies now figure prominently in several treatment modalities and are presented in a balanced fashion in many chapters of this book.

In mixing the first pigments for application to the canvas, the editors labored long over the composition of the table of contents and the choice of contributors. Accordingly, we decided to meld the works of clinicians from several disciplines with laboratory-based scientists actively researching neuroimaging, electrophysiology, molecular neuropathology, neurobiology, immunopathology and virology. To accomplish this, the book is divided into four sections: clinical parameters, neuropathology and etiopathogenesis, primary treatments, and symptomatic treatments based on advances in psychiatry, medicine and surgery. Cumulatively, these are areas that have permitted us to accomplish the goal of full longevity and modestly improved quality of life. In an attempt to keep abreast with developments in the field and to counter the possibility of becoming prematurely outdated, each chapter not only provides didactic coverage but also indicates recent trends and makes predictions for the future. Some sections are even more speculative and provide rationale for therapies not yet in vogue. The net result is a fresh, kaleidoscopic overview of multiple sclerosis from both the applied and basic standpoints – the balance between broad brush strokes and fine detail has been carefully weighed.

The compilation of this book has occupied the Editors and the contributors for more than two years. Particularly rewarding was the gradual realization by the Editors that the topics selected blended well and that the coverage is as complete as one can make it as of this date. Although our original palette began with and retained some authors from the book *Multiple Sclerosis: Pathology, Diagnosis and Management* by Hallpike, Adams and Tourtellotte (Chapman & Hall, London, 1983), more than 75% of the contributors are new to this volume and many cover topics that were not in existence in 1983.

We feel that any reader entering into a dialogue with this book will emerge refreshed, fulfilled and brimming with anticipation about what the next clinical trial will bring, when the viral/genetic pathogenesis relationship will be clarified, whether with etiology in hand we can design preventive and more effective primary treatments, and when more able symptomatic treatments will be discovered. We are not unaware that this will not be the last word on multiple sclerosis, but we are confident that, for several years to come, it will be regarded as the latest.

Cedric S. Raine, New York City, NY
Henry F. McFarland, Washington, DC
Wallace W. Tourtellotte, Los Angeles, CA

ABBREVIATIONS

AAO	age at onset
ACTH	adrenocorticotrophic hormone
ADCA	autosomal dominant cerebellar ataxia
ADEM	acute disseminated encephalomyelitis
AON	acute optic neuritis
APC	antigen-presenting cell
AR	at-risk
BAEP	brain stem auditory evoked potential
BBB	blood–brain barrier
bFGF	basic fibroblast growth factor
CDR	complement defining region
CFA	complete Freund's adjuvant
CNS	central nervous system
CNTF	ciliary neurotrophic factor
CSF	cerebrospinal fluid
CT	computerized tomography
DSS	disability status score
EAE	experimental allergic encephalomyelitis
EDSS	expanded disability status score
EIA	enzyme immunoassay
ERP	event-related potential
FS	functional symptoms
GFAP	glial fibrillary acidic protein
HAM	HTLV-1 associated myelopathy
HSMN	hereditary sensory and motor neuropathy
HSP	heat shock protein
HTLV-I	human T cell leukaemia virus type I
ICAM	intercellular cell adhesion molecule
IEF	isoelectric focusing
IFA	incomplete Freund's adjuvant
IFN	interferon
IGF	insulin-like growth factor
IL	interleukin
IM	intramuscular
IV	intravenous
LFA	lymphocyte function-associated antigen
LT	lymphotoxin
MAG	myelin-associated glycoprotein
MBP	myelin basic protein
MEP	magnetically evoked potential
MHC	major histocompatibility complex
MOG	myelin oligodendroglia glycoprotein
MP	methylprednisolone
MRI	magnetic resonance imaging
MS	multiple sclerosis
MSR	multiple stretch reflexes
MT	magnetization transfer
NAA	N-acetyl aspartase
NAR	not-at-risk
NMR	nuclear magnetic resonance
PBL	peripheral blood lymphocytes
PCD	programmed cell death
PDGF	platelet-derived growth factor
PET	positive emission tomography
PLP	proteolipid protein
PNS	peripheral nervous system
PVE	post-vaccinational encephalomyelitis
RAPD	relative afferent pupillary defect
RDA	representational difference analysis
SE	spin echo
SEP	somatosensory evoked potential
SLE	systemic lupus erythematosus
SPECT	single photon emission tomography
SSPE	subacute sclerosing pan-encephalitis
STIR	short term inversion recovery
TAL-H	transaldolase-H
TCR	T cell receptor
TE	echo time
TGF	transforming growth factor
TN	trigeminal neuralgia
TNF	tumour necrosis factor
TSP	tropical spastic paresis
VCAM	vascular cell adhesion molecule
VEP	visual evoked potential
VLA	very late antigen

NOTE ON TERMINOLOGY

The temporal course of multiple sclerosis has been the basis for classifying the disease. Existing terminology has included the following terms: relapsing-remitting (synonym: exacerbating-remitting), chronic-progressive (includes secondary-progressive and primary-progressive) and relapsing-progressive. The use of terminology has not been well standardized. The two prototypes are relapsing-remitting disease and primary-progressive disease, the latter referring to a chronic-progressive course from onset without preceding exacerbation. It is well known that the majority of patients with relapsing-remitting multiple sclerosis convert to a chronic-progressive course; in this circumstance the term secondary-progressive is applied. There had been controversy about whether patients with stepwise accumulation of neurological deficit without insidious progression between relapses should be classified as a relapsing-remitting or assigned to a separate category, relapsing-progressive. Also, it has been unclear whether patients with primary-progressive MS who have occasional acute attacks should be placed in a separate category such as the relapsing-progressive category.

Given the importance of MS classification to the selection of patients for clinical therapeutic trials, the Advisory Committee on Clinical Trials of the National Multiple Sclerosis Society (USA) undertook a survey to develop a consensus on definitions and terminology of the clinical course of multiple sclerosis. The results of this survey and recommendations of the committee were published in *Neurology*, 1996; 46: 970–911. Two hundred and fifteen members of the international MS clinical research community were surveyed; 125 (58%) completed the survey. There was a clear consensus on the definition of relapsing-remitting MS, primary-progressive MS, and secondary-progressive MS. It was decided that patients with relapsing-remitting MS with stepwise worsening of disability with clinical stability between attacks should be included in the relapsing-remitting category and not in the progressive MS category. As there was no consensus on the definition of relapsing-progressive MS, it was decided that this term should be abandoned, and a new term, progressive-relapsing MS, should be established for rare patients with MS who have superimposed acute relapses with or without full recovery in the context of progressively increasing disability.

Contributors to this volume address these issues in several chapters. Others use terminology that reflects the time-frame within which their contributions were prepared.

Brian G. Weinshenker, MD

PART ONE

CLINICAL PARAMETERS

1 CLINICAL FEATURES OF MULTIPLE SCLEROSIS

John N. Whitaker and
Galen W. Mitchell

1.1 Introduction

All of the attempts to understand the etiology and pathogenesis of multiple sclerosis (MS) for potential control, prevention or eradication, rely on an accurate diagnosis to recognize the disease. Beyond the certainty of the diagnosis itself is a determination of current disease activity and the extent of disability resulting from the disease. In order to appreciate the variables and heterogeneity of MS, these determinations require numerous factors to be considered, including:

1. the silence or expression of lesions in the central nervous system (CNS);
2. the monosymptomatic forms which may or may not evolve to MS;
3. the episodic and chronic features of neurological deficits underlying the subtyping of disease as well as the prognosis for disability and longevity;
4. the wide spectrum of disease intensity; and
5. the clinical and biological interpretation of test results from neuroimaging, cerebrospinal fluid (CSF) examination and electrodiagnosis.

Various aspects of these issues will be dealt with in the different chapters of this book. This introductory chapter is written to furnish a picture, really a snapshot, of a disorder that clinically affects over 350 000 persons in the United States alone, with the potential for enormous personal, family and societal costs. MS occurs unevenly, appearing to follow restrictions in geography, age, gender, race and ethnic group. These have generally been grouped into host factors of genetic susceptibility (Chapter 13) and environmental influences, which may be in part due to an infectious agent (Chapters 6, 7 and 8). Briefly, MS most commonly appears in young caucasian females living in cool, temperate climates.

1.2 Historical aspects

The distribution of MS is world-wide but very uneven. Fragmentary biographic accounts of MS date to the late fourteenth century [1] but the first recorded case is generally regarded as that of Sir Augustus Frederic D'Este (1794–1848), grandson of King George III of England, whose personal diary was accidentally discovered in 1940 and subsequently published [2]. The earliest clinicopathological descriptions of MS were those of Robert Carswell in 1838 and Jean Cruveilhier in 1841 [3]. However, it is Jean Martin Charcot, who probably became aware of the clinical disorder in the late 1850s [3], who furnished, in 1868, the first full clinical description of MS in a living patient. It is likely that Charcot collected less than 40 cases [4], but he initiated the process, still being addressed in this chapter and book, to delineate the clinical features and correlative tissue changes that define MS. The triad of intentional tremor, to be distinguished from the tremor at rest of Parkinson's disease, nystagmus and scanning dysarthria bear Charcot's name, but he was also aware of the spontaneous remissions of the disease [5]. A number of other clinicians and investigators made further contributions characterizing the disorder which was first reported in the United States in 1878 by Seguin (reviewed by Dejong [6]).

The concept of MS as an autoimmune disease originated with the production of experimental allergic encephalomyelitis (EAE) by inoculations of neural tissue [7, 8]. Discovery of an increase in CSF immunoglobulin level added to the focus on the role of the immune system and laboratory aids for clinical diagnosis [9]. Investigations of encephalitogenic proteins in the 1960s and 1970s were rapidly followed by unsuccessful pursuits to identify causative viral agents in the 1970s. Applications from the fields of immunology, glial and myelin biology, and molecular biology are the major basic science areas to drive the current research on MS. The therapeutic trials of new agents, which started in the late 1960s and grew rapidly in the 1980s, now dominate clinical research on MS. Magnetic resonance imaging (MRI) has had a shaping influence on the understanding of MS as a very dynamic disease in which multiple CNS lesions rarely reveal themselves and occur independently [10].

Multiple Sclerosis: Clinical and pathogenetic basis. Edited by Cedric S. Raine, Henry F. McFarland and Wallace W. Tourtellotte. Published in 1997 by Chapman & Hall, London. ISBN 0 412 30890 8.

1.3   Definition of the disease

Multiple sclerosis (MS) is an acquired primary demyelinating disease of the CNS in which myelin is the target of an autoimmune inflammatory process(es). Its clinical manifestations typically appear between 20 and 40 years of age with focal, multifocal, episodic and general neurological symptoms and signs. It has two clinical hallmarks. First is a temporal profile of symptoms and neurological deficits occurring in multiple episodes, designated as a relapse or exacerbation, followed by the disappearance of symptoms or restoration of function, known as a remission. By definition, a relapse lasts at least 24 hours and cannot be attributed to another cause, especially fever. The severity of a relapse is highly variable and relates to the area and volume of the CNS tissue damaged. A remission usually occurs more slowly than did the onset of the relapse and may be complete or incomplete. The gradual appearance of neurological deficits, referred to as progression, may be associated with or substituted for relapses and remissions, giving rise to different disease subtypes and courses (see Figure 1.1). It is the progressive deficit, which might also be viewed as the failure of remission, that accounts for disability and decline in quality of life.

The second hallmark is the dissemination of lesions anatomically within the CNS. The number of lesions that are reported by the affected patient or detected by the examiner is considerably less than can be demonstrated by cranial MRI (Chapter 3) or by evoked potentials (Chapter 4) recording responses to visual, auditory or somatosensory stimuli. The inflammatory demyelination of the CNS causing MS (Chapters 9 and 10) is reflected by quantitatively increased CSF immunoglobulin demonstrating restricted heterogeneity, or oligoclonality (Chapter 5). On the basis of whether one or both of these two clinical hallmarks are present and whether one or more paraclinical abnormalities can be demonstrated by cranial or spinal MRI, evoked potential or CSF testing, MS is diagnosed as clinically definite, probable or possible.

In order to place the description above in perspective, several other terms need to be defined. Demyelination refers to the acquired damage, whatever the cause, to apparently normal myelin, whereas dysmyelination is the term for disorders affecting genes of oligodendrocytes, and possibly other cells, encoding myelin proteins, enzymes and other factors important for myelinogenesis (Chapter 11). Primary demyelination implies that the myelin unit, comprised of the oligodendrocyte and CNS myelin sheath, is the pathogenic site of injury. MS is not the only human demyelinating disease though it is the most common (Table 1.1). In contrast, secondary demyelination occurs when the axonal components are damaged so that the requisite signal from the axolemma for myelin formation or maintenance is

Table 1.1   Primary demyelinating diseases of the central nervous system

Multiple sclerosis
  Relapsing-remitting (RR)
  Progressive-relapsing (PR)
  Primary-progressive (PP)
  Secondary-progressive (SP)
Fulminate demyelinating disease
  Marburg variant of multiple sclerosis
  Acute disseminated encephalomyelitis
Monosymptomatic demyelinating syndromes
  Optic neuritis (papillitis, retrobulbar neuritis)
  Acute transverse myelopathy
  Sacral myeloradiculitis
Demyelinating disease with restricted distribution
  Devic's syndrome (neuromyelitis optica)
  Balo's concentric sclerosis (tumor-like)
Para-infectious/post-infectious diseases
  Post-vaccinal/Post-infectious
  Acute hemorrhagic leukoencephalitis
Other diseases of myelin
  Infectious
  Toxic/metabolic
  Nutritional
  Damage by physical agents
  Genetic/inherited
  Miscellaneous

Modified after Traugott and Raine, 1984 [126] and Weinshenker, 1995 [127].

lost. Although the axon is relatively spared in MS, accounting for its designation as a primary demyelinating disease, the axon can also be affected, especially in later phases. CNS axonopathy appears to be an important component of chronic demyelination and progressive disease (Chapter 9 and 12).

1.4   Clinical criteria for the diagnosis of MS

The Schumacher criteria [11] link natural history and physical findings for the diagnosis of MS (Table 1.2). These criteria led to the designation of **clinically definite MS**, i.e. fulfilling the Schumacher criteria, probable MS and possible MS. **Probable MS** consisted of RR symptoms with only one neurologic sign commonly associated with MS (see below) or a documented single episode with signs of multifocal white matter disease with complete or partial recovery and no better explanation. **Possible MS** was defined as RR symptoms without documented signs or objective signs insufficient to establish more than one site of CNS involvement and no better explanation. While these criteria were replaced by others [12] which took into account the clinically silent and dynamic aspects of MS as well as CSF findings, the Schumacher criteria still form the basis for the recognition of the clinical grouping and natural history of MS (Figure 1.1).

Table 1.2 Schumacher criteria for diagnosis of multiple sclerosis

---

- Neurologic examination reveals objective abnormalities of CNS function
- History indicates involvement of two or more parts of CNS
- CNS disease predominantly reflects white matter involvement
- Involvement of CNS follows one or two patterns:
  - Two or more episodes, each lasting at least 24 hours and ≥ one month apart
  - Slow or stepwise progression of signs and symptoms over at least 6 months
- Patient 10–50 years old at onset
  Signs and symptoms cannot be better explained by other disease process

---

From Schumacher *et al.*, 1965 [11].

1.5 Clinical types and subtypes of MS based on temporal profile and intensity of disease

The multiplicity of neurological deficits, the relative admixture of relapses/remissions, with or without overall progression and the severity of disease leads to marked clinical heterogeneity of the population of individuals accurately diagnosed with MS. Categorization of MS cases into different subtypes has the primary goal of grouping patients for clinical recognition. In an effort to standardize the terminology used for MS subtypes, an international survey led to the following classification (Figure 1.1) [13]:

A Relapsing-remitting (RR) (Figure 1.1a); clearly defined disease relapses with full recovery or with

sequelae and residual deficit upon recovery. Periods between disease relapses are characterized by a lack of disease progression.

B Progressive-relapsing (PR) (Figure 1.1b); progressive disease from onset, with clear acute relapses, with or without full recovery, with periods between relapses characterized by continuing progression.

C Secondary-progressive (SP) (Figure 1.1c); initial RR disease course followed by progression with or without occasional relapses, minor remissions and plateaus.

D Primary-progressive (PP) (Figure 1.1d); disease progression from onset with occasional plateaus and temporary minor improvements.

In addition to this classification related to temporal profile and the possible combinations of relapses, remissions and progression, the same survey [13] addressed the accepted usage of terms to denote clinical severity. **Benign MS** is defined as disease which allows a patient to remain fully functional in all neurologic systems 15 years after onset of disease. **Malignant MS** is characterized by a rapid, progressive course, leading to significant disability in multiple neurologic systems or death in a relatively short time after disease onset. Furthermore, the pathological changes of MS may be clinically asymptomatic. There is as yet no clear explanation for this varying intensity of disease, but such should be considered in the ascertainment of cases of any epidemiological study of MS (Chapter 7).

1.6 Common diagnostic procedures and their added use in the diagnosis of MS

Cranial and spinal neuroimaging studies (Chapter 3), evoked potentials (Chapter 4) and CSF examination (Chapter 5) represent the major diagnostic tests, providing documentation to enhance the confidence of a clinical diagnosis of MS. The performance of cranial-spinal neuroimaging, specifically cranial MRI, and evoked potentials furnishes evidence for the multifocal, but possibly clinically silent, nature of lesions. CSF changes add the important information on the inflammatory basis of the lesions expressed clinically or detected by MRI and evoked potentials. Results of these testing methods have been incorporated into diagnostic criteria that more accurately express the certainty of diagnosis, especially the probable and possible types (Table 1.3). Although the diagnosis of MS is far easier and more certain with the availability of cranial MRI, a determination of disease activity and the disease progression remains difficult. Cranial MRI with enhancement (Chapter 3) and selected CSF results, primarily levels of myelin basic protein-like material [14], provide the best laboratory evidence of disease activity. Other

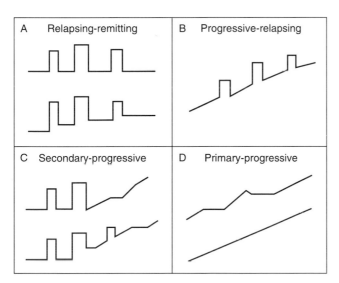

Figure 1.1 Four different courses of multiple sclerosis are graphically depicted. These are the relapsing-remitting (RR), progressive-relapsing (PR), secondary-progressive (SP) and primary-progressive (PP).

Table 1.3 Clinical and laboratory criteria for multiple sclerosis

Category	Minimum number		Paraclinical evidence[a]	CSF IgG[b]
	Relapses	CNS deficits		
Clinically	2	2		
definite	2	1	*and* 1	
Probable	2	1		
	1	2		
	1	1	*and* 1	
Laboratory-	2	1	*or* 1	+
supported	1	2		+
definite	1	1	*and* 1	+
Probable	2			+

[a] Cranial or spinal MRI or evoked potential abnormality not encompassed by the clinical neurological symptom or deficit.
[b] Oligoclonal IgG or increased index or synthesis rate of IgG.
After C.M. Poser *et al.*, 1983 [12].

changes on cranial MRI (Chapter 3) and an increase of urinary myelin basic protein-like material hold promise for detecting the failure of remission and progression of disease [15]. Since MS is clinically confined to the CNS, abnormal test results outside the CNS and CSF are major indications of an alternate diagnosis.

1.7 Clinical symptomatology

MS represents a complex clinical disorder with highly diverse signs and symptoms arising from CNS demyelination and the consequent slowed or blocked conduction in axons. Negative signs or symptoms, such as loss of vision, strength or sensation, are the typical manifestation (Table 1.4). The deficits themselves are etiologically nonspecific, so that an appreciation of their site(s) and combinations becomes critical for clinical interpretation, especially in the consideration of alter-

Table 1.4 Multiple sclerosis: symptoms at presentation and during course

Deficit reported	Presenting	During course
Visual/oculomotor	49[a]	100
Paresis	43	88
Paresthesias	41	87
Incoordination	23	82
Genito-urinary/Bowel	10	63
Cerebral	4	39

[a] Expressed as percentage. Since some patients had multiple symptoms, the total is greater than 100%.
After S. Poser *et al.*, 1979 [128].

Table 1.5 Paroxysmal disorders in multiple sclerosis

Tonic spasms and other involuntary movements
Trigeminal neuralgia
Diplopia
Episodic dysarthria and ataxia
Crossed paresthesia
Hemiataxia
Transient limb weakness
Neuralgic pain
Episodic pruritus

native diagnoses. In addition to the slowed or blocked axonal conduction, ectopic impulses and ephaptic transmission may exist in areas of demyelination (Chapter 12) with resultant positive signs or symptoms such as the paroxysmal syndromes (Table 1.5) and seizures. The mixture of positive and negative signs and symptoms provides the background for the highly varied and complicated clinical symptomatology.

1.7.1 SYMPTOMS AT ONSET OF DISEASE

In spite of the fact that demyelination may occur essentially anywhere within the CNS, the majority of patients have their initial symptoms in a relatively limited distribution (Table 1.4). The most common onset, in about 85%, temporally is with a relapse. The patient frequently presents with more than one symptom. While sensory disturbances, weakness or optic neuritis may occur in isolation, ataxia usually exists with a constellation of symptoms which may include vertigo, diplopia, weakness and sensory disturbances. Many times, the onset symptoms are also accompanied by more vague symptoms such as fatigue or malaise. Presentation with a predominately painful syndrome is uncommon and onset with aphasia, cognitive dysfunction, or more cortical manifestations is rare. For the 15% who have an insidious onset, the profile of PP or PR disease (Figure 1.1), a spastic and ataxic paraparesis predominates.

1.7.2 MAJOR SIGNS AND SYMPTOMS DURING THE COURSE OF MS

MS patients exhibit a wide spectrum of signs and symptoms, often related to the severity and form of their disorder (Table 1.4). Virtually all patients with long-standing or advanced disease have increased reflexes, spasticity, extensor plantar responses, weakness, ataxia, sensory loss, visual impairment and sphincter disturbances.

Weakness

The weakness may be mild, primarily manifested only with exertion and later in the day or when the ambient temperature is increased. In other patients, the weakness may be severe, precluding the use of the affected extremity. A typical pattern is asymmetrical leg weakness with the hand ipsilateral to the weaker leg showing diminished dexterity. It is uncommon for the patient to develop arm weakness without some degree of leg involvement, and almost never will a patient develop bilateral severe arm weakness without leg weakness. An occasional patient will develop an acute or subacute hemiparesis.

The weakness is usually associated with increased tone, increased muscle stretch reflexes (MSRs), extensor plantar responses, and in many cases the loss of superficial abdominal reflexes. The spasticity and increased MSRs are frequently more pronounced in the legs than the arms. Spasticity may contribute to fatigue in the ambulating patient, although, in the setting of severe weakness, the spasticity may be utilized to prevent buckling of the knees upon transfer or ambulation. Patients with moderate to severe lower extremity spastic weakness frequently have extensor spasms of the legs. These are usually painless spasms, which last several minutes and are induced by active or passive movement of the affected limb.

Sensory disturbances

Patients with established disease almost always note sensory disturbances. A careful clinical characterization of the reported sensory symptoms and documentation of an objective sensory deficit are often the critical step when dealing with the anxious or hysterical patient. Sensory symptoms may be reported as paresthesias, dysesthesias or distorted sensation. Tactile sensation may be diminished or altered with the patient perceiving that there is a film or light cloth over the skin in the affected area. Others report a tight or swollen sensation of a hand, foot or extremity. Some relate a girdle-like band around a limb or the trunk. At times, the band-like dysesthesia is severe, and when involving the chest, patients feel that they cannot breathe, and less commonly, relate early satiety with a band around the abdomen. Patients may complain of coldness, especially of the feet or legs, or less often, a warm or hot sensation of an extremity. On examination, vibratory loss in the lower extremities is the most common abnormality. Involvement of the cervical cord can cause profound sensory loss in both arms with pseudoathetosis and little sensory deficit in the legs. Proprioceptive and vibratory sensation loss may be dissociated. Patients with MS may surprise the examiner with little or no loss of pain in spite of the perception that the affected region is very numb. In other cases, pain and temperature are severely affected.

Facial sensory changes in the form of a trigeminal sensory neuropathy, separate from trigeminal neuralgia, may occur. The patient usually reports numbness of two or all divisions of the trigeminal nerve along with intraoral numbness. Facial hypalgesia and hypesthesia are expected.

Cerebellar dysfunction

The majority of patients do not present with cerebellar dysfunction. However, the development of signs and symptoms referable to the cerebellum is common in long-standing or severe disease. It is also unusual for a patient to develop an isolated cerebellar syndrome. More commonly, cerebellar signs occur with a multiplicity of other findings which usually include sensory disturbance, weakness and, possibly, brain stem signs. Severe cerebellar dysfunction is one of the most disabling features of MS. On this basis alone, patients may be totally dependent due to severe limb and truncal ataxia that precludes ambulation or even simple tasks such as feeding and self-hygiene. This is particularly true with severe upper extremity tremor, ataxia and dysmetria. Ataxic speech is relatively rare, and usually only heard in advanced disease. Patients with PP-MS frequently develop a spastic paraparesis with a cerebellar ataxic gait.

Visual impairment

Complaints related to decreased visual acuity and oculomotor dysfunction are very common in patients with MS. Their absence in the 'diagnosed' MS patient should raise questions about diagnostic accuracy. The most common findings usually take the form of an optic neuritis, nystagmus or internuclear ophthalmoparesis (Chapter 2).

1.7.3 PAROXYSMAL SYNDROMES

Patients with MS complain of a variety of transient symptoms (Table 1.6). Some of these are difficult to explain, while others are related to elevated body

Table 1.6 Genito-urinary and bowel dysfunction in multiple sclerosis

Bladder dysfunction
  Failure to store from spastic bladder
  Failure to empty
    Flaccid bladder
    Detrusor-sphincter dyssynergia
Sexual dysfunction
  Erectile impotence
  Anorgasmy
Bowel dysfunction
  Constipation
  Fecal urgency
  Fecal incontinence

temperature, relapses or ephaptic events. These ephaptic events, called paroxysmal syndromes, occur in 1–4% of MS patients and are usually attributed to lesions in the brain stem or spinal cord. These symptoms are usually intense, lasting seconds to minutes, and are stereotypic. The typical profile is for the patient to experience a cluster of these paroxysms for weeks to months, after which they spontaneously resolve. Paroxysmal symptoms may occur in isolation or as a manifestation of a relapse. Many of these are unique to MS and occasionally are the presenting symptom [16]. No associated changes in mental status occur, and EEGs taken during the episodes are normal [17]. A careful inquiry for the presence of these disorders is important since they can cause the patient significant discomfort or dysfunction and the majority respond to therapy with anticonvulsants.

Tonic spasms

These spasms begin in the limbs or trunk and spread upward or downward, at times crossing the midline. They last seconds to minutes and may occur spontaneously or be provoked by movement, tactile stimulation of a 'trigger zone', or hyperventilation [18]. Intense pain or an unpleasant sensation precedes or accompanies the spasms in the majority of patients. Tonic spasms may be differentiated from the typically painless flexor spasms, usually nocturnal and involving the legs, by the intensity of the pain and spasms and the stereotypic spread of the symptoms [18]. Also, in contrast to flexor spasms, these spasms do not correlate with the degree of underlying spasticity.

Trigeminal neuralgia

Trigeminal neuralgia (TN) occurs in 1–2% of MS patients [19]. The majority of patients have had MS for several years before developing the disorder, although TN may be the presenting symptom. As with non-MS patients, there are typical and atypical forms of TN. Typical TN involves abrupt, intense paroxysms of facial pain in the trigeminal distribution lasting not more than two minutes, separated by pain-free intervals. The maxillary or mandibular divisions of the nerve are most frequently involved, with a smaller subset of patients having both divisions affected. Simultaneous bilateral TN is highly suggestive of demyelinating disease, especially in the young adult. The pain in TN is often provoked by a minimal local stimulus to the affected side of the face. Atypical TN is similar to the TN just described except that there may be loss of the pain-free interval, with a continuous less intense pain persisting between the episodes, and the severe paroxysms of pain last longer, frequently several minutes.

Other paroxysmal sensory or painful symptoms

There are several other paroxysmal sensory or painful symptoms. These are frequently overlooked in the patient evaluation unless actively pursued. Examples include burning paresthesias or severe pain [17], aching pain [20], unpleasant quivering sensations [21], spontaneous Lhermitte's-like phenomena and itching [22, 23]. All of these episodes usually last seconds to a few minutes, except for the paroxysmal itching which may last as long as 30 minutes [22]. The sensory aberrations can affect any part of the body but more frequently involve the extremities, typically in areas where there is current or previous sensory loss. The paroxysmal itching sometimes occurs in a dermatomal distribution, especially over the shoulder and neck. It is very intense, often disturbing sleep, and sometimes associated with a burning or aching sensation or numbness. Most attacks occur spontaneously, but they may be precipitated by heat, movement or touch. Some patients find transient relief by pinching the affected sites.

Episodic dysarthria and ataxia

The attacks of paroxysmal dysarthria and ataxia usually last less than one minute, and may occur many times in one day [20, 24, 25]. The ataxia is cerebellar in character and may affect only the extremities on one side or be generalized, affecting the trunk and limbs. These symptoms may be severe with the speech uninterpretable and the patient falling with the ataxia. While the dysarthria and ataxia are always present, other symptoms may be associated including diplopia, numbness and weakness [20, 25]. The episodes may be precipitated by hyperventilation or anxiety [20, 24]. At times, this paroxysmal syndrome represents the presenting symptom of MS and provides a diagnostic dilemma. Consideration must be given to transient ischemic attacks in the vertebrobasilar system. Evidence of a demyelinating disorder in the evaluation, lack of a fixed deficit in spite of multiple attacks and the stereotypic nature of the event helps provide the correct diagnosis. In a young person without vascular risk factors, paroxysmal dysarthria and ataxia are highly suggestive of demyelinating disease.

Diplopia

In addition to diplopia accompanying dysarthria and ataxia, this symptom may occur in isolation, with the episodes lasting seconds to a few minutes, occurring up to 100 times a day [20]. Sometimes, there are clusters of episodes, cycling every few weeks.

Other paroxysmal syndromes

Other paroxysmal disorders include akinesia in one or more limbs lasting a few seconds and frequently recurring several times a day [20], weakness usually of a leg or hand lasting 10–20 seconds to a few minutes with resultant unexpected falls or dropping of objects [21], paroxysmal hemiataxia and crossed paraesthesia [20] and paroxysmal pelvic pain [26].

1.7.4 BLADDER, BOWEL AND SEXUAL DYSFUNCTION

Symptoms of bladder dysfunction are uncommon at presentation, but frequently develop with persistent disease, often correlating with the degree of disability, and in particular pyramidal tract dysfunction. Furthermore, urinary tract infections that frequently complicate the neurogenic bladder may contribute to increased lower extremity weakness and spasticity. They may also be life-threatening when urosepsis develops, especially in the patient treated with immunosuppressive agents. Bowel dysfunction in the form of constipation is common in debilitated patients. Fecal incontinence in the absence of diarrhea is unusual. The combination of psychologic, physical and endocrine factors contributes to sexual dysfunction in many MS patients. While varying degrees of erectile dysfunction are common in men, many retain the ability for ejaculation. Orgasms in females are usually preserved unless perineal sensory loss restricts arousal and stimulation. Overall, sexual activity is decreased or totally absent in over 50% of men and women. A more detailed discussion of symptoms, evaluation and treatment for bowel, bladder (Chapter 22) and sexual (Chapter 23) dysfunction is provided in later chapters.

1.7.5 NEUROBEHAVIORAL SYNDROMES

Virtually all recognizable neurobehavioral disorders have been noted in patients with MS (Chapter 21). At times, their occurrence appears unrelated to the pathophysiology of MS, while in others there are probable associations based on intracranial lesions or an increased prevalence in the MS population that is difficult to explain by random chance. The more common neurobehavioral abnormalities include depression, emotional lability, euphoria, dementia or cognitive impairment, and less frequently, bipolar disease, extreme anxiety and psychosis. Recognition of these disorders is important since some are readily treatable, thereby decreasing disability, social stress, unnecessary embarrassment and, overall, improving the patient's quality of life.

1.7.6 FATIGUE

Fatigue is an ill-defined state experienced by the majority of MS patients that is often present at or near the time of onset of disease and persists throughout the patient's course. It varies from mild to severely disabling. Most patients feel that the fatigue is exacerbated by exercise or with elevated body or ambient temperature. Fatigue is usually experienced in a diurnal pattern, being least in the first few hours after arising and greatest in the afternoon or evening. A short nap or brief period of rest may delay or relieve the fatigue. This pattern differs from the more constant feeling of fatigue described by the depressed patient.

The etiology of the fatigue is unknown but is probably multifactorial. Decreased efficiency of energy utilization due to weakness and spasticity may be contributory, but even those with very benign disease who have been relapse-free for years and have a normal examination may still complain of fatigue. Disturbances of sleep are three times higher in MS patients than in a control population and may contribute to fatigue, particularly when depression is also present [27]. The MRI lesions correlating best with sleep disturbance were in the right and left frontal white matter and the deep white matter of the right insula [27]. Polysomnographic studies show that MS patients have a reduction in sleep efficiency and more awakenings during sleep without changes in sleep latency or architecture [28]. Periodic leg movements, such as nocturnal flexor spasms correlating with MRI lesions in the cerebellum and brain stem [28], are more common in the MS patient but do not fully explain the sleep fragmentation. Other studies have demonstrated an association between fatigue, though not correlated with depression, and increased MRI lesions in the brain stem and midbrain [29]. Finally, patients with urinary frequency and nocturia suffer from interrupted sleep, sometimes arising to urinate frequently throughout the night.

1.7.7 THERMAL INFLUENCES

Many patients note increased fatigue, diffuse weakness or even focal neurological symptoms in the setting of elevated temperature with increased ambient temperature, during a febrile episode or with exercise with resultant elevated body temperature. It may be fever with infection, no longer permitting minor symptoms to be dismissed, that initially brings the MS patient to medical attention. When placed in a heat cabinet with air temperatures elevated to 55–60°C or a hot bath, MS patients often experience increasing disability and new deficits within 10–15 minutes [30, 31]. The heat-induced focal neurological deficits in MS patients were utilized in the 'hot bath test' which served as a diagnostic study for several years. The induced deficits were typically transient although a rare patient had persistent dysfunction. Some patients report increased fatigue, weakness or focal deficits lasting for days after significant heat exposure. The duration, but not the number, of relapses correlates with increased mean ambient and absolute maximum temperatures [32]. While moderate or cool temperatures are usually preferred by MS patients, exposure to cold may worsen function by increasing spasticity and muscle spasms.

1.7.8   PAIN

As an onset symptom, pain of varying intensity and type is recorded in 10–20% of patients [33–35] but is rare if common headaches and mild dysesthesia associated with sensory disturbances are excluded. Up to 65% of MS patients report acute or chronic pain during the course of their disease [35, 36] and 32% indicate that pain is one of their worst symptoms (Table 1.7). There is no clear relationship to age of disease onset and disability scores [33, 34]. The majority of pains reported are dysesthetic extremity pain, back pain, painful leg spasms and the paroxysmal pain syndromes. While pain was not associated with depression, it is increased in those with spasticity and myelopathy and in those showing poorer mental health and more social-role handicap [37]. Pain of musculoskeletal origin may also be noted, especially in severely disabled MS patients during rehabilitation [38].

In approximately 10% of MS patients with pain, this is acute and most commonly accompanies optic neuritis, the paroxysmal symptoms of trigeminal neuralgia or painful tonic spasms, a Lhermitte's sign or neuralgic extremity involvement. Optic neuritis frequently has an associated mild to moderate pain, which on occasion may be severe. This pain typically precedes the visual loss, is ipsilateral to the optic neuritis, is orbital or periorbital in location, increases

Table 1.7   Pain syndromes in multiple sclerosis

Acute pain
  Painful tonic spasms
  Trigeminal neuralgia
  Painful Lhermitte's sign
  Radicular pain
  Paroxysmal pain of limb, trunk or pelvis
Subacute pain
  Periorbital pain with optic neuritis
  Band-like dysesthesia
  Pressure palsies in the disabled (ulnar, median or
    peroneal)
Compression fracture related to treatment
Chronic pain
  Low back pain
  Limb dysesthesias
  Painful leg spasms
Other
  Headache

Modified from Moulin et al., 1988 [34].

with eye movement, and may sometimes be accompanied by a unilateral or generalized headache. Although headaches have been reported to be more common in MS patients than in controls [33], they are usually tension or migraine in type without a distinctive 'MS headache'. Headaches have also been associated with tumor-like giant plaque formation [39, 40] and with plaques of the brain stem [41] and periductal gray matter [36].

Lhermitte's sign, reported in a third of MS patients [42], is an electric shock-like feeling, tingling or a vibrating sensation, which occurs for a few seconds on neck flexion, travelling down the spine, sometimes into one or both legs, and less commonly, into the arm(s). This symptom rarely occurs in other conditions except subacute combined degeneration of the cord, neck trauma, radiation myelitis and prolapsed cervical disk [42]. Association with other signs and symptoms is variable, and Lhermitte's sign may occur in isolation without any other evidence of disease activity. As long suspected and confirmed by MRI, this sign results from lesions of the posterior columns of the cervical cord [43]. MS patients may develop radicular pain with sensory loss in a dermatomal distribution, suggestive of an acute monoradiculopathy [44, 45]. When the anterior nerve roots are involved, there may be loss of the appropriate reflex with weakness, fasciculations and atrophy developing over time. Study by MRI may reveal a spinal cord lesion, consistent with plaque, overlying and on occasion involving, the appropriate nerve root.

The frequency of chronic pain increases with advanced age and disease duration of longer than five years [33–35]. Chronic pain, most commonly associated with a myelopathy, develops in approximately 50% of patients and includes dysesthetic extremity pain (29%), back pain (14%), painful leg spasms (13%) and abdominal pain (2%). The back pain and painful leg spasms were more common in patients with increased disability. Chronic back pain is usually confined to the lower back, with occasional radiation into the hips or thighs, rarely below the knees. It is difficult to apportion the additive role of accompanying degenerative disease of the lumbar spine to the back pain. The abdominal pain, described as an aching, bloated periumbilical sensation with superimposed abdominal cramps, is more common in constipated patients and may be relieved by improved bowel habits.

In addition to this pain of neural origin, neurologic deficits, especially of the spinal cord, may alter pain perception in the MS patient so that pain is unappreciated, ignored or reported with variance or of less intensity than might be expected. Such sensory impairment may obscure direct and referred pain, such as appendicitis, ruptured bowel, myocardial ischemia or enlarging mass, and delay diagnosis and treatment.

Table 1.8 Less common neurological deficits in multiple sclerosis

Cerebral
    Aphasia [129]
    Hemiparesis [130]
    Seizure [131]
    Epilepsia partialis continua [132]

Diencephalon
    Sleep disturbances [27]
        Narcolepsy [133]
    Movement disorders [134]
        Dystonia [135]
        Hemiballism [136]
        Myoclonus
        Segmental myoclonus [137]
        Spasmodic torticollis [138]
        Bilateral ballism [139]
        Alternating paroxysmal dystonia [140]
        Trismus [141]
    Hypothermia [142]
    Ageusia [143]

Brain stem
    Locked-in state [144]
    Facial myokymia [145]
    Hemifacial spasm [146]
    Hearing loss [147]
    Cataplexy [148]
    Synkinetic movements
        Hiccups [149]
        Yawning
        Sighing
    Respiratory involvement [66]
    Cardiovascular [67]

Spinal cord
    Radicular pain [45]
    Noncommunicating syringomyelia [150]
    Propriospinal myoclonus [137]
    Spasmodic torticollis [151]

1.7.9 LESS COMMON BUT RELATED CLINICAL FEATURES

The typical symptoms and signs of MS at onset or during the course of disease (Table 1.4) may be associated with or replaced by less common and unusual neurological deficits (Table 1.8). While these less usual manifestations may be grouped anatomically, the clinical correlation with a specific anatomical lesion is imprecise. Recognition of the less common clinical features (Table 1.8) may, when they appear at onset, lead to an early and rapid diagnosis and, when they appear in the previously diagnosed MS patient, allay patient anxiety and obviate unnecessary testing.

1.8 Spinal cord demyelinating disorders

There are several syndromes that may occur as monosymptomatic demyelinating syndromes, sometimes with a restricted anatomical distribution (Table 1.1). Optic neuritis is dealt with in detail elsewhere (Chapter 2). As an initial event, a myelitis occurring in one of four different patterns or combinations represents another. The rate at which any of these groups goes on to develop MS and prognostic factors for such an outcome are usually the critical issues (Chapter 6).

Acute transverse myelopathy is characteristically a monophasic event producing a rapid onset of focal, bilateral corticospinal tract and ascending sensory tract deficits along with urinary and fecal retention. The rate at which this group goes on to develop MS varies widely, from 3% [46] to 80% [47], and some patients will show a relapsing disease confined to the spinal cord [48]. The presence of typical periventricular changes on cranial MRI [47] and of a partial rather than complete myelopathy appears to correlate best with the subsequent transition to MS. Similarly, **chronic progressive myelopathy**, in which motor system symptoms and signs usually predominate, may continue to show only a myelopathy [49] or may show dissemination clinically and by diagnostic testing [50]. **Sacral myeloradiculitis**, or Elsberg's syndrome, is characterized by acute urinary retention, sensory and motor deficits in the sacral dermatomes and CSF pleocytosis [51]. The prognosis is usually good, and the rarity of the condition makes the prognosis for development of MS unknown. In **Devic's syndrome** an acute transverse myelopathy is associated with bilateral optic neuritis in a number of temporal patterns. Patients with Devic's syndrome may be disabled from paraplegia and blindness but rarely show the typical patterns of MS (Figure 1.1).

1.9 Age of onset

The appearance of MS before age 16 or after age 60 is rare. Devic's syndrome, or neuromyelitis optica, with the combined optic neuritis and transverse myelopathy does not respect the age restrictions typical for MS. Those cases of MS with onset before age 16 have the same range of symptoms and signs as for those with the typical time of onset [52]. There is a more striking female predominance, the symptoms are predominantly afferent, affecting vision and sensation, and an RR course is usual [53]. The paraclinical tests of cranial MRI, evoked potentials and CSF abnormalities can be utilized as already mentioned [52, 54]. Nearly 10% of MS patients have onset of disease after age 50 [55] and approximately 1% after age 59 [56]. Older patients primarily show motor dysfunction, implying spinal cord involvement, more commonly have a progressive course without relapse, and have a more rapid development of disability than younger patients. CSF and evoked potentials are of high diagnostic yield, but the interpretation of the cranial MRI must take into account the presence of age-related microangiopathy.

1.10   The peripheral and autonomic nervous systems in MS

Although demyelination of the peripheral nervous system in MS patients may have a number of causes, including malnutrition [57], recognition of an involvement in MS could implicate other antigenic target(s) and influence the interpretation of electrodiagnostic test results. Decreased myelin sheath thickness and internode length have been noted [58] and hypertrophic changes of spinal nerve roots reported [59] in MS patients. Mild neurophysiological abnormalities have been detected in the sensory action potential of peripheral nerves with decreased velocity of the slow conducting myelinated nerve fibers, reduction in amplitude of the supernormal period [60] and prolongation of the relative refractory period [61]. While these morphological and physiological abnormalities may indicate the involvement of myelin or other components of the peripheral nervous system in MS, the peripheral nervous system in MS is typically uninvolved clinically [62] and the common electrodiagnostic measurements will be normal. There are, however, a small number of cases in which chronic idiopathic demyelinating polyneuropathy and CNS demyelination coexist with a range of coexpressed abnormalities from laboratory changes only to the full expression of both conditions [63–65]. There are insufficient numbers of these combined peripheral and central nervous system demyelinating diseases to determine if they are part of the continuum of MS or represent a different condition. Depending on the species involved and the immunogen, the peripheral nervous system, notably the spinal roots, may also be affected in experimental allergic encephalomyelitis.

While they may encompass the functional areas of the autonomic nervous system, the common bladder, bowel and sexual dysfunctions in MS are usually attributed to lesions of the spinal cord. Abnormalities of respiration [66] and cardiovascular [67] function may arise from lesions of the brain stem (Table 1.8). The clinical expression of other forms of autonomic dysfunction is rare, but sensitive testing, especially of cardiac conduction and sweating, detects a high incidence of abnormalities [68, 69]. It is possible that autonomic dysfunction contributes to the edema and skin changes of the feet in MS patients with spinal cord lesions or to some of the immune-mediated tissue damage in MS [69].

1.11   The accuracy of diagnosis

The following cardinal rules should always be obeyed when reaching a diagnosis of MS.

1. The majority of patients present with one or more of the signs of limb weakness, optic neuritis, para-esthesia, diplopia, ataxia, vertigo and disturbance of micturition.
2. Heat intolerance with or without precipitation of transient focal deficits, Lhermitte's sign in the absence of a herniated disk or trauma of the cervical spine, girdle-like dysthesias of the trunk and one of the paroxysmal syndromes (Table 1.5) rarely occur in the alternative diagnoses.
3. Although MS may occur in children, in those over age 60 and in a familial pattern, onset outside the ages of 20–50 and the existence of a strong family history with a clear pattern of inheritance is very uncommon.
4. MS patients rarely have rheumatological or constitutional symptoms, and their occurrence as well as any abnormality on blood testing (Table 1.9) should place the diagnosis of MS in doubt or raise the suspicion of a second disease or effect of medications.
5. Clinical features at onset which are uncommon in MS include aphasia, significant cognitive dysfunction, psychosis, extreme anxiety, a predominantly painful syndrome, and atypical features over the course of the disorder include hemianopic visual field defects, movement disorders, myelopathy without bowel or bladder involvement and persistence of a single lesion without evidence of more widespread demyelination.

In addition to adherence to these rules, there must be a keen awareness of the mimicking conditions and the acceptance that there is no single diagnostic test for MS; the entire composite of clinical features must be considered with a meticulous clinical history and examination. Optimally, the clinician should understand the relative importance, specificity and sensitivity of each symptom, sign and paraclinical study for each clinical form of MS, at varying points of time in the clinical course. The sensitivity, specificity and interpretation of the various paraclinical studies of MRI

Table 1.9   Laboratory blood tests in search of alternative diagnoses of the patient with apparent multiple sclerosis

---

Erythrocyte sedimentation rate or C-reactive protein
Antinuclear antibody titer and staining pattern
Vitamin B_{12} level
For fatigue: hemogram, chemical profile, thyroid function tests
In select patients as dictated by age, clinical symptomatology or risk factors:
    Angiotensin converting enzyme activity
    Anti-cardiolipin antibody
    Partial thromboplastin time, prothrombin time
    SS-A/Ro (Sjögren's syndrome antigen A)
    SS-B/La (Sjögren's syndrome antigen B)
    Lyme, brucella serology
    HTLV-1, HIV, VDRL serology
    Paraneoplastic autoantibodies
    Serum vitamin E level
    Plasma very long chain fatty acids

(Chapter 3), evoked potentials (Chapter 4) and CSF examination (Chapter 5) involved in the diagnosis are covered elsewhere in this book. Although variations temporally and by anatomical CNS deficits are the norm, the experienced clinician who follows acceptable criteria (Tables 1.2 and 1.3) and judiciously utilizes cranial and spinal MRI, CSF analysis and evoked potentials can make a positive and correct diagnosis in more than 95% of cases of MS. The symptomatic patient suspected to have MS but in whom the usual criteria cannot be met is often among the most anxious, but may be the most fortunate in having such little disease burden to preclude a confident diagnosis.

1.12 Differential diagnoses

Each of the dominant features of MS, especially that of anatomical dissemination in the CNS and over time, has its own differential diagnosis. The multifocal CNS lesions, typically presenting over hours to days, then partially or totally resolving over weeks to months can be seen with a variety of disorders, one of the most common being **systemic lupus erythematosus (SLE)**. Relapsing and remitting features and dominant neurological findings may occur in SLE, but the systemic symptoms of fever and weight loss and involvement of skin, joint and kidney, exclude MS unless a second disease is present. There are several neurological features of SLE that are atypical for MS. The most common CNS lupus manifestations are neuropsychiatric with dementia, psychosis, affective disorders and encephalopathies, all of which are uncommon in MS, especially as presenting symptoms. Chorea and peripheral nervous system (PNS) involvement, less commonly known features of SLE, are rare in MS. In spite of these clear differences, in patients with an optic neuritis and myelopathy the conditions may be clinically indistinguishable and not adequately separated by cranial MRI, CSF changes and evoked potentials. Fortunately, hematological and serological abnormalities of SLE are rare in the MS patient.

Patients with the **phospholipid antibody syndrome** may have multifocal CNS deficits from strokes as well as the common symptoms of vascular headaches, transient ischemic attacks and encephalopathies [70]. There is less chance of clinical confusion than with SLE, and the laboratory tests demonstrating the presence of anticardiolipin antibody and coagulopathy are negative in MS.

Behçet's disease is a rare, chronic, idiopathic, inflammatory disorder involving multiple organ systems, with a relapsing and remitting clinical course. The disease is characterized by oral and genital ulceration and uveitis, and the most common neurologic involvement is a focal meningoencephalitis with a tendency toward brain stem involvement [71]. Neurological manifestations include aseptic meningitis, strokes, transient ischemic attacks, cerebral venous thrombosis, seizures, confusional states, bulbar or pseudobulbar palsy, ocular palsies, pyramidal tract dysfunction, cerebellar ataxia and pseudotumor cerebri. A headache and fever, sometimes with associated meningeal signs, may occur with an exacerbation. Differentiation for MS is usually not a problem since the majority of neurological manifestations are clearly distinct from those expected in MS, the neurologic complications usually follow the systemic manifestations and there is a history or presence of mucocutaneous lesions. The greatest struggle to distinguish neuro-Behçet's disease from MS occurs in the patient with cranial neuropathies and transverse myelopathy and no mucocutaneous lesions. While visual impairment in neuro-Behçet's is usually due to uveitis, a retrobulbar neuritis can occur. CSF may show local synthesis of oligoclonal IgG [72], but the pleocytosis and elevated protein may be atypical for MS [14]. With cranial MRI, many patients show vascular abnormalities such as infarcts or cerebral venous thrombosis [73]. During the acute illness with CNS involvement, the expected cranial MRI in neuro-Behçet's patients will reveal multiple hyperintense lesions, less than 5 mm in diameter, scattered or confluent and mainly in the white matter on T2-weighted sequences. The changes may be distributed, in decreasing order, in the hemispheric white matter, brain stem, basal ganglia, thalamus or cortex [73]. More suggestive of the lesions of Behçet's disease than MS were the lack of predilection for periventricular white matter and the increased basal ganglia involvement.

Polyarteritis nodosa is a chronic systemic disease, much more common in older males, with necrotizing vasculitis of small and medium size arteries that may be clinically manifested in episodes, with infarction or hemorrhage of various organs, notably the kidney. The most common neurologic complications are of the PNS with polyneuropathies and mononeuritis multiplex; however, cranial nerve palsies and CNS involvement, which tends to appear after many months of systemic symptoms, in the form of encephalopathy, seizures and focal deficits, may also occur.

Primary granulomatous angiitis is a rare disease of uncertain etiology that predominantly, if not exclusively, involves the CNS [74]. This diagnosis should be considered in young adults who present with primary cognitive decline, confusion or aphasia and a cranial MRI suggestive of MS. Cranial MRI often reveals lesions suggestive of infarct; however, in some cases the abnormalities are limited to the periventricular white matter. There may be a moderate polymorphonuclear pleocytosis, but the CSF can be normal or show oligoclonal bands. The diagnosis of primary granulomatous angiitis requires cerebral angiography, and in some cases parenchymal brain biopsy [74].

Sjögren's syndrome is a common rheumatologic disorder characterized by the presence of two components of the triad of xerostomia, keratoconjunctivitis and another connective tissue disorder. Patients with primary Sjögren's syndrome complicated by CNS involvement have been described to have the clinical, CSF, evoked potentials and cranial MRI features of MS[75, 76]. The peak incidence of Sjögren's syndrome is in the fifth and sixth decades, and the common neurological complications are neuromuscular disorders and cranial neuropathies. Sjögren's syndrome mimicking MS must be rare, but it should be considered in the more elderly patient who also has rheumatological complaints, xerostomia or keratoconjunctivitis. The serological abnormalities of Sjögren's syndrome will also help in differentiating it from MS.

Sarcoidosis is an inflammatory disorder of unknown etiology, characterized by the presence of noncaseating epithelioid cell granulomas in multiple organs. Although the disease primarily involves the lungs, neurological manifestations occur in 5% of the patients[77] and, of the patients with neurological involvement, nearly half present with neurological symptoms[77]. These neurological manifestations are highly variable and include cranial neuropathies, aseptic meningitis, hydrocephalus, hypothalamic dysfunction, intracranial mass lesions, intraspinal mass lesions, diffuse encephalopathy, vasculopathy, seizures, peripheral neuropathy and myopathy[77]. The majority of these symptoms do not suggest the diagnosis of MS; however, affected patients are frequently of the appropriate age and may present with waxing and waning cranial neuropathies or brain stem symptoms suggestive of demyelinating disease. The optic nerve may be involved with subacute visual loss and some findings to suggest an optic neuritis. In others, the spinal cord is involved with a subacute or chronic myelopathy, with the former sometimes undergoing spontaneous relapses and remissions. Paraclinical studies may be beneficial, but again there is substantial overlap. In sarcoid patients with the typical changes of a CSF protein elevation above 100 mg/dl, a pleocytosis in excess of 30 and hypoglycorrhachia, a diagnosis of MS can be excluded. Unfortunately, CSF studies in sarcoidosis and MS may also be very similar, with a mild lymphocytosis, normal to elevated protein, elevated IgG, elevated IgG index and oligoclonal bands. Visual and brain stem auditory potentials are of little benefit since they are abnormal in about 30% of neurosarcoid patients without visual or brain stem symptoms[78]. When the MRI demonstrates meningeal involvement, hydrocephalus, hypothalamic lesions or enhancing mass lesions, sarcoidosis is strongly implicated. Unfortunately, the most common MRI abnormalities with neurosarcoidosis are periventricular and multifocal white matter lesions indistinguishable from those seen in MS[79]. Similarities are also present with spinal MRI[80, 81], although in some cases linear peripheral enhancement overlying the parenchymal involvement may more strongly suggest sarcoidosis[82]. The angiotensin converting enzyme (ACE) is elevated in the CSF of over half of patients with sarcoid, but may also be elevated in a small proportion of patients with pulmonary disease, MS[83], papillary ependymoma[84] and other CNS neoplasms[85] as well as CNS infections[83, 85]. The combination of diffuse pulmonary uptake on gallium scanning and elevated ACE yields a specificity of 83% to 99% for the diagnosis of sarcoidosis[86]. Further evidence of pulmonary involvement on the chest X-ray, hypercalcemia, hyperglobulinemia or anergy on skin testing will offer support for the diagnosis of sarcoid. An appropriate biopsy showing noncaseating epithelioid cell granulomas may be required in some patients.

Lyme disease is caused by the tick-borne spirochete *Borrelia burgdorferi*[87–89]. Neurological complications of the infection are common. A wide variety of neurological manifestations have been reported, with the more typical being meningitis, cranial neuritis and radiculoneuritis. In rare cases, a variety of CNS abnormalities has developed, including a spastic paraparesis and cerebellar ataxia[89–91]. In even more unusual cases these manifestations have occurred without the associated or preceding erythema chronicum migrans or arthritis[90]. It is these rare patients, along with those exhibiting a variety of potential cranial neuropathies, who could present a diagnostic dilemma. CSF examination of patients with the encephalomyelitic manifestations usually demonstrates an active lymphocytic pleocytosis, mild-to-moderate elevation in protein and a normal glucose. In patients with more chronic infections, elevation in intrathecal immunoglobulin synthesis, and even oligoclonal bands, may be present[89]. While the MRI may show evidence of vascular involvement[92], some images reveal signal abnormalities limited to the paraventricular white matter, quite indistinguishable from those of MS[91]. Fortunately, the anti-*Borrelia burgdorferi* antibodies which can usually be demonstrated in these patients are rare in patients with MS[93]. Lyme disease should be considered in areas where the spirochete and appropriate tick vectors are endemic.

The more problematic patients are those with **monoregional CNS involvement**, either with a relapsing or remitting clinical syndrome or the more common monophasic progressive course, as often seen in the primary progressive form of MS. These patients often present with an insidiously progressive spinal or spinal-cerebellar syndrome which appears clinically similar to several other CNS disorders. The availability of improved neuroimaging with MRI, evoked potentials to search for unexpressed multifocal CNS lesions and CSF testing for abnormalities of immunoglobulin has simplified the differential diagnosis for most of these disorders and MS. The MRI helps identify some of the mono-regional CNS lesions with a waxing and waning clinical course, such as arterial venous malformations or the unusual presentation of tumors or arachnoid cyst. MRI also helps identify many of the monoregional CNS lesions with a progressive course, including cervical spondylosis, craniovertebral anomalies such as the Chiari malformation, syringomyelia, arachnoid cyst, tumors or other masses. Subacute combined degeneration from vitamin B_{12} deficiency, HTLV-1 associated myelopathy and leukodystrophies, especially the female heterozygote with adrenoleukodystrophy or the male with adrenomyeloneuropathy, can be recognized with laboratory tests for vitamin B_{12} level and absorption, serology and very long chain fatty acids, respectively. Some of these disorders may also have a waxing or waning course or polyregional CNS symptoms as previously discussed.

1.13   Conversion disorders and MS

The array of neurological complaints offered by the hysterical patient and knowledge that patients with MS can present with or develop essentially any symptom attributable to a CNS lesion, often raises the question of MS in the hysterical patient. The transient sensory symptoms and the paroxysmal events seen in MS may add to the confusion. Much of the misdiagnosis in the past of hysteria as MS and vice versa was in an era when MS was not as well understood and modern paraclinical techniques of MRI, evoked potentials and CSF testing were not available. While not definitive, there are clinical features which help distinguish hysteria and MS. Patients with recent onset of MS usually provide an accurate and detailed history of a well-defined relapse, often followed by a remission of symptoms with periods of absent disease activity. The hysterical patient frequently presents with ill-defined symptoms that persist, often with a continual accumulation of new symptoms. When the symptoms do appear in discrete episodes, there are often psychosocial overlays which provide insight. Careful inquiry into the hysterical patient's symptoms often yields a symptom complex that is very nebulous, often defying lesion localization, and sometimes changing during the interview. Sometimes the hysterical patient is suggestible, with exaggerated symptoms that transcend the CNS and involve other aspects of the body. In contrast, in many MS patients, the more bizarre symptoms such as the ephaptic events must be carefully uncovered in the history, with some patients initially reluctant to reveal their existence. Finally, the predominantly painful syndromes so often noted in hysteria are uncommon at presentation with MS. These differentiating features between the patient populations

must be utilized with caution. An occasional patient with MS will develop hysterical tendencies and provide an exaggerated symptom complex.

1.14   Possible associated diseases

In spite of the plethora of aberrations reported in the immune system of patients with MS, the disorder tends to occur in isolation without overlapping syndromes common to other autoimmune disorders. In contrast to many autoimmune disorders, there are usually no stigmata of systemic disease and newly diagnosed patients usually appear quite healthy. Over the years anecdotal reports have suggested an association with many diseases, including myasthenia gravis, SLE, ankylosing spondylitis, scleroderma, ulcerative colitis and diabetes mellitus. In a population-based cohort of patients, an incidence analysis of autoimmune disorders and cancer revealed no statistically significant increased risk with MS[94].

1.15   Risk factors for relapse or progression

The acknowledged uncertainty of the etiology and pathogenesis of MS, the natural history of MS which involves spontaneous relapses and remissions, the natural human tendency to relate proximal though not necessarily causal events, the secondary gain and litigation have created an atmosphere in which many claims of causal association for a variety of factors in the precipitation of disease or induction of relapse or progression of MS must be addressed. There is a scarcity of prospective studies as indicated in the more extensive descriptions of risk factors (Chapter 8) and natural history (Chapter 6) presented elsewhere in this book.

One of the more controversial factors is **trauma**. Trauma is a common event in the population at large, and patients with MS are no exception. Furthermore, the disorder itself predisposes to trauma, with neurological deficits contributing to multiple falls. Rehabilitation of the patient with a spastic paraparesis after a leg or hip fracture may be quite difficult. There are numerous anecdotal cases cited in older articles and textbooks supporting trauma as a factor contributing to the onset or progression of MS[95]. The suggestion that trauma contributes to a relapse has been theoretically related to a disruption of the blood–brain barrier[96]. More recent prospective or retrospective studies have not confirmed a relationship of physical trauma to onset or deterioration of MS[97] or to disease activity[98]. Only following an electrical injury was there an increased frequency of relapse, and this did not achieve statistical significance. MS patients had two to three times more trauma than controls, but there was no association between the frequency of trauma and progression of disability [98]. There is no correlation between the occurrence of peripheral fractures and the onset of MS, relapse of MS, or final disability due to MS [99].

The population at highest risk for the development of MS are women of childbearing age. There is no evidence that the disease affects fertility and patients usually have normal pregnancies with healthy offspring. While patients with more malignant forms of MS or with severe disability usually defer bearing children, many women with MS desire families. Before 1950, the predominant belief was that pregnancy adversely affected the course of MS. Women with MS were commonly advised to avoid pregnancy, and pregnant patients sometimes underwent therapeutic abortions. In 1950, it was reported that pregnancy had no effect on the disease [100]. Several larger studies followed. An increased incidence of relapse post partum has been observed [101, 102]. Three other studies reported an improvement pre partum, worsening post partum, but no overall adverse effect on MS [103–105]. More recent prospective, controlled studies [106, 107] do not clarify the issue of increased relapses post partum. Most studies show little or no effect on the long-term course or disability related to the disease [107–109]. For women not desiring children, oral contraceptives are not contraindicated but should be used with care in patients requiring frequent antibiotics, anticonvulsants or other medications known to decrease their efficacy.

Infections and infectious agents have long been implicated in the pathogenesis of MS, its onset and its relapses. Several prospective studies suggest a correlation between infections and relapse of disease with common infections [110], especially after minor respiratory tract infections [111]. Chronic sinus infections were significantly associated with relapse [112]. The most likely mechanism for an association of viral infection and relapse of MS is the activation of the *in situ* CNS inflammatory lesion of MS by the host production of gamma interferon which, when administered intravenously in a clinical trial, precipitated relapses [113].

There have been several anecdotal cases of MS relapse following an **immunization**. These may have been related to increased symptoms due to a post-vaccination febrile response. Concerns over the possible deleterious effects of vaccinations have prompted many physicians to avoid elective immunizations in patients with MS. These concerns have been partially allayed by several studies. In MS patients vaccinated against influenza, measles and poliomyelitis [110], influenza [114] or swine influenza virus [115], there is no evidence of induction of a relapse. The effects on MS relapses will need to be continually evaluated as new immunogens continue to emerge. For example, isolated patients have experienced relapses after hepatitis vaccination, in both the authors' experience and that of others [116]. This may represent pure coincidence but merits observation.

The reported risk of MS progression or relapse following **surgical procedures or exposure to anesthetic agents** varies substantially. While the available data may not be considered definitive, it is difficult to detect an increase in complications related to the surgical procedure, anesthesia, postoperative infections, fever or other unidentified factors [98, 117–119]. On this basis, required surgery may generally be considered safe, but elective surgery should be contemplated carefully. Regarding anesthesia, it appears that general and local anesthetics have limited risk in the MS population. It is unclear if caution should be exercised with regional anesthesia in patients with severe myelopathic features, to avoid the possibility of hypotension.

Stress has been identified as a potential precipitating factor for the onset of MS and subsequent relapses. It is difficult to define and quantify stress, but several investigators have attempted to study the association of stress and MS. No apparent relationship has yet been established. Some studies have shown a relationship of MS symptoms or relapse to stress [120–122], but others have not [123]. In two prospective studies no relationship of stress to relapse could be uncovered [124, 125].

1.16 Counseling and management

The patient with newly diagnosed MS is usually filled with questions. The wisdom and accuracy used to address these questions are critical for the patient's understanding and adjustment to a highly variable and chronic disease. The most common questions relate to the type and severity of their disease (Figure 1.1 and Chapters 6 and 7), natural history (Chapter 6) for short- and long-term prognosis, recovery from deficits and the possible benefit of medications for symptoms or hastened recovery from a relapse (Chapters 18 and 23), risk factors that might be controlled (Chapter 8), risk of exposure to them by their relatives or friends, genetic implications in regard to childbearing plans or living children and relatives (Chapter 14), current information about etiology and pathogenesis (Chapters 7, 8 and 13–15), and the status of new (Chapter 18) or potential (Chapter 19 and 20) treatments. In providing this information for the interested patient and family, the informed clinician becomes a valued, principal physician in that patient's subsequent care.

ACKNOWLEDGMENTS

The clinical investigation related to what is described in this chapter was supported by the National Multiple Sclerosis Society, the National Institutes of Health and the Research Program of the Veterans Administration.

References

1. Medaer, R. (1979) Does the history of multiple sclerosis go back as far as the 14th century? *Acta Neurol. Scand.*, **60**, 189–92.
2. Firth, D. (1948) *The Case of Augustus D'Este*, vol. 1, London, Cambridge University Press.
3. Compston, A. (1988) The 150th anniversary of the first depiction of the lesions of multiple sclerosis. *J. Neurol. Neurosurg. Psychiatry*, **51**, 1249–52.
4. Fredrikson, S. and Kam-Hansen, S. (1989) The 150-year anniversary of multiple sclerosis: does its early history give an etiological clue? *Perspect. Biol. Med.*, **32**, 237–43.
5. Mann, R.J. (1973) Multiple sclerosis and three professors of pathologic anatomy. *Mayo Clin. Proc.*, **48**, 138–41.
6. DeJong, R.N. (1970) Multiple sclerosis. History, definition and general considerations, in *Handbook of Clinical Neurology* (eds P.J. Vinken and C.W. Bruyn), Amsterdam, Elsevier, pp. 45–62.
7. Rivers, T.M. and Schwentker, F.F. (1935) Encephalomyelitis accompanied by myelin destruction experimentally produced in monkeys. *J. Exp. Med.*, **61**, 689–702.
8. Kabat, D.A., Wolf, A. and Bezer, A.E. (1946) Rapid production of acute disseminated encephalomyelitis in rhesus monkeys by injection of brain tissue with adjuvants. *Science*, **104**, 363.
9. Kabat, E.A., Freedman, D.A., Murray, J.P. and Knaub, V. (1950) A study of the crystalline albumin, gamma globulin and total protein in the cerebrospinal fluid of one hundred cases of multiple sclerosis and in other diseases. *Am J. Med. Sci.*, **219**, 55–64.
10. Harris, J.O., Frank, J.A., Patronas, N., McFarlin, D.E. and McFarland, H.F. (1991) Serial gadolinium-enhanced magnetic resonance imaging scans in patients with early, relapsing-remitting multiple sclerosis: Implications for clinical trials and natural history. *Ann. Neurol.*, **29**, 548–55.
11. Schumacher, G.A., Beebe, G., Kebler, R.F. *et al.* (1965) Problems of experimental trials of therapy in multiple sclerosis. *Ann. NY Acad. Sci.*, **122**, 552–68.
12. Poser, C.M., Paty, D.W., Scheinberg, L.C. *et al.* (1983) New diagnostic criteria for multiple sclerosis: guidelines for research protocols. *Ann. Neurol.*, **13**, 227–31.
13. Lublin, F.D. and Reingold, S.C. (1996) Defining the clinical course of multiple sclerosis: results of an international survey. *Neurology*, **46**, 907–11.
14. Whitaker, J.N., Benveniste, E.N. and Zhou, S.R. (1990) Cerebrospinal fluid, in *Handbook of Multiple Sclerosis* (ed. S.D. Cook), New York, Marcel Dekker, pp. 251–70.
15. Whitaker, J.N., Kachelhofer, R.D., Bradley, E.L. *et al.* (1995) Urinary myelin basic protein-like material as a correlate of the progression of multiple sclerosis. *Ann. Neurol.*, **38**, 625–32.
16. Twomey, J.A. and Espir, M.L. (1980) Paroxysmal symptoms as the first manifestations of multiple sclerosis. *J. Neurol. Neurosurg. Psychiatry*, **43**, 296–304.
17. Espir, M.L.E. and Millac, P. (1970) Treatment of paroxysmal disorder in multiple sclerosis with carbamazepine (Tegretol). *J. Neurol. Neurosurg. Psychiatry*, **33**, 528–31.
18. Shibasaki, H. and Kuroiwa, Y. (1974) Painful tonic seizures in multiple sclerosis. *Arch. Neurol.*, **30**, 47–51.
19. Rushton, J.G. and Olafson, R.A. (1965) Trigeminal neuralgia associated with multiple sclerosis: report of 35 cases. *Arch. Neurol.*, **13**, 383–6.
20. Osterman, P.O. and Westerberg, C-E. (1975) Paroxysmal attacks in multiple sclerosis. *Brain*, **98**, 189–202.
21. Matthews, W.B. (1975) Paroxysmal symptoms in multiple sclerosis. *J. Neurol. Neurosurg. Psychiatry*, **38**, 617–23.
22. Osterman, P.O. (1979) Paroxysmal itching in multiple sclerosis. *Int. J. Dermatol.*, **18**, 626–7.
23. Yamamoto, M., Yabuki, S., Hayabara, T. and Otsuki, S. (1981) Paroxysmal itching in multiple sclerosis: a report of three cases. *J. Neurol. Neurosurg. Psychiatry*, **44**, 19–22.
24. Netsell, R. and Kent, R.D. (1976) Paroxysmal ataxic dysarthria. *J. Speech Hear. Disord.*, **41**, 93–109.
25. Miley, C.E. and Forster, F.M. (1974) Paroxysmal signs and symptoms in multiple sclerosis. *Neurology*, **24**, 458–61.
26. Miro, J., Garcia-Monco, C., Leno, C. and Berciano, J. (1988) Pelvic pain: an undescribed paroxysmal manifestation of multiple sclerosis. *Pain*, **32**, 73–5.
27. Clark, C.M., Fleming, J.A., Li, D. *et al.* (1992) Sleep disturbance, depression, and lesion site in patients with multiple sclerosis. *Arch. Neurol.*, **49**, 641–3.
28. Ferini-Strambi, L., Filippi, M., Martinelli, V. *et al.* (1994) Nocturnal sleep study in multiple sclerosis: correlations with clinical and brain magnetic resonance imaging findings. *J. Neurol. Sci.*, **125**, 194–7.
29. Müller, A., Wiedemann, G., Rohde, U., Backmund, H. and Sonntag, A. (1994) Correlates of cognitive impairment and depressive mood disorder in multiple sclerosis. *Acta Psychiatr. Scand.*, **89**, 117–21.
30. Guthrie, T.C. (1951) Visual and motor changes in patients with multiple sclerosis. A result of induced changes in environmental temperature. *Arch. Neurol. Psychiatry*, **65**: 437–51.
31. Edmund, J. and Fog, T. (1955) Visual and motor instability in multiple sclerosis. *Arch. Neurol. Psychiatry*, **73**, 316–23.
32. O'Reilly, M.A.R. and O'Reilly, P.M.R. (1991) Temporal influences on relapses of multiple sclerosis. *Eur. Neurol.*, **31**, 391–5X.
33. Moulin, D.E. (1989) Pain in multiple sclerosis. *Neurol. Clin.*, **7**, 321–31.
34. Moulin, D.E., Foley, K.M. and Ebers, G.C. (1988) Pain syndromes in multiple sclerosis. *Neurology*, **38**, 1830–4.
35. Stenager, E., Knudsen, L. and Jensen, K. (1991) Acute and chronic pain syndromes in multiple sclerosis. *Acta Neurol. Scand.*, **84**, 197–200.
36. Warnell, P. (1991) The pain experience of a multiple sclerosis population: a descriptive study. *Axone*, **13**, 26–8.
37. Archibald, C.J., McGrath, P.J., Ritvo, P.G. *et al.* (1994) Pain prevalence, severity and impact in a clinic sample of multiple sclerosis patients. *Pain*, **58**, 89–93.
38. Vermote, R., Ketelaer, P. and Carton, H. (1986) Pain in multiple sclerosis patients. A prospective study using the McGill Pain Questionnaire. *Clin. Neurol. Neurosurg.*, **88**, 87–93.
39. Sagar, H.J., Warlow, C.P., Sheldon, P.W.E. and Esiri, M.M. (1982) Multiple sclerosis with clinical and radiological features of cerebral tumor. *J. Neurol. Neurosurg. Psychiatry*, **45**, 802–8.
40. Nelson, M.J., Miller, S.L., McLain, L.W. Jr and Gold, L.H.A. (1981) Multiple sclerosis: large plaque causing mass effect and ring sign. *J. Comput. Assist. Tomogr.*, **5**, 892–4.
41. Butler, E.G. and Gilligan, B.S. (1989) Obstructive hydrocephalus caused by multiple sclerosis. *Clin. Exp. Neurol.*, **26**, 219–23.
42. Kanchandani, R. and Howe, J.G. (1982) Lhermitte's sign in multiple sclerosis: a clinical survey and review of the literature. *J. Neurol. Neurosurg. Psychiatry*, **45**, 308–12.
43. Gutrecht, J.A., Zamani, A.A. and Salgado, E.D. (1993) Anatomic-radiologic basis of Lhermitte sign in multiple sclerosis. *Arch. Neurol.*, **50**, 849–51.
44. Uldry, P.A. and Regli, F. (1992) Pseudoradicular limb pain in multiple sclerosis – magnetic resonance imaging in four cases. *Rev. Neurol.*, **148**, 692–5.
45. Ramirez-Lasspas, M., Tulloch, J.W., Quinones, M.R. and Snyder, B.D. (1992) Acute radicular pain as a presenting symptom in multiple sclerosis. *Arch. Neurol.*, **49**, 255–8.
46. Lipton, H.L. and Teasdall, R.D. (1973) Acute transverse myelopathy in adults. A follow-up study. *Arch. Neurol.*, **28**, 252–7.
47. Ford, B., Tampieri, D. and Francis, G. (1992) Long-term follow-up of acute partial transverse myelopathy. *Neurology*, **42**, 250–2.
48. Tippett, D.S., Fishman, P.S. and Panitch, H.S. (1991) Relapsing transverse myelitis. *Neurology*, **41**, 703–6.
49. Weinshenker, B.G., Gilbert, J.J. and Ebers, G.C. (1990) Some clinical and pathologic observations on chronic myelopathy: a variant of multiple sclerosis. *J. Neurol. Neurosurg. Psychiatry*, **53**, 146–9.
50. Paty, D.W., Blume, W.T., Brown, W.F., Jaatoul, N. *et al.* (1979) Chronic progressive myelopathy: investigation with CSF electrophoresis, evoked potentials, and CT scan. *Ann. Neurol.*, **6**, 419–24.
51. Komar, J., Szalay, M. and Dalos, M. (1982) Acute retention of urine due to isolated sacral myeloradiculitis. *J. Neurol.*, **228**, 215–17.
52. Sindern, E., Haas, J., Stark, E. and Wurster, U. (1992) Early onset MS under the age of 16 – clinical and paraclinical features. *Acta Neurol. Scand.*, **86**, 280–4.
53. Duquette, P., Murray, T.J., Pleines, J. *et al.* (1987) Multiple sclerosis in childhood: clinical profile in 125 patients. *J. Pediatr.*, **111**, 359–63.
54. Guilhoto, L.M.D.F., Osorio, C.A.M., Machado, L.R. *et al.* (1995) Pediatric multiple sclerosis report of 14 cases. *Brain Dev.*, **17**, 9–12.
55. Noseworthy, J., Paty, D., Wonnacott, T., Feasby, T. and Ebers, G. (1983) Multiple sclerosis after age 50. *Neurology*, **33**, 1537–44.
56. Hooge, J.P. and Redekop, W.K. (1992) Multiple sclerosis with very late onset. *Neurology*, **42**, 1907–10.
57. Hasson, J., Terry, R.D. and Zimmerman, H.M. (1958) Peripheral neuropathy in multiple sclerosis. *Neurology*, **8**, 503–10.
58. Pollock, M., Calder, C. and Allpress, S. (1977) Peripheral nerve abnormality in multiple sclerosis. *Ann Neurol*, **2**, 41–8.
59. Schoene, W.C., Carpenter, S., Behan, P.O. and Geschwind, N. (1977) 'Onion bulb' formations in the central and peripheral nervous system in association with multiple sclerosis and hypertrophic polyneuropathy. *Brain*, **100**, 755–73.
60. Shefner, J.M., Carter, J.L. and Krarup, C. (1992) Peripheral sensory abnormalities in patients with multiple sclerosis. *Muscle Nerve*, **15**, 73–6.
61. Hopf, H.C. and Eysholdt, M. (1978) Impaired refractory periods of peripheral sensory nerves in multiple sclerosis. *Ann. Neurol.*, **4**, 499–501.
62. Waxman, S.G. (1993) Peripheral nerve abnormalities in multiple sclerosis. *Muscle Nerve*, **16**, 1–5.
63. Mendell, J.R., Kolkin, S., Kissel, J.T. *et al.* (1987) Evidence for central nervous system demyelination in chronic inflammatory demyelinating polyneuropathy. *Neurology*, **37**, 1291–4.
64. Thomas, P.K., Walker, R.W., Rudge, P. *et al.* (1987) Chronic demyelinating peripheral neuropathy associated with multifocal central nervous system demyelination. *Brain*, **110**, 53–76.

65. Ormerod, I.E.C., Waddy, H.M., Kermode, A.G., Murray, N.M.F. and Thomas, P.K. (1990) Involvement of the central nervous system in chronic inflammatory demyelinating polyneuropathy: a clinical, electrophysiological and magnetic resonance imaging study. *J. Neurol. Neurosurg. Psychiatry*, 53, 789–93.

66. Howard, R.S., Wiles, C.M., Hirsch, N.P. *et al.* (1992) Respiratory involvement in multiple sclerosis. *Brain*, 115, 479–94.

67. Vita, G. Fazio, M.C., Milone, S. *et al.* (1993) Cardiovascular autonomic dysfunction in multiple sclerosis is likely related to brain stem lesions. *J. Neurol. Sci.*, 120, 82–6.

68. Senaratne, M.P., Carroll, D., Warren, K.G. and Kappagoda, T. (1984) Evidence for cardiovascular autonomic nerve dysfunction in multiple sclerosis. *J. Neurol. Neurosurg. Psychiatry*, 47, 947–52.

69. Karaszewski, J.W., Reder, A.T., Maselli, R., Brown, M. and Arnason, B.G.W. (1990) Sympathetic skin responses are decreased and lymphocyte beta-adrenergic receptors are increased in progressive multiple sclerosis. *Ann. Neurol.*, 27, 366–72.

70. Levine, S.R. (1994) Antiphospholipid syndromes and the nervous system. Clinical features, mechanisms, and treatment. *Semin. Neurol.*, 14, 168–78.

71. Nadeau, S.E. and Watson, R.T. (1993) Neurologic manifestations of vasculitis and collagen vascular syndromes, in *Clinical Neurology* (ed. R.J. Joynt), Philadelphia, Lippincott, pp. 1–166.

72. McLean, B.N., Miller, D. and Thompson, E.J. (1995) Oligoclonal banding of IgG in CSF, blood–brain barrier function, and MRI findings in patients with sarcoidosis, systemic lupus erythematosus, and Behçet's disease involving the nervous system. *J. Neurol. Neurosurg. Psychiatry*, 58, 548–54.

73. Wechsler, B., Dellisola, B., Vidailhet, M. *et al.* (1993) MRI in 31 patients with Behçet's disease and neurological involvement – prospective study with clinical correlation. *J. Neurol. Neurosurg. Psychiatry*, 56, 793–8.

74. Moore, P.M. and Cupps, T.R. (1983) Neurological complications of vasculitis. *Ann. Neurol.*, 14, 155–67.

75. Alexander, E.L., Malinow, K., Lejewski, J.E. *et al.* (1986) Primary Sjögren's syndrome with central nervous system disease mimicking multiple sclerosis. *Ann. Intern. Med.*, 104, 323–30.

76. Alexander, E.L., Beall, S.S., Gordon, B. *et al.* (1988) Magnetic resonance imaging of cerebral lesions in patients with Sjögren's syndrome. *Ann. Intern. Med.*, 108, 815–23.

77. Stern, B.J., Krumholz, A., Johns, C., Scott, P. and Nissim, J. (1985) Sarcoidosis and its neurologic manifestations. *Arch. Neurol.*, 42, 909–17.

78. Oksanen, V. (1986) Neurosarcoidosis: clinical presentation and course in 50 patients. *Acta Neurol. Scand.*, 73, 283–90.

79. Miller, D.H., Kendall, B.E., Barter, S. *et al.* (1988) Magnetic resonance imaging in central nervous system sarcoidosis. *Neurology*, 38, 378–83.

80. Kelly, R.B., Mahoney, P.D. and Cawley, K.M. (1988) MR demonstration of spinal cord sarcoidosis: report of a case. *Am. J. Neuroradiol.*, 9, 197–9.

81. Soucek, D., Prior, C., Luef, G., Birbamer, G. and Bauer, G. (1993) Successful treatment of spinal sarcoidosis by high-dose intravenous methylprednisolone. *Clin. Neuropharmacol.*, 16, 464–7.

82. Nesbit, G.M., Miller, G.M., Baker, H.L. Jr, Ebersold, M.J. and Scheithauer, B.W. (1989) Spinal cord sarcoidosis: a new finding at MR imaging with Gd-DTPA enhancement. *Radiology*, 173, 839–43.

83. Schweisfurth, H., Schioberg-Schiegnitz, S., Kuhn, W. and Parusel, B. (1987) Angiotensin I converting enzyme in cerebrospinal fluid of patients with neurological diseases. *Klin. Wochenschr.*, 65, 955–8.

84. Hidaka, C., Ehlers, M.R.W., Caldwell, P.B.R. and Herbert, J. (1991) Angiotensin-converting enzyme is a marker for papillary ependymomas. *Neurology*, 41, 131.

85. Oksanen, V., Fyhrquist, F., Somer, H. and Gronhagen-Riska, C. (1985) Angiotensin converting enzyme in cerebrospinal fluid: a new assay. *Neurology*, 35, 1220–3.

86. Nosal, A., Schleissner, L.A., Mishkin, F.S. and Lieberman, J. (1979) Angiotensin-I-converting enzyme and gallium scan in noninvasive evaluation of sarcoidosis. *Ann. Intern. Med.*, 90, 328–31.

87. Steere, A.C. (1989) Lyme disease. *N. Engl. J. Med.*, 321, 586–96.

88. Steere, A.C., Grodzicki, R.L. and Kornblatt, A.N. (1983) The spirochetal etiology of Lyme disease. *N. Engl. J. Med.*, 308, 733–40.

89. Halperin, J.J. (1995) Neuroborreliosis. *Am. J. Med.*, 98, S52–S59.

90. Reik, L., Burgdorfer, W. and Donaldson, J.O. (1986) Neurological abnormalities in Lyme disease without erythema chronicum migrans. *Am. J. Med.*, 81, 73–8.

91. Pachner, A.R., Duray, P. and Steere, A.C. (1989) Central nervous system manifestations of Lyme disease. *Arch. Neurol.*, 46, 790–5.

92. Kruger, H., Heim, E., Schuknecht, B. and Scholz, S. (1991) Acute and chronic neuroborreliosis with and without CNS involvement: a clinical, MRI, and HLA study of 27 cases. *J. Neurol.*, 238, 271–80.

93. Coyle, P.K. (1989) *Borrelia burgdorferi* antibodies in multiple sclerosis patients. *Neurology*, 39, 760–1.

94. Wynn, D.R., Rodriguez, M., O'Fallon, W.M. and Kurland, L.T. (1990) A reappraisal of the epidemiology of multiple sclerosis in Olmsted County, Minnesota. *Neurology*, 40, 780–6.

95. McAlpine, D. and Compston, N.D. (1952) Some aspects of the natural history of disseminated sclerosis. *Q. J. Med.*, 21, 135–67.

96. Poser, C.M. (1987) Trauma and multiple sclerosis. An hypothesis. *J. Neurol.*, 234, 155–9.

97. Bamford, C.R., Sibley, W.A., Thies, C. *et al.* (1981) Trauma as an etiologic and aggravating factor in multiple sclerosis. *Neurology (NY)*, 31, 1229–234.

98. Sibley, W.A., Bamford, C.R., Clark, K., Smith, M.S. and Laguna, J.F. (1991) A prospective study of physical trauma and multiple sclerosis. *J. Neurol. Neurosurg. Psychiatry*, 54, 584–9.

99. Siva, A., Radhakrishnan, K., Kurland, L.T. *et al.* (1993) Trauma and multiple sclerosis: a population-based cohort study from Olmsted County, Minnesota. *Neurology*, 43, 1878–82.

100. Tillman, A. (1950) The effect of pregnancy on multiple sclerosis and its management. *Res. Publ. Assoc. Res. Nerv. Ment. Dis.*, 28, 548–82.

101. Millar, J.H.D., Allison, R.S., Cheesman, E.A. and Merrett, J.D. (1959) Pregnancy as a factor influencing relapse in disseminated sclerosis. *Brain*, 82, 417–26.

102. Schapira, K., Poskanzer, D.C., Newell, D.J. and Miller, H. (1966) Marriage, pregnancy and multiple sclerosis. *Brain*, 89, 419–28.

103. Poser, S. and Poser, W. (1983) Multiple sclerosis and gestation. *Neurology*, 33, 1422–7.

104. Korn-Lubetzki, I., Kahana, E., Cooper, G. and Abramsky, O. (1984) Activity of multiple sclerosis during pregnancy and puerperium. *Ann. Neurol.*, 16, 229–31.

105. Ghezzi, A. and Caputo, D. (1981) Pregnancy: a factor influencing the course of multiple sclerosis. *Eur. Neurol.*, 20, 115–17.

106. Sadovnick, A.D., Eisen, K., Hashimoto, S.A. *et al.* (1994) Pregnancy and multiple sclerosis – a prospective study. *Arch. Neurol.*, 51, 1120–4.

107. Roullet, E., Verdier-Taillefer, M.H., Amarenco, P. *et al.* (1993) Pregnancy and multiple sclerosis: a longitudinal study of 125 remittent patients. *J. Neurol. Neurosurg. Psychiatry*, 56, 1062–5.

108. Weinshenker, B.G., Hader, W., Carriere, W., Baskerville, J. and Ebers, G.C. (1989) The influence of pregnancy on disability from multiple sclerosis: a population-based study in Middlesex County, Ontario. *Neurology*, 39, 1438–40.

109. Thompson, D.S., Nelson, L.M., Burns, A., Burks, J.S. and Franklin, G.M. (1986) The effects of pregnancy in multiple sclerosis: a retrospective study. *Neurology*, 36, 1097–9.

110. Sibley, W.A. and Foley, J.M. (1965) Infection and immunization in multiple sclerosis. *Ann. NY Acad. Sci.*, 122, 457–68.

111. Sibley, W.A., Bamford, C.R. and Clark, K. (1985) Clinical viral infections and multiple sclerosis. *Lancet*, 1, 1313–15.

112. Gay, D., Dick, G. and Upton, G. (1986) Multiple sclerosis associated with sinusitis: case-controlled study in general practice. *Lancet*, 1, 815–19.

113. Panitch, H.S., Hirsch, R.L., Schindler, J. and Johnson, K.P. (1987) Treatment of multiple sclerosis with gamma interferon: exacerbations associated with activation of the immune system. *Neurology*, 37, 1097–102.

114. Sibley, W.A., Bamford, C.R. and Laguna, J.F. (1976) Influenza vaccination in patients with multiple sclerosis. *J. Am. Med. Assoc.*, 236, 1965–6.

115. Myers, L.W., Ellison, G.W., Lucia, M. *et al.* (1977) Swine influenza virus vaccination in patients with multiple sclerosis. *J. Infect. Dis.*, 136 (Suppl.), S546–S554.

116. Herroelen, L., De Keyser, J. and Ebinger, G. (1991) Central-nervous-system demyelination after immunisation with recombinant hepatitis B vaccine. *Lancet*, 338, 1174–1175X.

117. Ridley, A. and Schapira, K. (1961) Influence of surgical procedures on the course of multiple sclerosis. *Neurology*, 11, 81–2.

118. Keschner, M. (1950) The effects of injury and illness on the course of multiple sclerosis. *Research Publications of the Association for Research into Nervous and Mental Disorders*, 28, 533–47.

119. Johnston, S.R.D., Burn, D.J. and Brooks, D.J. (1991) Peripheral neuropathy associated with lithium toxicity. *J. Neurol. Neurosurg Psychiatry*, 54, 1019–20.

120. Warren, S.A., Warren, K.G., Greenhill, S. and Paterson, M. (1982) How multiple sclerosis is related to animal illness, stress and diabetes. *Can. Med. Assoc. J.*, 126, 377–82.

121. Grant, I., Brown, G.W., Harris, T. *et al.* (1989) Severely threatening events and marked life difficulties preceding onset or exacerbation of multiple sclerosis. *J. Neurol. Neurosurg. Psychiatry*, 52, 8–13.

122. Franklin, G.M., Nelson, L.M., Heaton, R.K. *et al.* (1988). Stress and its relationship to acute exacerbations in multiple sclerosis. *J. Neurol. Rehab.*, 2, 27–11.

123. Pratt, R.T.C. (1951) An investigation of the psychiatric aspects of disseminated sclerosis. *J. Neurol. Neurosurg. Psychiatry*, 14, 326.

124. Nisipeanu, P. and Korczyn, A.D. (1993) Psychological stress as a risk factor for exacerbations in multiple sclerosis. *Neurology*, 43, 1311–12.

125. Rabins, P.V., Brooks, B.R., O'Donnell, P. *et al.* (1986) Structural brain correlates of emotional disorder in multiple sclerosis. *Brain*, 109, 585–97.

126. Traugott U. and Raine, C.S. (1984) The neurology of myelin diseases, in *Myelin* (ed. P. Morell), New York, Plenum, pp. 311–35.

127. Weinshenker, B.G. (1995) The natural history of multiple sclerosis, in, *Neurologic Clinics* (ed. J.P. Antel), Philadelphia, Saunders, pp. 119–46.

128. Poser, S., Wikstrom, J. and Bauer, H.J. (1979) Clinical data and the identification of special forms of multiple sclerosis in 1271 cases studied with a standardized documentation system. *J. Neurol. Sci.*, **40**, 159–68.

129. Achiron, A., Ziv, I., Djaldetti, R. *et al.* (1992) Aphasia in multiple sclerosis – clinical and radiologic correlations. *Neurology*, **42**, 2195–7.

130. Cowan, J., Ormerod, I.E.C. and Rudge, P. (1990) Hemiparetic multiple sclerosis. *J. Neurol. Neurosurg. Psychiatry*, **53**, 675–80.

131. Thompson, A.J., Kermode, A.G., Moseley, I.F., Macmanus D.G. and McDonald, W.I. (1993) Seizures due to multiple sclerosis – seven-patients with MRI correlations. *J. Neurol. Neurosurg. Psychiatry*, **56**, 1317–20.

132. Hess, D.C. and Sethi, K.D. (1990) Epilepsia partialis continua in multiple sclerosis. *Int. J. Neurosci.*, **50**, 109–11.

133. Younger, D.S., Pedley, T.A. and Thorpy, M.J. (1991) Multiple sclerosis and narcolepsy: possible similar genetic susceptibility. *Neurology*, **41**, 447–8.

134. Mao, C.C., Gancher, S.T. and Herndon, R.M. (1988) Movement disorders in multiple sclerosis. *Mov. Disord.*, **3**, 109–16.

135. Coleman, R.J., Quinn, N.P. and Marsden, C.D. (1988) Multiple sclerosis presenting as adult onset dystonia. *Mov. Disord.*, **3**, 329–32.

136. Riley, D. and Lang, A.E. (1988) Hemiballism in multiple sclerosis. *Mov. Disord.*, **3**, 88–94.

137. Kapoor, R., Brown, P., Thompson, P.D. and Miller, D.H. (1992) Propriospinal myoclonus in multiple sclerosis. *J. Neurol. Neurosurg. Psychiatry*, **55**, 1086–8.

138. Plant, G.T., Kermode, A.G., Du Boulay, E.P. and McDonald, W.I. (1989) Spasmodic torticollis due to a midbrain lesion in a case of multiple sclerosis. *Mov. Disord*, **4**, 359–62.

139. Masucci, E.F., Saini, N. and Kurtzke, J.F. (1989) Bilateral ballism in multiple sclerosis. *Neurology*, **39**, 1641–2.

140. Lugaresi, A., Uncini, A. and Gambi, D. (1993) Basal ganglia involvement in multiple sclerosis with alternating side paroxysmal dystonia. *J. Neurol.*, **240**, 257–8.

141. D'Costa, D.F., Vania, A.K. and Millac, P.A. (1990) Multiple sclerosis associated with trismus. *Postgrad. Med. J.*, **66**, 853–4.

142. Geny, C., Pradat, P.F., Yulis, J. *et al.* (1992) Hypothermia, Wernicke encephalopathy and multiple sclerosis. *Acta Neurol. Scand.*, **86**, 632–4.

143. Combarros, O., Miro, J. and Berciano, J. (1994) Ageusia associated with thalamic plaque in multiple sclerosis. *Eur. Neurol.*, **34**, 344–6.

144. Seeldrayers, P.A., Borenstein, S., Gerard, J.M. and Flament-Durand, J. (1987). Reversible capsulo-tegmental locked-in state as first manifestation of multiple sclerosis. *J. Neurol. Sci.*, **80**, 153–61.

145. Jacobs, L., Kaba, S. and Pullicino, P. (1994) The lesion causing continuous facial myokymia in multiple sclerosis. *Arch. Neurol.*, **51**, 1115–19.

146. Telischi, F.F., Grobman, L.R., Sheremata, W.A., Apple, M. and Ayyar, R. (1991) Hemifacial spasm. Occurrence in multiple sclerosis. *Arch. Otolaryngol.*, **117**, 554–6.

147. Mustillo, P. (1984) Auditory deficits in multiple sclerosis: a review. *Audiology*, **23**, 145–64.

148. D'Cruz, O.F., Vaughn, B.V., Gold, S.H. and Greenwood, R.S. (1994) Symptomatic cataplexy in pontomedullary lesions. *Neurology*, **44**, 2189–91.

149. Chang, Y.Y., Wu, H.S., Tsai, T.C. and Liu, J.S. (1994) Intractable hiccup due to multiple sclerosis: MR imaging of medullary plaque. *Can. J. Neurol. Sci.*, **21**, 271–2.

150. Ransohoff, R.M., Whitman, G.J. and Weinstein, M.A. (1990) Non-communicating syringomyelia in multiple sclerosis: detection by magnetic resonance imaging. *Neurology*, **40**, 718–21.

151. Klostermann, W., Vieregge, P. and Kompf, D. (1993) Spasmodic torticollis in multiple sclerosis – significance of an upper cervical spinal cord lesion. *Mov. Disord.*, **8**, 234–6.

2 OPTIC NEURITIS

Shirley H. Wray

The linkage between idiopathic optic neuritis and multiple sclerosis (MS) is firmly established. In the majority of patients, optic neuritis is due to demyelination, whether or not clinically apparent MS is present. Optic neuritis is predominantly a disease of young adults. In the New England region of the US, the incidence of optic neuritis in adult women exceeds that in men by a ratio of 1.8:1. The mean age of onset in women is 30.2 years (range 9–55 years, median 29 years). In men, the mean age of onset is 31.1 years (range 16–60 years, median 32 years) [1]. The condition is rare in children [2, 3], in whom it is usually post- or para-infectious, often simultaneously bilateral and generally characterized by a good visual prognosis [4]. Children have a comparatively low risk (35%) of developing MS [5]. Optic neuritis in patients 40–50 years of age behaves similarly to the disorder in younger adults (18–39 years of age). In patients over 50 years of age, optic neuritis can be a misleading diagnosis since other disorders, particularly ischemic optic neuropathy, commonly cause acute or subacute visual loss.

2.1 Symptoms

A triad of symptoms heralds an acute attack of optic neuritis: loss of vision, ipsilateral eye pain and dyschromatopsia. The initial attack is unilateral in 70% of adult patients and bilateral in 30% [6]. Associated visual symptoms are movement- and sound-induced phosphenes [7–9], obscuration of vision in bright light and Uhthoff's symptom. [10, 11–13] In asymptomatic patients, mild dyschromatopsia, temporal pallor of the optic disc and slits in the nerve fiber layer detected on a routine eye examination are clear signs of the disease. Subclinical cases are also detectable electrophysiologically by delay of the P 100 potential latency on the visual evoked potential test [14]. They are also detectable post mortem, as demyelination of the optic nerve [15].

2.1.1 LOSS OF VISION

Decreased visual acuity as an isolated symptom occurs in 58% of optic neuritis cases [6]. The rate at which vision fails may be very rapid, within hours (29%); fast, within

Table 2.1 Visual acuity (VA) in 108 eyes with acute isolated optic neuritis at the onset, at maximum loss of acuity and at 8 weeks

	Initial (%)	Maximum (%)	At 8 weeks (%)
20/15–20/60	52	34	74
20/70–NLP	48	66	25
20/200–NLP	38	54	20

NLP, No light perception.

From Wray *et al.*, 1995 [1], with permission.

1–2 days (20%); slow, within 3–7 days (23%); or even slower, within 1–2 weeks (7%). Within 7 days of the onset, the visual acuity may be less than 20/60 in 52% of eyes, 20/70 to 20/100 in 48% and worse than 20/200 in 38%. A significant number of eyes continue to lose vision down to an acuity of 20/200 or worse before stabilizing (Table 2.1) [1]. Chronic progressive demyelinating optic neuropathy, characterized by slowly progressive visual loss without remission, is a rare variant of optic neuritis. A further variant of chronic progressive demyelinating optic neuropathy is characterized by slowly progressive loss of visual acuity punctuated by acute episodes of more profound visual loss and incomplete restoration of vision after each exacerbation.

2.1.2 EYE PAIN

The incidence of ipsilateral eye pain in unilateral optic neuritis ranges from 53% to 88% [1, 6]. In one study, 115 optic neuritis patients (62%) complained of pain during an attack in or behind the involved eye. In 39 (21%) it occurred only with eye movements. In 19 (16%) pain preceded a decrease in visual acuity. Headache in the involved eye region was reported by 40 patients (22%) and generalized headache by 24 (13%) [6]. Typically, the pain is experienced as a dull ache or sinus pain, with or without tenderness of the globe. It reaches maximum severity within 24–36 hours and resolves spontaneously within 48–72 hours. Persistent pain for 7 days is highly atypical and should prompt a search for other causes of optic neuropathy.

Multiple Sclerosis: Clinical and pathogenetic basis. Edited by Cedric S. Raine, Henry F. McFarland and Wallace W. Tourtellotte. Published in 1997 by Chapman & Hall, London. ISBN 0 412 30890 8.

The cause of the eye pain is unknown. It does not correlate with the severity of visual loss, with the absence of optic disc swelling (which implies retrobulbar optic neuritis), with enlargement of the optic nerve or with localization of the demyelinating plaque in the intracanalicular region [16].

2.1.3   DYSCHROMATOPSIA

Impaired color vision, dyschromatopsia, is always present in optic neuritis, characterized by a reduced vividness of saturated colors [6, 14, 17]. In color terminology, saturation refers to the purity of color, and desaturation is the degree to which a color is mixed with white. Some patients shown a red target characterize the sensation as darker, i.e. red is shifted toward amber, whereas others say the color is bleached or lighter, i.e. red is shifted towards orange. In the absence of a macular lesion, color desaturation is a highly sensitive indicator of optic nerve disease.

2.1.4   MOVEMENT- AND SOUND-INDUCED PHOSPHENES

Movement phosphenes in MS optic neuritis must be distinguished from phosphenes of retinal origin which are a prelude to retinal detachment. In optic neuritis phosphenes occur almost exclusively with horizontal eye movement, are best perceived in a dark or dimly lit room with the eyes closed, and appear as a very brief flash of light lasting only 1 or 2 seconds even if lateral gaze is maintained. Repeated eye movements cause temporary lulling of the phosphenes with reappearance after several minutes' rest. They occur unilaterally and ipsilateral to the affected eye before, during and/or after an attack, and last for as long as 9 months [7]. Rarely, they may occur 6 months after full recovery, when the visual acuity is 20/20 and fundoscopy is normal.

Phosphenes can also be precipitated by sudden noise when the patient is resting in the dark [8, 9]. They occur transiently in disease of the eye or of the optic nerve, including optic neuritis and compressive optic neuropathy.

2.1.5   OBSCURATION OF VISION IN BRIGHT LIGHT

Obscuration of vision in bright light is a symptom of acute optic neuritis. Patients with chronic optic neuritis in fact see better in dim light. In MS patients the variability of seeing in different lighting conditions is related to the luminance of the background, with vision becoming more impaired as background luminance increases [10]. This luminance-dependent variability is not due to visual fatigue of the type reported in optic neuritis, but rather to a fluctuating interference in the transmission of visual signals along a demyelinated visual pathway [18, 19].

2.1.6   UHTHOFF'S SYMPTOM

Uhthoff's symptom, episodic transient obscuration of vision with exertion, occurs in isolated optic neuritis [11, 12] and in MS [13]. The incidence of Uhthoff's symptom in optic neuritis is approximately 50%. Sixteen per cent of patients develop it within 2 weeks of the onset of visual loss and 58% within 2 months. Such patients may experience a long period free of the symptom, e.g. 3–32 months, followed by the return of episodes without a recurrent attack of optic neuritis [12].

Typically, the visual obscuration is provoked by 5–20 minutes of brisk exercise. Acuity becomes blurred and colors desaturated. After a rest period of 5–60 minutes or up to 24 hours, vision returns to normal. Exertion is not however the only provoking factor for Uhthoff's symptom. Hot baths or showers account for 27.5% of cases and hot weather for another 27.5% (Table 2.2) [12]. In optic neuritis patients, Uhthoff's symptom is a bad prognostic sign: it correlates significantly with the presence of multifocal white matter lesions on brain MRI ($P < 0.025$) and an increased risk of conversion to clinical MS within a mean follow-up of 3.5 years ($P < 0.01$). Uhthoff's symptom also correlates with a higher incidence of recurrent optic neuritis [12].

2.2   History

To make a diagnosis of optic neuritis a meticulous history must be taken and it must document:

1. the mode of onset and rate of progression of visual loss;
2. the location, character and severity of pain;
3. symptoms that indicate involvement of structures adjacent to the optic nerve, for example, the nasal

Table 2.2   Factors provoking Uhthoff's symptom

Factor	No. of patients	%
Physical exertion	21	52.5
Hot bath or shower	11	27.5
Hot weather	11	27.5
Stress, anxiety, anger	5	12.5
Tired, end of day	4	1.0
Hot food or drink	3	7.5
Cooking	2	5.0
Other specific activity[a]	3	7.5

[a] Working a cash register, playing the trumpet and reading (1 patient each).

From Scholl et al., 1991 [12], with permission.

sinuses, the olfactory nerve, the chiasm and/or the pituitary gland; and

4. a complete symptomatic inquiry for previous disease of the eye and/or central nervous system (CNS) for symptoms suggestive of demyelinating disease.

A medical history should include details of all medications, particularly those that can produce optic nerve or retinal toxicity (including ethambutol, isoniazid, phenothiazines and anti-neoplastic agents). Drug and alcohol use, recent head and eye trauma (and the medico-legal details), as well as stress and psychiatric disorder(s) must also be recorded.

2.3 Clinical signs

The clinical signs of optic neuritis mirror those of optic nerve disease. They are as follows.

- Visual acuity (distance and near) – reduced
- Dyschromatopsia
- Contrast sensitivity – impaired
- Stereo-acuity – reduced
- Visual field – generalized depression, central, paracentral and cecocentral scotoma
- Afferent pupillary defect
- Optic disc(s) – hyperemia and acute swelling.

2.3.1 VISUAL ACUITY

Subnormal visual acuity must be assessed by measuring **best corrected** (i.e. best refracted) visual acuity. A pinhole can be used for a reasonable approximation of best corrected visual acuity. Visual acuity at distance is measured with a Snellen chart (normal 6/6 m; 20/20 ft). In the fractional denotation, e.g. 6/60 metric (20/200 conventional), the numerator 6 (or 20) stands for the testing distance (in meters or feet), and the denominator 60 (or 200) stands for the test letter's size normally seen at that denominator distance. Near acuity is measured with a near card (Jaeger chart). Bifocals or near spectacles must be worn by presbyopes (who have difficulty with accommodation) when testing near vision.

2.3.2 DYSCHROMATOPSIA

Acquired color vision abnormalities in red/green perception usually imply optic neuropathy. Color vision defects can be detected clinically using Hardy–Rand–Ritler or Ishihara pseudoisochromatic plates. More sensitive testing can be achieved with the Farnsworth–Munsell 100 Hue test. Using this test the author detected dyschromatopsia in all 23 cases (30 eyes) with optic neuritis, compared to 12/23 cases (13 eyes) tested with Ishihara plates. Dyschromatopsia was present

when visual acuity had recovered to 20/40 or better[17].

2.3.3 CONTRAST SENSITIVITY

Most patients with recovered optic neuritis and 20/20 Snellen acuity insist that vision in the affected eye(s) is imperfect[20]. Using psychophysical tests, such as contrast sensitivity measurements, investigators have been able to detect the hidden visual loss[21–23] (for review see [24]). One important outcome of this research is that optic neuritis patients who have difficulty seeing and 20/20 vision are protected from misdiagnosis as non-organic cases of functional amblyopia.

Low contrast letter wall charts provide the clinician with an easy method for measuring contrast sensitivity. Pelli–Robson low contrast letter charts discriminate normal from abnormal peak contrast function (a mid-range spatial frequency), and provide reproducible results[25]. The measurement of peak contrast sensitivity is an extremely effective indicator of subclinical optic neuritis. However, the test is not useful in differentiating optic neuritis from maculopathies, and because it is a subjective test, it is of no value in distinguishing organic from non-organic factitious visual loss.

2.3.4 STEREO-ACUITY

The Titmus polaroid 3-D vectograph stereo-acuity test is recommended for both children and adults with optic neuritis. Individuals with normal 20/20 vision in each eye, and binocular fixation (no manifest strabismus), have an average stereopsis of 40 seconds of arc. Stereo-acuity is reduced as acuity decreases down to 20/200, at which level monocular and binocular responses become identical. The value of a normal stereo-acuity in the presence of impaired Snellen acuity indicates either that the Snellen acuity is incorrect or that the patient is claiming poor acuity and the visual loss is factitious.

2.3.5 VISUAL FIELD

In acute optic neuritis, the cardinal field defect is a widespread depression of sensitivity, particularly pronounced centrally as a cecocentral scotoma (Figure 2.1). An isolated central scotoma is atypical in demyelination; this pattern is more typical of Leber's hereditary optic atrophy or of a toxic-nutritional optic neuropathy. In unilateral cases of optic neuritis plotting the field of the contralateral eye is particularly important since the detection of a subtle temporal depression may indicate the presence of a sellar mass. A finding of generalized depression, paracentral scotomas or scattered nerve fiber bundle defect(s) between 5 degrees and 20 degrees from fixation may indicate sequelae of prior demyelinating optic neuropathy.

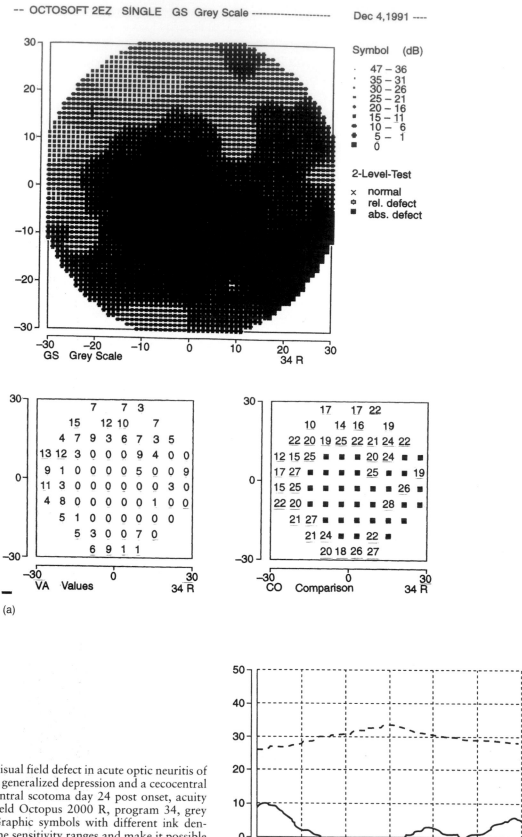

Figure 2.1   Typical visual field defect in acute optic neuritis of the right eye showing generalized depression and a cecocentral scotoma. (a), Cecocentral scotoma day 24 post onset, acuity 20/200 OD. Static field Octopus 2000 R, program 34, grey scale presentation. Graphic symbols with different ink densities correspond to the sensitivity ranges and make it possible to topologically identify sensitivity distribution. Light areas indicate higher sensitivity values, dark areas lower sensitivity values. (b), Octosoft 2EZ-3D profile zero meridian, showing cecocentral scotoma profile of static field shown in (a).

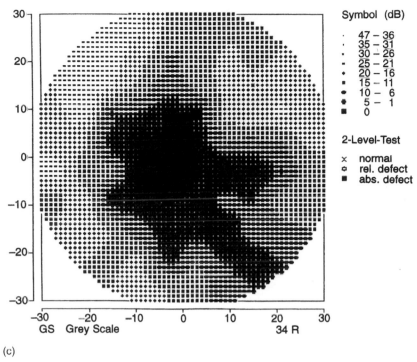

(c)

Figure 2.2 Resolving cecocentral scotoma day 30 post onset, acuity 20/70 OD.

2.3.6 AFFERENT PUPILLARY DEFECT

Unless there is an optic nerve lesion in the fellow eye from previously unrecognized optic neuritis, a unilateral relative afferent pupil defect (RAPD) will be present in the symptomatic neuritic eye. Normal pupillary response consists of prompt, symmetric constriction (miosis) on exposure to light or on near convergence. Diminished response to a direct light stimulus, combined with a normal consensual pupillary response following stimulation of the contralateral eye, characterize the RAPD. The best way to elicit the RAPD is to perform a swinging flashlight test [26]. To perform this test the examiner should maintain a rhythmic equal time alternation of the light from one eye to the other to avoid asymmetric retinal bleach [27].

An afferent pupil defect can be assessed even if one pupil is unreactive due to mydriatics, miotics, oculomotor palsy or trauma. In such cases, when performing the swinging flashlight test, the direct and consensual responses of the single reactive pupil must be compared. The reactive pupil's direct light response reflects the afferent function of the ipsilateral eye; its consensual response reflects the afferent function of the contralateral eye.

A unilateral afferent pupillary defect can be roughly quantified by the use of graded neutral density filters. By placing a neutral filter in front of the normal eye, the examiner can effectively eliminate the relative afferent defect by 'balancing' the visual loss in the two eyes. The filter density needed to balance the pupil defect is a measure of the loss of input to the affected eye and can be compared to earlier measurements for evidence of progression of the disease process [28, 29]. In acute optic neuritis, the incidence of the RAPD is 44–76%. In recovered optic neuritis, the incidence drops to 17–55% [6]. In the absence of a maculopathy, the RAPD is a highly sensitive sign of an ipsilateral optic nerve lesion and can be seen in an eye with 20/20 vision.

2.3.7 THE OPTIC DISC

The appearance of the optic disc in acute optic neuritis is normal in 64%, swollen (papillitis; Figure 2.2) in 23%, blurred and/or hyperemic in 18% and blurred with peripapillary hemorrhages in 2%. Temporal pallor occurs in 10% suggesting a preceding attack of optic neuritis in the same eye. In recovered optic neuritis, 6 months after the first attack, a normal disc is present in 42% of eyes, temporal pallor in 28% and total disc pallor in 18%. In MS in remission, optic pallor is present in 38% of eyes [30].

2.3.8 THE RETINA

Two retinal signs are associated with optic neuritis and MS: retinal venous sheathing due to periphlebitis retinae and defects in the retinal nerve fiber layer.

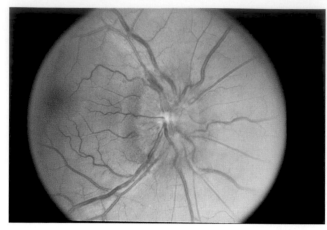

Figure 2.3   Color fundus photograph of a swollen left optic disc in a patient with acute demyelinating optic neuritis and 20/100 acuity.

Retinal venous sheathing, characterized by deposits of a small, round or ill-defined confluent white exudate along a peripheral vein usually associated with vitreous cells, is present in 28% of patients with isolated optic neuritis. In a systematic study of 50 patients presenting with acute optic neuritis, retinal vascular abnormalities and/or signs of inflammation were found in 14 patients: fluorescein leakage in 10, perivenous sheathing in 6, cells in the vitreous in 6, and in the anterior chamber in 4. In 2 patients, cells in the media were seen without retinal changes. After a mean follow-up of 3.5 years, MS had developed in 8/14 patients with retinal vascular abnormalities and/ or evidence of inflammation and in 5/32 without these features. The difference is significant (P < 0.02) [31].

Retinal venous sheathing in the MS eye occurs as an apparently isolated asymptomatic condition, usually in both eyes [32–34]. The condition can resolve completely and then recur. Some investigators have concluded that virtually all MS patients develop venous sheathing at some point in their lifetime [35]. Others have reported an incidence of only 10% in the MS population they studied, and associate venous sheathing pre-eminently with progressive MS [36]. In this group of patients sheathing remained unchanged for periods varying from 5 to 11 months, with an extreme of up to 2 years.

The connection between venous sheathing and demyelination is important. The occurrence of peri-venular abnormalities in a region free of myelin and oligodendrocytes shows that vascular changes in MS can occur independently of contiguous demyelination and in fact may be the primary event in the formation of a new lesion. The finding of retinal venous sheathing in a patient in whom a diagnosis of optic neuritis or MS is suspected but not confirmed is of diagnostic significance.

Atrophy of the nerve fiber layer precedes the appearance of obvious optic atrophy and occurs in all types of optic neuropathy regardless of etiology. In the MS eye, insidious atrophy of retinal nerve fibers occurs without visual symptoms of optic nerve dysfunction [37]. Defects in the retinal nerve fiber layer due to axonal atrophy are seen in optic neuritis and MS as slits in the nerve fiber striations in the arcuate fiber bundles. The incidence of retinal slits in MS is as high as 70% and when slits are seen in the normal eye of a patient with contralateral optic neuritis, they constitute evidence for a second subclinical optic nerve lesion [38].

2.4   Differential diagnosis

Errors in the diagnosis of optic neuritis can be minimized if the neurologist is alert to discrepancies in the clinical picture presented. These include unusual features in the onset or course; for example, the absence of pain or onset over 50 years of age, failure to remit and/ or the presence of neurological abnormalities in the upper cranial nerves not attributable to MS.

2.4.1   UNILATERAL OPTIC NEURITIS

The differential diagnosis of unilateral optic neuritis includes ischemic optic neuropathy, rhinogenous optic neuritis from sinus disease, Lyme borreliosis optic neuropathy, syphilis, HIV-associated optic neuropathies and non-organic factitious visual loss (for review see [39]).

2.4.2   SIMULTANEOUS OR SEQUENTIAL BILATERAL OPTIC NEURITIS

When optic neuritis strikes both eyes, simultaneously or sequentially, the disorder must be distinguished from Devic's disease, immune mediated optic neuropathy, nutritional amblyopia, Jamaican optic neuropathy, Leber's hereditary optic neuropathy and functional blindness (for review see [39]).

Devic's disease, neuromyelitis optica, is an inflammatory CNS demyelinating disease which is considered to be a variant of MS [40, 41]. Devic's affects both eyes simultaneously or sequentially in children, in young adults, and in the elderly, and is accompanied by transverse myelitis within days or weeks. The condition is rare in the US. An updated clinical profile of neuromyelitis optica and the prognostic implications of a single attack in two patients has recently been reported together with a review of 43 cases from the literature [42]. The data show that the presenting symptom is bilateral optic neuritis in 36% of patients, unilateral optic neuritis in 40%, transverse myelitis in 13%, and simultaneous optic neuritis and transverse myelitis in 11%. The interval between development of optic neuritis and transverse myelitis ranges from simultaneous onset to 7 weeks; in 60% of patients, the interval is less than one week. The severity of the optic neuritis tends to correlate with the severity of the transverse myelitis. In most patients the visual deficit is bilateral (91%) and usually severe, with unilateral or bilateral blindness in 58%. Eighty-four per cent of cases have an abnormal cerebrospinal fluid (CSF) during the acute stage of the illness: 62% of these cases have elevated CSF protein and 61% CSF pleocytosis. The reported neurological outcome indicates that 70% of the patients improve neurologically, 14% have a poor outcome and 16% die in the acute stage. Predictors of a poor outcome are older age, high CSF pleocytosis and severe myelitis. Forty-two per cent of patients have a recurrence of demyelinating disease after the initial recovery, consistent with a diagnosis of MS.

2.5 Imaging plaques

Before the use of brain CT and MRI, the presence of CSF pleocytosis and oligoclonal immunoglobulin provided paraclinical evidence of the dissemination of lesions and met the criteria for the diagnosis of laboratory-supported MS in isolated optic neuritis. They indicated an increased risk of progression to MS [43].

Brain and orbit CT scans are used to eliminate a compressive lesion or to evaluate the nasal sinuses. In optic neuritis the CT can show transient enlargement and contrast enhancement of the affected nerve [44]. Brain MRI, with and without gadolinium, is more sensitive than CT for imaging multifocal plaques in the white matter. MRI abnormalities of this type occur in 56–72% of adult patients with isolated optic neuritis [12, 45–47] and in 90–98% of patients with clinically definite MS [48, 49].

Modification of the brain imaging technique using the STIR sequence (an inversion recovery sequence with a short inversion time) and a surface coil specially designed for orbit imaging, increases the diagnostic potential of visualizing plaques in the optic nerve(s). Using this technique investigators examined 37 adult patients (25 women and 12 men) with known optic neuritis [16]. Twenty-nine patients (78%) had isolated optic neuritis; 8 (21%) had probable or definite MS. Focal high-signal MRI lesions were detected in 84% of symptomatic and 20% of asymptomatic optic nerves. The mean longitudinal extent of the lesions measured 1 centimeter. Lesion sites were classified as: (a) anterior, when the lesion was in continuity with the nerve head and did not extend beyond midorbit; (b) intraorbital, when it extended from midorbit to the optic canal; (c) intracanalicular, when it was within the optic canal; (d) intracranial, when that portion of the optic nerve was involved; and (e) chiasmal, when the chiasm was affected. Lesions frequently struck more than one site in

Table 2.3 Frequency of MR lesions at each site in 44 symptomatic optic nerves

Site	Frequency of involvement	
	No.	%
Anterior	20/44	45
Mid-intraorbital	27/44	61
Intracanalicular	15/44	34
Intracranial	2/44	5
Optic chiasm	1/44	2

From Miller *et al.*, 1988 [16], with permission.

continuity. Table 2.3 shows the frequency of lesions at each site in the symptomatic optic nerves. The retrobulbar segment was most commonly involved, with an incidence of 61% in the mid-intraorbital region. No additional lesions were seen with gadolinium-enhanced MRI, although in one patient gadolinium demonstrated intracranial nerve and chiasmal involvement that was not visible with the STIR sequence.

2.6 Prognosis

2.6.1 VISUAL RECOVERY

Although irreversible optic nerve damage occurs in 85% of optic neuritis patients [20], the prognosis for the recovery of Snellen acuity is good: 65–80% of cases regain an acuity of 20/30 or better. Forty-five per cent of these cases recover rapidly within the first four months; 35% recover normal or near normal acuity at 1 year; and 20% fail to make any significant improvement.

In a multicenter study to evaluate visual recovery, following a trial of steroid therapy – the optic neuritis treatment trial (ONTT) – visual function was assessed after a 6- and 12-month follow-up period (Table 2.4). The three arms of the trial were:

1. intravenous (IV) methylprednisolone (MP) (Solumedrol 250 mg every 6 hours) for 3 days followed by oral prednisone (Deltasone 1 mg/kg body weight per day, rounded to the nearest 10 mg) for 11 days;
2. an oral prednisone group (Deltasone 1 mg/kg body weight per day) for 14 days; and
3. a placebo group.

Results showed that in the group receiving IV MP followed by oral prednisone visual function recovered faster than in the placebo group; this was particularly true for the reversal of visual field defects ($P = 0.001$). However, IV MP followed by oral prednisone did not improve visual outcome after 1 year and the outcome in the oral prednisone group did not differ from that in the placebo group [50, 51].

Table 2.4 Median visual function scores at 1 year by treatment group

Test	Placebo (n = 133)	IV MP and OP[a] (n = 137)	P[b]	OP[a] (n = 139)	P[b]
Visual acuity (Snellen equivalents)	20/16	20/16	0.68	20/16	0.25
Pelli–Robson contrast sensitivity (chart line number)	14	14	0.59	14	0.71
Humphrey visual field (mean deviation in dB)	−1.45	−1.63	0.75	−1.90	0.41
Farnsworth–Munsell 100 Hue color vision (error score)	79.9	76.0	0.15	71.1	0.37

[a] IV MP, intravenous methylprednisolone; OP, oral prednisone.
[b] P values are for Wilcoxon rank-sum tests, adjusted by baseline visual acuity, comparing each treatment group with placebo group.

Adapted from Beck et al. 1993 [51].

2.6.2 RECURRENT OPTIC NEURITIS

In the author's patient population in New England, optic neuritis recurred in 33% (33/101) of unilateral monosymptomatic optic neuritis patients (36% women, 25% men) in one or the other eye during an 8-year follow-up period. In 81 unselected patients with a first attack of acute monosymptomatic optic neuritis, the incidence of recurrent attacks was significantly greater in patients with Uhthoff's symptom (18 of 40 or 47.5%) than in patients without Uhthoff's symptom (4 of 41 or 10%) (P = 0.00017) [18]. The high incidence of recurrent optic neuritis in patients with Uhthoff's symptom is of prognostic value and accords with other published data.

In the ONTT 18 patients (13%) in the IV MP followed by oral prednisone group, 39 (30%) in the oral prednisone group, and 20 (16%) in the placebo group had at least one new episode of optic neuritis in either eye during the 6–24 months of follow-up (Table 2.5). Analysis of the length of time to the first new episode of optic neuritis in either eye demonstrated that the rate of new episodes was significantly higher in the oral prednisone group (P = 0.02). This was an unexpected finding that prompted the investigators, in 1993, to issue a warning to physicians that oral prednisone alone is contraindicated in the treatment of optic neuritis [50–52].

2.6.3 CONVERSION TO MULTIPLE SCLEROSIS

The probability that an individual with optic neuritis will develop MS is high. Nearly half of the patients will convert to MS in 15 years [53]. At the lower end of risk, several studies suggest a conversion rate of one-third to one-half and at the higher end, of 60%, 71% and even higher. In the ONTT definite MS developed within the first 2 years in 8% (134 patients) of the IV MP followed by prednisone group, in 16% (129 patients) of the oral prednisone group and 18% (126 patients) of the placebo group. However, the beneficial effect of the intravenous steroid regimen appeared to lessen after the first two years of follow-up [54] and by the third year after treatment, the rate of developing definite MS appeared similar in all treatment groups (Table 2.6).

Brain MRI now provides the means to assess the risk of conversion to clinical MS. In the ONTT abnormal scans with multifocal white matter lesions were present in 46.9% of the patients and the MRI proved to be a powerful predictor of MS. Patients in the placebo group, with two or more periventricular white matter lesions

Table 2.5 Patients who had new attacks of optic neuritis within 2 years of study entry

Event	Placebo (n = 126)	IV MP and OP[a] (n = 134)	OP[a] (n = 129)
Affected eye	13 (10.3%)	13 (9.7%)	22 (17.1%)
Contralateral eye	10 (7.9%)	8 (6.0%)	22 (17.1%)
Either eye	20 (15.9%)	18 (13.4%)	39 (30.2%)
Relative risk (95% confidence interval)[b]		0.79 (0.42–1.50)	2.01 (1.15–3.51)

n = number of patients.

[a] IV MP, intravenous methylprednisolone; OP, oral prednisone.
[b] Each treatment group compared with placebo group.

Modified from Trobe, 1994, [52], with permission.

Table 2.6 Cumulative percentage of patients with clinically definite multiple sclerosis by treatment group

Time period	Placebo (%) (n = 126)	IV MP and OP[a] (%) (n = 134)	OP[b] (%) (n = 129)
6 mth	7.4	3.1	7.2
1 yr	13.4	6.4	10.5
2 yr	17.7	8.1	15.6
3 yr	21.3	17.3	24.7
4 yr[b]	26.9	24.7	29.8

n = number of patients.

[a] IV MP, intravenous methylprednisolone; OP, oral prednisone.
[b] Four-year follow-up is not yet complete for all patients.

Adapted from Beck, R.W. (1995) The optic neuritis treatment trial: three-year follow-up results. *Arch. Ophthalmol.*, 113, 136.

measuring at least 3 mm in size had a 36% chance of developing MS after two years; patients with one signal abnormality had a 17% chance of converting to MS; and those with no abnormality had only a 3% chance [55]. Intravenous MP followed by oral prednisone had its greatest impact on delaying the early development of MS in patients whose MRI scans were most abnormal. Among patients with two or more signal abnormalities, the two-year development of MS was reduced from 36% to 16%; in those with one abnormality, from 17% to 11%. In those without signal abnormalities, the incidence of MS was so low (3%) that the therapeutic efficacy could not be determined (Table 2.7).

The delay in conversion to MS for up to 24 months after a single 3-day course of IV MP followed by oral prednisone is a highly important observation. Prior to this report, the only agents found to alter the natural history of the relapsing–remitting (RR) form of MS were gamma interferon which increased the rate of new clinical attacks, and COP I and interferon beta-1b which reduced the number of attacks. Critical points raised are: first, that this study was only partially blinded and patients assigned to the in-hospital IV MP followed by prednisone therapy group knew that they had received high-dose MP, and secondly, that although the statistical analyses are thorough, the actual number of patients in whom MS developed was small: 18 in the placebo group, 19 in the oral prednisone group and 10 in the IV MP group. Nevertheless, the statistical difference was larger than typically seen in clinical trials, and it was found in patients with a variety of demographic features and from all 15 recruitment centers [56].

2.7 Conclusion

Progress in medicine is based on research. Research conclusions ultimately rest on experimentation involving human subjects. After decades of uncertainty, guidelines for the treatment of the commonest herald symptom of MS, optic neuritis, are now in place. Patients who fit the ONTT profile of acute unilateral idiopathic optic neuritis should now be informed of the association between optic neuritis and MS, and a brain MRI to establish the risk of conversion to clinical MS should be performed. The MRI distinguishes two groups of patients: Group I – MRI normal, and Group II – MRI positive, based on the presence of multifocal periventricular white matter lesions consistent with demyelinating disease.

A US/Canadian multicenter, randomized, double-blind, placebo-controlled clinical trial will, over the next three years, take us further along the research road helping us determine whether Biogen's recombinant human interferon beta product, avonex (interferon beta-1a) is beneficial in delaying the onset of clinically definite MS in Group II subjects who have experienced a first attack of optic neuritis and who are at high risk for MS based on the presence of multiple brain MRI signal abnormalities. All patients to be enrolled in the study will initially receive IV MP followed by oral prednisone therapy, within 14 days of symptom onset. Subjects with bilateral optic neuritis will be ineligible for study participation, but other patients who have a monosymptomatic attack affecting the spinal cord, brain stem or cerebellum will be eligible to take part.

Table 2.7 Proportion of patients with MRI signal abnormalities who developed one or more neurological events other than optic neuritis within 2 years of study entry

MRI periventricular signal abnormalities > 3 mm at study entry	Placebo	IV MP and MP OP[a]	OP[a]
None	2/62 (3.2%)	2/65 (3.1%)	6/75 (8.0%)
One	2/12 (16.7%)	2/18 (11.1%)	1/7 (14.3%)
Two or more	14/39 (35.9%)	6/37 (16.3%)	12/37 (32.4%)

[a] IV MP, intravenous methylprednisolone; OP, oral prednisone.

Adapted from Beck *et al.*, 1993 [54].

The multicenter study shares the goal of all carefully thought through biomedical research: to improve diagnostic, therapeutic and prophylactic procedures but at the same time, and just as important, advance our understanding of the pathogenesis of recurrent disease. In this case it is the pathogenesis of demyelinating disease, one of the most elusive and significant problems in neurology.

References

1. Wray, S.H., Scholl, G.B. and Giffen, C. (1996) Optic neuritis and gender. *In preparation*.
2. Kennedy, C. and Carroll, F.D. (1960) Optic neuritis in children. *Arch. Ophthalmol.*, **63**, 747.
3. Riikonen, R. (1989) The role of infection and vaccination in the genesis of optic neuritis and multiple sclerosis in children. *Acta Neurol. Scand.*, **80**, 425.
4. Kennedy, C. and Carter, S. (1961) Relation of optic neuritis to multiple sclerosis in children. *Pediatrics*, **28**, 377.
5. Riikonen, R., Donner, M. and Erkkila, H. (1988) Optic neuritis in children and its relationship to multiple sclerosis: a clinical study of 21 children. *Dev. Med. Child Neurol.*, **30**, 349.
6. Nikoskelainen, E. (1975) Symptoms, signs and early course of optic neuritis. *Acta Ophthalmol.*, **53**, 254.
7. Davis, F.A., Bergen, D., Schauf, C. *et al.* (1976) Movement phosphenes in optic neuritis: a new clinical sign. *Neurology* **26**, 1100.
8. Lessell, S. and Cohen, M.M. (1979) Phosphenes induced by sound. *Neurology*, **29**, 1524.
9. Page, N.G.R., Bolger, J.P. and Sanders, M.D. (1982) Auditory evoked phosphenes in optic nerve disease. *J. Neurol. Neurosurg. Psychiatry*, **45**, 7.
10. Patterson, V.H., Foster, D.H. and Heron, J.R. (1980) Variability of visual threshold in multiple sclerosis: effect of background luminance on frequency of seeing. *Brain*, **103**, 139.
11. Perkin, G.D. and Rose, F.C. (1976) Uhthoff's syndrome. *Br. J. Ophthalmol.*, **60**, 60.
12. Scholl, G.B., Song, H-S. and Wray, S.H. (1991) Uhthoff's symptom in optic neuritis: Relationship to magnetic resonance imaging and development of multiple sclerosis. *Ann. Neurol.*, **30**, 180.
13. Uhthoff, W. (1889) Untersuchungen uber die bei der multiplen Herdsklerose vorkommenden Augenstorungen. *Arch. Psychiatry*, **21**, 303.
14. Engell, T., Trojaborg, W. and Raun, N.E. (1987) Subclinical optic neuropathy in multiple sclerosis. A neuro-ophthalmological investigation by means of visually evoked response, Farnsworth–Munsell 100 Hue test and Ishihara test and their diagnostic value. *Acta Ophthalmol.*, **65**, 735.
15. Ulrich, J. and Groebke-Lorenz, W. (1983) The optic nerve in multiple sclerosis: a morphological study with retrospective clinico-pathological correlations. *Neuro-Ophthalmology*, **3**, 149.
16. Miller, D.H., Newton, M.R., van der Poel, J.C. *et al.* (1988) Magnetic resonance imaging of the optic nerve in optic neuritis. *Neurology*, **38**, 175.
17. Griffin, J.F. and Wray, S.H. (1978) Acquired color vision defects in retrobulbar neuritis. *Am. J. Ophthalmol.*, **86**, 193.
18. McDonald, W.I. and Sears, T.A. (1970) The effects of experimental demyelination on conduction in the central nervous system. *Brain*, **93**, 583.
19. Rasminsky, M. and Sears, T.A. (1972) Internodal conduction in undissected demyelinated nerve fibers. *J. Physiol.*, **227**, 323.
20. Fleishman, J.A., Beck, R.W., Linares, O.A. *et al.* (1987) Deficits in visual function after resolution of optic neuritis. *Ophthalmology*, **94**, 1029.
21. Regan, D., Silver, R. and Murray, T.J. (1977) Visual acuity and contrast sensitivity in multiple sclerosis – hidden visual loss; an auxiliary diagnostic test. *Brain*, **100**, 563.
22. Lorance, R.W., Kaufman, D.O., Wray, S.H. *et al.* (1987) Contrast visual testing in neurovisual diagnosis. *Neurology*, **37**, 923.
23. Regan, D. (1984) Visual psychophysical tests in the diagnosis of multiple sclerosis, in *The Diagnosis of Multiple Sclerosis* (ed. C.M. Poser), New York, Thieme-Stratton, P. 64.
24. Hess, R.F. and Plant, G.T. (1986) The psychophysical loss in optic neuritis: spatial and temporal aspects, in *Optic Neuritis* (eds R.F. Hess and G.T. Plant), Cambridge, Cambridge University Press, p. 109.
25. Rubin, G.S. (1988) Reliability and sensitivity of clinical contrast sensitivity tests. *Clin. Vision Sci.*, **2**, 169.
26. Levatin, P. (1959) Pupillary escape in disease of the retina or optic nerve. *Arch. Ophthalmol.*, **62**, 768.
27. Thompson, H.S. and Jiang, M.Q. (1987) Letter to the editor. *Ophthalmology*, **94**, 1360.
28. Fineberg, E. and Thompson, H.S. (1979) Quantitation of the afferent pupillary defect, in: *Neuro-Ophthalmology Focus* (ed. J.L. Smith), New York, Masson, p. 25.
29. Thompson, J.S., Corbett, J.J. and Cox, T.A. (1981) How to measure the relative afferent pupillary defect. *Surv. Ophthalmol.*, **26**, 39.
30. Zeller, R.W. (1967) Ocular findings in the remission phase of multiple sclerosis. *Am. J. Ophthalmol.*, **64**, 767.
31. Lightman, S., McDonald, W.I., Bird, A.C. *et al.* (1987) Retinal venous sheathing in optic neuritis: its significance for the pathogenesis of multiple sclerosis. *Brain*, **110**, 405.
32. ter Braak, J.G. and Herwaarden, A. (1933) Ophthalmo-encephalomyelitis. *Klin. Monatsbl. Augenheilk.*, **91**, 316.
33. Rucker, C.W. (1944) Sheathing of the retinal veins in multiple sclerosis. *Mayo Clin. Proc.*, **19**, 176.
34. Rucker, C.W. (1947) Retinopathy of multiple sclerosis. *Trans. Am. Ophthalmol. Soc.*, **45**, 564.
35. Engell, T. and Andersen, P.K. (1982) The frequency of periphlebitis retinae in multiple sclerosis. *Acta Neurol. Scand.*, **65**, 601.
36. Bamford, C.R., Ganley, J.P., Sibley, W.A. *et al.* (1978) Uveitis, perivenous sheathing and multiple sclerosis. *Neurology*, **28**, 119.
37. Frisen, L. and Hoyt, W.F. (1974) Insidious atrophy of retinal nerve fibers in multiple sclerosis. *Arch. Ophthalmol.*, **92**, 91.
38. Feinsod, M. and Hoyt, W.F. (1975) Subclinical optic neuropathy in multiple sclerosis. *J. Neurol. Neurosurg. Psychiatry*, **38**, 1109.
39. Wray, S.H. (1994) Optic neuritis, in: *The Principles and Practices of Ophthalmology: the Harvard System* (eds D.M. Albert and F.A. Jakobiec), vol. 4, Philadelphia, Saunders, p. 2539.
40. Devic, E. (1894) Myelite subaigue compliquée de névrite optique. *Bull. Méd. (Paris)*, **8**, 1033.
41. Gault, F. (1894) De la neuromyelite optique aigue. Lyons, Thesis.
42. Whitham, R.H. and Brey, R.L. (1985) Neuromyelitis optica: two new cases and review of the literature. *J. Clin. Neuro-Ophthalmol.*, **5**, 263.
43. Sandberg-Wollheim, M. (1978) Optic neuritis: cerebrospinal fluid findings and clinical course, in *XXIII Concilium Ophthalmologicum, Kyoto* (eds K. Shimizu and J.A. Oosterhuis), International Congress Series No. 450, Amsterdam, Excerpta Medica, p. 347.
44. Howard, C.W., Osher, R.H. and Tomsak, R.L. (1980) Computed tomographic features in optic neuritis. *Am. J. Ophthalmol.*, **89**, 699.
45. Ormerod, I.E.C., McDonald, W.I., du Boulay, E.P. *et al.* (1986) Disseminated lesions at presentation in patients with optic neuritis. *J. Neurol. Neurosurg. Psychiatry*, **49**, 124.
46. Jacobs, L., Kinkel, P.R. and Kindel, W.R. (1986) Silent brain lesions in patients with isolated optic neuritis. A clinical and nuclear magnetic resonance imaging study. *Arch. Neurol.*, **43**, 452.
47. Frederiksen, J.L., Larsson, H.B., Henriksen, O. *et al.* (1989) Magnetic resonance imaging of the brain in patients with acute monosymptomatic optic neuritis. *Acta Neurol. Scand.*, **80**, 512.
48. Ormerod, I.E.C., Miller, D.H., McDonald, W.I. *et al.* (1987) The role of NMR imaging in the assessment of multiple sclerosis and isolated neurological lesions: a quantitative study. *Brain*, **110**, 1579.
49. Paty, D.W., Oger, J.J.F., Kastrukoff, L.F. *et al.* (1988) MRI in the diagnosis of MS: a prospective study with comparison of clinical evaluation, evoked potentials, oligoclonal banding and CT. *Neurology*, **38**, 180.
50. Beck, R.W., Cleary, P.A., Anderson, M.M. Jr *et al.* (1992) A randomized, controlled trial of corticosteroids in the treatment of acute optic neuritis. *N. Engl. J. Med.*, **326**, 581–8.
51. Beck, R.W. and Cleary, P.A. (1993) Optic neuritis treatment trial: one-year follow-up results. *Arch. Ophthalmol.*, **111**, 773.
52. Trobe, J.D. (1994) Managing optic neuritis: results of the optic neuritis treatment trial. *Focal Points*, **XII** (2), s.2, 1–10.
53. Rizzo, J.F. and Lessell, S. (1988) Risk of developing multiple sclerosis after uncomplicated optic neuritis: a long-term prospective study. *Neurology*, **38**, 185.
54. Beck, R.W., Cleary, P.A., Trobe, J.D. *et al.* and the Optic Neuritis Study Group (1993) The effect of corticosteroids for acute optic neuritis on the subsequent development of multiple sclerosis. *N. Engl J. Med.*, **329**, 1764.
55. Beck, R.W., Arrington, J., Murtagh, F.R., Cleary, P.A. and Kaufman, D.I. (1993) Brain magnetic resonance imaging in acute optic neuritis – experience of the optic neuritis study group. *Arch. Neurol.*, **50**, 841.
56. Silberberg, D.H. (1993) Corticosteroids and optic neuritis (Editorial). *N. Engl. J. Med.*, **329**, 1808.

3 IMAGING IN MULTIPLE SCLEROSIS

David H. Miller

In recent years, improvements in imaging have made a major contribution in the evaluation of multiple sclerosis (MS). This chapter will consider these developments. It will largely concentrate on magnetic resonance imaging (MRI), which has had by far the greatest impact, but first will briefly review the contribution of CT, PET and SPECT.

3.1 Computerized tomography (CT) scanning

Except for the occasional very large plaques detected using radio-isotope brain scanning, CT was the first imaging modality to demonstrate the lesions of MS in life. An early study with brain CT demonstrated atrophy in 4 and discrete low attenuation lesions in the cerebral white matter in 7 of 19 patients with definite or probable MS [1]. It was later noted that some lesions enhanced following the administration of intravenous iodinated contrast media. Enhancing lesions, indicating breakdown of the blood–brain barrier, occurred more often during clinical relapses, and their detection was increased by performing delayed scanning after high doses of contrast [2].

3.2 Positron emission tomography (PET)

PET can study cerebral blood flow and metabolism *in vivo*. An early study in MS reported a generalized reduction in cerebral blood flow and oxygen usage in both the cerebral cortex and deep white matter, which correlated with atrophy on CT [3]. There are a number of drawbacks of PET: (i) it is expensive and has a limited availablity; (ii) a relatively low resolution limits the study of individual MS lesions; (iii) exposure to radiation limits the opportunities to follow changes over time. These problems maybe partly circumvented with the recent developments of MR techniques for monitoring regional changes in cerebral blood oxygenation and flow.

3.3 Single photon emission tomography (SPECT)

Although its spatial resolution is poor, SPECT is cheaper and more widely available than PET, and provides an alternative method for assessing cerebral blood flow. SPECT studies in MS have looked at the relationship between lesion site and metabolism on the one hand and cognitive deficits on the other [4]. Neither PET nor SPECT has a role in the diagnosis of MS.

3.4 Magnetic resonance imaging (MRI)

This section starts with a brief resumé of NMR theory followed by a description of the sequences commonly used to evaluate MS. The use of MRI in MS is then considered with repect to diagnosis, understanding the mechanisms of functional impairment and monitoring treatment.

3.4.1 NMR THEORY

The principles of nuclear magnetic resonance (NMR) were first described in 1946 by Bloch and Purcell. For many years, NMR applications were limited to physics and chemistry. The production of MR images from humans required the construction of large-bore magnets with strong and homogeneous magnetic fields, together with developing a method for spatial localization of acquired NMR signals. This was not achieved until 1980.

Conventional MR images are derived from the NMR signals of mobile hydrogen nuclei (protons) which are abundant in the water and fat of living organisms. In the central nervous system, different tissues, normal or pathological, are discriminated largely by differences in the density and macromolecular environment of their mobile water protons, and hence MS plaques are depicted with remarkable sensitivity.

Multiple Sclerosis: Clinical and pathogenetic basis. Edited by Cedric S. Raine, Henry F. McFarland and Wallace W. Tourtellotte. Published in 1997 by Chapman & Hall, London. ISBN 0 412 30890 8.

3.4.2 MRI SEQUENCES IN THE EVALUATION OF MULTIPLE SCLEROSIS

The first report of unenhanced MRI in MS was from the Hammersmith Hospital in London [5], and it included a comparison with CT scanning: in 10 patients there were 131 brain lesions seen on MRI and only 19 on CT. This study used an inversion recovery sequence, in which lesions appeared as regions of low signal compared to higher signal normal brain. It soon became apparent that T2-weighted spin echo (SE) sequences, which reveal MS lesions as areas of high signal, detected even more plaques [6]. Not surprisingly, MRI has totally superseded CT as a method for imaging MS lesions, whether for diagnosis or to monitor the course of the disease. It provides a quantum increase in sensitivity, and unlike CT, it can be safely repeated on many occasions.

T2-weighted conventional SE is still widely used for diagnostic imaging in cases of suspected MS, although it is increasingly being replaced by fast or turbo SE, a sequence which produces images of a similar character, but in a fraction of the time [7]. A recent study found that a fast Fluid Attenuated Inversion Recovery (fast FLAIR) sequence detected substantially more MS lesions than conventional SE [8]. Fast FLAIR combines heavy T2-weighting (giving high signal lesions compared to normal brain) with suppression of signal from CSF (on conventional T2-weighted SE sequences, CSF has moderate or high signal, which can lead to difficulty in visualizing periventricular or subcortical plaques). Further studies are needed to determine whether fast FLAIR should replace fast or conventional SE as the 'gold standard' unenhanced sequence in evaluating MS.

Using paramagnetic gadolinium chelates to reduce the T1 relaxation time of water protons, some MS lesions display contrast enhancement. Gadolinium enhancement implies an abnormal blood–brain barrier, and is a characteristic feature of new, inflammatory lesions. It is demonstrated on T1-weighted sequences. Enhancing lesions are demonstrated much more frequently on MRI than CT, and there are more enhancing lesions during clinical relapses than in remission [9]. The standard dose of a gadolinium chelate is 0.1 mmol/kg intravenously, and in serial studies its use considerably increases the number of new, active lesions detected when compared to a T2-weighted sequence alone [10]. This is because in many new enhancing areas there is either no corresponding change on the T2-weighted scan, or the change is too subtle to be sure that it is real. Higher doses of gadolinium chelates (e.g. 0.3 mmol/kg) detect still more enhancing lesions, as can the use of a magnetization transfer prepared T1-weighted SE sequence with conventional doses. These approaches are not required for routine diagnostic studies, but may have a role in future therapeutic trials using MRI to monitor outcome – serial gadolinium enhanced scanning using standard doses is already being widely used in this context.

3.4.3 DIAGNOSIS

Brain MRI demonstrates multifocal white matter abnormalities in over 95% of patients with clinically definite MS [6]. The characteristic findings are of multiple white matter lesions (seen as high signal areas on proton density or T2-weighted sequences) predominantly around the lateral ventricles in an irregular and asymmetrical pattern, but also frequently involving the brain stem and cerebellum (Figure 3.1). Lesions at the corticomedullary junction are not uncommon and may be helpful in the distinction of MS from subcortical arteriosclerotic encephalopathy (Binswanger's disease) in which the U-fibres are spared. Lesions in the corpus callosum are best visualized on sagittal images [11]; this site is frequently involved in MS but not in vascular disease. Lesions are often irregular in shape, although ovoid or round lesions also occur and are characteristic. In brains scanned post mortem, areas of signal change on MRI have generally corresponded with chronic plaques demonstrated histopathologically [6].

MRI in diagnosis (the Poser criteria)

The diagnosis of MS is essentially a clinical one, requiring the demonstration of characteristic symptoms and signs of lesions disseminated within central nervous system white matter in both time and space. MRI is not always necessary but is often of great assistance in making the diagnosis earlier and with more confidence than would otherwise be possible. The most commonly used diagnostic criteria are those of the Poser Committee [12]. Using these, a patient aged 10–59 years, who has had two attacks characteristic of MS at least one month apart

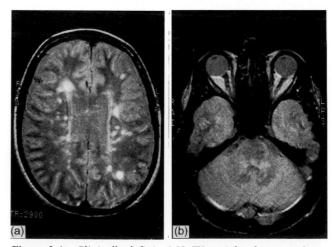

Figure 3.1 Clinically definite MS. T2-weighted images showing (a) multifocal periventricular and discrete cerebral white matter lesions and (b) lesions in the floor of the fourth ventricle.

Table 3.1 MRI and the Poser criteria

	MRI	Poser classification
Two attacks: clinical evidence of two lesions	+	CDMS
	–	CDMS
Two attacks: clinical evidence of one lesion	+	**CDMS**
	–	CPMS
One attack: clinical evidence of one lesion	+ (with new lesions developing)	CPMS
	–	Not diagnostic
One attack: clinical evidence of one lesion + CSF OCBs	+ (with new lesions developing)	LSDMS
	–	Not diagnostic

Situations in which a positive MRI scan permits a more certain diagnosis are shown in bold type.

and who on clinical examination has evidence of two separate lesions, can be diagnosed as having clinically definite disease, providing there is no better alternative explanation. Paraclinical evidence of one of the lesions, such as characteristic abnormalities on MRI or evoked potential recordings, may be used. Therefore, in young adult patients who have had two or more attacks but have clinical evidence of only one lesion, the finding of multiple MRI abnormalities characteristic of MS allows a definite diagnosis (Table 3.1).

In patients who present with an acute clinically isolated syndrome (e.g. optic neuritis, or an internuclear ophthalmoplegia or a partial spinal cord syndrome), the finding of characteristic MRI abnormalities is not immediately diagnostic because indistinguishable abnormalities can occur in the less common monophasic demyelinating disorder, acute disseminated encephalomyelitis (ADEM) [13]. If follow-up MRI after more than one month reveals new lesions, a diagnosis of clinically probable MS can be made, even in the absence of further clinical events. If, in addition, oligoclonal bands are present in the cerebrospinal fluid, the diagnosis is then laboratory-supported definite MS. If MRI was not performed during the acute episode, a later scan with contrast may be useful: enhancement of a lesion suggests recent inflammation (see below), which if present implies dissemination in time and therefore a diagnosis of MS rather than ADEM. This hypothesis still requires clinical verification, although there is evidence from unenhanced serial MRI in ADEM that lesions tend to resolve, and new lesions do not develop [13].

Differential diagnosis

White matter lesions are seen in many disorders other than MS (Table 3.2). They are commonly found in healthy subjects with advancing age, where they are

Table 3.2 MRI white matter abnormalities

Condition	MRI features
Multiple sclerosis	Multifocal, asymmetrical, periventricular lesions
ADEM	Can be identical to MS. Symmetrical cerebral, basal ganglia or cerebellar lesions in some
Ageing	Usually less extensive than MS. Discrete lesions. Little posterior fossa involvement
Behçet's syndrome	Prominent brain stem involvement
Cerebrovascular disease	Large lesions of arterial territories involving cortex as well as small lesions. Smooth periventricular lesions
Decompression sickness	Focal subcortical lesions? Any difference from healthy controls
Fat embolism	High signal lesions on T1-weighted images, high or low signal on T2-weighted
HIV encephalitis	Patchy or punctate white matter lesions, commonly involving basal ganglia. Diffuse pattern in AIDS dementia complex
HTLVI-associated myelopathy	Usually few supratentorial lesions only
Hydrocephalus	Diffuse smooth periventricular high signal
Irradiation	Diffuse periventricular and subcortical lesions
Leucodystrophies	Various patterns of extensive symmetrical white matter abnormalities; atrophy
Migraine	A few more discrete lesions than age-matched controls
Mitochondrial encephalopathy	Diffuse abnormalities as well as stroke-like lesions
Motor neuron disease	Symmetrical high signal involving pyramidal tracts, especially internal capsules
Neurosarcoidosis	Can be identical to MS but also large parenchymal lesions, prominent basal involvement and diffuse meningeal enhancement
Phenylketonuria	Periventricular and subcortical changes
Progressive multifocal leucoencephalopathy	Large focal lesions
Subacute sclerosing panencephalitis	Few scattered white matter lesions
Systemic lupus erythematosus	Mainly subcortical lesions; lesions involving arterial territories
Trauma	Variable

Common causes are shown in bold type.

caused by small-vessel disease [14]. Several criteria to increase the specificity for MS have been developed. The Fazekas criteria require the presence of at least three lesions on brain MRI and that at least two of the following three features are also present: a lesion abutting the body of the lateral ventricles, an infratentorial lesion, and a lesion > 6 mm in diameter. An evaluation of 1500 patients using these criteria, of whom 134 were judged clinically to have MS, yielded a sensitivity of 81% and specificity of 96% for the diagnosis [15].

While a careful consideration of the clinical context and pattern of MRI abnormalities often enables a diagnosis (Figure 3.2), there are a number of relapsing-remitting and inflammatory disorders, most notably neurosarcoidosis and the vasculitides, that can be particularly hard to distinguish from MS. In these disorders, certain imaging features can assist the distinction:

1. In systemic lupus erythematosus, the white matter lesions are often predominantly subcortical rather than the periventricular predominance usually seen in MS.

2. The most common neurological syndromes in Behçet's disease implicate the brain stem, and MRI findings reflect this – although cerebral white matter lesions occur, they are usually few in number, but there can be extensive brain stem pathology, including swelling and enhancement acutely and atrophy in chronic lesions (Figure 3.3).

3. In sarcoidosis, periventricular lesions may be indistinguishable from those of MS, but there may also be prominent meningeal enhancement, especially around the base of the brain, particularly in the region of the chiasm and hypothalamus (Figure 3.4), such a finding being incompatible with MS.

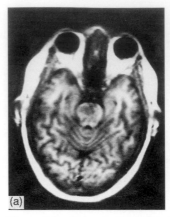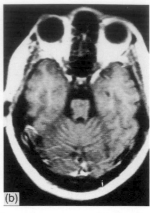

Figure 3.3   Behçet's disease. (*a*) Inversion recovery image of a 38-year-old female with an acute brain stem syndrome. There is extensive altered signal and swelling in the midbrain; (*b*) follow-up MRI 5 years later reveals marked midbrain atrophy; the patient was now severely disabled in spite of immunosuppression during the intervening years. (Reproduced from S.P. Morrissey *et al.*, *European Neurology*, 33, 287–93 (1993), with permission of S. Karger AG, Basle.)

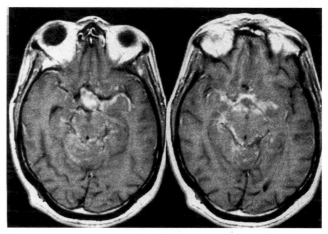

Figure 3.4   Neurosarcoidosis. T1-weighted images reveal gadolinium enhancement of basal meninges and nodular thickening in the chiasmatic region; the patient presented with an optic neuropathy. (Reproduced from D.H. Miller and W.I. McDonald, Neuroimaging in multiple sclerosis, *Clinical Neuroscience*, 2, 215–24 (1994), with permission of Wiley-Liss, Inc., a subsidiary of John Wiley & Sons, Inc.)

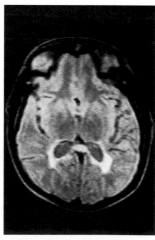

Figure 3.2   Adrenomyeloneuropathy. This 40-year-old male presented with progressive spastic paraparesis. T2-weighted image reveals symmetrical abnormalities in the posterior cerebral white matter. The diagnosis was confirmed by the subsequent finding of elevated very long chain fatty acids.

Nevertheless, no MRI finding is pathognomonic of MS, and imaging appearances, no matter how characteristic they may be, should never be used alone to establish a diagnosis of MS – the clinical context and age of the patient must always be considered.

Newer MR techniques to improve specificity

Magnetization transfer (MT) imaging is a method for studying the pool of water protons which are bound to macromolecules; thus it provides an indication of the amount of tissue structure. A high MT ratio implies dense structure and is seen in normal white matter. Individual MS lesions reveal a wide range of MT ratios varying from slight to marked reductions compared to normal white matter [16]. In a group comparison, there are quantitative differences between vascular and demyelinating lesions [17, 18]. The abnormalities of MT ratios are generally less severe in vascular disease, suggesting better tissue preservation than in MS. This is consonant with post-mortem studies of elderly individuals in whom the ubiquitous cerebral MRI white matter abnormalities have been associated with vascular ectasia and dilated perivascular spaces, but only rarely with more severe tissue disruption such as infarction [14]. This contrasts with the complete demyelination and often substantial axonal loss seen in chronic MS plaques [19]. In addition, white matter lesions in MS are more likely to appear hypointense on T1-weighted SE scans than lesions due to vascular disease [20] and hypointense lesions on T1-weighted scans have a lower MT ratio than isointense lesions [21].

Proton MR spectroscopy studies metabolites other than water which contain mobile protons. In the brain, the major metabolites seen on long echo time (TE) spectroscopy are N-acetyl aspartate, choline-containing compounds, creatine/phosphocreatine and lactate. On short TE spectroscopy, other detectable metabolites include myoinositol, glutamate/glutamine and alanine. Although lipid protons are abundant in myelin, they are relatively immobile and therefore barely visible in healthy white matter. An intrinsic limitation of spectroscopy is spatial resolution – because of the relatively low concentration (millimolar) of the metabolites, large volumes (usually 4–8 ml) need to be studied in order to obtain adequate NMR signals. A variety of metabolic abnormalities are seen in different white matter pathologies (Table 3.3; Figures 3.5, 3.6), but the diagnostic role

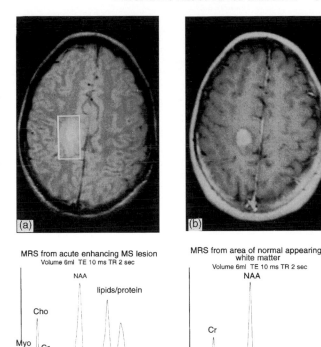

Figure 3.5 Acute MS lesion: T2-weighted (*a*) and gadolinium enhanced T1-weighted (*b*) MRI and short TE proton spectra of the lesion (*c*) and normal appearing white matter (*d*). The lesion is enhancing and its spectrum reveals large lipid peaks at 0.9 and 1.3 ppm. (Myo, myoinositol; Cho, choline-containing compounds; Cr, creatine/phosphocreatine; NAA, N-acetyl aspartate.)

of spectroscopy has been limited because of long acquisition times, difficulties with quantification and the low specificity of many of the abnormalities reported.

Spinal cord

Until recently, MR imaging of the spinal cord was slow, and motion artefacts as well as limited resolution hampered the detection of small MS plaques. With the newer multi-array receiver coils and fast or turbo SE pulse sequences it is now possible to obtain high resolution T2-weighted sagittal images of the whole spinal cord in under 6 minutes. Such an approach has detected lesions in 75% of MS patients [22] (Figure 3.7). Spinal MRI is of particular diagnostic value in the presence of a normal brain MRI where the finding of multiple intrinsic cord lesions provides paraclinical evidence of dissemination in space – since performing systematic spinal studies in our unit, we have seen 20

Table 3.3 Proton MR spectroscopy abnormalities in different pathologies

	NAA	Cho	Cr	Lac	Lip	Myo
Acute MS plaques	D	I	N	I	I	I
Chronic MS plaques	D	N	N	N	N	I
Systemic lupus erythematosus	D	N	N	N	N	N
Metachromatic leucodystrophy	D	N	N	I	N	I
Adreno-leucodystrophy	D	I	N	I	I	N
Canavan's disease	I	D	N	N	N	N
Phenylketonuria	N	N	D	N	N	N
Spinocerebellar degeneration	D	D	N	N	N	N

Abbreviations: NAA, N-acetyl aspartate; Cho, choline containing compounds; Cr, creatine/phosphocreatine; Lac, lactate; Lip, lipid; Myo, myoinositol; I, increased; D, decreased; N, normal.

MRS of cerebellar white matter
in MS patient
(no ataxia) v control
Volume 3.5ml TE 135 ms TR 2.135 sec

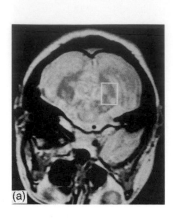

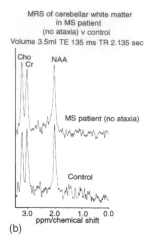

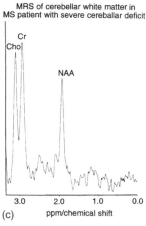

MRS of cerebellar white matter in
MS patient with severe cereballar deficit

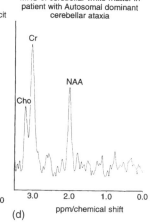

MRS of cerebellar white matter in
patient with Autosomal dominant
cerebellar ataxia

Figure 3.6 Proton MRS of cerebellar white matter: (a) MRI shows region studied; (b) spectrum from non-ataxic MS patient; (c) spectrum from ataxic MS patient; (d) spectrum from patient with autosomal dominant cerebellar ataxia (ADCA). NAA is reduced in the ataxic MS patient and the patient with ADCA. The Cho peak is also reduced in the ADCA patient. (Abbreviations as Figure 3.5.)

patients thought likely to have MS on clinical grounds, in whom brain MRI was normal or revealed only minor non-specific abnormalities but intrinsic cord lesions were present. Spinal imaging is also valuable in older patients, since cord lesions do not develop with ageing *per se* in the way that brain lesions do.

The cord lesions in MS seen at post mortem are usually small, and this observation is confirmed *in vivo* – most MRI detectable lesions do not involve more than one segment on sagittal images, and there is only partial cross-sectional involvement on axial images. This pattern corresponds with the clinical picture of spinal relapses of MS which characteristically produce a patchy or partial deficit, e.g spinothalamic sensory loss with preserved pyramidal function. By contrast, in post-infectious acute transverse myelitis and the acute myelopathy associated with systemic lupus erythematosus, the acute clinical deficit is usually complete, and MRI reveals lesions

extending over many segments. A recent follow-up study of patients presenting with a clinically isolated acute cord syndrome found that further clinical manifestations allowing a diagnosis of MS were seen in 4 of 8 patients with an intrinsic cord lesion less than one segment, and in none of 6 patients with longer lesions [23].

The presentation with a progressive myelopathy has an extensive differential diagnosis, including MS, and modern MRI is the investigation of choice. High resolution MRI is superior to myelography in demonstrating compressive lesions. It is also an excellent screening investigation for spinal arteriovenous malformations. Axial sequences may reveal signal changes in the lateral columns in motor neuron disease (abnormalities in corticospinal tracts in the brain are also seen)

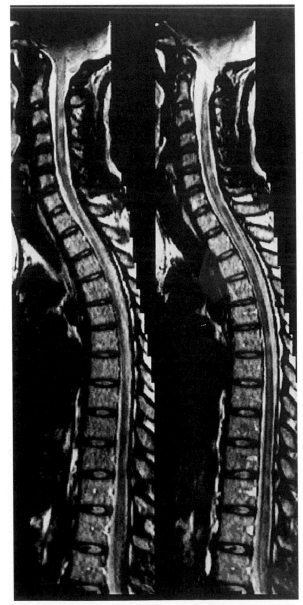

Figure 3.7 Multiple sclerosis. Sagittal T2-weighted images reveal multiple, small, high signal lesions within the cord.

and in the posterior column in vitamin B$_{12}$ deficiency. In HTLV-1 associated myelopathy, focal lesions of the sort seen in MS are not described, but diffuse atrophy is present. The diagnostic capability of spinal MRI is still evolving, and further improvements in resolution should be seen with new coil designs and new sequences such as magnetization transfer gradient echo, fast FLAIR and 3D fast SE.

Optic nerve

An attack of optic neuritis occurs in most MS patients at some stage and is the presenting symptom in 20%. MRI detects lesions within the optic nerve with high sensitivity, using either the short tau inversion recovery (STIR) pulse sequence [24] or frequency-selective fat suppression techniques [25] to reduce the signal intensity of orbital fat (Figure 3.8). Optic nerve MRI is not required for diagnosis when the characteristic clinical findings of acute unilateral optic neuritis are present, but may be of value in atypical cases, especially those with progressive visual loss; in such patients a tumour involving the anterior visual pathways must be ruled out. High resolution images of the optic nerves can be obtained using orbital multi-array coils and a fat-suppressed fast SE sequence, with an in-plane resolution of 0.4 mm and 3 mm thick slices [26]. Such resolution is of value in the diagnosis of patients with acute or subacute visual loss. In anterior ischaemic optic neuropathy, MRI is normal during the acute phase, although high signal develops after several months (probably due to Wallerian degeneration in the nerve), whereas in optic neuritis there is abnormal signal in both acute and chronic lesions. In tobacco–alcohol amblyopia the nerves

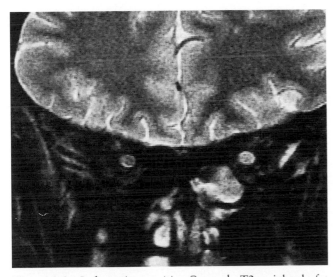

Figure 3.8 Left optic neuritis. Coronal, T2-weighted, fat suppressed, high resolution image reveals high signal within the left optic nerve. Also note the normal ring-like appearance of the optic nerve sheath on both sides.

appear normal. In Leber's hereditary optic neuropathy there is signal change within the optic nerves in chronic lesions, although this tends to spare the anterior portion of the nerves; the nerves also appear atrophic. In benign intracranial hypertension, there is a marked increase in thickness of the optic nerve sheath.

3.4.4 UNDERSTANDING THE MECHANISMS OF FUNCTIONAL IMPAIRMENT

MRI presents an unrivalled opportunity to study the pathological evolution of MS *in vivo*. The absence of known side-effects allows repeat examinations at frequent intervals. Serial MRI studies, in combination with clinical and electrophysiological observations, are providing new insights into the pathophysiological basis of functional impairment in MS. Studying acute lesions provides insights into the mechanisms of relapse and remission, and evaluation of chronic lesions will help to elucidate the causes of irreversible disability.

Acute lesions

In early relapsing-remitting and secondary-progressive MS, new lesions develop much more frequently than the occurrence of clinical activity [27, 28]. An early event in most new lesions is gadolinium enhancement indicating breakdown of the blood–brain barrier [29]. Enhancement may occur prior to signal change appearing on T2-weighted images, indicating that blood–brain barrier breakdown might be the initial event in lesion formation. Enhancement has been correlated with histologic activity, the most consistent feature being inflammation with perivascular lymphocytes and extensive macrophage infiltrates [30].

Another early event in the formation of large new cerebral plaques is the appearance of mobile lipid peaks on short TE proton MR spectroscopy [31]. These are present during the initial phase of gadolinium enhancement and gradually resolve over 4–8 months; it is likely that they represent myelin breakdown products. Thus, gadolinium enhancement and proton MR spectroscopy respectively provide an indication of inflammation and demyelination in new lesions (Figure 3.5).

Gadolinium enhancement usually lasts for about one month, but in rare instances lasts less than 2 weeks or more than 3 months. During this period, the area of signal change on unenhanced T2-weighted images increases in size, probably due to enlargement of the region of inflammation and demyelination and to surrounding vasogenic oedema. As the blood–brain barrier impairment reverses, the lesion shrinks but usually leaves a residual abnormality, probably representing an area of persistent demyelination and gliosis. The majority of cerebral gadolinium enhancing lesions are asymptomatic, but they occur more commonly during clinical relapse [32]. In a study of acute optic neuritis the phase of gadolinium leakage in the symptomatic lesion was associated with acute visual loss and a reduced amplitude of the visual evoked potential (VEP), both of which reversed one month later at which time gadolinium leakage had also ceased [33]. This evolution occurred in the face of a persistent delay in the latency of the VEP, indicating that demyelination was present throughout. Thus, remyelination, which can be extensive in the early stages of MS [34] is unlikely to have accounted for the functional recovery seen in these patients. The observations suggest that blood–nerve barrier breakdown and inflammation *per se* probably contribute to the acute reversible deficits seen in MS.

Chronic lesions

The total lesion load, as measured from conventional T2-weighted brain scans, bears little or no relationship to the degree of disability. This is due to a number of factors. First, inaccuracies in the methods of measuring lesion load. Secondly, lesion location, a small lesion in a clinically eloquent area being potentially much more disabling than a large lesion in a less critical area (although one might still expect an overall association of lesion load with disability in that the greater the lesion load, the more likely is the chance of lesions occurring in strategic locations). Thirdly, pathophysiological heterogeneity of lesions which all look the same on conventional MR images. The latter factor is important. Irreversible disability in MS is likely to be due either to failure of conduction in persistently demyelinated fibres, or to axonal loss, which in some long-standing lesions can be profound [19]. The ability of demyelinated fibres to conduct impulses probably depends upon the formation of sodium channels along the internodal membrane, and there is currently no MR method for demonstrating this process. However, there are a number of quantitative MR parameters which are potential markers of axonal loss. The hypothesis that axonal loss is an important cause of irreversible disability has been supported by five recent studies using such approaches.

1. T2 relaxation curve analysis revealed more biexponential lesions (indicating an expanded extracellular space and by inference tissue loss) in secondary progressive MS compared to benign disease [35].
2. Lesion magnetization transfer ratio decreases correlate with disability [17].
3. Increases in hypointense lesion area on T1-weighted images correlate with increases in disability over a 2-year period [36].
4. The presence of spinal cord atrophy is associated with greater disability [22].
5. The concentration of cerebellar white matter N-acetyl aspartate (NAA) on proton spectroscopy is reduced in patients with severe ataxia but not in non-ataxic patients [37].

All five markers correlated more strongly with disability than did the conventional MRI lesion load. However, some caution is necessary. The first four approaches are in essence detecting **tissue** loss – while this could be loss of axons (and myelin), it might be loss of myelin alone. The functional consequences of these two types of tissue loss may be very different. Quantification of NAA is more specific, since in the adult brain it is almost exclusively contained within neurons. However, reversible reductions in NAA have been seen in acute lesions [31], indicating that factors other than axonal loss may affect the concentration of NAA. Data from experimental allergic encephalomyelitis suggest that mitochondrial dysfunction may be sufficient to reduce the concentration of NAA [38]. The demonstration of a persistent reduction of NAA on serial evaluation of lesions probably does indicate axonal loss [39], and this has been demonstrated in the cerebellum of MS patients with permanent and severe ataxia [37]. Confirmation that axonal loss causes a reduction in NAA also comes from the finding of reduced cerebellar concentrations in patients with autosomal dominant cerebellar ataxia, a disorder in which neuronal loss in the cerebellum is known to occur [37] (Figure 3.6).

In future, longitudinal studies are needed using these and other putative markers of tissue/axonal loss to elucidate more fully the relationships between pathology and the development of irreversible disability in MS.

3.4.5   MONITORING TREATMENT

The traditional method for assessing the efficacy of new therapies in MS is to conduct a controlled clinical trial using clinical endpoints, most often relapse rate or change in disability. Given the natural tendency of the disease to remit spontaneously, and the slow rate at which disabilities accumulate, such trials, in order to be definitive, require large numbers of patients (several hundred) to be studied over several years. Therefore it is natural to look for an alternative laboratory marker of disease activity.

There are two requirements for an ideal laboratory marker: first, it should be more sensitive than clinical monitoring, allowing efficacy to be assessed rapidly and in small numbers of patients; secondly, it should be predictive of the subsequent clinical course. The status of MRI in relation to these criteria is now presented, followed by discussion of how MRI might best be used in current clinical trials.

Sensitivity

Serial unenhanced T2-weighted brain MRI at monthly intervals in patients with early relapsing-remitting MS reveals new or enlarging lesions five to ten times more often than the occurrence of clinical relapses [27]. A similar level of activity is seen in patients who have entered the secondary-progressive phase of the disease [28]. In these patient groups, gadolinium enhancement doubles the number of detectable active (i.e new, enlarging or enhancing) lesions [10], and if monthly scanning with and without enhancement is performed over one year, an average of 20 active lesions per patient will be seen. However, in those with progressive disease from onset (primary-progressive MS), an average of only three active lesions per patient per year will be seen [28], and monthly scanning in this group of patients has little merit.

Predictive value in clinically isolated syndromes

Between 50 and 70% of patients presenting with a clinically isolated syndrome suggestive of MS (optic neuritis, acute partial myelitis and brain stem syndromes such as internuclear ophthalmoplegia) already have asymptomatic cerebral white matter lesions on MRI. Several groups have now reported follow-up findings after 2–5 years [40–44]. If brain MRI is normal, the risk of progressing to clinically definite MS is low (about 5% after 5 years); if there are multiple white matter lesions the risk is much greater (65% after 5 years in one study [43]). Furthermore, a correlation has emerged between the *number* of lesions at presentation and the subsequent risk for MS [40, 43, 44] – after 5 years, Morrissey *et al.* [43] found that 85% with four or more lesions had gone on to develop MS. These findings are relevant for counselling individual patients, and suggest that MRI should be used to select the most appropriate patients for trials of therapies aimed at preventing the evolution from an isolated syndrome to clinically definite disease.

The predictive value of MRI for subsequent disability is less clear. One report demonstrated a moderate correlation between MRI lesion load at presentation and disability after 5 years ($r = 0.6$) [45]. However, less than 10% of the patient cohort had developed severe disabilities at 5 years, and much longer follow-up is required to assess definitively the risks in a disease that usually runs its course over two or three decades.

Predictive value in established multiple sclerosis

In established disease, the crucial question is: what is the predictive value of MRI for future disability? In many early studies, little or no correlation emerged in longitudinal studies comparing brain MRI and clinical features. This disappointing state of affairs has several likely explanations.

1. Most brain lesions do not cause symptoms.
2. There are inaccuracies in quantifying both clinical and MRI parameters.
3. Short follow-up studies of a few months are not sufficient for showing meaningful changes in disability.
4. There is pathophysiological heterogeneity of lesions which all appear the same on conventional images.

More encouragingly, three recent studies with longer follow-up have reported correlations. In nine relapsing-remitting patients followed monthly for 2–3 years, logistic regression analysis revealed a significant effect of the number and area of enhancing brain lesions on both the onset and continuation of clinical worsening as measured by the expanded disability status score (EDSS) [32]. A second report followed 18 patients for 1 year, with brain MRI initially weekly and later at monthly intervals [46]; a positive correlation of low magnitude was observed between the cumulative number of new MRI lesions and deterioration in disability. A larger study of a heterogeneous cohort of 281 patients revealed a weak but statistically significant correlation ($r = 0.13$) between the number of new and enlarging lesions on a T2-weighted scan and increase in disability over 2–3 years [47].

These associations are still weak, and in addition the relationship between short-term MRI activity – as seen for example on monthly gadolinium enhanced scans for 6 months) – and long-term disability is uncertain. Further follow-up studies are needed, using the recent improvements in MR techniques for lesion detection and pathological characterization discussed in earlier sections. It is to be hoped that more convincing correlations will then emerge.

Role of MRI in clinical trials in established multiple sclerosis

How might MRI be used in clinical trials? Two roles emerge: first is to screen new therapies, using MRI as the primary measure of efficacy; second is to use MRI as a secondary outcome measure in large scale clinical trials in which disability is the primary outcome.

Because of the high level of lesion activity, MRI **screening studies** are most useful in early relapsing-remitting or secondary-progressive patients. Two study designs may be considered: crossover or parallel groups. Using monthly MRI it has been calculated that a 60% reduction in active lesions should be detectable using a 1 month baseline followed by a 6 month treatment phase in a parallel-design, placebo-controlled study of 2×40 patients [48]. This parallel design is a sound approach to screening new drugs, and a number have already been evaluated in this way. Nevertheless, because of the marked variation in lesion activity between patients, parallel designs still need substantial numbers of patients. Intra-patient variation in activity over time is also considerable, though less than inter-patient variation. Thus, crossover designs provide a more powerful form of MRI monitoring [48, 49].

A double crossover strategy is better avoided where there is uncertainty as to the duration of a persistent treatment effect after stopping treatment, and this is almost always the case when evaluating MS treatments. A single crossover study uses the patient as their own control, with a period of baseline scanning followed by the treatment phase. One criticism of this approach is that the scan rater is unblinded. A more serious concern is that a positive result is due to selection bias, patients entering the study during an active clinical and MRI phase of the disease and subsequently regressing towards the mean. Serial MRI for 4 years or more years in a cohort of relapsing-remitting patients at the NIH has elucidated the variations in MRI activity with time and their relationship to clinical changes [32, 50]. Statistical analysis of these data suggest that a screening period of at least 6 months reduces the chances of regression toward the mean. The demonstration in 14 of the NIH patients of a reduction in the mean number of gadolinium enhancing lesions by over 80% when comparing the first 6 months of interferon beta-1b treatment with the preceding 7 months of screening [51] is persuasive evidence of the value of such an approach.

In summary, screening studies with monthly scanning for 6–12 months using either a single crossover or parallel groups design are of particular value in relapsing-remitting or secondary-progressive MS. The results of such studies should provide a rational basis for deciding whether to proceed with the expense and effort involved in a full scale clinical trial – a positive effect on MRI activity would establish the case for proceeding, while a negative result would argue against. Because of the uncertain relationship between clinical and MRI activity in established MS, the definitive outcome should still be disability.

In large scale **definitive clinical studies** of 2–3 years' duration, measurement of total brain lesion load at 6–12-monthly intervals is indicated, the value of this approach having been emphasized by the striking results of the North American interferon beta-1b study [52]. In that study, lesions were outlined manually by a single, experienced rater. This approach is the only one validated in a large scale trial, and can reasonably be seen as the current 'gold standard' – implicit is a belief that the eye of an experienced observer is the surest way of defining MRI lesions. However, the manual outlining technique has inherent limitations: it is time-consuming, depends on a single rater (inter-rater reproducibility is poor), and has a large subjective element. There is good deal of work in progress to develop more automated and objective computer assisted techniques for lesion segmentation. One approach applies a global threshold to moderately T2-weighted scans; another applies a focal threshold to individual lesions. These techniques have been reported in preliminary studies to improve reproducibility of lesion load measurements compared to full manual outlining, but they are time-consuming and still require considerable manual editing. The use of multiparametric image data looks a promising way for more rapid and automated separation of lesions from normal brain, but validation studies are needed.

In order to ascertain the longer-term effects of therapy on lesion activity, there is a case for more frequent (monthly) scanning of a subgroup of patients, either throughout the 2–3 years of the trial or perhaps 6 months at the start and end of the study. Finally, if the predictive value of the putative MR markers for axonal loss is confirmed, implementation of these techniques will be important in future studies. Of these, unenhanced T1-weighted SE imaging is the easiest technique to implement in multicentre studies. Standardization of techniques across centres for magnetization transfer imaging, spectroscopy and quantification of spinal cord area is more problematic, and at present such approaches are best confined to centres with a particular interest.

3.5   Conclusion

MRI plays a key role in the assessment of patients with MS. Brain MRI is the single most useful investigation during diagnostic work-up, and recent technical advances have made spinal MRI a very useful tool in the evaluation of patients with undiagnosed myelopathies or where MS is thought likely on clinical grounds but brain MRI is normal. Potential MR markers of inflammation, demyelination and axonal loss are helping to elucidate the mechanisms of acute relapse and irreversible disability. In relapsing-remitting and secondary-progressive disease, serial MRI at monthly intervals is increasingly being used to evaluate new therapies. Because the relationship between short-term MRI activity and long-term disability is uncertain, definitive trials should continue to have primary clinical endpoints.

ACKNOWLEDGEMENTS

The Multiple Sclerosis NMR Research Unit at The Institute of Neurology in London uses a 1.5T GE Signa scanner provided by The Multiple Sclerosis Society of Great Britain and Northern Ireland. The spinal cord and optic nerve images were obtained using multi-array coils and fast spin echo sequences, both provided by General Electric Medical Systems.

References

1. Cala, L.A. and Mastaglia, F.L. (1976) Computerized axial tomography in multiple sclerosis. *Lancet*, **1**, 689.
2. Vinuela, F.V., Fox, A.J., Debrun, G.M. *et al.* (1982) New perspectives in computed tomography of multiple sclerosis. *Am. J. Roentgenol.*, **139**, 123–7.
3. Brooks, D.J., Leenders, K.L., Head, G. *et al.* (1984) Studies on regional cerebral oxygen utilization and cognitive function in multiple sclerosis. *J. Neurol. Neurosurg. Psychiatry*, **47**, 1182–91.
4. Pozzilli, C., Passafiume, C., Bernadi, S. *et al.* (1991) SPECT, MRI and cognitive function in multiple sclerosis. *J. Neurol. Neurosurg. Psychiatry*, **54**, 110–15.
5. Young, I.R., Hall, A.S., Pallis, C.A. *et al.* (1981) Nuclear magnetic resonance imaging of the brain in multiple sclerosis. *Lancet*, **318**, 1063–6.
6. Ormerod, I.E.C., Miller, D.H., McDonald, W.I. *et al.* (1987) The role of NMR imaging in the assessment of multiple sclerosis and isolated neurological lesions: a quantitative study. *Brain*, **110**, 1579–616.
7. Thorpe, J.W., Halpin, S.F., MacManus, D.G. *et al.* (1994) A comparison between fast spin echo and conventional spin echo in the detection of multiple sclerosis lesions. *Neuroradiology*, **36**, 388–92.
8. Rydberg, J.N., Hammond, C.A., Grimm, R.C. *et al.* (1994) Initial experience in MR imaging of the brain with a fast Fluid-attenuated Inversion-Recovery pulse sequence. *Radiology*, **193**, 173–80.
9. Grossman, R.I., Gonzales-Scarano, F., Atlas, S.W. *et al.* (1986) Multiple sclerosis: gadolinium enhancement in MR imaging. *Radiology*, **169**, 117–22.
10. Miller, D.H., Barkhof, F. and Nauta, J.J.P. (1993) Gadolinium enhancement increases the sensitivity of MRI in detecting disease activity in multiple sclerosis. *Brain*, **116**, 1077–94.
11. Gean-Marton, A.D., Venzia, L.G., Marton, K.I. *et al.* (1991) Abnormal corpus callosum: a sensitive and specific indicator of multiple sclerosis. *Radiology*, **180**, 215–21.
12. Poser, C.M., Paty, D.W., Scheinberg, L. *et al.* (1983) New diagnostic criteria for multiple sclerosis: guidelines for research protocols. *Ann. Neurol.*, **13**, 227–31.
13. Kesselring, J., Miller, D.H., Robb, S.A. *et al.* (1990) Acute disseminated encephalomyelitis. MRI findings and the distinction from multiple sclerosis. *Brain*, **113**, 291–302.
14. Kirkpatrick, J.B. and Hayman, L.A. (1987) White-matter lesions in MR imaging of clinically healthy brains of elderly subjects: possible pathological basis. *Radiology*, **162**, 509–11.
15. Offenbacher, H., Fazekas, F., Schmidt, R. *et al.* (1993) Assessment of MRI criteria for a diagnosis of MS. *Neurology*, **43**, 905–9.
16. Dousset, V., Grossman, R., Ramer, K.N. *et al.* (1992) Experimental allergic encephalomyelitis and multiple sclerosis: lesion characterisation with magnetisation transfer imaging. *Radiology*, **182**, 483–91.
17. Gass, A., Barker, G.J., Kidd, D. *et al.* (1994) Correlation of magnetization transfer ratio with clinical disability in multiple scerosis. *Ann. Neurol.*, **36**, 62–7.
18. Wong, K.T., Grossman, R.I., Boorstein, J.M. *et al.* (1995) Magnetization transfer imaging of periventricular hyperintense white matter in the elderly. *Am. J. Neuroradiol.*, **16**, 253–8.
19. Adams, C.B.T. (1989) *A Colour Atlas of Multiple Sclerosis and Other Myelin Disorders*, London, Wolfe Medical Publications.
20. Uhlenbrock, D. and Sehlen, S. (1989) The value of T1-weighted images in the differentiation between MS, white matter lesions, and subcortical arteriosclerotic encephalopathy (SAE). *Neuroradiology*, **31**, 203–12.
21. Hiehle, J.F., Grossman, R.I., Ramer, K.N. *et al.* (1995) Magnetization transfer effect in MR-detected multiple sclerosis lesions: comparison with gadolinium-enhanced spin-echo images and nonenhanced T1-weighted images. *Am. J. Neuroradiol.*, **16**, 69–77.
22. Kidd, D., Thorpe, J.W., Thompson, A.J. *et al.* (1993) Spinal cord MRI using multi-array coils and fast spin echo. II. Findings in multiple sclerosis. *Neurology*, **43**, 2632–7.
23. Campi, A., Filippi, M., Comi, G. *et al.* (1995) Acute transverse myelopathy: spinal and cranial MR study with clinical follow-up. *Am. J. Neuroradiol.*, **16**, 115–23.
24. Miller, D.H., Newton, M.R., van der Poel, J.C. *et al.* (1988) Magnetic resonance imaging of the optic nerve in optic neuritis. *Neurology*, **38**, 175–9.
25. Lee, D.H., Simon, J.H., Szumowski, J. *et al.* (1991) Optic neuritis and orbital lesions: lipid suppressed chemical shift imaging. *Radiology*, **179**, 543–6.
26. Gass, A., Barker, G.J., MacManus, D.G. *et al.* (1995) High resolution magnetic resonance imaging of the anterior visual pathway in patients with optic neuropathies using fast spin echo and phased array local coils. *J. Neurol. Neurosurg. Psychiatry*, **58**, 562–9.
27. Willoughby, E.W., Grochowski, E., Li, D.K.B. *et al.* (1989) Serial magnetic resonance scanning in multiple sclerosis: a second prospective study in relapsing patients. *Ann. Neurol.*, **25**, 43–9.
28. Thompson, A.J. Kermode, A.G., Wicks, D. *et al.* (1991) Major differences in the dynamics of primary and secondary progressive multiple sclerosis. *Ann. Neurol.*, **29**, 53–62.
29. Miller, D.H., Rudge, P., Johnson, G. *et al.* (1988) Serial gadolinium enhanced magnetic resonance imaging in multiple sclerosis. *Brain*, **111**, 927–39.
30. Katz, D., Taubenberger, J.K., Cannella, B. *et al.* (1993) Correlation between magnetic resonance imaging findings and lesion development in multiple sclerosis. *Ann. Neurol.*, **34**, 661–9.
31. Davie, C.A., Hawkins, C.P., Barker, G.J. *et al.* (1994) Serial proton magnetic resonance spectroscopy in acute multiple sclerosis lesions. *Brain*, **117**, 49–58.
32. Smith, M.E., Stone, L.A., Albert, P.S. *et al.* (1993) Clinical worsening in multiple sclerosis is associated with increased frequency and area of gadopentate dimeglumine enhancing magnetic resonance imaging lesions. *Ann. Neurol.*, **33**, 480–9.
33. Youl, B.D., Turano, G., Miller, D.H. *et al.* (1991) The pathophysiology of optic neuritis: an association of gadolinium leakage with clinical and electrophysiological deficits. *Brain*, **114**, 2437–50.
34. Prineas, J.W., Barnard, R.O., Kwon, E.E. *et al.* (1993) Multiple sclerosis: remyelination of nascent lesions. *Ann. Neurol.*, **33**, 137–51.
35. Filippi, M., Barker, G.J., Horsfield, M.A. *et al.* (1994) Benign and secondary progressive multiple sclerosis: a preliminary quantitative MRI study. *J Neurol.*, **241**, 246–51.
36. van Waldeveen, M.A.A., Barkhof, F., Hommes, O.R. *et al.* (1995) Correlating MR imaging and clinical disease activity in multiple sclerosis: relevance of hypointense lesions on short TR/TE ('T1-weighted') spin-echo images. *Neurology*, **45**, 1684–90.
37. Davie, C.A., Barker, G.J., Webb, S. *et al.* (1994) Proton magnetic resonance spectroscopy (MRS) study of cerebellar dysfunction in multiple sclerosis. *J. Neurol.*, **341** (Suppl. 1), S151.
38. Brenner, R., Munro, P.M.G., Williams, S.C.R. *et al.* (1993) Abnormal neuronal mitochondria: a cause of reduction in Na in demyelinating disease. *Society of Magnetic Resonance in Medicine, 12th Annual Meeting, Abstracts*, **1**, 281.
39. Arnold, D.L., Reiss, G.T., Matthews, P.M. *et al.* (1994) Use of proton magnetic resonance spectroscopy for monitoring disease progression in multiple sclerosis. *Ann. Neurol.*, **36**, 76–82.
40. Lee, K.H., Hashimoto, S.A., Hooge, J.P. *et al.* (1991) Magnetic resonance imaging of the head in the diagnosis of multiple sclerosis: a prospective 2-year follow up with comparison of clinical evaluation, evoked potentials, oligoclonal banding, and CT. *Neurology*, **41**, 657–60.
41. Jacobs, L., Munschauer, F.E. and Kaba, S.E. (1991) Clinical and magnetic resonance imaging in optic neuritis. *Neurology*, **41**, 15–19.
42. Ford, B., Tampieri, D. and Francis, G. (1992) Long term follow up of acute transverse partial myelopathy. *Neurology*, **42**, 250–2.
43. Morrissey, S.P., Miller, D.H., Kendall, B.E. *et al.* (1993) The significance of brain magnetic resonance imaging abnormalities at presentation with clinically isolated syndromes suggestive of multiple sclerosis. *Brain*, **116**, 135–46.
44. Beck, R.W., Cleary, P.A., Trobe, J.D. *et al.* (1993) The effect of corticosteroids for acute optic neuritis on the subsequent development of multiple sclerosis. *N. Engl. J. Med.*, **329**, 1764–9.
45. Filippi, M., Horsfield, M.A., Morrissey, S.P. *et al.* (1994) Quantitative brain MRI lesion load predicts the course of clinically isolated syndromes suggestive of multiple sclerosis. *Neurology*, **44**, 635–41.
46. Khoury, S.J., Guttmann, C.R.G., Orav, E.J. *et al.* (1994) Longitudinal MRI in multiple sclerosis: correlation between disability and lesion burden. *Neurology*, **44**, 2120–4.
47. Filippi, M., Paty, D.W., Kappos, L. *et al.* (1995) Correlations between changes in disability and T2-weighted brain MRI activity in multiple sclerosis: a follow-up study. *Neurology*, **45**, 255–60.
48. Nauta, J.J.P., Thompson, A.J., Barkhof, F. and Miller, D.H. (1994) Magnetic resonance imaging in monitoring the treatment of multiple sclerosis patients: statistical power of parallel-groups and crossover designs. *J. Neurol. Sci.*, **122**, 6–14.
49. McFarland, H.F., Frank, J.A., Albert, P.S. *et al.* (1992) Using gadolinium – enhanced magnetic resonance imaging lesions to monitor disease activity in multiple sclerosis. *Ann. Neurol.*, **32**, 758–66.
50. Albert, P.S., McFarland, H.F., Smith, M.E. and Frank, J.A. (1994) Time series for modelling counts from a relapsing-remitting disease: application to modelling disease activity in multiple sclerosis. *Stat. Med.*, **13**, 453–66.
51. Stone, L.A., Frank, J.A., Albert, P.S. *et al.* (1995) The effect of beta interferon on blood brain barrier disruptions demonstrated by contrast enhanced MRI in relapsing remitting multiple sclerosis. *Ann. Neurol.*, **37**, 611–19.
52. Paty, D.W. and Li, D.K.B., UBC MS/MRI Study Group, IFNB Multiple Sclerosis Study Group (1993) Interferon beta-1b is effective in relapsing-remitting multiple sclerosis. II. MRI analysis results of a multicenter, randomized, double-blind, placebo-controlled trial. *Neurology*, **43**, 662–7.

4 EVOKED POTENTIALS IN MULTIPLE SCLEROSIS

Marc R. Nuwer

Over the past 20 years, evoked potentials (EPs) have proved themselves a useful test to diagnose multiple sclerosis (MS). These tests also have served in research into the pathophysiology of demyelination and as an adjunct in MS therapeutic trials.

EPs are sensitive, objective and highly reproducible. They can detect **clinically silent lesions**, i.e. physiologic changes not accompanied by physical signs or symptoms. Silent lesions can provide evidence of a second or third lesion in early clinical MS. This can help make the diagnosis of MS. The tests are objective because they require no patient participation beyond lying quietly or watching a visual display screen. A patient cannot substantially alter the test results. The EP tests are scored in a standard manner, leaving little room for subjective error by the reader. The tests yield identical reproducible values from day to day and year to year as long as the conditions of the testing are well controlled. EPs are readily quantified to 2–3 significant figures, aiding the comparison of a patient's results to the age-matched controls, and aiding statistical testing of research hypotheses.

The physiology underlying EPs is well understood, including the effect of demyelination [1–5]. Classical demyelination causes delayed axonal conduction or even complete conduction blocks across the demyelinated region. EPs are the electrical potentials (voltages) evoked by brief sensory stimuli. Axonal volleys generating EPs are conducted along the peripheral and central nervous system pathways associated with the stimulated sensory modality. These nervous system signals become delayed or blocked when crossing through a patch of demyelination. In that case the EPs generated beyond the demyelination are abnormal because they are delayed, attenuated or absent. Substantial knowledge already exists about the locations of EP generator sites around the nervous system. With this knowledge, the EP reader can determine the approximate level of the nervous system at which a delay or a block probably has occurred. In turn this result allows the clinician to locate where the nervous system has been impaired in an individual patient. When multiple sites of impairment

occur, EP tests can help identify the first site of impairment, but are not able to count the number of sites impaired. Often they cannot detect further sites along the conduction pathway after the first impaired region encountered. EPs mainly test a few specific portions of the nervous system: the central visual pathways, the brain stem auditory pathways and the posterior column/medial lemniscus/internal capsule sensory pathways. There is not yet any reliable EP testing of the spinothalamic or cerebellar pathways. EP testing of the pyramidal tract motor pathways has been developed. These central motor conduction velocity tests are available clinically in some countries, but not yet in others such as the US [6–8].

EPs are useful in many other areas of neurologic practice beyond MS. Brain stem auditory EPs can screen for hearing impairment [9]. All three EP modalities (visual, auditory and somatosensory) are useful in evaluating comatose patients, allowing quantified assessment of degree of impairment [10–11], and help in assessing locations of lesions. Many hereditary degenerative neurologic conditions cause specific patterns of changes in various EP peaks, which occasionally provide clues differentiating between some of these conditions [12]. EPs are used to monitor in the operating room, allowing for identification of nervous system impairment early enough to correct the impairment before it becomes permanent [13]. The presence of normal EPs despite severe symptoms can help confirm conversion hysteria or malingering. EPs can also help separate peripheral from central localization of impairment, and separate spinal from intracranial localization for a variety of sensory disorders. In the latter circumstances, EPs' usefulness is analogous to deep tendon reflexes when they are used to separate central from peripheral motor pathway disorders.

4.1 Visual evoked potentials

Visual evoked potentials (VEPs) can be evoked either by a strobe flash or by a checkerboard pattern reversal device.

Multiple Sclerosis: Clinical and pathogenetic basis. Edited by Cedric S. Raine, Henry F. McFarland and Wallace W. Tourtellotte. Published in 1997 by Chapman & Hall, London. ISBN 0 412 30890 8.

The flash technique was described first [14], but the pattern reversal VEP technique was subsequently found to be more sensitive for detecting demyelinating lesions [15]. The pattern is typically a checkerboard of black and white squares, in which each white square becomes black and each black square becomes white twice each second. This is accomplished on a digital video screen or with a mirror and galvinometer. The subject is tested one eye at a time in a darkened room. Recordings are made at the occipital scalp and the latency to a large positive electrical polarity peak is measured at 90–200 msec after each checkerboard reversal. About 100 separate stimulus presentations are performed with their results averaged together to reduce random background 'noise' such as EEG and EKG. This positive polarity peak, seen usually at 100 msec, is called P100 (Figure 4.1). It represents the culmination of a series of neurological events, beginning with axonal conduction along the optic nerve, chiasm and optic tract to the lateral geniculate body. From there a second axonal volley travels up the optic radiations, passing directly through the posterior periventricular white matter for rather long distances, and eventually reaching the occipital cortex. Substantial additional processing occurs within the occipital cortex for 30–50 msec after the axonal volley arrives there. Finally a large surface positive electrical potential is generated from the striate cortex. This is detectable at the occipital scalp as the P100 peak.

Impairment in MS occurs at several sites along this pathway. The optic nerve is often the site of demyelination, but the optic tract and especially the periventricular white matter are also often involved, as recently demonstrated by elegant neuroimaging techniques. Demyelination at the periventricular optic radiations may be a major contributor to P100 delays in some patients, whereas optic neuritis is the principal site of VEP impairment in others. Pre-chiasmatic optic nerve lesions can be separated from the post-chiasmatic lesions by testing the two eyes separately. Interocular discrepancies in P100 latencies are usually attributed to lesions at the optic nerve, for obvious anatomical reasons.

VEPs are more sensitive to demyelination than even a careful clinical examination of visual function [16–18]. When visual EPs were compared with careful clinical examination in 198 MS patients, there was never an abnormality in the neuro-ophthalmologic examination when the visual EP was normal [17]. Various clinical examinations were often normal when the visual EP was abnormal. When the visual EP was abnormal 96% of patients had normal visual fields by confrontation, 55% had normal visual fields by formal testing, 74% had normal pupillary responses, 39% had normal appearance of the optic fundus, and there was no red desaturation in 27% of patients carefully tested.

The checkerboard reversal pattern VEP technique is abnormal in almost all patients who have a clear history of optic neuritis. In a summary of various reports in the medical literature, Chiappa [18] noted that about 90% of patients with optic neuritis showed abnormal pattern VEPs, with the percentage closer to 100% in many of the individual research reports. When there was no clinical evidence for optic neuritis, the VEPs were still abnormal in 51% of 715 MS patients [19–43] (Table 4.1).

VEPs tend to worsen monotonically. Once a lesion has occurred and the VEP has become delayed, only small degrees of improvement occur even over many years [44]. Because of this, VEPs can help to establish whether an episode of suspicious visual changes many years ago was indeed due to an episode of optic neuritis. This is of clinical value in trying to establish a diagnosis of MS. In a patient presenting with a single spinal cord or brain stem lesion VEP studies may determine whether optic neuritis has occurred at any time in the past years. Finding such a second, visual system lesion has helped in establishing many a diagnosis of MS.

Table 4.1 Rates of abnormalities for evoked potentials in MS: aggregate results of 26–31 separate research series

	Pattern visual	Brain stem auditory	Somatosensory
Number of patients	1950	1006	1006
Number of research series	26	26	31
Rates of EP abnormality (%):			
Definite MS	85	67	77
Probable MS	58	41	67
Possible MS	37	30	49
Asymptomatic patients[a]	51	38	42
All patients	63	46	58 (upper extremity) 76 (lower extremity)

[a] Asymptomatic for the sensory modality or nervous system region being tested.

From Chiappa, 1990 [18].

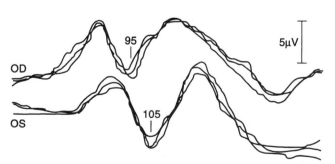

Figure 4.1 Visual evoked potentials to checkerboard reversal stimulation. The OS P100 latency of 105 msec is 10 msec longer than the P100 OD. Such an asymmetry in latency is pathognomonic of optic neuritis OS. (Courtesy of UCLA EP Lab.)

Some other disorders can also affect VEP latencies. Some hereditary degenerative neurologic conditions (e.g. Friedreich's ataxa)[12,45], as well as B_{12} deficiency[46], neurosyphilis[47] and other disorders[48] can slow P100 latencies. Occasionally these latter conditions produce mild interocular P100 latency differences, but a large interocular latency difference is almost always due to the demyelination of optic neuritis, so that finding establishes that demyelination caused the VEP abnormality. Sometimes demyelination causes symmetrical P100 delays by bilaterally symmetric demyelination. Finding bilaterally symmetrical P100 delays is considered confirmatory for an abnormality but nonspecific for the particular type of pathology.

The VEP is about twice as sensitive as MRI for detecting demyelinating lesions in the optic nerves, chiasm and optic tracts[49–51]. In searching for a second lesion in patients with known optic neuritis, brain MRI is more sensitive than VEP of the unaffected eye[52]. In patients with early MS, MRI has been compared to VEPs in several studies. Brain MRI was abnormal in 46–62% of patients in these studies, whereas VEP was abnormal in 44–46% of these patients[51,53,54]. Multimodality EP testing had a higher yield of abnormalities. For patients with acute or chronic spinal cord lesions being evaluated for a diagnosis of MS, brain MRI has a higher yield of abnormalities (56–82%) than did VEP (7–28%) when compared[55].

VEPs are also helpful in clarifying the nature of signal enhancing lesions, by helping to separate MS from the dozen occasional causes of MRI lesions mimicking MS[56].

VEPs can help study the physiology of demyelination. VEP latencies and amplitudes are affected by heat and by medications that alter conduction across a demyelinated plaque. Heat alters VEPs in MS[57–59], in a way analogous to the clinical Uhthoff's phenomenon or the hot bath test. Using VEP, these heat effects can be measured precisely. Hyperventilation can improve the VEP, causing some improved amplitudes and even shorter latencies[60]. This corresponds to previous observations that hyperventilation, alkalosis and hypocalcemia can bring about transient improvements in MS clinical deficits. The calcium channel blocker verapamil[61] and the potassium channel blocker 4-aminopyridine[62] can also substantially improve VEPs transiently in some MS patients.

Overall, checkerboard reversal pattern VEPs are of established value as an aid in the clinical evaluation of patients when diagnosis of MS is under consideration. The finding of abnormalities in these visual pathways is common in MS, even in patients with no other clinical indications of central visual pathway impairment. VEPs are more sensitive than MRI in detecting optic neuritis. These tests are useful in clarifying whether a previous visual event was optic neuritis, and in looking for visual pathway impairment in patients with single brain stem or spinal cord lesions.

4.2 Brain stem auditory evoked potentials

Signals from brain stem auditory generators can be detected at the scalp. These signals represent activation of brain stem pathways after presentation of a 100 μsec click sound through earphones. Pathways involved are probably those associated with the ability to localize an auditory stimulus in space, rather than those used for speech or tone discrimination. Neurons generating the brain stem auditory EP (BAEP) are located in the pons and midbrain. These tests detect lesions only if the lesion lies at least in part in the specific brain stem pathways tested. They fail to detect lesions at or below the medulla, or at the thalamus and above. But these tests are so sensitive that they can detect a fraction of a millisecond delay when it does lie in the specific brain stem pathways tested.

The VIIIth cranial nerve is the generator of wave I, the first peak in the brain stem auditory EP. This wave I peripheral potential is a valuable indicator that the click stimulus has been adequately processed by the cochlea and other peripheral parts of the auditory pathway. Wave I is almost always normal in MS patients who have no additional hearing disorder. The four succeeding BAEP waves are labeled II–V (Figure 4.2). They arise from the brain stem itself. Wave II is generated around the cochlear nucleus at the caudal pons. Wave III arises around the superior olive and trapezoid body in the central pons. Waves IV and V probably arise from regions around the lateral lemniscus bilaterally, as axonal volleys travel rostrally toward the inferior colliculus. Central nervous system lesions can be localized by observing which waves are disrupted or delayed. Lateralizing a lesion is straightforward for lower pontine lesions. The laterality of lesions is more difficult to assess at the lower midbrain or upper pons.

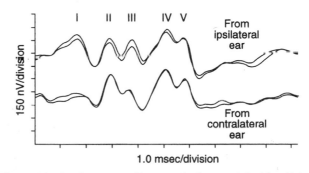

Figure 4.2 Brain stem auditory evoked potentials, identifying the five main peaks. (Reproduced with permission from Nuwer *et al.*, 1994[146].)

The typical abnormalities found in MS patients include: (a) a prolongation of waves II–V, measured by the I–V interpeak latency; (b) a loss of amplitude of wave V, measured by V/I amplitude ratio; and (c) disappearance of V. Figure 4.3 shows an example of various degrees of brain stem auditory EP abnormalities in MS patients.

Other types of neurologic disorders can also affect the brain stem auditory EPs. These include tumors [63, 64] and ischemia [64], and some hereditary degenerative neurological disorders [12]. As such, BAEP abnormalities cannot be considered pathognomonic of MS. Rather, these abnormalities indicate a lesion located at a pontine or low midbrain level.

Internuclear ophthalmoplegia is the clinical sign correlating best with BAEP abnormalities. This is because both are readily disrupted by mid-pontine plaques. Other brain stem signs have a lesser degree of correlation. Vertigo, dysarthria and dysphagia have a

Table 4.2 Correlation between degree of brain stem auditory EP abnormality and MS patient signs and symptoms

Correlation with change in BAEPs	Signs/symptoms
History	
0.41	Diplopia
0.23	Dysphagia
0.16	Vertigo
0.12	Hearing impairment
0.10	Dysarthria
0.03	Facial sensory impairment
Physical signs	
0.39	Ocular dysmetria or gaze paresis
0.32	Nystagmus
0.29	Facial weakness
0.25	Dysarthria
0.23	Facial sensory loss
0.21	Slow tongue movements
0.09	Other brain stem signs
0.04	Subjective hearing threshold

Changes in BAEP, correspond best to signs and symptoms of oculomotor impairment.

From Nuwer *et al.*, 1988 [145].

rather mediocre to low correlation with abnormalities of these EPs (Table 4.2).

Chiappa has summarized the aggregate results from a variety of research reports in the medical literature [18] which included 1006 MS patients [32, 34, 66–89]. Among these patients, 46% had abnormal brain stem auditory EPs (Table 4.1) Among patients having no history or physical signs of brain stem abnormalities, 38% had BAEP abnormalities. Abnormality rates in individual studies varied between 21% and 55%. The abnormalities found in such asymptomatic patients represent clinically silent lesions detected by these EP techniques.

Brain stem auditory EPs have repeatedly been found to be more sensitive than MRI for detecting pontine lesions [90–93]. Brain MRI is more sensitive than BAEP in patients undergoing an evaluation to diagnose MS. Among three studies directly comparing the two tests, brain MRI was abnormal among 68–83% of patients, whereas BAEP testing was abnormal among 41–50% of patients [54, 65, 92].

Overall, BAEP testing seems an appropriate clinical tool to confirm that cranial nerve or other signs or symptoms are due to central, brain stem impairment as opposed to impairment along the peripheral pathways. The test is sensitive to impairment at the pons and lower midbrain. For that specific purpose, it is more sensitive than brain MRI. For the general setting of evaluating possible MS patients, brain MRI has a higher yield of abnormality.

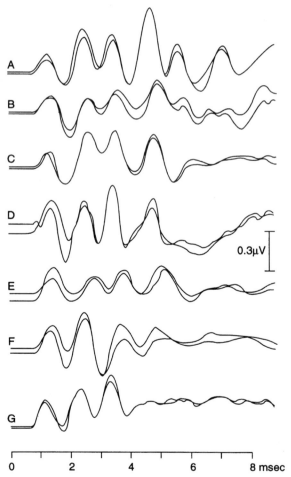

0.3μV

0   2   4   6   8 msec

Figure 4.3 Examples of various degrees of abnormality in waves IV and V in the brain stem auditory EP test in MS. The upper EP traces are less affected, and the lower traces are more affected. Demyelination causes some prolongation of latencies, with loss of amplitude and eventual absence of peaks II–V. (Reproduced with permission from Nuwer *et al.*, 1988 [145].)

4.3   Somatosensory evoked potentials

Somatosensory testing is initiated by brief electrical stimuli delivered to the median nerve at the wrist or the posterior tibial nerve at the ankle. Recordings are taken at several levels, the first over the brachial plexus or the lumbar spinal cord. More rostral recordings are made at the neck and scalp. These recordings follow the sensory nerve volleys as they travel progressively more rostrally, entering the central nervous system tracts. The pathways subserving somatosensory evoked potentials (SEPs) are the posterior column, medial lemniscus and internal capsule. There are no satisfactory EPs for testing the spinothalamic pathways.

For median nerve EPs, the principal peaks are the N9 generated at the brachial plexus, the N13 from mid-cervical spinal cord, the P14 from cervicomedullary junction, the N18 from nearby the thalamus, and finally the N20 from the postcentral primary somatosensory cortex (Figure 4.4). For the posterior tibial nerve EPs, the principal peaks are the N8 from the sciatic nerve at the rostral popliteal fossa, the N22 from the lumbar spinal cord and P37 from the primary somatosensory cortex. Additional posterior tibial nerve somatosensory EP peaks can be detected sometimes over the rostral cervical spinal cord or brain stem.

Peak latency and amplitude abnormalities can help determine the anatomic level of disruption along these sensory pathways. This localizing ability of EP tests is useful in MS, where diagnosis requires finding lesions in separate locations. Localization is also helpful in other neurologic evaluations in which approximate localization is valuable.

Chiappa[18] has summarized the results from an aggregate of several published clinical studies which describe the rate of abnormality for median nerve somatosensory EPs in MS patients[29, 32, 34, 35, 44, 74, 77, 79, 94–115]. Median nerve EP abnormalities were seen in 42% of MS patients who had *no* signs or symptoms of sensory systems impairment, as well as abnormalities in 75% of patients who *did* have signs or symptoms of appropriate sensory abnormalities. Posterior tibial nerve SEPs have revealed a slightly greater rate of finding clinically silent abnormalities (Table 4.1).

Various other neurologic disorders can also affect the SEPs. Peripheral neuropathy and other peripheral disorders can affect the peripheral conduction velocities. Fortunately, these peripheral effects can be removed from the analysis of central nervous system conduction by subtracting away the latencies of the peripheral N9 or N22 peaks seen over the brachial plexus or lumbar spinal cord. A variety of hereditary and degenerative neurologic conditions[12] can slow central conduction latencies in sensory pathways. Some acquired metabolic disorders such as B_{12} deficiency also can slow central

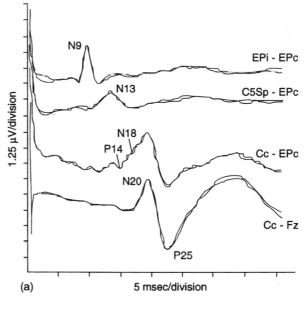

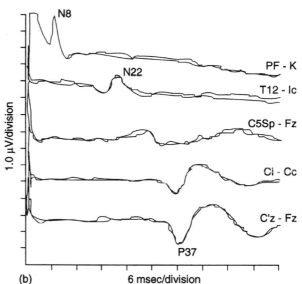

Figure 4.4 Examples of the peaks seen in normal short latency median nerve (*a*) and posterior tibial nerve (*b*) somatosensory EP testing. Recording sites EPi and EPc are at shoulders; C5Sp and T12 over the spine; PF, K and Ic at the popliteal fossa, knee and iliac crest; Ci, Cc, C'z and Fz on the scalp. The several standard peaks are identified here. (Reproduced with permission from Nuwer *et al.*, 1994[147].)

somatosensory conduction[116]. Focal lesions due to ischemia, tumors, myelopathy associated with spondylosis and other focal disorders can disrupt conduction along the central portions of the somatosensory pathways. As such, information from SEPs must be integrated with other clinical information in order to assess whether EP changes are due to MS as opposed to other neurologic disorders.

Brain MRI is more sensitive than either median nerve SEP or posterior tibial nerve SEP alone in MS. In one direct comparison in 46 suspected or confirmed MS cases, 25 (54%) had abnormal median nerve SEPs, 33 (72%) had abnormal posterior tibial nerve SEPs, whereas 34 (74%) had an abnormal brain MRI scan [65]. In another study of 60 patients with definite, probable or possible MS, 29 (48%) had abnormal median nerve SEPs, 37 (61%) had abnormal posterior tibial nerve SEPs, whereas 50 (83%) had an abnormal brain MRI [92]. Similar results were seen for cervical MRI in 46 patients with spinal cord syndromes being evaluated for MS [55]. In that study, 31/46 (67%) of patients had an abnormal cervical MRI, whereas 26/46 (57%) had abnormal SEPs.

Overall, SEPs provide a useful tool for detecting clinically silent lesions which contribute to the diagnosis of MS. They provide a sensitive way to assess the spinal cord pathways, which can complement other testing such as brain MRI.

4.4 Multimodality evoked potential testing

The three evoked potential modalities have been compared to each other, to MRI and to cerebral spinal fluid findings in MS. This literature is useful for understanding which modality is most sensitive for various clinical presentations as well as in MS overall. Such comparisons can also be helpful in planning strategies for research studies, such as therapeutic trials.

Chiappa [18] has summarized the aggregate results of 26–31 original research reports which studied the abnormality rates for the three EP modalities [19–44, 66–89, 94–115] (Table 4.1). Among these studies, abnormality rates were highest for pattern visual EPs and lowest for brain stem auditory EPs. Somatosensory EPs had abnormality rates nearly as good as VEPs, even exceeding the latter's rate in the possible and probable MS category. Lower extremity SEPs from peroneal and posterior tibial nerves seem to be abnormal more often than median nerve SEPs. Some users believe that posterior tibial nerve EPs are actually more sensitive than visual EPs in routine clinical practice. Silent lesions, i.e. EP abnormalities despite no signs or symptoms in that sensory modality, are seen in one-third to one-half of the patients studied in these reports.

Among patients with an established diagnosis of MS, SEPs are the most likely to be abnormal. In one study [117] of all three EP modalities in 101 patients with chronic progressive MS, pattern VEPs were abnormal in 75%; BAEPs in 48%; and median nerve SEPs in 93%. Typical criteria for abnormality were used, which are shown in Table 4.3. In most of these patients the EPs were abnormal but not completely absent. This latter fact is important if one wishes to

Table 4.3 Evoked potentials found among 101 patients with chronic progressive MS (left and right sides scored separately)

Pattern visual EPs	
Median P100 latency	119 msec (normal < 105)
No. normal	50/202 (25%)
present but abnormal	132/202 (65%)
absent	20/202 (10%)
Median P100 amplitude	4.0 μV
Brain stem auditory EPs	
Median I–V inter-peak latency	4.4 msec (normal < 4.6)
Median V/I amplitude ratio	64% (normal > 50%)
No. normal	105/202 (52%)
V present but abnormal	24/202 (12%)
V absent	63/202 (32%)
all peaks absent	2/202 (1%)
Median nerve somatosensory EPs	
No. normal	15/202 (7%)
No. N9 absent	0/202
N13 absent	70/202 (35%)
N20 absent	115/202 (57%)
P40 absent	1/202
Median N20 latency	26 msec
N20 amplitude	0.8 μV
P40 latency	48 msec
P40 amplitude	5.0 μV

Small adjustments to normal limits for individual patients were made for age, gender and height (details not shown here). Absent peaks were excluded from median latency determination here. Somatosensory normal limits were N20–N9 < 10.5 msec, N20–13 < 7.0 msec, and N13–N9 < 4.3 msec; absolute latencies of N20 or P40 were not used when assessing normality.

From Nuwer *et al.*, 1987 [117].

follow changes in EPs over time, both for any improvement or any deterioration.

How useful are EPs in providing diagnostic information in patients being evaluated to rule out MS? Hume and Waxman [118] recently reported their findings for a 2½ year follow-up study in 222 patients initially suspected of having MS. During follow-up, 48/222 (22%) patients eventually developed clinically definite MS. Among these 48 patients, 90% had abnormal EPs at the time of their initial clinical evaluation. In 65% of these 48 patients, the EPs had provided positive diagnostic evidence of a silent lesion previously unsuspected by the clinician or the patient. In 25% of these 48 patients, the EPs provided confirmatory information only. Among these same 48 patients the VEPs were positive in 53%, SEPs in 26% and the BAEPs in 13%. The visual EP was the only one of the EP tests to be positive in 14 patients (30% of the patients who developed definite MS); the somatosensory in 5 (11%); and the brain stem auditory in none. In that same study, 18 of the original 222 patients eventually received a diagnosis other than MS. Among these patients, evoked potentials were generally normal.

Abnormal EPs were encountered in a few patients with other disorders, e.g. an abnormal VEP in a patient with vasculitis. Overall, the false positive rate for EPs appeared to be about 13% in this rule-out MS diagnostic paradigm, compared to a 65% true positive rate. The types of abnormalities encountered also differed, with EP findings of very asymmetric VEP latencies seen only among MS patients.

In that same study, Hume and Waxman looked at disease progression in patients initially evaluated for possible MS. They found a 71% chance of clinical deterioration over $2\frac{1}{2}$ years if the patient had abnormal EPs, whereas there was only a 16% chance of clinical deterioration over the same time span if the patient had normal EPs. Several CSF measures were not so accurate in predicting deterioration.

The sensitivity of MRI has been compared to EPs in MS. Multimodality EP testing is abnormal about as often as MRI among patients with definite or probable MS [50, 54, 65, 90, 92–93, 118–119]. Either type of test finds abnormalities in approximately 70% of patients undergoing diagnostic evaluation. Multimodality EP testing was found to be slightly more sensitive than MRI in several series [50, 54, 65, 92]. Brain stem auditory EPs were more sensitive than MRI for detecting lesions in the pons [90, 93]. Visual EPs were more sensitive than MRI for detecting optic neuritis. Some published reports have evaluated how well these tests find *multiple* abnormalities, thereby confirming a multifocal disorder. MRI can show multiplicity of lesions more effectively than multimodal EPs [50, 93]. In the Hume and Waxman [118] study following 222 rule-out MS patients for $2\frac{1}{2}$ years, MRI and multimodal EPs were equally effective for predicting which patients would eventually be diagnosed as MS or have a deteriorating clinical course. Similar results were found by Lee *et al.* [53] among 200 patients.

The likelihood of an MS diagnosis was enhanced by use of EPs alone in 7/25 (28%) of patients studied by Gilmore *et al.* [65]. In the same study, brain MRI results alone made the diagnosis more likely in 4/25 (16%). Among the remaining 14/25 (56%) patients, the EPs and the MRI both made the diagnosis more likely by providing evidence of additional lesions and abnormalities typical of demyelinating disease. In a larger patient group studied by the same authors, EPs found a second, silent lesion in 21/58 (36% of patients).

In comparison to oligoclonal banding and similar CSF changes, multimodal EPs were slightly more likely to be abnormal in early or possible MS [53, 113, 120–123], although specific results did vary among reports.

Finally, it is appropriate to look at the comparative resource utilization of EPs and MRI. Such data are available in the US Medicare Fee Schedule, which allows 29.12 relative value units (RVUs) for brain MRI, and 29.42 each for cervical and thoracic MRI. In contrast, all four evoked potential tests together are valued at 8.66 RVUs. This includes 1.24 RVUs for VEP, 3.31 RVUs for four extremity SEP and 4.11 RVUs for BAEP. In this relative value assessment of resource utilization, all four EP tests cost less than one-third as much as one brain MRI, or one-tenth the cost of combined brain, cervical and thoracic MRI.

Most investigators have concluded that the two types of tests are complementary, one assessing anatomy and the other assessing physiology. Each has its own niche in the MS diagnostic evaluation paradigm.

4.5 Magnetically evoked motor potentials

Neurons in the cerebral cortex can be depolarized and discharged by applying electrical stimulation. This can be done at surgery, and it can also be done through an intact skull as an outpatient procedure. Considerable voltage is need to drive electrical currents from the scalp through the skull to the cortex, e.g. 300–400 volts. In outpatients, such electrical stimulation is painful.

An ingenious solution to this painful situation has been devised. A powerful magnetic device held at the scalp can set up a brief but extremely intense magnetic field which spreads readily into the cerebral cortex. The skull is a resistor for electrical currents, but it is not a resistor for a magnetic field, which passes unimpeded through the skull. According to the standard principles of electromagnetism, a fluctuating magnetic field invariably creates an electrical potential. The same principle applies for standard electric generators. By delivering a brief intense magnetic pulse over the scalp, an electric current is created in the cerebral cortex strong enough to discharge the neurons there. The technique can be designed to discharge only the cells in a particular one square centimeter or so under the location of the magnetic stimulator. Various specific cortical regions can be stimulated by precisely locating the magnetic stimulator coil over the scalp.

The magnetic technique was popularized a decade ago by Barker *et al.* [124, 125]. Before that, investigators in MS and other neurological disorders had used transcranial electrical stimulation to study motor pathways [126, 127]. Recordings were made at muscles or large peripheral nerves. The studies using this transcranial electrical technique in MS had demonstrated marked prolongation of central motor conduction times in most MS patients tested [6–8]. With the advent of magnetic cortical stimulation, the clinical feasibility of the technique improved greatly. Nearly all clinicians studying motor pathway stimulation now use the magnetic techniques.

Central motor pathway conduction is impaired by a variety of neurologic disorders. Several studies have demonstrated a high rate of central motor conduction time delays in MS [6–8, 128–132]. The rate of abnormality is even higher for lower extremity recording than for the upper extremity.

In one study, magnetically evoked motor potentials (MEPs) were compared to multimodality sensory evoked potentials (VEP, BAEP, SEP) and also to MRI testing [132]. In that study 68 patients clinically suspected of having MS were tested. Among the 40/68 (59%) eventually diagnosed as having MS, the MRI was positive in 88%, MEP 83%, VEP 67%, SEP 63% and BAEP 42%. The MEP was abnormal also among one-third of the patients who eventually received other CNS diagnoses or no clear diagnosis. Among 10% of the MS patients, the MRI was normal but the neurophysiological tests were abnormal, confirming a CNS disorder. The paraclinical indicators as a whole were important for finding silent second lesions in 17/40 (43%) of the patients eventually diagnosed with MS. On overall diagnostic sensitivity for finding silent lesions, the multimodality sensory evoked potentials were best, followed by MRI then MEP. If sensory evoked potentials were broken out by each individual modality, MRI and MEP had better sensitivities.

Central motor conduction tests can also demonstrate abnormalities in other neurologic disorders. In motor neuron disease, slowed central motor conduction was found among 13/15 patients in one study [133] and 8/11 patients in another [134], whereas SEPs were normal. Among patients with hereditary motor and sensory neuropathy (HMSN) patients had delayed central conduction when they had clinical signs of pyramidal disease. The degrees of delay differed in different specific disorders, presumably corresponding to different pathophysiology in different subtypes of HMSN [135].

Magnetically evoked central motor conduction tests should be considered a test available to search for clues in diagnosing MS, and in the differential diagnosis of other possible central motor disorders.

4.6   Use of evoked potentials in MS therapeutic trials

Evoked potentials are useful as a measurement tool for MS therapeutic trials. Testing can be repeated annually or semi-annually. The costs associated with such testing are reasonable. Visual testing seems to be the best for use of therapeutic trials, because of its ease of measurement. In one large trial of azathioprine and steroids, visual and median nerve middle latency sensory EPs had approximately equal statistical significance in demonstrating efficacy. They were superior to BAEPs in predicting and confirming the clinical outcome of that study [117]. VEPs do not require the

annoying somatosensory electrical shocks on the wrist. The SEPs take twice as long to perform compared to VEPs. The somatosensory short latency EPs, using peaks between 13 and 22 msec, are often unsatisfactory for therapeutic trials because they are often absent in a patient who would enter a trial. Middle latency somatosensory peaks are essentially preserved in all patients and are therefore more useful in therapeutic trials, [117], but most laboratories are not familiar with these SEPs.

EP use in therapeutic trials is commensurate with the recommendations of the Ad Hoc Working Group on the Design of Clinical Studies to Assess Therapeutic Efficacy in Multiple Sclerosis [136]. In that report it was stated: 'the unpredictability of the clinical course of MS makes it necessary for the investigator to be particularly critical in choosing methods for assessing the changes in patients relative to any putative therapy . . . the frequent occurrence of lesions in clinically silent areas provides part of the impetus for seeking to include laboratory parameters in modern therapeutic trials . . . determinations that seem to be potentially most useful at the time of writing include visual evoked response (and several immunological tests).' Such a use of EPs has been demonstrated in at least one well-designed thorough study of EPs in a therapeutic trial [117]. MRI has become a highly recommended and desirable test modality for following patients through therapeutic trials. The quantifiable aspects of MRI testing include the amount of plaque load and the number of plaques seen. However, quantifying these requires considerable sophistication, cost, time and effort. The sensitivity of MRI seems superior to EPs for this purpose, because the MRIs cover a much greater volume of deep white matter. Yet, in many trials the visual EPs may yield the same general outcome data in a sensitive, objective, reproducible way. In this author's opinion, VEPs are the more cost-effective alternative of the two approaches, appropriate for use in many MS therapeutic trials.

Some skepticism has been voiced about the usefulness of EPs in monitoring the course of MS disease activity, since EPs often remain quite abnormal even when the MS becomes relatively inactive. This is actually, however, an advantage of EPs since they tend to worsen in a monotonic fashion. EPs can detect the physiologic remnants of a new plaque that appeared during the months or years between baseline and follow-up testing.

The EP results provide additional clinical information beyond what can easily be determined by physical examination or detailed history. This is because the EPs tend to pick up many silent lesions that are not reflected in the physical examination or history.

The specific research methods for using EPs in therapeutic trials are important. There are appropriate ways in which to carry out the study, and other ways in which the EP testing may be of little or no benefit. This is especially important in the test scoring. The EPs should be scored as the actual latency values. Test–retest differences ought to be reassessed by direct, careful comparison of the actual EP traces themselves, rather than by separate scoring of the individual traces. In this way, the reader can make sure that the scoring is based on exactly the same portion of the EP peaks when separate repetitions are scored. Direct comparison substantially reduces the year-to-year variability. Statistics with EPs should use latency values and year-to-year comparisons in the therapeutic trial should be analyzed with parametric statistics. This is superior to simple scoring as better/worse/unchanged, changed/unchanged or normal/abnormal as has unfortunately been used in many reports of EPs in therapeutic MS trials. The latter simple techniques are not powerful statistically, defeating the goals of quantified study.

EPs have been valuable in two therapeutic trials, worth presenting here as examples. In a study of azathioprine, antilymphocyte globulin and steroids, visual, brain stem auditory and short latency median nerve somatosensory EPs were performed at the beginning and end of the 15-month treatment course [137]. EP changes were scored as better, worse, or unchanged. The authors found that the auditory and short latency somatosensory EP tests were difficult to interpret because of the complexity of the multiple peaks and absent peaks. The visual pattern reversal EPs deteriorated in their control group, but were more stable ($P = 0.06$) in the immunosuppressed group. A small clinical improvement was seen in the treatment group, compared to the control group, although this was not statistically significant. In this study, the VEPs were better at detecting changes than the other modalities and the VEPs showed a probable therapeutic effect even when the clinical data otherwise showed a trend that did not reach a statistical significance.

In the UCLA study of azathioprine with or without steroids in a three-year, double-blind, placebo-controlled therapeutic trial in chronic progressive MS, EPs substantially outperformed routine physical examination and disability scales in predicting the study outcome [117]. Visual, brain stem auditory and median nerve middle latency somatosensory EPs were followed annually for three years. Treatment-related visual and somatosensory EP changes became statistically significantly different one year before group differences were detected by the Standard Neurological Examination scores. These changes are illustrated in Figure 4.5. The statistical significance at each year is shown. For the VEPs, the probability of a treatment-related difference was good even at year 1 in this three-year study. By year 2 the significance of the difference had grown to $P = 0.02$, and by year 3 to $P = 0.002$, with the double-drug-treated group seeming to be stable over the course of this therapeutic trial. The statistical significance of this VEP difference was substantially greater in degree than was true for the Standard Neurological Examination score, which only reached the $P = 0.04$ level of statistical significance by the study's third year. The statistical significance of EP changes also was substantially greater than for differences seen using other clinical scales. EPs were considered to be a sensitive, objective measurement useful in MS therapeutic trials.

By way of comparison, in that same study the EPs were evaluated using simple better/worse/unchanged criteria. When the visual EPs were analyzed using 10 msec, 7 msec or 5 msec criteria for 'change', the

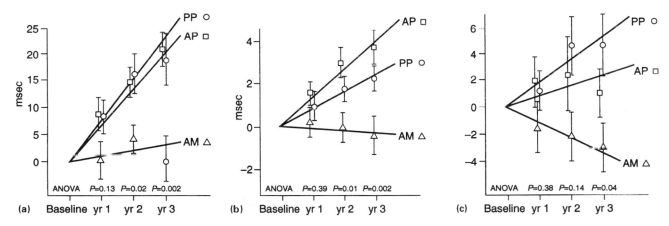

Figure 4.5 Effects of azathioprine and steroids on (a) VEP, (b) SEP and (c) on a standard neurological examination score, during a 3-year study in 57 patients. The three drug treatment groups are shown (AP, azathioprine, AM, azathioprine plus steroids, PP, placebo only). In each case increasing scores represent worsening. Statistical significance is shown above each horizontal axis. These data show that the AM group remained stable or even had slightly improved scores for each type of measurement. Error bars represent the standard error of the mean. Overall, the statistical significance of the group differences can be seen earlier and more strongly in the EP data. (Reproduced with permission from Nuwer et al., 1987 [117].)

group differences using a χ^2 analysis did not quite reach statistical significance. The lesson is that EPs in a therapeutic trial must be applied by taking advantage of the quantified nature of actual latency values, rather than the statistically much less powerful and much less effective better/worse/unchanged, or normal/abnormal or changed/unchanged types of qualitative schemes for scoring.

Other studies have also looked at EPs during MS therapeutic trials. Most have not found EPs to be helpful, although many failed to use EPs in the quantified manner described above. In some other studies the treatment used probably was not effective, and the EP results were therefore quite correct in reporting that there was no effect. For example, hyperbaric oxygen tests in MS did not change EPs [138, 139]. High-dose methylprednisolone was found to cause no change in any three EP modalities when retested at 1 week or at 1 month despite some clinical improvement in some patients [140]. Several steroid regimens were compared by La Mantia *et al.* [141]. Their EP changes paralleled clinical changes seen at 6 months. In interferon trials, EPs did confirm the clinical positive findings [142]. In that study EP changes were said to parallel exacerbations with some fluctuations independent of the clinical course, although details of EP testing were not actually described. Studies of plasmapheresis found that EPs tended to corroborate clinical changes found in four reports [97, 114, 143, 144].

Overall, EPs seem to be a reasonable and cost-effective tool for clarifying and adding statistical significance in MS therapeutic trials. They are useful especially when applied in a careful, quantified manner and analyzed with parametric statistics.

4.7 Conclusions

Evoked potentials can measure very accurately the conduction latencies along macular central visual pathways, mid-brain stem auditory pathways and the large fiber somatosensory lemniscal system. Detection of subclinical impairment, and objective confirmation of symptoms or equivocal signs, can help a clinician establish the diagnosis of multiple sclerosis. New magnetic techniques are now available to test the pyramidal tracts.

Multimodality EP testing is abnormal in nearly all patients with definite MS. Visual EP alone is abnormal in 85% of patients with definite MS. However, somatosensory EPs are slightly more sensitive than visual EPs in early possible MS. Brain stem auditory EPs are the least sensitive modality in MS. These tests all have valuable roles in the assessment of many patients in whom the diagnosis of possible MS is being considered.

In MS therapeutic trials, visual EPs can provide a quick and cost-effective tool that is sensitive to progression or stability of MS over one or several years. These tests of physiology can complement neuroimaging and serologic tests in the clinical and scientific study of MS.

References

1. Waxman, S.G. (1981) Clinicopathological correlations in multiple sclerosis and related diseases, in *Demyelinating Disease: Basic and Clinical Electrophysiology* (eds S.G. Waxman and J.M. Ritchie), New York, Raven Press, pp. 169–82.
2. Waxman, S.G. and Ritchie, J.M. (1981) Electrophysiology of demyelinating disease: future directions and questions, in *Demyelinating Disease: Basic and Clinical Electrophysiology* (eds S.G. Waxman and J.M. Ritchie), New York, Raven Press, pp. 511–14.
3. Raminsky, M. (1981) Hyperexcitability of pathologically myelinated axons and positive symptoms in multiple sclerosis, in (1981) *Demyelinating Disease: Basic and Clinical Electrophysiology* (eds S.G. Waxman and J.M. Ritchie), New York, Raven Press, pp. 289–98.
4. Sears, T.A. and Bostock, H. (1981) Conduction failure in demyelination: is it inevitable?, in *Demyelinating Disease: Basic and Clinical Electrophysiology* (eds S.G. Waxman and J.M. Ritchie), New York, Raven Press, pp. 357–76.
5. Sedgwick, E.M. (1983) Pathophysiology and evoked potentials in multiple sclerosis, in *Multiple Sclerosis: Pathology, Diagnosis and Management* (eds J.F. Hallpike *et al.*), Baltimore, MD, Williams and Wilkins, pp. 177–201.
6. Mills, K.R. and Murray, N.M.F. (1985) Corticospinal tract conduction time in multiple sclerosis. *Ann. Neurol.*, 18, 601–5.
7. Hess, C.W., Mills, K.R., Murrays, N.M.F. and Schriefer, T.N. (1987) Magnetic brain stimulation: central motor conduction studies in multiple sclerosis. *Ann. Neurol.*, 22, 744–52.
8. Cowan, J.M.A., Rothwell, J.C., Dick, J.P.R. *et al.* (1984). Abnormalities in central motor pathway conduction in multiple sclerosis. *Lancet* ii, 304–7.
9. Starr, A., Amlie, R.N., Martin, W.H. and Sanders, S. (1977) Development of auditory function in newborn infants revealed by auditory brain stem potentials. *Pediatrics*, 60, 831–9.
10. Cant, B.R., Hume, A.L., Judson, J.A. and Shaw, N.A. (1986) The assessment of severe head injury by short-latency somatosensory and brain-stem auditory evoked potentials. *Electroencephalogr. Clin. Neurophysiol.*, 65, 188–95.
11. Karnaze, D.S., Marshall, L.F., McCarthy, C.S., Klauber, M.R. and Bickford, R.G. (1982) Localizing and prognostic value of auditory evoked responses in coma after closed head injury. *Neurology*, 32, 299–302.
12. Nuwer, M.R., Perlman, S.L., Packwood, J.W. and Kark, R.A.P. (1983) Evoked potential abnormalities in the various inherited ataxias. *Ann. Neurol.*, 13, 20–7.
13. Nuwer, M.R. (1986) *Evoked Potential Monitoring in the Operating Room*, New York, Raven Press.
14. Richey, E.T., Kooi, K.A. and Tourtellotte, W.W. (1971) Visually evoked responses in multiple sclerosis. *J. Neurol. Neurosurg. Psychiat.*, 34, 275–80.
15. Halliday, A.M., McDonald, W.I. and Mushin, J. (1972) Delayed visual evoked response in optic neuritis. *Lancet*, i, 982–5.
16. Kupersmith, M.J., Nelson, J.I., Seiple, W.H., Carr, R.E. and Weiss, P.A. (1983) The 20/20 eye in multiple sclerosis. *Neurology*, 33, 1015–20.
17. Brooks, E.B. and Chiappa, K.H. (1982) A comparison of clinical neuro-ophthalmological findings and pattern shift visual evoked potentials in multiple sclerosis, in *Clinical Applications of Evoked Potentials in Neurology* (eds J.J. Courjan, F. Mauguiere and Revol, M.), New York, Raven Press, pp. 453–7.
18. Chiappa, K.H. (1990) *Evoked Potentials in Clinical Medicine*, 2nd edn, New York, Raven Press.
19. Halliday, A.M., McDonald, W.I. and Mushin, J. (1973) Delayed pattern evoked responses in optic neuritis in relation to visual acuity. *Trans. Ophthalmol. Soc. UK*, 93, 314–24.
20. Halliday, A.M., McDonald, W.I. and Mushin, J. (1973) Visual evoked response in the diagnosis of multiple sclerosis. *Br. Med. J.*, iv, 661–4.
21. Asselman, P., Chadwick, D.W. and Marsden, C.D. (1975) Visual evoked responses in the diagnosis and management of patients suspected of multiple sclerosis. *Brain*, 98, 261–82.
22. Hume, A.L. and Cant, B.R. (1976) Pattern visual evoked potentials in the diagnosis of multiple sclerosis and other disorders. *Proc. Austr. Assoc. Neurol.*, 13, 7–13.

23. Celesia, G.G. and Daly, R.F. (1977) Visual electroencephalographic computer analysis (VECA). *Neurology*, **27**, 637–41.
24. Matthews, W.B., Small, D.G., Small, M. and Pountney, E. (1977) Pattern reversal evoked visual potential in the diagnosis of multiple sclerosis. *J. Neurol. Neurosurg. Psychiatry*, **40**, 1009–14.
25. Cant, B.R., Hume, A.L. and Shaw, N.A. (1978) Effects of luminance on the pattern visual evoked potential in multiple sclerosis. *Electroencephalogr. Clin. Neurophysiol.*, **45**, 496–504.
26. Duwaer, A.L. and Spekreijse, H. (1978) Latency of luminance and contrast evoked potentials in multiple sclerosis patients. *Electroencephalogr. Clin. Neurophysiol.*, **45**, 244–58.
27. Shahrokhi, F., Chiappa, K.H. and Young, R.R. (1978) Pattern shift visual evoked responses: two hundred patients with optic neuritis and/or multiple sclerosis. *Arch. Neurol.* **35**, 65–71.
28. Tackmann, W., Strenge, H., Barth, R. and Sojka-Raytscheff, A. (1979) Diagnostic validity for different components of pattern shift visual evoked potentials in multiple sclerosis. *Eur. Neurol.*, **18**, 243–8.
29. Trojaborg, W. and Petersen, E. (1979) Visual and somatosensory evoked cortical potentials in multiple sclerosis. *J. Neurol. Neurosurg. Psychiatry*, **42**, 323–30.
30. Chiappa, K.H. (1980) Pattern shift visual, brainstem auditory, and short-latency somatosensory evoked potentials in multiple sclerosis. *Neurology*, **30** (7 part 2), 110–23.
31. Diener, H.C. and Scheibler, H. (1980) Follow-up studies of visual potentials in multiple sclerosis evoked by checkerboard and foveal stimulation. *Electroencephalogr. Clin. Neurophysiol.*, **49**, 490–6.
32. Purves, S.J., Low, M.D., Galloway, J. and Reeves, B. (1981) A comparison of visual brainstem auditory, and somatosensory evoked potentials in multiple sclerosis. *Can. J. Neurol. Sci.*, **8**, 15–19.
33. Kjaer, M. (1980) Visual evoked potentials in normal subjects and patients with multiple sclerosis. *Acta Neurol. Scand.*, **62**, 1–13.
34. van Buggenhout, E., Ketelaer, P. and Carton, H. (1982) Success and failure of evoked potentials in detecting clinical and subclinical lesions in multiple sclerosis patients. *Clin. Neurol. Neurosurg.*, **84**, 3–14.
35. Walsh, J.C., Garrick, R., Cameron, J. and McLeod, J.G. (1982) Evoked potential changes in clinically definite multiple sclerosis: a two year follow up study. *J. Neurol. Neurosurg. Psychiatry*, **45**, 494–500.
36. Wilson, W.B. and Keyser, R.B. (1980) Comparison of the pattern and diffuse-light visual evoked responses in definite multiple sclerosis. *Arch. Neurol.*, **37**, 30–4.
37. Lowitzsch, K., Kuhnt, U., Sakmann, Ch. *et al.* (1976) Visual pattern evoked reponses and blink reflexes in assessment of MS diagnosis. *J. Neurol.*, **213**, 17–32.
38. Mastaglia, F.L., Black, J.L. and Collins, D.W.K. (1976) Visual and spinal evoked potentials in the diagnosis of multiple sclerosis. *Br. Med. J.*, ii, 732.
39. Hennerici, M., Wenzel, D. and Freund, H-J. (1977) The comparison of small-size rectangle and checkerboard stimulation for the evaluation of delayed visual evoked response in patients suspected of multiple sclerosis. *Brain*, **100**, 119–36.
40. Collins, D.W.K., Black, J.L. and Mastaglia, F.L. (1978) Pattern reversal visual evoked potential. *J. Neurol. Sci.*, **36**, 83–95.
41. Nilsson, B.Y. (1978) Visual evoked responses in multiple sclerosis: comparison of two methods for pattern reversal. *J. Neurol. Neurosurg. Psychiatry*, **41**, 499–504.
42. Wist, E.R., Hennerici, M. and Dichgans, J. (1978) The Pulfrich spatial frequency phenomenon: a psycholophysical method competitive to visual evoked potentials in the diagnosis of multiple sclerosis. *J. Neurol. Neurosurg. Psychiatry*, **41**, 1069–77.
43. Rigolet, M.H., Mallecourt, J., LeBlanc, M. and Chain, F. (1979) Etude de la vision des couleurs et des potentiels évoqués dans diagnostic de la sclérose en plaques. *J. Fr. Ophthalmol.*, **2**, 553–60.
44. Matthews, W.B. and Small, D.G. (1979) Serial recording of visual and somatosensory evoked potentials in multiple sclerosis. *J. Neurol. Sci.*, **40**, 11–21.
45. Mamoli, B., Graf, M. and Toifl, K. (1979) EEG, pattern-evoked potentials and nerve conduction velocity in a family with adrenoleukodystrophy. *Electroencephalogr. Clin. Neurophysiol.*, **47**, 411–19.
46. Krumholz, A., Weiss, H.D., Goldstein, P.J. and Harris, K.C. (1981) Evoked responses in vitamin B-12 deficiency. *Ann. Neurol.*, **9**, 407–9.
47. Lowitzsch, K. and Westhoff, M. (1980) Optic nerve involvement in neurosyphilis: diagnostic evaluation by pattern-reversal visual evoked potentials (VEP). *EEG EMG*, **11**, 77–80.
48. Streletz, L.J., Chambers, R.A., Bae, S.H. and Israel, H.L. (1981) Visual evoked potentials in sarcoidosis. *Neurology*, **31**, 1545–9.
49. Martinelli, V. Comi, G., Filippi, M. *et al.* (1991) Paraclinical tests in acute-onset optic neuritis: basal data and results of a short follow-up. *Acta Neurol. Scand.*, **84**, 231–6.
50. Farlow, M.R., Markand, O.N., Edwards, M.K., Stevens, J.C. and Kolar, O.J. (1986) Multiple sclerosis: magnetic resonance imaging, evoked responses, and spinal fluid electrophoresis. *Neurology*, **36**, 828–31.
51. Paty, D.W., Oger, J.J.F., Kastrukoff, L.F. *et al.* (1988) MRI in the diagnosis of MS: a prospective study with comparison of clinical evaluation, evoked potentials, oligoclonal banding and CT. *Neurology*, **38**, 180–5.
52. Frederiksen, J.L., Larsson, H.B.W., Olesen, J. and Stigsby, G. (1991) MRI, VEP, SEP, and biothesiometry suggest monosymptomatic acute optic neuritis to be a first manifestation of multiple sclerosis. *Acta Neurol. Scand.*, **83**, 343–50.
53. Lee, K.H., Hashimoto, S.A., Hooge, J.P. *et al.* (1991) Magnetic resonance imaging of the head in the diagnosis of multiple sclerosis: a prospective 2-year follow-up with comparison of clinical evaluation, evoked potentials, oligoclonal banding, and CT. *Neurology*, **41**, 657–60.
54. Giesser, B.S., Kurtzberg, D., Vaughan, H.G. *et al.* (1987) Trimodal evoked potentials compared with magnetic resonance imaging in the diagnosis of multiple sclerosis. *Arch. Neurol.*, **44**, 281–4.
55. Miller, D.H., McDonald, W.I., Blumhardt, L.D. *et al.* (1987) Magnetic resonance imaging in isolated noncompressive spinal cord syndromes. *Ann. Neurol.*, **22**, 714–23.
56. McDonald, W.I. (1988) The role of NMR imaging in the assessment of multiple sclerosis. *Clin. Neurol. Neurosurg.*, **90**, 3–9.
57. Persson, H.E. and Sachs, C. (1980) VEPs during provoked visual impairment in multiple sclerosis, in *Evoked Potentials* (ed. C. Barber), Baltimore, MD, University Park Press, pp. 575–579.
58. Regan, D, Murray, T.J. and Silver, R. (1977) Effect of body temperature on visual evoked potential delay and visual perception in multiple sclerosis. *J. Neurol. Neurosurg. Psychiatry*, **40**, 1083–91.
59. Bajada, S., Mastaglia, F.L., Black, J.L. and Collins, D.W.K. (1980) Effects of induced hyperthermia on visual evoked potentials and saccade parameters in normal subjects and multiple sclerosis patients. *J. Neurol. Neurosurg. Psychiatry*, **43**, 849–52.
60. Davies, H.D., Carroll, W.M. and Mastaglia, F.L. (1986) Effects of hyperventilation on pattern-reversal visual evoked potentials in patients with demyelination. *J. Neurol. Neurosurg. Psychiatry* **49**, 1392–6.
61. Gilmore, R.L., Kasarskis, E.J. and McAllister, R.G. (1985) Verapamil-induced changes in central conduction in patients with multiple sclerosis. *J. Neurol. Neurosurg. Psychiatry*, **48**, 1140–6.
62. Jones, R.E., Heron, J.R., Foster, D.H., Snelgar, R.S. and Mason, R.J. (1983) Effects of 4-aminopyridine in patients with multiple sclerosis. *J. Neurol. Sci.*, **60**, 353–62.
63. House, J.W. and Brackmann, D.E. (1979) Brainstem audiometry in neurotologic diagnosis. *Arch. Otolaryngol.*, **105**, 305–9.
64. Brown, R.H. Chiappa, K.H. and Brooks, E.G. (1981) Brainstem auditory evoked responses in 22 patients with intrinsic brainstem lesions: implications for clinical interpretations. *Electroencephalogr. Clin. Neurophysiol.*, **51**, 38.
65. Gilmore, R.L., Kasarskis, E.J., Carr, W.A. and Norvell, E. (1989) Comparative impact of paraclinical studies in establishing the diagnosis of multiple sclerosis. *Electroencephalogr. Clin. Neurophysiol.*, **73**, 433–42.
66. Robinson, K. and Rudge, P. (1975) Auditory evoked responses in multiple sclerosis. *Lancet*, i, 1164–6.
67. Robinson, K. and Rudge, P. (1977) Abnormalities of the auditory evoked potentials in patients with multiple sclerosis. *Brain*, **100**, 19–40.
68. Robinson, K. and Rudge, P. (1977) The early components of the auditory evoked potential in multiple sclerosis. *Progr. Clin. Neurophysiol.*, **2**, 58–67.
69. Robinson, K. and Rudge, P. (1980) The use of the auditory evoked potential in the diagnosis of multiple sclerosis. *J. Neurol. Sci.*, **45**, 235–44.
70. Stockard, J.J. and Rossiter, V.S. (1977) Clinical and pathologic correlates of brain stem auditory response abnormalities. *Neurology*, **27**, 316–25.
71. Lacquanti, F., Benna, P., Gilli, M., Troni, W. and Bergamasco, B. (1979) Brain stem auditory evoked potentials and blink reflex in quiescent multiple sclerosis. *Electroencephalogr. Clin. Neurophysiol.*, **47**, 607–10.
72. Mogensen, F. and Kristensen, O. (1979) Auditory double click evoked potentials in multiple sclerosis. *Acta Neurol. Scand.*, **59**, 96–107.
73. Chiappa, K.H., Harrison, J.L., Brooks E.B. and Young, R.R. (1980) Brainstem auditory evoked responses in 200 patients with multiple sclerosis. *Ann. Neurol.*, **7**, 135–43.
74. Green, J.B., Price, R. and Woodbury, S.G. (1980) Short-latency somatosensory evoked potentials in multiple sclerosis. Comparison with auditory and visual evoked potentials. *Arch. Neurol.*, **37**, 630–3.
75. Hausler, R. and Levine, R.A. (1980) Brain stem auditory evoked potentials are related to interaural time discrimination in patients with multiple sclerosis. *Brain Res.*, **191**, 589–94.
76. Stockard, J.J. and Sharbrough, F.W. (1980) Unique contributions of short-latency somatosensory evoked potentials in patients with neurological lesions. *Progr. Clin. Neurophysiol.*, **7**, 231–63.
77. Tackmann, W., Strenge, H., Barth, R. and Sojka-Raytscheff, A. (1980) Evaluation of various brain structures in multiple sclerosis with multi-modality evoked potentials, blink reflex and nystagmography. *J. Neurol.*, **224**, 33–46.
78. Fischer, C., Blanc, A., Mauguiere, F. and Courjon, J. (1981) Apport des potentiels évoqués auditifs précoces au diagnostic neurologique. *Rev. Neurol. (Paris)*, **137**, 229–40.
79. Khoshbin, S. and Hallett, M. (1981) Multimodality evoked potentials and blink reflex in multiple sclerosis. *Neurology*, **31**, 138–44.
80. Parving, A., Elbering, C. and Smith, T. (1981) Auditory electrophysiology. Findings in multiple sclerosis. *Audiology*, **20**, 123–42.

81. Shanon, E., Himmelfarb, M.Z. and Gold, S. (1981) Pontomedullary vs pontomesencephalic transmission time. A diagnostic aid in multiple sclerosis. *Arch. Otolaryngol.*, **107**, 474–5.

82. Barajas, J.J. (1982) Evaluation of ipsilateral and contralateral brainstem auditory evoked potentials in multiple sclerosis patients. *J. Neurol. Sci.*, **54**, 69–78.

83. Elidan, J., Sohmer, H., Gafni, M. and Kahana, E. (1982) Contribution of changes in click rate and intensity on diagnosis of multiple sclerosis by brainstem auditory evoked potentials. *Acta Neurol. Scand.*, **65**, 570–85.

84. Green, J.B., Walcoff, M. and Lucke, J.F. (1982) Phenytoin prolongs far-field somatosensory and auditory evoked potentials interpeak latencies. *Neurology*, **32**, 85–8.

85. Prasher, D.K., Sainz, M., Gibson, W.P.R. and Findley, L.J. (1982) Binaural voltage summation of brain stem auditory evoked potentials: an adjunct to the diagnostic criteria for multiple sclerosis. *Ann. Neurol.*, **11**, 86–91.

86. Tackmann, W. and Ettlin, T. (1982) Blink reflexes elicited by electrical, acoustic and visual stimuli. II. Their relation to visual-evoked potentials and auditory brain stem evoked potentials in the diagnosis of multiple sclerosis. *Eur. Neurol.*, **21**, 264–9.

87. Hutchinson, M. Blandford, S. Glynn, D. and Martin, E.A. (1984) Clinical correlates of abnormal brainstem auditory evoked responses in multiple sclerosis. *Acta Neurol. Scand.*, **69**, 90–5.

88. Kayamori, R., Dickins, S., Yamada, T. and Kimura, J. (1984) Brainstem auditory evoked potential and blink reflex in multiple sclerosis. *Neurology*, **34**, 1318–23.

89. Koffler, B., Oberascher, G. and Pommer, B. (1984) Brain-stem involvement in multiple sclerosis: a comparison between brain-stem auditory evoked potentials and the acoustic stapedius reflex. *Neurology*, **231**, 145–7.

90. Baum, K., Scheuler, W., Hegerl, U. *et al.* (1988) Detection of brainstem lesions in multiple sclerosis: comparison of brainstem auditory evoked potentials with nuclear magnetic resonance imaging. *Acta Neurol. Scand.*, **77**, 283–8.

91. Comi, G., Canal, N., Martinelli, V. *et al.* (1987) Comparison between magnetic resonance imaging and other techniques in 39 multiple sclerosis patients. *Rivista Neurol.*, **57**, 44–7.

92. Comi, G., Martinelli, V., Medaglini, S. *et al.* (1989) Correlation between multimodal evoked potentials and magnetic resonance imaging in multiple sclerosis. *Neurology*, **236**, 4–8.

93. Culter, J.R., Aminoff, M.J. and Brant-Zawadzki, M. (1986) Evaluation of patients with multiple sclerosis by evoked potentials and magnetic resonance imaging: a comparative study. *Ann. Neurol.*, **20**, 645–8.

94. Abbruzzese, G., Abbruzzese, M., Favale, E. *et al.* (1980) The effect of hand muscle vibration on the somatosensory evoked potential in man: an interaction between lemniscal and spinocerebellar inputs? *J. Neurol. Neurosurg. Psychiatry*, **43**, 433–7.

95. Anziska, B., Cracco, R.Q., Cook, A.W. and Feld, E.W. (1978) Somatosensory far field potentials: studies in normal subjects and patients with multiple sclerosis. *Electroencephalogr. Clin. Neurophysiol.*, **45**, 602–10.

96. Chiappa, K.H., Choi, S. and Young, R.R. (1980) Short latency somatosensory evoked potentials following median nerve stimulation in patients with neurological lesions. *Progr. Clin. Neurophysiol.*, **7**, 264–81.

97. Dau, P.C., Petajan, J.H., Johnson, K.P. *et al.* (1980) Plasmapheresis in multiple sclerosis: preliminary findings. *Neurology*, **30**, 1023–8.

98. Dorfman, L.J., Bosley, T.M. and Cummins, K.L. (1978) Electrophysiological localization of central somatosensory lesions in patients with multiple sclerosis. *Electroencephalogr. Clin. Neurophysiol.*, **44**, 742–53.

99. Eisen, A. and Nudleman, K. (1979) Cord to cortex conduction in multiple sclerosis. *Neurology*, **29**, 189–93.

100. Eisen, A. and Odusote, K. (1980) Central and peripheral conduction times in multiple sclerosis. *Electroencephalogr. Clin. Neurophysiol.*, **48**, 253–65.

101. Eisen, A., Stewart, J., Nudleman, K. and Cosgrove, J.B.R. (1979) Short-latency somatosensory responses in multiple sclerosis. *Neurology*, **29**, 827–34.

102. Eisen, A., Paty, D., Purves, S. and Hoirch, M. (1981) Occult fifth nerve dysfunction in multiple sclerosis. *Can. J. Neurol. Sci.*, **8**, 221–5.

103. Eisen, A., Purves, S. and Hoirch, M. (1982) Central nervous system amplification: its potential in the diagnosis of early multiple sclerosis. *Neurology*, **32**, 359–64.

104. Ganes, T. (1980) Somatosensory evoked response and central afferent conduction times in patients with multiple sclerosis. *J. Neurol. Neurosurg. Psychiatry*, **43**, 948–53.

105. Kazis, A., Vlaikidis, N., Xafenias, D., Papanastasiou, J. and Pappa, P. (1982) Fever and evoked potentials in multiple sclerosis. *J. Neurol.*, **227**, 1–10.

106. Kjaer, M. (1980) The value of brainstem auditory, visual and somatosensory evoked potentials and blink reflexes in the diagnosis of multiple sclerosis. *Acta Neurol. Scand.*, **62**, 220–36.

107. Mastaglia, F.L., Black, J.L., Edis, R. and Collins, D.W.K. (1978) The contribution of evoked potentials in the functional assessment of the somatosensory pathway. *Clin. Exp. Neurol.*, **15**, 279–98.

108. Matthews, W.B. and Esiri, M. (1979) Multiple sclerosis plaque related to abnormal somatosensory evoked potentials. *J. Neurol. Neurosurg. Psychiatry*, **42**, 940–2.

109. Namerow, N.S. (1968) Somatosensory evoked response in multiple sclerosis patients with varying sensory loss. *Neurology*, **18**, 1197–204.

110. Namerow, N.S. (1970) Somatosensory recovery functions in multiple sclerosis patients. *Neurology*, **30**, 813–17.

111. Noel, P. and Desmedt, J.E. (1980) Cerebral and far-field somatosensory evoked potentials in neurological disorders involving the cervical spinal cord, brainstem, thalamus and cortex. *Progr. Clin. Neurophysiol*, **7**, 205–30.

112. Small, D.G., Matthews, W.B. and Small, M. (1978) The cervical somatosensory evoked potential (SEP) in the diagnosis of multiple sclerosis. *J. Neurol. Sci.*, **35**, 211–24.

113. Trojaborg, W., Bottcher, J. and Saxtrup, O. (1981) Evoked potentials and immunoglobulin abnormalities in multiple sclerosis. *Neurology* **31**, 866–71.

114. Weiner, H.L. and Dawson, D.M. (1980) Plasmapheresis in multiple sclerosis: preliminary study. *Neurology*, **30**, 1029–33.

115. Larrea L.G. and Mauguiere, F. (1988) Latency and amplitude abnormalities of the scale far-field P14 to median nerve stimulation in multiple sclerosis. A SEP study of 122 patients recorded with a non-cephalic reference montage. *Electroencephalogr. Clin. Neurophysiol.*, **71**, 180–6.

116. Fine, E.J. and Hallet, M. (1980) Neurophysiological study of subacute combined degeneration. *J. Neurol. Sci.*, **45**, 331–6.

117. Nuwer, M.R., Packwood, J.W., Myers, L.W. and Ellison, G.W. (1987) Evoked potentials predict the clinical changes in multiple sclerosis drug study. *Neurology*, **37**, 1754–61.

118. Hume, A.L. and Waxman, S.G. (1988) Evoked potentials in suspected multiple sclerosis: diagnostic value and prediction of clinical course. *J. Neurol. Sci.*, **83**, 191–210.

119. Guerit, J.M. and Argile, A.M. (1988) The sensitivity of multimodal evoked potentials in multiple sclerosis. A comparison with magnetic resonance imaging and cerebrospinal fluid analysis. *Electroencephalogr. Clin. Neurophysiol.*, **70**, 230–8.

120. Bartel, D.R. Markand, O.N. and Kolar, O.J. (1983) The diagnosis and classification of multiple sclerosis: evoked responses and spinal fluid electrophoresis. *Neurology*, **33**, 611–17.

121. Miller, J.R., Burke, A.M. and Bever, C.T. (1983) Occurrence of oligoclonal bands in multiple sclerosis and other CNS diseases. *Ann. Neurol.*, **13**, 53–8.

122. Cosi, V., Citterio, A., Battelli, G. *et al.* (1987) Multimodal evoked potentials in multiple sclerosis: a contribution to diagnosis and classification. *Ital. J. Neurol. Sci.* (Suppl. 6), 109–12.

123. Ganes, T., Brautaset, N.J., Nyberg-Hansen, R. and Vandvik, B. (1986) Multimodal evoked response and cerebrospinal fluid oligoclonal immunoglobulins in patients with multiple sclerosis. *Acta Neurol. Scand.*, **73**, 472–6.

124. Barker, A.T., Jalinous, R. and Freeston, I.L. (1985) Non-invasive magnetic stimulation of human motor cortex. *Lancet*, **2**, 1106–07.

125. Barker, A.T., Freeston, I.L., Jalinous, R. and Jarratt, J.A. (1986) Clinical evaluation of conduction time measurements in central motor pathways using magnetic stimulation of the human brain. *Lancet*, **i**, 1325–6.

126. Merton, P.A. and Morton, H.B. (1980) Stimulation of the cerebral cortex in the intact human subjects. *Nature*, **285**, 227.

127. Merton, P.A. Morton, H.B., Hill, D.K. and Marsden, C.D. (1982) Scope of a technique for electrical stimulation of human brain, spinal cord and muscle. *Lancet*, **ii**, 596–600.

128. Hess, C.W., Mills, K.R. and Murray, N.M.F. (1986) Measurement of central motor conduction in multiple sclerosis by magnetic brain stimulation. *Lancet*, **ii**, 596–600.

129. Ingram, D.A., Thompson, A.J. and Swash, M. (1988) Central motor conduction in multiple sclerosis: evaluation of abnormalities revealed by transcutaneous magnetic stimulation of the brain. *J. Neurol. Neurosurg. Psychiatry*, **51**, 487–94.

130. Jones, S.M.J., Streletz, L.J., Raab, V.E. *et al.* (1991) Lower extremity motor evoked potentials in multiple sclerosis. *Arch. Neurol.*, **48**, 944–8.

131. Mayr, N., Baumgartner, C., Zeitlhofer, J. and Deecke, L. (1991) The sensitivity of transcranial cortical magnetic stimulation in detecting pyramidal tract lesions in clinically definite multiple sclerosis. *Neurology*, **41**, 566–9.

132. Ravnborg, M., Liguori, R., Christiansen, P., Larsson, H. and Sørenson, P.S. (1992) The diagnostic reliability of magnetically evoked motor potentials in multiple sclerosis. *Neurology*, **42**, 1296–301.

133. Hugon, J., Lubeau, M., Tabaraud, F. *et al.* (1987) Central motor conduction in motor neuron disease. *Ann. Neurol.*, **22**, 544–6.

134. Berardelli, A., Inghilleri, M., Formisano, R., Accornero, N and Manfredi, M. (1987) Stimulation of motor tracts in motor neuron disease. *J. Neurol. Neurosurg. Psychiatry*, **50**, 732–7.

135. Claus, D., Waddy, H.M., Harding, A.E., Murray, N.M.F. and Thomas, P.K. (1990) Hereditary motor and sensory neuropathies and hereditary spastic paraplegia: a magnetic stimulation study. *Ann. Neurol.*, **28**, 43–9.

136. Brown, J.R., Beebe, G.W., Kurtzke, J.F. *et al.* (1979) The design of clinical studies to assess the therapeutic efficacy in multiple sclerosis. *Neurology*, **29** (9, part 2), 1–23.

137. Mertin, J., Rudge, P., Kremer, M. *et al.* (1982) Double-blind controlled trial of immunosuppression in the treatment of multiple sclerosis. Final report. *Lancet*, **ii**, 351–4.

138. Neiman, J., Nilsson, B.Y., Barr, P.O. and Perkins, D.J.D. (1985) Hyperbaric oxygen in chronic progressive multiple sclerosis: visual evoked potentials and clinical effects. *J. Neurol. Neurosurg. Psychiatry*, **48**, 497–500.

139. Harpur, G.D., Suke, R., Bass, B.H. *et al.* (1986) Hyperbaric oxygen therapy in chronic stable multiple sclerosis: double-blind study. *Neurology*, **36**, 988–91.

140. Smith, T., Zeeberg, I. and Sjo, O. (1986) Evoked potentials in multiple sclerosis before and after high-dose methylprednisolone infusion. *Eur. Neurol.*, **25**, 67–73.

141. La Mantia, L., Riti, F., Milanese, C. *et al.* (1994) Serial evoked potentials in multiple sclerosis bouts. Relation to steroid treatment. *Ital. J. Neurol. Sci.*, **15**, 333–40.

142. Sipe, J.C., Knobler, R.L., Braheny, S.L. *et al.* (1984) A neurologic rating scale (NRS) for use in multiple sclerosis. *Neurology*, **34**, 1368–72.

143. Khatri, B.O., McQuillen, M.P., Harrington, G.J., Schmoll, D. and Hoffmann, R.G. (1985) Chronic progressive multiple sclerosis: double-blind controlled study of plasmapheresis in patients taking immunosuppressive drugs. *Neurology*, **35**, 312–19.

144. Gordon, P.A., Carroll D.J., Etches, W.S. *et al.* (1985) A double-blind controlled pilot study of plasma exchange versus sham apheresis in chronic progressive multiple sclerosis. *Can. J. Neurol. Sci.*, **12**, 39–44.

145. Nuwer, M.R., Packwood, J.W., Ellison, G.W. and Meyers, L.W. (1988) A parametric scale for BAEP latencies in multiple sclerosis. *Electroencephalogr. Clin. Neurophysiol.*, **71**, 33–9.

146. Nuwer, M.R., Aminoff, M., Goodin, D., Matsuoka, S. *et al.* (1994) IFCN recommended standards for brain-stem auditory evoked potentials. *Electroencephalogr. Clin. Neurophysiol.*, **91**, 12–17.

147. Nuwer, M.R., Aminoff, M., Desmedt, J. *et al.* (1994) IFCN recommended standards for short latency somatosensory evoked potentials. *Electroencephalogr. Clin. Neurophysiol.*, **91**, 6–11.

5 MULTIPLE SCLEROSIS CEREBROSPINAL FLUID

*Wallace W. Tourtellotte and
Hayrettin Tumani*

5.1 Introduction

Progress has been made in the past decade in laboratory aids (magnetic resonance imaging, evoked potentials, CSF and blood) to support the clinical diagnosis and to follow the course of patients with MS [1].

Neuropathologically MS is a disease with multifocal areas of primary demyelination (loss of myelin sheath with relative sparing of axons), mostly in the white matter, associated with a polyphasic chronic inflammatory reaction [2]. Magnetic resonance imaging (MRI) can locate *in vivo* multiple areas of demyelination in the white matter (plaques) [3]. Additionally, MRI with gadolinium enhancement can further classify plaques on the basis of breaks in the blood–brain barrier, presumably associated with acute demyelinating activity related to inflammation [4–6]. Evoked potentials can detect central conduction slowing and blockage in demyelinated areas. The CSF examination can predict chronic inflammation in plaques.

Particularly attractive to clinical neurochemists and immunologists is examination of MS CSF, a lacuna of the extracellular space of the central nervous system (CNS) [7] (Figure 5.1). Solutes, such as IgG and albumin, found in the extracellular space of the CNS, sink into the CSF space of 150 ml which turns over about three times per day. Accordingly, an examination of CSF constituents can be reflective of the content of the extracellular space of the CNS in health and disease [8]. The greatest attraction of a CSF examination in MS is that it can reflect an inflammatory condition of the brain.

Over the past decade we have prepared 11 reviews on clinical aspects of MS and the reaction found in the CSF [9–18]. In each review reference lists were presented to document facts and controversies; to avoid repetition, in this chapter only key references will be cited.

The information about MS CSF in this chapter will be divided into five broad areas:

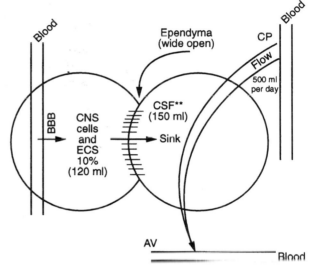

Figure 5.1 Cerebrospinal fluid (CSF) is a lacuna of the extracellular space of the central nervous system. AV, arachnoid villi. BBB, blood–brain barrier; CNS, central nervous system, CP, choroid plexus. *Neurons, astrocytes, oligodendroglia, microglia, endothelium, inflammatory cells (lymphocytes, plasma cells synthesizing Ig, macrophages, activated microglia, cytokines); **lacuna of CNS extracellular space (ECS).

1. the CSF profile indicative of MS;
2. issues about MS CSF;
3. perspectives;
4. post-lumbar puncture (LP) headaches;
5. methodology.

In our experience, after a clinical work-up of a patient for the diagnosis of MS, which includes a history and physical, mental and neurologic examinations as well as blood/urine laboratory tests to rule out other diseases or complications (antinuclear antibodies, erythrocyte sedimentation rate, angiotensin converting enzyme, syphilitic serology, *Borrelia burgdorferi* IgG and IgM specific antibody index, HIV-1, HTLV-I, HHV-6, HSV IgG antibody index) we recommend a brain MRI with gadolinium enhancement. The

Multiple Sclerosis: Clinical and pathogenetic basis. Edited by Cedric S. Raine, Henry F. McFarland and Wallace W. Tourtellotte. Published in 1997 by Chapman & Hall, London. ISBN 0 412 30890 8.

spinal cord and optic nerve should also be imaged with and without gadolinium if clinical information so indicates. This is followed by evoked potentials testing; and then we recommend a lumbar puncture for CSF examination with matched serum. Only a laboratory which has been credentialled to do CSF cell counts, glucose analysis, albumin and IgG analyses, as well as oligoclonal IgG banding, should be used.

5.2   CSF profile indicative of clinically definite MS

The CSF profile indicative of clinically definite MS is not pathognomonic but it occurs in almost every patient with clinically definite MS and eliminates most other diseases. It is a manifestation of a modestly active chronic inflammatory reaction within the blood–brain barrier. If this profile is not found in a patient suspected of MS, the diagnosis should be questioned and an alternative explanation sought for the symptoms and signs. Alternatively, the MS patient could have a complication.

5.2.1   THE PROFILE

Appearance

MS CSF is crystal clear except in cases of transverse myelitis which produces a block of the spinal subarachnoid space. In this case, the CSF can appear yellow and can clot (Froin's syndrome) [8].

CSF dynamics

The pressure is normal, except when transverse myelitis has resulted in a block of the spinal subarachnoid space. When a blocked subarachnoid space is entered by lumbar puncture, the fluid flows for a few milliliters and then a dry tap follows [8].

It is recommended that an MRI be performed prior to the lumbar puncture in cases suspected of a spinal subarachnoid block. If the MRI shows a block or partial block, we do not recommend a lumbar puncture. It has been reported that reducing the CSF pressure below a block can worsen neurologic symptoms and signs [19]. If a CSF examination is needed for diagnostic purposes, it can be obtained by a cisternal route.

Cytology

A total leukocyte count of 5 cells/μl (mean (M) ± 2 s.d.) or more is abnormal and found in 34% of MS cases. A cell count > 50 is very rare (P < 0.001) and makes multiple sclerosis unlikely. In such a case, other diseases should be considered, or the patient has MS with a complication. The differential count (Wright's stain) is

normal: plasma cells are not increased and there are no polymorphonuclear cells. Total leukocyte and differential cell counts show no relationship to relapse, but there is a tendency to lower cell counts the longer the duration of MS. The cell count is modestly proportional to elevated intrathecal IgG synthesis rates [20].

Glucose

CSF and matched blood are best obtained in the fasting state; the normal ratio of CSF to blood concentration is 0.6 [8]. The ratio is not elevated even if the patient has hyperglycemia. When the ratio is low, a complication of MS should be considered.

Albumin

Dynamic studies with intravenously injected radiolabeled albumin [21] have shown that the albumin in CSF is exclusively derived from the blood. Albumin is synthesized only in the liver, and is not catabolized within the CNS. The absolute concentration of CSF albumin, the major CSF protein, depends on many factors including its blood concentration, blood–CSF barrier integrity, rate of CSF flow, age of the patient and the volume of CSF drawn [11, 22–24]. By analyzing albumin in CSF and serum and calculating the albumin CSF/serum quotient or albumin leakage rate by our formula it is possible to assess the overall integrity of the blood–brain–CSF barrier (BBCB) to mid-size proteins such as albumin and IgG [21, 23]. Figure 5.2 shows that the albumin CSF/serum quotient and our trans-BBCB albumin leakage rate correlate nearly perfectly (r = 0.99).

An **albumin concentration in the CSF** more than 34 mg/dl (M ± 2 s.d.) is abnormal and present in 23% of

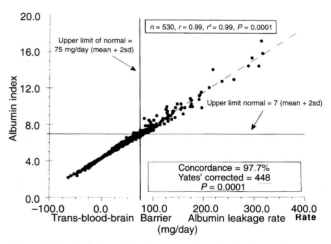

Figure 5.2 Relationship between albumin index and trans-blood–brain barrier albumin leakage rate. All patients were classified as clinically definite MS using the Poser *et al.* criteria [1]. See text for calculation of albumin index and leakage formula. (Reproduced from *Journal of Neuroimmunology*, **46**, 185–92 (1993) with permission.)

cases of clinically definite MS only if the serum albumin concentration is normal, 3.6–5.6 g/dl (M ± s.d.). An albumin concentration of more than 65 mg/dl, is very rare ($P < 0.001$) [15].

The **albumin CSF/serum** (Q_{ALB}) **quotient** is age-dependent [25, 26]. The upper reference limit (M ± 2 s.d.) for the first 10 ml of lumbar fluid is 5.0 (if < 15 years of age), 6.5 (if 16–40 years of age), 8 (if 40–60 years of age), and 8–9 (if > 60 years of age). Most patients with MS have albumin quotient values below the upper reference limit. An albumin quotient higher than 7 is present in 12% of cases of clinically definite MS. A value higher than 14 in MS is very rare ($P < 0.001$), and makes MS unlikely [23].

Sample calculation:

$$Q_{ALB} = \left(\frac{ALB_{CSF}}{ALB_{serum}} \right) \times 1000.$$

If CSF albumin equals 30 mg/dl and serum albumin = 4600 mg/dl, then

$$Q_{ALB} = \left(\frac{30}{4600} \right) \times 1000 = 6.5.$$

The **trans-BBCB albumin leakage rate** in mg/day =

$$\left(ALB_{CSF} - \frac{ALB_{serum}}{230} \right) \times 5$$

where albumin in the CSF (mg/dl) is corrected for natural leakage of albumin from sera to CSF by subtracting albumin in the serum (mg/dl) divided by 230 (230 is a ratio constant derived from normal individuals, Alb_{serum}/Alb_{CSF}). Multiplication by 5 converts the corrected CSF albumin content to mg/day since 5 dl of CSF is formed on average per day [27]. More than 75 mg/day is abnormal; it occurs in 23% of clinically definite MS patients. More than 275 mg/day is very rare in MS ($P < 0.001$) [10, 17].

Sample calculation:
If CSF albumin is 30 mg/dl and serum albumin 4600 mg/dl, then trans-BBB albumin leakage =

$$\left(30 - \frac{4600}{230} \right) \times 5 = 50 \text{ mg/day.}$$

Total protein

Total protein concentration in the CSF of more than 54 mg/dl is abnormal and presents in 23% of MS cases but a value of more than 110 mg/dl is very rare in MS ($P < 0.001$) [20]. The significance of an elevated CSF total serum protein is the same as for albumin, described above, i.e. it is a marker of the BBCB integrity. We consider total protein measurement archaic, and it should be replaced by evaluation of albumin in CSF and serum which is more reliably determined [10].

Intrathecal IgG synthesis

IgG is synthesized by only one cell type in the body, namely the plasma cell [28]. In health there are no plasma cells in the brain [29]. A normal IgG concentration in the CSF is determined by the concentration in the blood [11, 23], by the natural permeability of the relatively open endothelial capillary tight junctions primarily located in the choroid plexus [22] and by the CSF turnover [24, 30]. Hence, an abnormally elevated IgG concentration in the CSF can be the result of an elevated blood IgG concentration, breaks in the BBCB endothelial tight junctions and/or choroid plexus epithelium tight junctions, and reduced CSF turnover. Additionally, CSF IgG can be elevated by synthesis of IgG by plasma cells inside the BBCB after B lymphocytes are recruited in CNS disease and mature there to plasma cells. If after correction of CSF IgG concentration for high serum IgG concentration as well as leakage of IgG across the BBCB, there is an excess of CSF IgG, then intrathecal IgG synthesis is occurring [21]. Accordingly, intrathecal IgG synthesis calculations are a marker for plasma cells secreting IgG inside the BBCB, i.e. evidence of inflammation in the CNS. In MS this inflammation is most frequently located at active plaque edges [31]. The detection of an intrathecal synthesis of IgG requires an approach that will discriminate between blood-derived and brain-derived fractions in CSF. Quantitative approaches are based on calculations of the CSF/serum quotients [10, 21, 24, 26, 32]. The quotients can also be used for intrathecal synthesis of other immunoglobulin classes (IgA, IgM) and organism-specific antibodies [24, 33].

The most popular formulas, namely IgG index [34], IgG synthesis rate [35], both linear approaches, and IgG_{Loc}, a non-linear approach [24], are of similar clinical sensitivity in MS (for details about the formula and comparison with our rate formula see [24]). The correlation between the IgG index, the IgG synthesis rate (mg/24h) and the IgG_{Loc} (mg/dl) is good to near perfect in cases with normal blood–CSF barrier function, common in MS (Figures 5.3–5.5). A comparison of all three formulas is illustrated in Table 5.1. Additionally, they are roughly proportional to the cerebral plaque burden detected by MRI [36]. If the patient has received ACTH or corticosteroids, it will reduce both IgG synthesis rate and index for about 3 months [35].

Longitudinal studies have shown that intrathecal IgG synthesis rate and IgG index modestly decrease with duration of the disease [37].

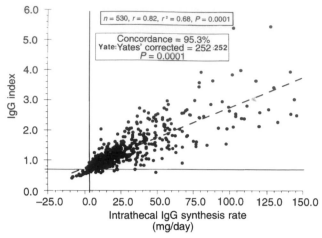

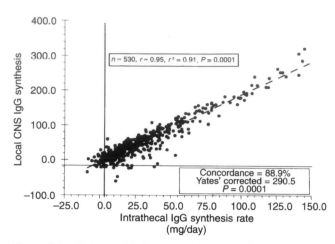

Figure 5.3   Relationship between IgG index and intrathecal IgG synthesis rate formula. All patients were classified as clinically definite MS using the Poser criteria [1]. See text for calculation of IgG index and synthesis rate. (Reproduced from *Journal of Neuroimmunology*, **46**, 185–92 (1993) with permission.)

Figure 5.5   Relationship between Schuller and Sagar formula and intrathecal IgG synthesis rate formula. All patients were clinically classified as clinically definite MS according to the Poser criteria [1]. See text for calculation of IgG index and synthesis rate. (Reproduced from *Journal of Neuroimmunology*, **46**, 185–92 (1993) with permission.)

IgG concentration in the CSF of > 8 mg/dl (M ± 2 s.d.) is present in 89% of cases of clinically definite MS. It is considered meaningful only if the serum IgG concentration is normal and there is no abnormal BBCB dysfunction, i.e. albumin quotient, < 9 (M ± 2 s.d.), and/or trans-BBCB albumin leakage < 75 mg/day (M ± 2 s.d.) [17].

The measurement of **CSF IgG alone** is of limited value, since its concentration can be influenced by several factors already mentioned. To distinguish between intrathecal IgG synthesis versus blood-derived IgG from hypergammaglobulinemia and/or blood–CSF

barrier dysfunction, it is necessary to correct for the latter two conditions. The CSF/serum quotient for IgG corrects for variations in serum IgG. To correct for the individual variations related to BBCB dysfunction, the CSF/serum IgG quotient is divided by the CSF/serum albumin quotient. This formula is referred to as the IgG index.

$$IgG\ index\ =\ \frac{CSF\ IgG}{Serum\ IgG}\ divided\ by\ \frac{CSF\ albumin}{Serum\ albumin}$$

A value of more than 0.73 (M ± 2 s.d.) is abnormal and present in 92% of clinically definite MS cases, while an index more than 4 is very rare ($P < 0.001$) [38].

Sample calculation
If CSF IgG = 20 mg/dl, CSF albumin = 40 mg/dl, serum albumin = 4600 mg/dl and serum IgG = 1000 mg/dl, then

$$IgG\ index\ =\ \frac{20}{1000}\ divided\ by\ \frac{40}{4600}\ =\ 2.3.$$

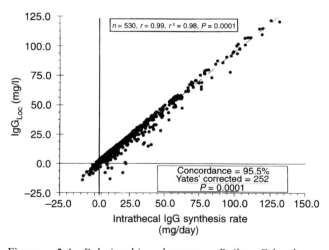

Figure 5.4   Relationship between Reiber–Felgenhauer IgG$_{LOC}$ and intrathecal IgG synthesis rate formula. All patients were classified as clinically definite MS using the Poser criteria [1]. See text for calculation of IgG index and synthesis rate. (Reproduced from *Journal of Neuroimmunology*, **46**, 185–92 (1993) with permission.)

An abnormal **intrathecal IgG synthesis** rate of more than 6 mg/day (M ± 2 s.d.) is present in 92% of clinically definite MS cases; but a value of more than 130 is very rare ($P < 0.001$) [17].

The formula for intrathecal IgG synthesis rate (mg/day) is [35]:

$$= \left[\left(IgG_{CSF} - \frac{IgG_{serum}}{369} \right) - \left(Alb_{CSF} - \frac{Alb_{serum}}{230} \right) \times \left(\frac{IgG_{serum}}{Alb_{serum}} \right) (0.43) \right] \times 5$$

Intrathecal IgG synthesis represents the IgG in mg/day in the CSF derived from extravascular sources, i.e. synthesized inside the BBCB, where IgG_{CSF} is the IgG concentration (mg/dl) in the patient's CSF; IgG_{serum} is the patient's serum IgG concentration (mg/dl); 369 is a ratio constant that quantitatively determines the proportion of CSF IgG normally passing by filtration from the serum into the CSF through natural leaks in the BBCB. It is the quotient of the average normal serum IgG concentration divided by the average normal CSF IgG concentration. Thus, $IgG_{serum}/369$ is the IgG that is expected to cross the normal BBCB from the serum to the CSF, based on the patient's serum IgG concentration. Alb_{CSF} is the albumin concentration (mg/dl) in the patient's CSF; Alb_{serum} is the patient's serum albumin concentration (mg/dl); 230 represents a constant that determines the proportion of CSF albumin normally passing by filtration from the serum into the CSF through natural leaks in the BBCB. It is the quotient of the average normal serum albumin concentration divided by the average normal CSF albumin concentration.

Thus,

$$Alb_{CSF} - \left(\frac{Alb_{serum}}{230} \right)$$

represents the excess CSF albumin that has crossed a dysfunctioned BBCB. This term is then multiplied by

$$\left(\frac{IgG_{serum}}{Alb_{serum}} \right) \times 0.43$$

to convert the excess CSF albumin to excess CSF IgG (on a molar basis) that has crossed the damaged barrier with the albumin, assuming passive transport of one mole of IgG for one mole of albumin. To calculate the daily intrathecal IgG synthesis rate (mg/day), this entire equation is then multiplied by 5 to convert from concentration in mg/dl to mg/day, since 5 dl of CSF is formed each day on average. This formula has been validated in normal humans by a radioisotope two-compartment study[35].

Sample calculation
If CSF IgG = 20 mg/dl, CSF albumin = 40 mg/dl; serum albumin = 4600 mg/dl and serum IgG = 1000 mg/dl, then the intrathecal IgG synthesis rate, mg/day =

$$\left[\left(20 - \frac{1000}{369} \right) - \left(40 - \frac{4600}{230} \right) \times \left(\frac{1000}{4600} \right) (0.43) \right]$$
$$\times 5 = 67 \, mg/day$$

Using the graphical approach, Reiber and Felgenhauer[24] empirically discovered a non-linear relation between Q_{IgG} and Q_{Alb}, particularly in cases with BBCB dysfunction (Figure 5.6.). The Q_{IgG} changes in a non-linear function with increasing Q_{Alb}, displaying the shape of a hyperbolic function. The Reiber and Felgenhauer formula IgG_{Loc} is based on this non-linear relation. **Loc** is synthesis of IgG locally inside the blood–brain–CSF barrier.

$$IgG_{Loc} (mg/dl) = (Q_{IgG} - Q_{Lim(IgG)}) \times IgG_{serum}$$

Q_{IgG} is the CSF/serum quotient of IgG; the factor $Q_{Lim(IgG)} = 0.93 \times ((Q_{Alb})^2 + 6 \times 10^{-6}) - 1.7 \times 10^{-3}$; Q_{Alb} is the CSF/serum quotient of albumin.

This factor represents the upper border line or **limit** (hyperbolic function) of the reference range discriminating between blood- and brain-derived CSF IgG.

Sample calculation
If CSF IgG = 20 mg/dl, serum IgG = 1000 mg/dl, CSF albumin = 40 mg/dl, serum albumin = 4600 mg/dl, then

$$
\begin{aligned}
Q_{IgG} &= 20 \times 10^{-3}, \\
Q_{Alb} &= 8.7 \times 10^{-3}, \\
Q_{Lim(IgG)} &= 8.4 \times 10^{-3}, \text{ and} \\
IgG_{Loc} &= [20 \times 10^{-3} - 8.4 \times 10^{-3}] \times 1000 \, mg/dl \\
IgG_{Loc} &= 11.6 \, mg/dl
\end{aligned}
$$

A value of more than 0.1 mg/dl is abnormal and present in 70% of clinically definite MS cases[24]. Figures 5.6 and 5.7 demonstrate the above formula graphically.

The locally synthesized CSF IgG (IgG_{Loc}) can also be expressed as a percentage of the total CSF IgG concentration, defined as intrathecal fraction (IgG_{IF}) in per cent.

$$IgG_{IF} = [IgG_{Loc}/CSF \, IgG] \times 100$$

IgG_{IF} = 58% in the above sample calculation.

The search for **unique CSF oligoclonal IgG bands** is a very different, nonquantitative way to detect intrathecal IgG synthesis by plasma cells. This is a very popular request of neurologists because CSF oligoclonal IgG bands are more frequently abnormal than the quantitative formulae. Unfortunately, the methodology has not been standardized between laboratories. This is to be contrasted with determination of albumin and IgG for

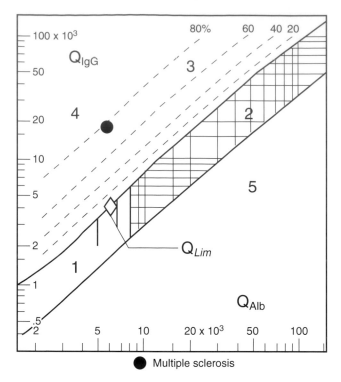

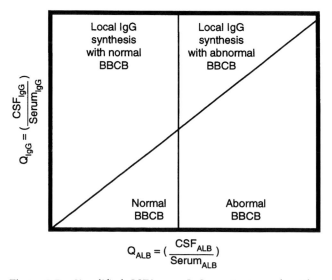

Figure 5.6 CSF/serum quotient diagram for IgG according to Reiber and Felgenhauer [23]. Q_{IgG}, CSF/serum IgG quotient; Q_{Alb}, CSF/serum albumin quotient (BBCB marker); Q_{lim}, upper border line of the reference range discriminating between blood- and brain/choroid plexus-derived CSF IgG. *1*, Normal results, i.e. no intrathecal IgG synthesis and intact BBCB function; *2*, abnormal blood–CSF barrier function and no intrathecal IgG synthesis (e.g. Guillain–Barré-syndrome); *3*, intrathecal IgG synthesis and abnormal BBCB function (e.g. bacterial meningitis); *4*, intrathecal IgG synthesis and intact BBCB function; *5*, values below the lower hyperbolic line indicate methodological or pre-analytical error.

Figure 5.7 Simplified CSF/serum IgG quotient graph with a non-linear discriminating line and result patterns. The Y axis shows increasing values for Q_{IgG} and the X axis shows increasing values for Q_{Alb}. The four areas represent the possible result patterns. BBCB, blood–brain–CSF barrier.

calculation of intrathecal IgG synthesis formulae where the methodology utilizing laser nephelometry is reliable and valid.

The methodology for IgG oligoclonal bands should include a comparison of the same exact amount of CSF and serum IgG (we use 0.5 μg) utilizing isoelectric focusing in polyacrylamide gel followed by immunofixation of the heavy chains of IgG and silver staining to a standardized endpoint [39]. This method can reveal five different banding patterns in the cathodic region pH > 8:

1. no unique cathodic bands in CSF;
2. unique CSF restricted cathodic oligoclonal bands;
3. cathodic CSF oligoclonal bands with identical bands in serum, but less intense than CSF;
4. identical banding pattern in CSF and serum;
5. monoclonal bands in CSF and serum of the same intensity.

Only patterns 2 and 3 represent intrathecal synthesis. A single unique distinct band found in the CSF and not in serum is considered abnormal [39]. More than one such band is present in 97% of clinically definite MS cases [11, 17]. The average number of bands in a clinically definite MS patient is 13 ± 9 (M ± 2 s.d.) and is not related to magnitude of intrathecal IgG synthesis rate [17]. Each patient who has CSF oligoclonal bands has a unique pattern [40]; it is our notion that IgG banding pattern is genetically determined.

Combining intrathecal IgG synthesis formulae and unique CSF oligoclonal IgG bands If the number of cases with abnormal intrathecal IgG synthesis rate and oligoclonal bands are summated more than 99% of clinically definite MS cases show intrathecal IgG synthesis [11] (see Table 5.1).

Intrathecal synthesis of antibodies against measles, rubella and varicella zoster (MRZ reactions)

The intrathecal oligoclonal IgG fractions consist of many different specific antibodies. The most frequent intrathecally synthesized virus-specific antibodies in the CSF of MS patients are those against measles (79%), rubella (70%), varicella zoster (62%) and herpes simplex (36%) [41]. The combination of the measles, rubella and/or varicella zoster antibodies, referred to as the MRZ reaction, is found in 94% of MS cases [24]. The intrathecal MRZ reaction is not seen in acute CNS infections, such as neurosyphilis, neurotuberculosis, neuroborreliosis or neurocysticercosis, but it can be present in autoimmune diseases with CNS involvement (neurolupus; chronic, late stages of some infectious diseases). Therefore, the intrathecal MRZ reaction can be considered as an indicator for chronic inflammatory CNS disease, about as sensitive in MS as intrathecal oligoclonal IgG but more specific than intrathecal IgG synthesis formulae [42]. The origin of these intrathecal

Table 5.1 Intrathecal IgG synthesis; indices, formulae, MRZ antibody index and unique CSF oligoclonal IgG bands

Formula	Unit	Quantitative function	Basis	Disease	False positivity	Sensitivity for MS (%)
IgG index	None	> 0.73	Theoretical	Wide spectrum of neuro-diseases	Yes, if Q_{Alb} very abnormally elevated	92
Intrathecal IgG synthesis rate	mg/day	> 6 mg/day	Radioactive clearance studies in CSF in relation to serum	Wide spectrum of neuro-diseases	Yes, if Q_{Alb} very abnormally elevated	92
IgG$_{(Loc)}$	mg/dl	See Figures 5.6, 5.7	Empirical laws of diffusion	Wide spectrum of neuro-diseases	No	92
Unique IgG CSF oligoclonal bands which are not present in serum	Cathodic	By our method[a] 1 band is significant	Plasma cells secrete IgG of different isoelectric points, inside BBCB cathodic bands are unique	Wide spectrum of neuro-diseases	Bad technology can cause false positive and false negative	97
MRZ IgG antibody index	None	> 1.5	Empirical	MS	see S.5.2.1 (MRZ reaction)	94
Combine intrathecal IgG syn rate, MRZ and unique CSF oligoclonal bands	–	–	–	–	–	> 99

[a] Technique is important: 0.5 µg of IgG of neat CSF and matched serum is diluted and simultaneously isoelectrophoresed (amphogels pH 4–9) then immunofixed with antibody IgG heavy chain and silver stained to a standard endpoint.

BBCB, blood–brain–CSF barrier; MRZ, varicella zoster; CSF, cerebrospinal fluid.

specific antibodies remains uncertain, and there is no strong evidence supporting a relationship to the etiology of MS, since a *de novo* replication of the corresponding viral genome has not been found [43, 44]. In the literature, they are referred to as 'polyspecific activation', 'nonsense response', 'side-product' or 'bystanders' of the ongoing immune response [42, 45]. The intrathecal specific antibody tests have gained further clinical relevance through improvement of the sensitivity of the evaluation techniques, as well as by correction for any BBCB dysfunction [33]. The relevance of the intrathecal polyspecific immune response has been confirmed by detection of virus specific oligoclonal IgG, mainly measles, rubella and zoster, using a sensitive antigen-mediated capillary blot technique [45].

It has occurred to us that MRZ common infections of childhood which induce life-long immunities could be related to the finding of a high prevalence of MRZ antibodies in the CSF in MS. Is it possible that any inflammation such as that found in active plaques could recruit memory T cells, and after activation they result in secretion of specific antibodies into the extracellular space, which sink into the CSF?

Myelin basic protein

This protein is unique to the myelin sheath, and its presence or its fragments, which include epitope (69–89 amino acids), in CSF can be used as an index of active demyelination [46, 47]. A value more than 0.16 ng/ml (M + 2 s.d.) turns out to be present in 80% of patients with acute MS and 40% of chronic progressive MS but very few patients with stable MS. A result greater than 4 ng/ml is highly suggestive of a rapid rate of myelin degradation, as in a recent exacerbation of MS. Results of 1–3 ng/ml are consistent with a slower rate of myelin degradation or with recovery from an acute flare of demyelination. Levels of 1–3 ng/ml are seen in patients with MS whose acute attack is greater than one week old and in some patients with chronic active MS. Less than 5% of patients with inactive MS have values greater than 1 ng/ml range. Results less than 1 ng/ml indicate a lack of rapid demyelination [48].

The test is not specific for MS but may be positive in some degree in any disease with major demyelination. This includes optic neuritis and transverse myelitis, as well as other diseases where there is major destruction of myelin but in which demyelination is not the primary process, e.g. radiation necrosis, cerebrovascular accidents, head trauma, intrathecal chemotherapy [48].

MBP-like material, as an index of CNS myelin breakdown regardless of cause [49], may predict response to therapy, e.g. steroids [50]. Frequent sampling of CSF, however, is not desirable. Measurements of MBP-like material in alternative fluids, such as urine, have not shown a direct correlation between urinary MBP-like material and disease activity or an effect of treatment in MS [51]. On the other hand, Whitaker *et al.* did show a correlation with the number of lesions and total lesion burden determined by T2-weighted MRI [52]. Further, they found that urinary MBP-like material rose more in the placebo group than in the interferon beta-1b treatment groups. The highest level was found in the placebo-treated patients with a transition from the relapsing-remitting phase to the chronic progressive phase [52], and now HHV-6 (sections 5.3.2 and 5.3.9).

Negative constituents

Negative CSF cultures for micro-organisms as well as negative tests for neural antigens and microbial antibodies are an important part of the CSF profile indicative of MS. In spite of numerous studies, no persuasive elevation of antibodies indicative of acute infection has been found, except for the simultaneous intrathecal synthesis of antibodies to measles, rubella, varicella zoster and herpes simplex [42] and anti-myelin basic protein [53, 54].

5.2.2   TEMPORAL STABILITY OF THE MS CSF PROFILE

More than two decades of serial longitudinal testing of CSF and matched blood from clinically definite MS patients has revealed a temporal stability of this profile with two exceptions: a tendency for CSF leukocytes [20] and elevated intrathecal IgG synthesis rate to decrease the longer the disease duration [37]. Further, an elevated intrathecal IgG synthesis rate can be reduced toward normal by administration of ACTH or corticosteriods [35]. On the other hand, the CSF oligoclonal IgG band pattern persists even though the total CSF IgG is significantly reduced. Additionally, utilizing a two-dimensional electrophoresis method from the same longitudinal collection shows temporal invariance and clonal uniformity of Ig kappa and lambda generated spots [40].

Based on this information, persistence of the MS CSF profile on serial CSF examinations over years is supportive of the diagnosis of MS.

The intrathecal IgG synthesis rate of 30 mg/day, the average synthesis rate for an MS patient, is dynamic and staggering. We have calculated that 5×10^9 fully activated plasma cells sinking all their IgG into the CSF are needed to perform this feat. If the plasma cells in the brain have a half-life of a couple of days, as is the case for the core immune system, B cells have to be recruited at the rate of 2.5×10^9 per day.

Accordingly, we speculate that IgG synthesis intrathecally is driven by a specific antigen which is constantly present, to obtain this level of immunoactivity. It is also our notion that there is a negative feedback of IgG synthesis to plasma cells to keep the rate of synthesis at a steady state for any given patient. Is it possible that a putative MS virus is located in an MS plaque which is categorized as active?

5.2.3   VALIDITY AND RELIABILITY OF THIS PROFILE

The steady-state kinetics utilizing ^{131}I-labeled IgG (serum to CSF) have been established in MS patients [21]. From these data we constructed an intrathecal IgG synthesis rate formula which could predict the results of the isotope study (section 5.2.2). Hence, it is not necessary to use radioactive IgG to detect and determine the intrathecal IgG synthesis rate. To calculate the synthesis rate, IgG index or IgG (Loc), it is necessary to know the IgG and albumin concentrations in the CSF and matched serum.

The intrathecal IgG synthesis formulae correlate well with each other [10] (Figures 5.3–5.5). Further, even though the Schuller and Sagar formula [32a] is faulted by not including a serum albumin factor, a factor which turns out to be normal in MS patients without complications, there is an excellent correlation with the IgG synthesis rate formula (see Figure 5.5). Accordingly, the cardinal element of the CSF profile indicative of MS, namely intrathecal IgG synthesis, has a consensus from different investigators.

In the recently reported multi-center cyclosporine A clinical trial which included 353 MS patients with CSF analyses from 12 major neurologic centers in the USA (out of 557 total cases), strict clinical criteria were used to enter only clinically definite MS patients [55]. It turned out after selection on clinical grounds that 97% had white matter lesions on MRI while 100% had a CSF profile indicative of clinically definite MS as outlined above. The correlation between total MRI lesion area in various regions of the brain and clinical disability, instrumented neurologic function measurement, evoked potentials, intrathecal IgG synthesis rate and unique CSF IgG oligoclonal bands from 60 patients was investigated [36]. The cerebral plaque area on MRI was positively correlated with the intrathecal IgG synthesis rate (Figure 5.8), impaired performance on a neuropsychological test battery and abnormal visual evoked potentials, but not with the number or pattern

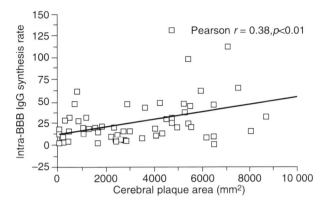

Figure 5.8 Intra blood–brain CSF barrier (BBCB) rate (mg/day) versus cerebral (axial) plaque area per case. (Reproduced from Baumhefner *et al.*, 1990 [36], by permission of the Editors of *Archives of Neurology*.)

of oligoclonal IgG bands. This is the first time a convincing correlation with intrathecal IgG synthesis rate has been reported. The number and pattern of oligoclonal bands did not correlate with intrathecal IgG synthesis rate, as stated above.

According to Reiber and Felgenhauer [23], their new formula, $IgG_{(Loc)}$, represents a non-linear function and can be applied to all cases, no matter how severe the BBCB dysfunction may be. There are further advantages of the IgG_{Loc} formula. First, it is applicable to the calculation of intrathecal synthesis of larger sized immunoglobulins (IgA_{Loc} and IgM_{Loc}) Secondly IgG_{Loc} can be expressed as a percentage of the CSF IgG concentration, and this is compatible with the graphical evaluation, where simultaneous information is given about any intrathecal inflammatory response and any blood–CSF–brain-barrier dysfunction [23]. The Committee of the European Concerted Action for Multiple Sclerosis recommends in its recent consensus report the use of non-linear formulae or graphs for the interpretation of intrathecal IgG synthesis, as the linear approaches can lead to false positive intrathecal IgG synthesis rate in cases with BBCB dysfunction, e.g. in early bacterial meningitis and Guillain–Barré syndrome [56]. However, in normal or modest BBCB leakage, as is usually the case for MS, both linear and non-linear approaches are of similar clinical sensitivity.

In spite of the above evidence, Lefvert and Link [38] and Hirsche and van der Helm [57] prefer to utilize intrathecal IgG synthesis based on the IgG index. Their results indicated that the IgG index was more discriminatory for MS and that the precision of determining the index was much higher than other intrathecal IgG synthesis formulae. It is our position that the good correlation between the intrathecal IgG synthesis rate and the IgG index should cast doubt on their restricted point of view. (Figures 5.3–5.5 give the correlation between the various formulae.)

5.2.4 DO OTHER DISEASES HAVE A CSF PROFILE SIMILAR TO MS?

A borderline elevated rate of intrathecal IgG synthesis and IgG index with none or one IgG oligoclonal band, a cardinal characteristic of the CSF profile indicative of MS, can occur rarely in individuals rated normal by history and neurologic examination. This information comes from the author's laboratory and it is not a procedural error. Accordingly, we believe that rarely a normal individual has intrathecal IgG synthesis, evidence of secreting plasma cells inside the BBCB.

Intrathecal IgG synthesis can be present in 30–50% of other CNS inflammatory conditions as well as 5–10% of non-inflammatory neurologic diseases, usually of known etiology. The CNS inflammatory conditions include: subacute sclerosing panencephalitis (SSPE), HAM (HTLV-1), Behçet's syndrome, occasionally progressive multifocal leukoencephalopathy, transverse myelitis, neurosyphilis, Lyme disease and yaws, chronic phase of CNS infection (bacteria, parasites, toxoplasmosis, cysticercosis, trypanosomiasis), mycoses, viruses (HIV-1 and herpes simplex encephalitis), postinfectious and postvaccinal vasculomyelinopathies and CNS vasculitides such as systemic lupus erythematosus. The neurological conditions which provoke an inflammatory response include cerebrovascular disease, brain tumor, CNS lymphoma and many others [11].

From this long list of diseases which produce intrathecal IgG synthesis, a by product of inflammation containing secretory plasma cells inside the blood–CSF–brain barrier, it has to be concluded that intrathecal IgG synthesis (intrathecal IgG synthesis formulae and/or CSF oligoclonal bands) *per se* is not discriminatory for MS. Unfortunately, many clinicians exclusively use CSF oligoclonal IgG bands as the only discriminator to support the diagnosis of MS, a laboratory test which has not been standardized from one laboratory to another.

Fortunately, the discriminating process can be enhanced if the CSF profile indicative of MS is used [14]. Patients with MS are not likely to have pleocytosis (more than 50 leukocytes per µl) ($P = 0.001$) or more than a few CSF polymorphonuclear cells. A low glucose CSF/serum ratio is never found in MS patients unless there is a complication, or the fluid was not drawn during steady-state conditions between CSF and blood. Fasting assures this steady state. If there is a marked elevation of the albumin quotient > 10 or CSF total protein > 100 mg/dl when the serum total protein concentration is normal, or a CSF albumin elevation > 65 mg/dl when the serum albumin concentration is normal, or a trans-BBCB albumin leakage of > 75 mg/day, then there are only three chances out of 1000 that the patient has MS. Furthermore, an intrathecal IgG synthesis rate > 130 mg/day or IgG index more than 4 are also very rare in MS ($P < 0.003$). Also of importance are negative CSF cultures for micro-organisms, and negative CSF serological monospecific reactions for various infectious diseases, such as syphilis, measles, rubella, HIV-1, Lyme disease and HTLV-1, whereas intrathecal synthesis of polyspecific viral antibodies index such as measles, zoster and rubella reaction (MRZ) are a common feature in MS [33]. In addition, intrathecal IgG synthesis (formulae, MRZ reaction and/or CSF IgG oligoclonal bands) should persist on subsequent examinations when inflammation is due to MS. On the other hand, intrathecal IgG synthesis formulae can be significantly lowered for several months by ACTH and/or corticosteroids but unique CSF IgG bands do not disappear [35]. In addition, there is a tendency for intrathecal IgG synthesis to fall the longer the patient lives [37], but oligoclonal IgG bands remain.

5.2.5 HOW TO USE THE CSF PROFILE IN CLINICAL ROUTINE

Our recommendation regarding a judicious use of the CSF profile to diagnose or exclude MS, and to monitor disease activity, is summarized in the algorithm shown in Figure 5.9.

5.3 Issues and perspectives

Despite the breadth of accounting by many investigators of the CSF profile indicative of MS presented above, there exists an agenda of unanswered issues that go to the heart of the MS CSF profile. Discussion of the most recent of these follows.

5.3.1 CYTOLOGY, B AND T CELLS

The low level of CSF pleocytosis is to be contrasted with the high counts of leukocytes in the CNS [29], yet there is evidence that the CSF cells in MS are abnormal. In the CSF the percentage of T lymphocytes which express CD3 marker account for 80% versus 65% in the blood, whereas the percentage of T helper (CD4$^+$) and T suppressor/cytotoxic (CD8$^+$) cells is equivalent to that found in blood, about a 2:1 ratio [58]. The percentage of B cells in the CSF is approximately the same as blood, 16–18% [59]. There has been no consistent change in T or B lymphocyte subsets in MS patients during exacerbation or in the chronic progressive phase of MS [58, 60], so the CSF cell profile in MS appears to be of little clinical value.

There is an unconfirmed report that an increased percentage of lymphocytes in the MS CSF are in the G1 phase of the proliferative cycle during all stages of disease activity [61]. Along this same line a pronounced

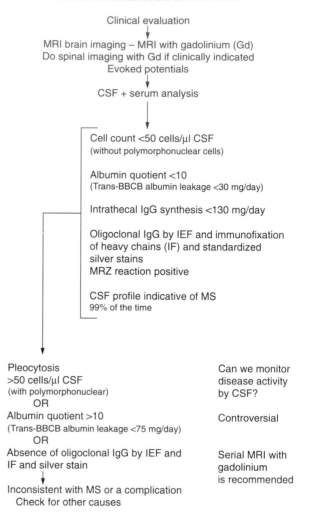

Figure 5.9 Multiple sclerosis evaluation algorithm. BBCB, blood–brain–CSF barrier; IEF, isoelectric focusing; IF, immunofixation.

B-cell response has been found in CSF from MS patients, of a much higher degree than in acute septic meningoencephalitis, against CNS autoantigens, myelin and myelin basic protein [62]. This could be an important concomitant of demyelination. Whether MBP-reactive B cells contribute to demyelination or arise as a secondary phenomenon in responses to myelin breakdown products is yet to be determined [63].

In vitro studies show that in patients with MS large numbers of cells in CSF produce antibodies against a variety of myelin antigens (MBP, proteolipid protein, myelin oligodendrocyte protein, myelin associated protein). Such cells are strongly enriched in CSF, but are not specific for MS. The pathogenetic role of the myelin-autoreactive cells might be promoting demyelination and presenting antigens to T cells [64]. Also, increased numbers of T cells producing cytokines have been found in CSF and blood from MS patients [64].

The subtype T-helper 1 cells (TH1) produce the proinflammatory cytokines (interleukin 2, interferon gamma, lymphotoxin), while the other subtype (TH2) is associated with the immune-modulating or counteracting cytokines (interleukin 4, 5, 6, 10, TGF beta). The TH1 response appears to be pathogenetically more relevant [65]. TH2 associated products, such as TGF beta, and other immune-modulating substances such as interferon beta, are considered to be possible therapeutic agents [66, 67].

5.3.2 SPECIFICITY OF INTRATHECAL IgG SYNTHESIS AND MRZ REACTION AND PRELIMINARY HUMAN HERPES VIRUS 6 RESULTS

An enigma in MS patients is that the specificity of intrathecal IgG synthesis (formulae and oligoclonal bands) is unknown, despite the fact that it occurs in large quantities, is temporally and clonally stable, is present in more than 99% of clinically definite MS patients, and is lowered but not eradicated by ACTH or corticosteroids (Figure 5.10). When ACTH or corticosteroids are stopped, intrathecal IgG synthesis rebounds [17, 35]. Because of these facts, it is unreasonable to believe, as has been proposed, that intrathecal IgG synthesis is non-sense [68, 69], i.e. no specificity, with polyclonal IgG synthesis replicating the patient's immune history. The grand clue to the etiology of MS may be revealed if we solve this enigma.

Additionally, it has been suggested that there are several explanations for failure to detect specific antibody in MS CSF IgG [70]. Is it possible that it is due to poorly suppressed clonal stimulation from a large assortment of antigens? This proposal is favored by the known immunoregulatory defect in MS of diminished suppressor T cell function [71]. Or could it be that the

appropriate antigen has not been examined in a sufficiently sensitive assay?

Is it possible that the antibody present may exist in an aggregated or complex form with antigens preventing detection of its presence? This is suggested by the studies of several workers [53, 54, 72–74].

Numerous searches have been made to determine the specificity of the CSF IgG [11, 70]. The most prevalent candidates in descending order are measles, rubella and herpes zoster [42].

The simultaneous intrathecal synthesis of polyspecific viral antibodies, most likely not a cause of multiple different diseases, is strongly indicative of a chronic inflammatory disease. The MRZ reaction is not seen in any acute infectious CNS disease, where intrathecal oligoclonal IgG bands are expected to be present [42, 45]. Therefore, the MRZ reaction, although most likely not related to etiopathogenesis, can be considered as a somewhat specific test with confirmatory relevance.

On the other hand, Challoner reported plaque-associated expression of human herpes virus 6 (HHV-6) in multiple sclerosis brain tissue [75]. Accordingly, using matched CSF and serum, we determined the HHV-6 antibody index. This index is a type of measurement of the activity of intrathecal plasma cells which are synthesizing antibodies to HHV-6 utilizing an ELISA method [48].

The HHV-6 specific antibody index is as follows:

$$\left(\frac{\text{HHV-6 Ig in CSF}}{\text{Total Ig in CSF}} \right) \div \left(\frac{\text{HHV-6 Ig in serum}}{\text{Total Ig in serum}} \right)$$

our cut-off was 3 s.d. above our normal value. We found 50% of patients with optic neuritis only, 70% of patients with clinically definite multiple sclerosis had an elevated value and 11% of normal patients.

It is our conviction that we must standardize a method for measuring mg of specific IgG antibody per ml in the CSF and serum or we will not know the importance of specific antibodies reported in ELISA units in MS CSF and serum. With determination of mg of specific IgG antibody/ml in CSF and serum, the intrathecal IgG synthesis rate formula can be utilized to determine the percentage of the total intrathecal IgG synthesis which is specific. For example, in SSPE, 25% of the total intrathecal IgG synthesis rate is due to specific antibody to measles, the etiological agent of SSPE [76].

5.3.3 WHY IS MS CSF IgG BANDED ON ELECTROPHORESIS?

Studies by Tourtellotte have dealt with affinity column-purified serum monoclonal antibodies specific for a melanoma antigen [77]. Application of isoelectric focusing on polyacrylamide gel followed by immuno-

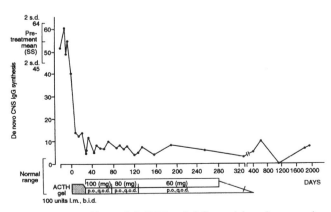

Figure 5.10 Effect of ACTH gel followed by alternate-day prednisone on *de novo* CNS IgG synthesis rate (intrathecal BBCB IgG synthesis) in an MS patient. (Reproduced from Tourtellotte *et al.*, 1980a [35] by permission of the Editors of *Neurology*.)

fixation for heavy chain IgG and silver staining revealed numerous bands, all of which had antibody potency. Hence a clone of plasma cells produces oligoclonal antibody protein. We surmise that the CSF oligoclonal pattern of an MS patient which is temporally invariant over years could be produced by a clone or a few clones of plasma cells. We speculate that the bands are antibodies to a single antigen, as were the affinity-purified monoclonal antibodies specific for melanoma antigen. Further, it has been shown that only 20% of the IgG oligoclonal bands in SSPE react with total measles antigens [76].

What is the chemical basis of the oligoclonal bands? There exists a paucity of studies to answer this question. It has been reported in 1985 that addition of neuraminidase-treated MS CSF characterized by IgG oligoclonal bands yielded additional subfractions, whereas endoglycosidases D or H showed only weak effects [78]. The findings suggest that the specific removal of oligosaccharide residues from immunoglobulins changed their charge, producing heterogeneous subfractions with isoelectricfocusing. More studies along this line need to be carried out.

It is our proposal that the oligoclonal bands found in MS are comparable to fingerprints: each patient has his own pattern which is genetically determined. Each synthesized IgG band pattern for a patient could be specific for the same antigen. When the MS brain is inflamed, it evolves to a chronic type of inflammation, manifested by the presence of plasma cells and their oligoclonal IgG secretion. The main evidence for this proposal comes from a longitudinal study of CSF and matched blood from MS patients taken at intervals of several times per year up to 12 years (Figure 5.10). Utilizing two-dimensional electrophoresis we found that patients' oligoclonal band pattern very rarely changes, and never disappears with time [40].

5.3.4 EFFECTS OF BLOODY TAP ON INTRATHECAL IgG SYNTHESIS

We found that contamination of normal CSF with as little as 0.2% serum gave a significantly elevated intrathecal IgG synthesis rate (mg/day) and IgG index; this is equivalent to a CSF erythrocyte count of about 5000 per mm^3. When CSF erythrocyte counts were below 1000 per mm^3, there was no effect [79]. Further, we found that a final concentration of $>2\%$ serum was necessary to obliterate unique CSF oligoclonal bands found in multiple sclerosis CSF.

Additionally, a serum contamination of 0.5% was required to elevate the trans-BBB albumin leakage rate. Accordingly, it is necessary to accomplish a lumbar puncture which does not introduce blood into the CSF sample. If one sees blood in the initial sample withdrawn, we recommend the following: replace the stylet, wait for 1 minute by the clock, then withdraw 16 drops or 1 ml. Repeat waiting for 1 minute and withdrawal of 1 ml for a total of five times. If the fluid is not crystal clear continue this procedure until it is. Fluid can appear pink tinted with as few as 200 erythrocytes/mm^3. Submit the cleared CSF for intrathecal IgG synthesis (rate and oligoclonal bands).

5.3.5   IgA AND IgM INTRATHECAL SYNTHESIS

IgG has been purified from MS CSF and sera and analyzed by two-dimensional electrophoresis. The heavy chains were similar in CSF and serum, whereas the CSF light chains were completely dissimilar to matched serum. These studies indicate a major limited diversity of clonal patterns and compartmentalized intrathecal synthesis of IgM. Further, there was clonal stability of patterns up to 12 years after the onset of

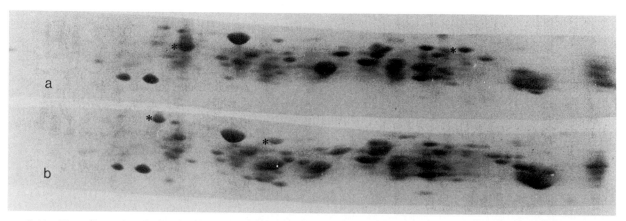

Figure 5.11   Two-dimensional electrophoresis (2-DE) Ig kappa and lambda light chains generated from CSF from an MS patient: (*a*) patient's baseline; (*b*) after 12 years. Similarity of pherograms proves temporal and clonal stability of MS CSF Ig. (Reproduced from *Journal of Experimental Medicine*, **163**, 41–53 (1986), figure 2, with permission.)

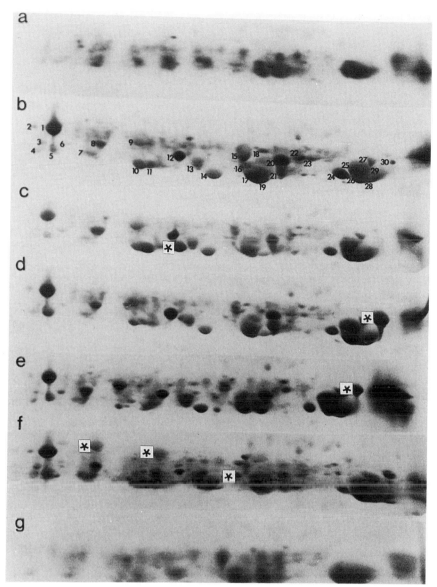

Figure 5.12 Two-dimensional electrophoresis (2-DE) of Ig kappa and lambda light chains. (*a*) Ig isolated from four regions of an MS brain (two sections from each cerebral hemisphere containing one or several plaques of demyelination), (*b–e*) and of autologous CSF (*f*) and serum (*g*). CSF and serum Ig were isolated as described [80]. For Ig isolation from brain, tissue was solubilized by a modification of the procedure of [147]. Approximately 3 grams of tissue from each brain region was used and the Ig was isolated using 102 ml PAS for each affinity purification. Only the light (L) chain regions of the 2-DE gels are shown. The L chain region in (*b*) was chosen as prototype for comparison with the L chains of CSF and the other three brain regions from which IgG was isolated (*c–e*). The numbers in (*b*) indicate prominent L chain spots. The asterisks in (*c–f*) indicate spots that differ substantially in intensity from the prototype (*b*). The CSF L chain complex shown in (*f*) is CSF obtained from this patient 5 years before death. Autolysis time for the control brain (*a*) was 18 hours, and the autolysis time for the MS brain (*c–e*) was 12 hours (Reproduced from *Journal of Experimental Medicine*, **163**, 41–53 (1986), figure 4, with permission.)

MS (Figure 5.11). The restricted clonal pattern and its stability was proposed as a consequence of B cell stimulation by disease-related antigen(s) with limited complexity [80].

For a given brain, we have also found regional stability of the IgG light chain pattern (Figure 5.12). Additionally, the light chain pattern was nearly identical to the patient's own CSF obtained premortally, but very different from the matched serum, indicating compartmentalization of the synthesis of IgG inside the BBCB. These data support the hypothesis that solutes such as IgG synthesized in the brain by plasma cells are secreted into the extracellular space of the brain (Figure 5.1), and sink into an ever-flowing CSF. Accordingly, the MS CSF IgG is reflective of the IgG in the brain or it is a barometer of the state of immunologic activation of CNS plasma cells and/or their number [81, 82].

IgA

Mingioli *et al.*, utilizing a radioimmunoassay on unconcentrated CSF, found an average value of CSF IgA in normal subjects of 1.3 µg per ml with a 95% confidence interval of 0.32–5.5 µg per ml; 22% of MS patients had an elevated IgA/total protein ratio [83].

These results have been confirmed by Sindic *et al.* [84], who obtained similar normal values using a particle-counting immunoassay and an IgA-index =

$$\left(\frac{CSF_{IgA}}{Serum_{IgA}} \right) \div \left(\frac{CSF_{albumin}}{Serum_{albumin}} \right)$$

Eighteen per cent of clinically definite MS patients were positive. They found that intrathecal synthesis of IgA was mostly dimeric and that IgA1 remained the predominant class [84].

IgA has been purified from MS CSF and sera [80]; it was analyzed by two-dimensional electrophoresis. MS CSF IgA alpha chain spots overlapped in mobility with serum alpha chains; however, a portion of the alpha chain complex in CSF was shifted cathodically, forming discrete spots. On the other hand, the CSF light chains of IgA were completely dissimilar to those of serum. These studies indicated major limited diversity and compartmentalized intrathecal synthesis of IgA in MS. There was clonal stability of patterns up to 12 years after the onset of disease. The restricted clonal pattern and its stability was proposed as a consequence of B cell stimulation by disease-related antigen(s) with limited epitope complexity.

IgA analysis is of little value for the laboratory supported diagnosis of MS.

IgM

Mingioli *et al.* used a radioimmunoassay on unconcentrated CSF fluid from normal subjects [83]. The mean value of IgM in CSF was 51 ng/ml with a range of 9 to 395 ng/ml. This same group [85] found 48% of clinically definite MS patients to have an abnormally elevated CSF IgM/albumin value along with 5% of patients with other neurological diseases and 6% of normal subjects; 40% of the MS patients with normal CSF IgG/albumin had an elevated CSF IgM value; and 51% of the patients with a high IgG value had a high IgM. ACTH treatment had no effect on CSF IgM, but it did lower the CSF IgG value. The IgM fraction did not contain measles antibodies.

Other researchers have shown that MS patients had a high IgM index =

$$\left(\frac{CSF_{IgM}}{Serum_{IgM}} \right) \div \left(\frac{CSF_{albumin}}{Serum_{albumin}} \right)$$

whereas none of the patients with a history of MS exceeding 15 years had an abnormal index. In addition, 5% of clinically definite MS patients had a high IgM/albumin ratio without an increase in IgG index =

$$\left(\frac{CSF_{IgG}}{Serum_{IgG}} \right) \div \left(\frac{CSF_{albumin}}{Serum_{albumin}} \right)$$

or the presence of unique CSF IgG oligoclonal bands. Further, 10% of stroke patients also had a high ratio [86].

Utilizing the ELISA technology, it was found that 70% of patients with acute aseptic meningitis and 10% of MS patients had an elevated IgM index in the presence of a normal IgG and IgA index. It was concluded that determination of the IgM index should be performed in suspected inflammatory CNS disorders [87].

IgM has been purified from MS CSF and sera and it was analyzed by two-dimensional electrophoresis. The µ-chains were similar in CSF and serum, whereas the CSF light chains were completely dissimilar to those from matched serum. These studies indicate a major limited diversity of clonal patterns and compartmentalized intrathecal synthesis of IgM. There was clonal stability of the patterns up to 12 years after the onset of MS. The restricted clonal pattern and its stability was proposed as a consequence of B cell stimulation by disease-related antigen(s) with limited epitope complexity [80].

IgM analysis is of little value for the laboratory supported diagnosis of MS.

5.3.6   FREE KAPPA AND LAMBDA LIGHT CHAINS

The presence of free light chains has been widely interpreted as signifying persistent intense stimulation by antigen or by a mitogenic factor inside the BBCB. The resulting hyperstimulation of B cells and their differentiated products leads to a desynchronization of light and heavy chain assembly and the release of light chain fragments into the extracellular space of the brain from where they diffuse into the CSF [18, 88–96]. The first report studied MS CSF for free light chains and found them by IEF to be mainly in the pH range of 3.5–6.4. In 8 of 9 MS patients free light chains were found, but none in the corresponding sera, supporting the hypothesis that they are synthesized in the CNS. A predominance of free lambda chains was found, as well as oligoclonal bands, indicating additional heterogeneity.

A study of 38 MS patients for free light chains (kappa and/or lambda) in the CSF by Vakaet and Thompson [97] showed only five of them with one band of kappa free light chains, and 33 with one or more bands of lambda free light chains. The 33 MS patients with 1 or more bands of lambda free light chains were compared with 33 control MS patients who did not have free light chains but who showed only an oligoclonal pattern of gamma-globulins in their CSF. They found that the number of free lambda light chains correlated with the number of white blood cells in the CSF, and also found that they correlated inversely with the time interval between the last relapse and the date of the lumbar puncture, and with the duration of the disease. They proposed that the presence of free lambda light chains in the CSF indicated that recent antigenic stimulation had occurred within the MS CNS. Furthermore, the inverse correlation of the number of lambda free light chains with the duration of the disease suggested a pathologic expression of the 'burning out' phenomenon of the MS process.

An immunopathological study [98] suggests a correlation between the histological activity of a plaque and the excess of free light chains found in the CSF. In all plaques and nonplaque areas examined, an excess of light over heavy chains was found. The light chain excess was greatest in recent plaques. In contrast to the ratio in the CSF, a predominance of kappa light chains (kappa/lambda ratio 1.7) was found in both plaque and nonplaque areas. When a particular light chain was found in the perivascular region of the plaque, it tended to predominate in the plaque substance as well. The preponderance of either kappa or lambda light chains in some plaques suggested that clones of B cells might be proliferating within them. A nonspecific mitogenic effect might be expected to lead to more heterogeneous light chain proliferation.

It has been suggested that an increase of free kappa chains may become a sensitive or a more specific test of CSF humoral abnormalities [99]. Work needs to be done on the antibody nature of the free light chains.

In alternative fluids, free kappa light chain levels in urine have been shown to correlate with disease activity in relapsing-remitting MS in 7 of 8 patients. They were elevated during periods of clinically active disease and decreased during stable disease [100]. In the chronic progressive form of MS, serial analyses of free kappa light chain levels did not reveal a strong correlation with extended disability status scale (EDSS) scores or MRI changes [101].

Thus, free light chain analysis is of little value for the laboratory supported diagnosis of MS. It is our proposal that the MS brain inflammatory reaction never 'sleeps', as manifested by the temporal invariance and clonal uniformity of intra-BBCB IgG [40]. A reminder: the average MS patient synthesizes 30 mg/day of IgG intrathecally. Since the CSF turns over about three times a day, plasma cells are active enough to replenish this bulk removal of IgG via the arachnoid villi.

5.3.7 IMMUNE COMPLEXES

Tissue-deposited and circulating immune complexes are found in a variety of human diseases and may contribute to disease pathogenesis. Isolation of immune complexes and identification of the antigenic constituent is a potential means of identifying putative disease-related antigens. For example, an analysis of immune complexes from two patients with progressive rubella panencephalitis showed that complexes from both serum and CSF contained antibody directed against rubella virus. Serum complexes were also shown to contain rubella antigen [102].

Work on immune complexes in MS has been reviewed [18, 103, 104]. In general antibody–antigen complexes have been detected in MS CSF, where they may occur independently of the serum level. Immune complexes have been reported in MS serum in 10–70% of cases, but the levels are low compared with immunological disorders, such as systemic lupus erythematosus. The frequency of immune complexes in MS CSF was 10–57%. There are a few reports that correlate CSF immune complexes with relapsing-remitting and progressive disease [105, 106].

More specifically, lipid or lipid-associated myelin-membrane antigens may be present in immune complexes found in the sera of MS patients [107]. Along the same lines, others have shown that the circulating immune MBP was a component of complexes in some MS sera [105].

A report of the correlation of free antibody to MBP with exacerbations of MS, and bound antibody to MBP with chronic progressive stages of MS, is of considerable interest [53, 54]. Isolated immune complexes from the CSF of MS patients and controls showed the following: MS complexes contained antibody to HSV (13 cases), measles virus (8 cases), CMV (5 cases) and rubella virus (5 cases). In some complexes, HSV or CMV antigen was detected along with antibody. MBP or antibody to MBP was found in the complexes of 7 patients with MS and 2 patients with other neurological diseases. Serum complexes containing antibody reactive with galactocerebroside and ganglioside were present in 12 patients with MS and 3 with other neurological diseases. More than 60% of the MS group had IgM and IgA serum complexes, including 5 patients with very high IgA levels [108].

Another investigator [104] isolated and characterized immune complexes from the CSF of 12 individuals (6 with exacerbations of MS and 6 with other neurological or psychiatric disease). Three MS patients had complexed HSV-1 viral antigen and antibody; 3 patients had complexed MBP. Two MS patients and 1 with hypoxic encephalopathy had complexed antibody directed against brain glycolipids. CSF complexes were distinct from serum complexes, suggesting intrathecal IgG synthesis.

More work needs to be done to identify the antibody and antigen nature of MS CSF complexes, but from this review immune complexes are of little value for the laboratory supported diagnosis of MS.

5.3.8 COMPLEMENT

CSF complement components in MS patients have been shown to be increased in proportion to the increase in immunoglobulins, and some patients exhibit elevations in intrathecal complement synthesis. Immunoassays of CSF complement components are slightly increased or decreased in other studies. Since macrophages in other organs have been shown to synthesize complement, it is reasonable that complement can be produced locally by macrophages in the MS brain [18, 103].

The levels of C3 in serum and CSF from MS patients did not differ from the levels in a control group, whereas the levels of C4 in MS serum were elevated and the C4 levels in MS CSF reduced [109]. A low level of C4 in CSF correlated significantly with the occurrence of CSF immune complexes. Activation products of C4 and C3 in serum were seen in 11 of 32 patients, appearing significantly more frequently among patients with circulating immune complexes. No C4 or C3 activating products could be identified in CSF. Because of the absence of C3 activation products, the authors concluded that there was no evidence of complement activation and therefore no reason to suspect an accelerated inflammatory reaction. They postulated that low CSF C4 might be the result of receptor binding of C4 and immune complexes since the latter were simultaneously elevated in the CSF.

Using an immunoradiometric assay to measure the concentration of the terminal component of complement (C9) in CSF and plasma from 35 patients with MS and 55 controls with other neurological diseases, a study reported in *The Lancet* showed there was a highly significant reduction in CSF C9 concentration with multiple sclerosis ($0.26 \pm 0.02\,\mu g/ml$) compared with controls ($1.52 \pm 0.20\,\mu g/ml$) [110]. Plasma C9 levels were within normal range, suggesting that C9 was being 'consumed' within the CNS, presumably by formation of complexes which then bind to oligodendroglia membrane, or the myelin sheath. Since 90% of MS patients had a reduction, measurement of C9 seemed to be more useful as an aid to the clinical diagnosis than the IgG index. Reduced CSF C9 concentration in patients with MS implies C9 consumption due to formation of membrane attack complexes, which could mediate myelin damage and cause more widespread but reversible loss of function, accounting for the transient symptoms characteristic of the disease. An Editorial

appeared in the same issue [111] commenting on this discovery with regard to the importance of methodological detail. Until this is addressed, the significance cannot be determined.

More work needs to be done on CSF complement as precise and sensitive methods become available, but to date there is little value for the laboratory supported diagnosis of MS.

5.3.9 CYTOKINES AND INTERFERONS

According to Peter *et al.* [112] serum and CSF levels of IL-2, sIL-2R, TNFα and IL-1β in chronic progressive MS lacked clinical utility.

Interleukin 1 (IL-1) activates lymphocytes and plays a role in initiating an immune response [113]. It was found to be increased in the CSF of MS patients [114].

Interleukin 2 (IL-2) and sIL-2R, a growth factor to T cells, is released by activated cells such as T cells, B cells and macrophages. Elevations in serum and/or CSF have been found in a few MS patients [115, 116].

Interleukin 6 (IL-6) inhibits production of TNFα [117]. IL-6 is sometimes elevated in the CSF of patients with MS [114, 118].

Tumor necrosis factor alpha (TNFα) is a known potent mediator of inflammation [113, 119–121] and there is evidence to implicate TNFα in the pathogenesis of MS [114, 118]. It has been reported [122] that TNFα was elevated in the CSF of 53% of patients with chronic progressive MS. The levels correlated with the degree of disability and rate of neurologic determination.

Another potent mediator of inflammation is interferon gamma. It has been reported [123] that 30 of 30 CSF samples from patients with MS had detectable levels. It was also found that MS blood mononuclear cells produced significantly more TNFα than controls when stimulated *in vitro* with concanavalin A.

In the search for disease activity and predictive markers in the blood of MS patients, promising results have been recently reported from studies with cytokines and adhesion molecules [124–127]. Significant increases in TNFα mRNA expression in peripheral blood mononuclear cells 4–6 weeks prior to relapse in relapsing-remitting MS were demonstrated using semiquantitative PCR [126]. A similar pattern was observed for lymphotoxin mRNA expression. At the same time, transforming growth factor β (TGFβ) and interleukin 10 mRNA levels declined [126]. A significant increase of circulating intercellular adhesion molecule 1 (cICAM-1) levels in serum of MS patients was present at the time of relapse (799 ng/ml vs 449 ng/ml; $P < 0.001$), whereas the highest serum levels for circulating tumor necrosis factor receptor (cTNF-R p60) occurred 4 weeks after the onset of the relapse (1.8 ng/ml at relapse vs 2.3 ng/ml 4 weeks after a relapse; $P < 0.001$) [124]. Further studies and long-term trials are needed to confirm these intriguing findings. Although not specific or diagnostic for MS, cytokine and adhesion molecule levels in the blood of MS patients open a new door for frequent monitoring and therapeutic interventions. The diagnosis of MS, however, still first necessitates a CSF analysis.

5.3.10   IS THE CSF PROFILE INDICATIVE OF MS HELPFUL IN THE DIAGNOSIS OF EARLY MS?

The first series of MS patients obtained from the national cooperative ACTH trial were relapsing and remitting patients with modest disability (average Kurtzke EDSS score of 3.5) [128]. The frequency and degree of intrathecal IgG synthesis were the same as in more recent studies with chronic progressive patients with moderate to severe disability (average EDSS score of 5.4) [10] (Figures 5.3, 5.4, 5.5). There is a paucity of CSF analyses after the first symptom; it is our impression that intrathecal IgG synthesis is well established prior to the first symptom.

While the diagnostic significance of CSF markers is well established in the diagnosis of MS, the utility of CSF analysis in the prognostic evaluation of patients with acute optic neuritis (AON) is still controversial. Intrathecal oligoclonal IgG (OI) in CSF of patients with AON has been reported to be associated with higher risk of developing MS in some studies [129–131]. According to other researchers a significant predictive value of CSF analyses was not found [132, 133]. Many studies compared the utility of MRI and intrathecal OI and found a higher prognostic value of MRI [94, 134–136]. However, the diagnostic sensitivity of OI depends very much on the technique used [112], and prevalences ranging from 38% to 69% have been reported for patients with AON [94, 132].

In a recent study (Tumani *et al.*, in preparation), the prognostic value of multiple baseline CSF and serum markers was evaluated, including the MRZ reaction as well as HHV-6 specific antibody index, in patients with AON who were clinically followed up for 4 years as part of the multi-center optic neuritis treatment trial (ONTT) [137]. Correlation of the CSF markers with progression to MS and with baseline MRI results was performed. Thirty-six paired CSF and serum samples obtained prior to treatment were analyzed for albumin and IgG by nephelometry to calculate intrathecal IgG synthesis, for oligoclonal IgG (OI) by isoelectric focusing (IEF) and immunofixation, and MRZ and HHV-6-specific antibody indices by enzyme immunoassay (EIA). The blood–brain–CSF barrier function was determined by the CSF/serum albumin quotient. Baseline magnetic resonance imaging (MRI) scanning was performed by a standard protocol. We found no abnormalities in the BBCB to albumin.

Fifty per cent of patients with AON developed MS in 4 years. Of the patients who developed MS, the MRI was positive at baseline in 77%. If OI and MRI were positive at baseline, 83% developed MS. If OI, MRZ and MRI were positive at baseline 86% developed MS. If the OI, MRZ and MRI were negative at baseline, only 16% developed MS. Accordingly, we recommend a CSF and matched blood examination to determine the CSF profile indicative of MS, as detailed in section 5.2.

Further, we have preliminary data that 50% of AON patients at baseline had a significant elevation (cut-off 3 s.d. above our laboratory average) of their HHV-6-specific antibody index, a type of quantitation of specific IgG synthesized by plasma cells located intrathecally.

5.3.11   WHAT HAVE WE LEARNED FROM 2-D ELECTROPHORESIS?

Elevated CSF IgG and oligoclonal IgG bands on electrophoresis are valuable clinical markers for B cell proliferation in the brains of patients with MS [40]. Using two-dimensional (2-D) electrophoresis, it has been established that the humoral immune response in MS brain is characterized by finite clonal complexity for the major Ig classes. An important question is whether this immune response is clonally stable or varies with time, related to the development of new lesions and random entry of B cells into the MS brain. To investigate this, serial electrophoretic studies on CSF obtained from 19 patients with MS were performed; the intervals ranged from 7 to 12 years with a mean of 8 years. These analyses included studies of IgG, IgA and IgM, and revealed that the humoral immune response in MS is clonally stable up to 12 years, the oldest serial specimen in the collection (Figure 5.10). Spontaneous fluctuations or reduction in CSF IgG levels by drugs did not qualitatively affect B cell clonal proliferation.

It has been asserted that intrathecal IgG synthesis in MS is non-sense antibody because the spectrotypes of IgG isolated from different regions of MS brains differ [68, 69]. Factors other than clonal heterogeneity could account for differences found using one-dimensional analysis, so we utilized 2-D electrophoresis (2-DE). Plasma cell clonal products resolve into unique and well-resolved spots by 2-DE; the method is uniquely suitable for analysis of restricted immune responses. Accordingly, IgG from 11 regions of three MS brains was isolated and the 2-DE patterns were compared [40]. The similarity of the 2-DE patterns in a given brain indicates unequivocally that major clones are distributed uniformly, although some clones are more prominent in some brain areas. IgA and IgM isolated from the same areas also showed similar patterns. Furthermore, the patterns of light and heavy chains in brain regions differed from serum, but were similar to the autologous CSF, providing new evidence that CSF IgG in MS derives from synthesis *in situ* (Figure 5.11). The results indicate that, once initiated, B cell clonal proliferation to plasma cells persists indefinitely and is qualitatively little altered at a clonal level over time, even when CSF IgG levels change or are altered by drugs. The above-mentioned results are consistent with the allotype and idiotype hypothesis of Ig production in MS and conflict with non-sense antibody proposals of the origin and nature of CNS *in situ* synthesized Ig in MS.

In view of the fact that 2-DE resolves the secretion of plasma cells into unique and well-resolved spots, in contrast to one-dimensional analysis, in which a band is an overlay of several or a multitude of plasma cell clone Ig secretions, we have addressed the following question: will 2-DE of CSF and autologous serum be of value for diagnosis and for evaluating putative treatments? We have found the procedures used by Walsh and Tourtellotte [40] too complex and time-consuming to be used in clinical laboratories.

5.3.12 SHOULD THE CSF PROFILE BE INCLUDED AS AN OUTCOME ASSESSMENT IN CLINICAL TRIALS?

A major task in MS clinical trials is *objectively* evaluating new putative therapies. We recommend that the CSF profile indicative of MS as proposed in this chapter be a major secondary rational assessment in clinical trials designed to evaluate a primary treatment.

The reader is reminded that a component of the immunological under-pinning of the MS inflammatory reaction is plasma cells. The IgG synthetic activity of the intrathecal plasma cells can be quantified by our intrathecal IgG synthesis rate formula (mg/day), and this is a continuous process which is temporally and clonally stable. The average MS patient synthesizes 30 mg of IgG per day inside the BBCB. It is our notion that eradicating intrathecal IgG synthesis in MS should be the ultimate outcome of a successful treatment, even though we do not know what causes the synthesis and we do not know whether it is favorable or adverse to oligodendrocytes or the myelin sheath. It is our opinion that intrathecal IgG synthesis is the best marker for brain inflammation, no matter what causes the inflammation.

There are four mechanisms to decrease the number of plasma cells in the MS brain.

1. Decrease the number of circulating B cells and/or the helper T cell; e.g. using immunosuppressive/cyto-toxic agents.
2. Decrease the ability of immune cells to pass across the BBCB; e.g. with anti-inflammatory agents such as corticosteroids or ACTH.
3. Down-regulate brain inflammation in MS; e.g. with COP-I or beta interferon.
4. Eradicate the cause of MS; e.g. using beta interferon as an anti-viral agent.

There is no question that ACTH and corticosteroids decrease the intrathecal IgG synthesis rate, but they do not eradicate oligoclonal bands. However, in almost all cases the IgG synthesis rate increases to pre-treatment values after a variable time of weeks to months [17, 35]. Intrathecal administration of corticosteroids can be more effective than parenteral or oral administration.

ACTH has been shown to improve function after a relapse [128]. It is our proposal that ACTH and corticosteroids are effective because MS brain inflammation is down-regulated, and hence the environment of the demyelinated axon is normalized, allowing the nerve fibers to conduct better. Good evidence for down-regulation is that there is a decrease in the intrathecal IgG synthesis rate, a product of intrathecal plasma cells (Figure 5.10) [35].

Based on the hypothesis that MS is an autoimmune disease, as is experimental allergic encephalitis (EAE), numerous clinical trials have been designed utilizing immunosuppressive-cytotoxic regimens such as cyclo-phosphamide, azathioprine, Ara-C (parenteral and intrathecal), CCNU, BCNU, 5-FU, cyclosporine A and CNS irradiation [138–140]. None reduced the IgG synthesis rate and all have marginal clinical efficacy.

Leustatin, another immunosuppressant-cytotoxic agent shown to be dramatically effective in a 1-year pilot clinical trial, lowered the intrathecal IgG synthesis rate [141].

COP-I, a proposed blocker of antigen-presenting cells, which is effective in relapsing-remitting MS, but not in chronic-progressive MS, does not lower the intrathecal IgG synthesis rate [139].

Interferon beta 1a, a natural antivirotic which has been shown to be effective in MS, decreases the intrathecal IgG synthesis rate and down-regulates a number of immunologic parameters (Rudick, personal communication).

Another rationale for the inclusion of intrathecal IgG synthesis (rate and bands) in clinical trials is based on the use of CSF in monitoring therapy in infectious diseases in which an effective treatment is known. For example, in neurosyphilis the CSF parameters become normal after treatment [142] and if normalization does not occur, high-dose penicillin will result in normal parameters. If MS is due to an infectious disease, it is expected that an effective treatment would eradicate intra-BBCB IgG synthesis, as it does in neurosyphilis. Further, if MS is due to auto-immunity, and we had a treatment to eradicate the auto-immunity process, signs of chronic inflammation of the brain (intrathecal IgG synthesis) would be eradicated.

In summary, it is our recommendation that the MS CSF profile be utilized as a major secondary outcome measure in clinical trials (primary measures are clinical effectiveness). The cardinal aspect of the profile is intrathecal IgG synthesis. Nobody questions the source – intrathecal plasma cells; hence, normalization of intrathecal IgG synthesis is evidence that the polyphasic chronic inflammation of the MS brain is no longer present.

Further, a persistently normal intrathecal IgG synthesis would be important evidence that the goal of primary MS therapy has been achieved. It is our opinion that if a patient shows clinical improvement but no down-regulation of the MS inflammatory reaction, then the protocol needs to be evaluated.

5.3.13 OTHER CONSTITUENTS

There have been numerous investigations of other constituents in MS CSF (e.g. that by Tourtellotte [11], table 4, p. 120, and Whitaker *et al.* [70]. Often a standard micro-chemical or biological method has been applied to determine whether significant abnormalities in the CSF existed. As long as the etiopathogenesis of MS is unknown, we endorse this approach.

5.4 Post-lumbar puncture headache

A multitude of factors involved in the etiology of the post-lumbar puncture headache (PPH) have been surveyed [143]. That study indicated several factors to be of prime importance, including needle size, gender and age. We and others found that a lumbar puncture headache incidence of 36% was the same in patients with MS as with other neurologic disease (OND) and normal individuals [144]

Subsequently a study was designed to evaluate more precisely the effect of needle size on the production of the PPH [145]. One hundred consecutive healthy paid volunteers who were rated normal on physical and neurological examinations were included in the study. Sixty were male and 40 were female. Their average age was 23.2 years, with a range of 20–41 years. Members of each successive pair of incoming volunteers were randomly assigned to have a spinal tap with either the 22 gauge (O.D. 0.71 mm) needle group or the 26 gauge (O.D. 0.46 mm) needle group. The punctures were performed with the subjects in the left lateral recumbent position, without local anesthesia or sedation; subjects remained recumbent for 1 hour post-puncture.

Twenty ml of CSF were withdrawn by means of a 5 ml syringe from each subject With the aid of a stopwatch, the withdrawal rate was 1 ml per minute. The needle was never left indwelling for more than 25 minutes and not for less than 21 minutes.

It was found that, while there was a 75% incidence of some type of complaint in both needle groups, 'major' complaints were one-third more frequent in the 22 gauge group. The incidences of postural headaches in the 22 and 26 gauge needle groups were 36% and 12%, respectively. Furthermore, none of the postural head-

aches produced by the 26 gauge needle was severe, whereas 44% of headaches in the 22 gauge needle group were severe. Nausea was associated with 72% of the postural headaches in the 22 gauge group, but only 33% in the 26 gauge group. Backaches were also more frequent in the 22 gauge group (72% versus 56%), the difference being close to statistical significance. Females were found to suffer postural headaches significantly more frequently than males (40% versus 13%).

It is our recommendation, based on this information, that smaller gauge needles be used to obtain MS CSF.

5.5 CSF methodology

Data are no better than the methods used to obtain them. Accordingly, the standardized methods used in our laboratory were highlighted in our chapter in the book edited by Poser *et al.* [13], and since then the details of the isoelectric focusing procedure have been published [39]. In addition to the reliable, valid and sensitive methods, perfectly normal individuals have been used as the gold standard, always removing 20 ml of CSF by syringe at the rate of 1 ml per minute, the same collection procedure used for MS patients. Note that all of the MS patients used to obtain the cut-off points in the MS CSF profile come from pre-treatment randomized clinical trials:

1. ACTH vs. placebo [128];
2. azathioprine vs. methylprednisolone vs. placebo [146];
3. cyclosporin A vs. placebo [55].

These are near-perfect sources of patients for the clinical chemists to calculate meaningful fiducial limits and correlations, since all patients studied fit the most stringent of clinical criteria, and there was standardized methodology for removal of CSF and matched blood [1].

Collection

The amount of CSF collected should be standardized. Routinely, 20 ml is collected using a 25 gauge needle. Before the fluid is aliquoted for analysis the fluid must be well mixed.

Cell counts and differential

This procedure has been detailed elsewhere [20].

Albumin and IgG determinations

Nephelometry is used to quantitate albumin and IgG by analyzing increases in turbidity, measured by increasing scatter of laser light. The interaction of specific antibodies in the reagent with the antigen from the sample results in the formation of antigen–antibody complexes which are rendered insoluble by the presence of precipitating reagents. Most modern nephelometers compare the rate of formation of antigen–antibody complexes (determined by computer analysis of laser light scatter data) to that of known antigenic standards in order to measure precisely the protein antigens present in moderate concentrations.

Detection and quantification of unique CSF oligoclonal bands

The application of isoelectric focusing (IEF), immunoglobulin G (IgG) immunofixation and silver staining for the analysis of unconcentrated CSF and sera is described [39]. These methods have been standardized and applied to IgG oligoclonal band analysis. The sensitivity of the procedure was 0.3 µg IgG. Optimum results were obtained with 0.5 µg IgG in 5–20 µl application volumes. Equal quantities of CSF and serum IgG analyzed by IEF in 55 normal individuals showed comparable intensities and isoelectric points in both body fluids.

This IEF method can reveal three different banding patterns:

1. no unique bands in CSF;
2. CSF restricted oligoclonal bands and none in serum;
3. CSF oligoclonal bands identical to, but less intense than, those found in serum.

Only (2) and (3) are considered evidence for unique CSF oligoclonal bands, evidence that plasma cells are synthesizing IgG intrathecally.

5.6 Perspective

In our view, the long-term goals of clinical chemists who study MS CSF are fivefold.

1. We must continue to search for other constituents to make the profile more discriminative.
2. Based on the assumption that the etiology of MS is hidden in the antibody nature of IgG intrathecally synthesized, the search must continue for this antibody specificity. If found, the profile would be considered the basis for the diagnosis of MS, rather than an aid to diagnosis.
3. Even in the present state of knowledge about the CSF profile indicative of MS, we recommend that it be incorporated in MS clinical trials. Furthermore, if we could make an early laboratory diagnosis of MS, i.e. a diagnosis as soon as possible after the first symptoms, we could, with confidence, ethically include a type of MS patient with the least amount of irreversible damage in randomized clinical trials.

Reminder: the MS CSF profile indicative of clinically definite MS establishes that a modest chronic active inflammation exists inside the BBB. Accordingly, ideal outcome measures of a clinical randomized trial of this type would be normalization of intrathecal IgG synthesis, that is to say, eradication of intrathecal plasma cells. For example, in neurosyphilis, a sufficient amount of penicillin will eradicate the synthesis.

4. The need for standardization of CSF methodology is indicated.
5. Cytokines and adhesion molecules in blood and/or CSF are promising paraclinical markers to assess disease activity after the diagnosis of MS has been established. As mediators and immunoregulators of the inflammatory processes in multiple sclerosis, they reflect the ups and downs of the underlying inflammatory process and represent an important laboratory tool for frequent disease activity monitoring. Furthermore, their role as therapeutic agents is under investigation by many multi-center treatment trials.

ACKNOWLEDGMENTS

We acknowledge the assistance of Diane C. Guntrip in the preparation of the manuscript.

References

1. Poser, C.M., Paty, D.W., McDonald, W.I., Scheinberg, L. and Ebers, G.C. (1984) *The Diagnosis of Multiple Sclerosis*, New York, Thieme-Stratton.
2. Adams, C.W.M. (1983) The general pathology of multiple sclerosis: morphological and chemical aspects of the brain, in *Multiple Sclerosis: Pathology, Diagnosis and Management* (eds J.F. Hallpike, C.W.M. Adams and W.W. Tourtellotte), Baltimore, MD, Williams and Wilkins, pp. 203–40.
3. Sanders, V., Conrad, A.J. and Tourtellotte, W. (1993) On classification of post-mortem multiple sclerosis plaques for neuroscientists. *J. Neuroimmunol.*, **46**, 207–16.
4. Grossman, R.I., Gonzalez-Scarano, F., Atlas, S.W., Galetta, S. and Silberberg, D.H. (1986) Multiple sclerosis: gadolinium enhancement in MR imaging. *Radiology*, **161**, 721–5.
5. Kermode, A.G., Tofts, P.S., Thompson, A.J. (1990) Heterogeneity of blood–brain barrier changes in multiple sclerosis: an MRI study with gadolinium-DTPA enhancement. *Neurology*, **40**, 229–35.
6. Miller, D.H., Rudge, P., Johnson, G. *et al.* (1988) Serial gadolinium enhanced magnetic resonance imaging in multiple sclerosis. *Brain*, **111**, 927–39.
7. Tschirgi, I.D. (1960) Chemical environment of the central nervous system, in *Handbook of Physiology. A Critical, Comprehensive Presentation of Physiological Knowledge and Concepts* (eds J. Field, H. Magoun and V. Hall), Baltimore, MD, Williams and Wilkins for American Physiological Society, Washington, DC.
8. Fishman, R.A. (1992) *Cerebrospinal Fluid in Diseases of the Nervous System*, Philadelphia, Saunders.
9. Baumhefner, R.W., Tourtellotte, W., Paty, D. *et al.* (1986) Peripheral, cerebrospinal fluid and CNS immune cell subset and functional alterations in multiple sclerosis, in *Immunotherapies in Multiple Sclerosis* (eds O. Hommes, J. Mertin and W. Tourtellotte), Suffolk, UK, Stuart Phillips Publications, St Edmundsbury Press, pp. 335–80.
10. Syndulko, K., Tourtellotte, W., Conrad, A., Izquierdo, G., Multiple Sclerosis Study Group, Alpha Interferon Study Group and and Azathioprine Study Group (1993) Trans-blood–brain-barrier albumin leakage and comparisons of intrathecal IgG synthesis calculations in multiple sclerosis patients. *J. Neuroimmunol.*, **46**, 185–92.
11. Tourtellotte, W.W. (1985) The cerebrospinal fluid in multiple sclerosis. In *Handbook of Clinical Neurology, 3* (eds P. Vinken, G.W. Bruyn, H. Klawans and J. Koetsier), Amsterdam, Elsevier, vol. 47, pp. 79–130.

12. Tourtellotte, W.W. (1987) Cerebrospinal fluid profile indicative of clinical definite multiple sclerosis: a proposal, facts, issues, opportunities and perspective, in *Advances in CSF Protein Research and Diagnosis* (ed. E.J. Thompson), Lancaster, MTP Press, pp. 17–34.

13. Tourtellotte, W.W. and Walsh, M.J. (1984) Cerebrospinal fluid profile in multiple sclerosis, in *The Diagnosis of Multiple Sclerosis* (eds C.M. Poser, D.W. Paty, L. Scheinberg, W.I. McDonald and G.C. Ebers), New York, Thieme-Stratton, pp. 165–78.

14. Tourtellotte, W.W., Walsh, M.J., Baumhefner, R.W., Staugaitis, S. and Shapshak, P. (1988) The current status of multiple sclerosis intra-blood–brain barrier IgG synthesis. *Ann. NY Acad. Sci.*, **436**, 52–67.

15. Tourtellotte, W.W., Staugaitis, S., Walsh, M.J. *et al.* (1985) The basis of intra-blood–brain barrier IgG synthesis. *Ann. Neurol.*, **17**, 21–7.

16. Tourtellotte, W., Baumhefner, R., Shapshak, P. and Osborne, M. (1987) The status of intra-blood–brain-barrier IgG synthesis in multiple sclerosis. *Riv. Neurol.*, **57**(3), 236–8.

17. Tourtellotte, W.W., Baumhefner, R.W., Syndulko, K. *et al.* (1988). The long march of the cerebrospinal fluid profile indicative of clinical definite multiple sclerosis; and still marching. *J. Neuroimmunol.*, **20**, 217–27.

18. Walsh, M.J., Tourtellotte, W.W. and Potvin, A.R. (1983) Central nervous system immunoglobulin synthesis in neurological disease. Quantitation, specificity, and regulation, in *Neurobiology of Cerebrospinal Fluid* (ed. J. Wood), New York, Plenum Press, vol. 2, pp. 331–68.

18a. Walsh, M.J., Tourtellotte, W.W. and Potvin, J.H. (1983) The cerebrospinal fluid in multiple sclerosis, in *Multiple Sclerosis: Pathology, Diagnosis and Management* (eds J.F. Hallpike, C.W.M. Adams and W.W. Tourtellotte), London, Chapman and Hall, pp. 275–358.

19. Wong, M.C., Krol, G. and Rosenblum, M.K. (1992) Occult epidural chloroma complicated by acute paraplegia following lumbar puncture. *Ann. Neurol.*, **31** (1), 110–12.

20. Tourtellotte, W.W. (1970) Cerebrospinal fluid in multiple sclerosis, in *Handbook of Clinical Neurology* (eds P. Vinken and G.W. Bruyn), Amsterdam, North Holland, vol. 9, pp. 324–82.

21. Tourtellotte, W.W., Potvin, A.R., Fleming, J.O. *et al.* (1980) Multiple sclerosis: measurement and validation of central nervous system IgG synthesis rate. *Neurology*, **30**, 240–4.

22. Brightman, M.W. (1965) The distribution within the brain of ferritin injected into cerebrospinal fluid compartments. II. Parenchymal distribution. *Am. J. Anat.*, **117**, 193–220.

23. Reiber, H. and Felgenhauer, K. (1987) Protein transfer at the blood cerebrospinal fluid barrier and the quantitation of the humoral immune response within the central nervous system. *Clin. Chim. Acta*, **163**, 319–28.

24. Reiber, H. (1994) Flow rate of cerebrospinal fluid (CSF). A concept common to normal blood–CSF barrier function and to dysfunction in neurological diseases. *J. Neurol. Sci.*, **122**, 189–203.

25. Blennow, K., Fredman, P., Wallin, A. *et al.* (1993) Protein analyses in cerebrospinal fluid. II. Reference values derived from healthy individuals. *Eur. Neurol.*, **33** (2), 129–33.

26. Tibbling, G., Link, H. and Ohman, S. (1977) Principles of albumin and IgG analyses in neurological disorders. *Scand. J. Clin. Lab. Invest.*, **37**, 385–90.

27. Cutler, J.W.P., Page, L., Galicich, J. and Watters, G.V. (1968) Formation and absorption of cerebrospinal fluid in man. *Brain*, 707–20.

28. Myers, C.D. (1991) Role of B cell antigen processing and presentation in the humoral immune response. *FASEB J.*, **5**, 2547–53.

29. Prineas, J.W. (1985) The neuropathology of multiple sclerosis, in *Handbook of Clinical Neurology*, **3**, (eds P. Vinken, G. Bruyn, H. Klawans and J. Koetsier), vol. 47, *Demyelinating Diseases*, Amsterdam, Elsevier, pp. 213–57.

30. Reiber, H. (1994) The hyperbolic function: a mathematical solution of the protein flux/CSF flow model for blood–CSF barrier function. *J. Neurol. Sci.*, **126**, 243–5.

31. Simpson, J.F., Tourtellotte, W.W., Kokmen, E. *et al.* (1969) Fluorescent protein tracing in multiple sclerosis brain tissue. *Arch. Neurol.*, **20**, 373–7.

32. Schuller, E. and Sagar, H. (1981) Local synthesis of CSF immunoglobulins. A neuroimmunological classification. *J. Neurol. Sci.*, **51**, 361–70.

32a. Schuller, E. and Sagar, H.J. (1983) Central nervous system IgG synthesis in multiple sclerosis. *Acta Neurol. Scand.*, **67**, 365–71.

33. Reiber, H. and Lange, P. (1991) Quantification of virus-specific antibodies in cerebrospinal fluid and serum: sensitive and specific detection of antibody synthesis in brain. *Clin. Chem.*, **37**, 1153–60.

34. Link, H. and Tibbling, G. (1977) Principles of albumin and IgG analysis in neurological disorders. III. Evaluation of IgG synthesis within the central nervous system in multiple sclerosis. *Scand. J. Clin. Lab. Invest.*, **37**, 397–401.

35. Tourtellotte, W.W., Baumhefner, R.W., Potvin, A.R. *et al.* (1980) Multiple sclerosis de novo CNS IgG synthesis: effect of ACTH and corticosteroids. *Neurology*, **30**, 1155–62.

36. Baumhefner, R.W., Tourtellotte, W.W., Syndulko, K. *et al.* (1990) Quantitative multiple sclerosis plaque assessment with magnetic resonance imaging. Its correlation with clinical parameters, evoked potentials and intra-blood–brain-barrier IgG synthesis. *Arch. Neurol.*, **47**, 19–26.

37. deCastro, P., Baumhefner, R.W., Syndulko, K. and Tourtellotte, W.W. (1990) Longitudinal intra-BBB IgG synthesis rate: temporal and clonal stability of intra-BBB IgG synthesis lasting up to eighteen years in patients with multiple sclerosis. *Ann. Neurol.*, **28** (2), 253.

38. Lefvert, A.K. and Link, H. (1985) IgG production within the central nervous system: a critical review of proposed formulae. *Ann. Neurol.*, **17**, 13–20.

39. Staugaitis, S.M., Shapshak, P., Tourtellotte, W.W., Lee, M.M. and Reiber, H.O. (1985) Isoelectric focusing of unconcentrated cerebrospinal fluid: application to ultrasensitive analysis of oligoclonal immunoglobulin-G. *Electrophoresis*, **6**, 287–91.

40. Walsh, M.J. and Tourtellotte, W.W. (1986) Temporal invariance and clonal uniformity of brain and cerebrospinal IgG, IgA and IgM in multiple sclerosis. *J. Exp. Med.*, **163**, 41–53.

41. Felgenhauer, K., Schadlich, H., Nekic, M. and Ackermann, R. (1985) Cerebrospinal fluid virus antibodies. A diagnostic indicator for multiple sclerosis. *J. Neurol. Sci.*, **71**, 292–9.

42. Felgenhauer, K. and Reiber, H. (1992) The diagnostic significance of antibody specificity indices in multiple sclerosis and herpes virus induced diseases of the nervous system. *Clin. Invest.*, **70**, 28–37.

43. Godec, M., Asher, D., Murray, R. *et al.* (1992) Absence of measles, mumps, and rubella viral genomic sequences from multiple sclerosis brain tissue by polymerase chain reaction. *Ann. Neurol.*, **32** (3), 401–4.

44. Nicoll, J., Kinrade, E. and Love, S. (1992) PCR-mediated search for herpes simplex virus DNA in sections of brain from patients with multiple sclerosis and other neurological disorders. *J. Neurol. Sci.*, **113** (2), 144–51.

45. Sindic, C., Monteyne, P. and Laterre, E. (1994) The intrathecal synthesis of virus-specific oligoclonal IgG in multiple sclerosis. *J. Neuroimmunol.*, **54**, 75–80.

46. Cohen, S.R., Brooks, B.R., Herndon, R.M. and McKhann, G.M. (1980) A diagnostic index of active demyelination: myelin basic protein in cerebrospinal fluid. *Ann. Neurol.*, **8**, 25–31.

47. Whitaker, J.N. and Herman, P.K. (1988) Human myelin basic protein peptide 69–89: immunochemical features and use in immunoassay of cerebrospinal fluid. *J. Neuroimmunol.*, **19**, 47–57.

48. Peter, J. (1993–1994) *Use and Interpretation of Tests in Neuroimmunology*, 2nd edn, Specialty Laboratories Inc., 2211 Michigan Avenue, Santa Monica, CA 90404–3900, pp. 179–81.

49. Whitaker, J., Lisak, R., Bashir, R. *et al.* (1980) Immunoreactive myelin basic protein in the cerebrospinal fluid in neurological disorders. *Ann. Neurol.*, **7** (1), 58–64.

50. Whitaker, J.K., Layton, B., Herman, P.K. *et al.* (1993) Correlation of myelin basic protein-like material in cerebrospinal fluid of multiple sclerosis patients with their responses to glucocorticoid treatment. *Ann. Neurol.*, **33**, 10–17.

51. Whitaker, J., Williams, P., Layton, B.E. *et al.* (1994) Correlation of clinical features and findings on cranial magnetic resonance imaging with urinary myelin basic protein like material in patients with multiple sclerosis. *Ann. Neurol.*, **35** (5), 577–85.

52. Whitaker, J., Kachelhofer, R., Bradley, E. *et al.* (1995) Urinary myelin basic protein-like material as a correlate of the progression of multiple sclerosis. *Ann. Neurol.*, **38**, 625–32.

53. Warren, K.G. and Catz, I. (1993) Autoantibodies to myelin basic protein within multiple sclerosis central nervous system tissue. *J. Neurol. Sci.*, **115**, 169–76.

54. Warren, K.G. and Catz, I. (1993) Increased synthetic peptide specificity of tissue-CSF bound anti-MBP in multiple sclerosis. *J. Neuroimmunol.*, **43**, 87–96.

55. The Multiple Sclerosis Study Group (1990) Efficacy and toxicity of cyclosporine in chronic progressive multiple sclerosis: a randomized, double-blind, placebo-controlled clinical trial. *Ann. Neurol.*, **27**, 591–605.

56. Andersson, M., Alvarez-Cermeno, J., Benardi, G. *et al.* (1994) Cerebrospinal fluid in the diagnosis of multiple sclerosis: a consensus report. *J. Neurol. Neurosurg. Psychiatry*, **57**(8), 897–902.

57. Hirsche, E.A.H. and van der Helm, H.J. (1987) Rate of synthesis of IgG within the blood–brain barrier and the IgG index compared in the diagnosis of multiple sclerosis. *Clin. Chem.*, **33**, 113–14.

58. Hauser, S.L., Reinherz, E.L., Hoban, C.J., Schlossman, S.F. and Weiner, H.L. (1983) Immunoregulatory T-cells and lymphocytoxic antibodies in active multiple sclerosis: weekly analysis over a six month period. *Ann. Neurol.*, **13**, 418–25.

59. Bamborschke, S. and Heiss, W.D. (1987) Cerebrospinal fluid and peripheral blood leukocyte subsets in acute inflammation of the CNS. *J. Neurol. Sci.*, **79**, 1–2.

60. Reder, A.T. and Arnason, B.G.W. (1985) Immunology of multiple sclerosis, in *Handbook of Clinical Neurology*, **3** (eds P. Vinken, G. Bruyn, H. Klawans and J. Koetsier), vol. 47, *Demyelinating Diseases*, Amsterdam, Elsevier, pp. 337–95.

61. Noronha, A.B.C., Richman, D.P. and Arnason, B.G.W. (1980) Detection of in vivo stimulated cerebrospinal fluid lymphocytes by flow cytometry in patients with multiple sclerosis. *N. Engl. J. Med.*, **303**, 713–17.

62. Olsson, T., Baig, S., Höjeberg, B. and Link, H. (1989) Antimyelin basic protein and antimyelin antibody producing cells in multiple sclerosis. *Ann. Neurol.*, **27**, 132–6.

63. Calder, V., Owen, S., Watson, C., Feidmann, M. and Davison, A. (1989) MS: a localized immune disease of the central nervous system. *Immunol. Today*, **10** (3), 99–103.

64. Olsson, T. (1994) Multiple sclerosis: cerebrospinal fluid. *Ann. Neurol.*, **36** (Suppl.), S100–S102.

65. Olsson, T. (1992) Cytokines in neuroinflammatory disease: role of myelin autoreative T cell production of interferon-gamma. *J. Neuroimmunol.*, **40**, (2–3), 211–18.

66. IFNβ Multiple Sclerosis Study Group and University of British Columbia MS/MRI Analysis Group (1993) Interferon beta-1b is effective in relapsing remitting multiple sclerosis: I Clinical results of a multicenter, randomized, double-blind, placebo-controlled trial. *Neurology*, **43**, 655–61.

67. Rowe, P. (1994) Clinical potential for TGF-beta. *Lancet*, **344**, 72–3.

68. Mattson, D.H., Roos, R.P. and Arnason, B.G.W. (1980) Isoelectric focusing of IgG eluted from multiple sclerosis and subacute sclerosing panencephalitis brains. *Nature*, **287**, 335–7.

69. Mattson, D.H., Roos, R.P. and Arnason, B.G.W. (1981) Comparison of agar gel electrophoresis and isoelectric focusing in multiple sclerosis and subacute sclerosing panencephalitis. *Ann. Neurol.*, **9**, 34–41.

70. Whitaker, J.N., Benveniste, E.N. and Zhou, S. (1990) Cerebrospinal fluid, in *Handbook of Multiple Sclerosis* (ed. S. Cook), New York, Marcel Dekker, pp. 251–70.

71. Reder, A.T., Antel, J.P., Oger, J.J.-F. *et al.* (1984) Low T8 antigen density of lymphocytes in active multiple sclerosis. *Ann. Neurol.*, **16**, 242–9.

72. Warren, K.G. and Catz, I. (1986) Diagnostic value of cerebrospinal fluid anti-myelin basic protein in patients with multiple sclerosis. *Ann. Neurol.*, **20**, 20–5.

73. Panitch, H.S., Hooper, C.J. and Johnson, K.P. (1980) CSF antibody to myelin basic proteins: measurement in patients with multiple sclerosis and subacute sclerosing panencephalitis. *Arch. Neurol.*, **37**, 206–9.

74. Bashir, R.M. and Whitaker, J.N. (1980) Molecular features of immunoreactive myelin basic protein in cerebrospinal fluid of persons with multiple sclerosis. *Ann. Neurol.*, **7**, 50–7.

75. Challoner, P., Smith, K., Parker, J. *et al.* (1995) Plaque-associated expression of human herpes virus 6 in multiple sclerosis. *Proc. Natl Acad. Sci.*, **92**, 7440–4.

76. Conrad, A., Chiang, E.Y., Andeen, L. *et al.* (1994) Quantitation of intrathecal measles virus IgG synthesis rate: subacute sclerosing panencephalitis and MS. *J. Neuroimmunol.*, **54**, 99–108.

77. Tourtellotte, W.W., Shapshak, P., Staugaitis, S.M. and Saxton, R.E. (1984) Hypothesis: multiple sclerosis cerebrospinal fluid IgG multiple bands are derived from one or a few IgG secretor cell clones, in *Experimental Allergic Encephalomyelitis. a Useful Model for Multiple Sclerosis* (eds E. C.J. Alvord, M.W. Kies and A.J. Suckling), New York, Alan R. Liss, pp. 371–8.

78. Kleine, T.O. and Haak, B. (1985) Heterogeneous oligoclonal pattern of CSF immunoglobulins analyzed by isoelectrofocusing on polyacrylamide gels: due to different oligosaccharide content?, in *Protides of the Biological Fluids* (ed. H. Peeters), New York, Pergamon Press, pp. 217–18.

79. Peter, J.B., Bowman, R.L. and Bowman, R.L.J. (1987) Blood or plasma contamination of CSF: effect on CNS IgG synthesis rate and IgG index. *Am. J. Clin. Pathol.*, **87**(3), 422.

80. Walsh, M.J., Tourtellotte, W.W., Roman, J. and Dreyer, W. (1985) Immunoglobulin G, A, and M-clonal restriction in multiple sclerosis cerebrospinal fluid and serum-analysis by two-dimensional electrophoresis. *Clin. Immunol. Immunopathol*, **35**, 313–27.

81. Tourtellotte, W.W. and Parker, J.A. (1966) Multiple sclerosis: correlation between IgG in cerebrospinal fluid and brain. *Science*, **154**, 1044–6.

82. Tourtellotte, W.W. and Parker, J.A. (1967) Some spaces and barriers in postmortem multiple sclerosis, in *Progress in Brain Research* (eds A. Lajtha and D.H. Ford), Amsterdam, Elsevier, vol. 29, pp. 493–522.

83. Mingioli, E.S., Strober, W., Tourtellotte, W.W. *et al.* (1978) Quantitation of IgG, IgA and IgM in the CSF by radioimmunoassay. *Neurology.*, **28**, 991–5.

84. Sindic, C., Delacroix, D., Vaerman, J., Laterre, E.C. and Masson, P.L. (1984) Study of IgA in the cerebrospinal fluid of neurological patients with special reference to size, subclass and local production. *J. Neuroimmunol.*, **7**, 65–75.

85. Williams, A.C., Mingioli, E.S., McFarland, H.F., Tourtellotte, W.W. and McFarlin, D.E. (1978) Increased CSF IgM in multiple sclerosis. *Neurology*, **28**, 996–8.

86. Sindic, C., Cambiaso, C., Depré, A., Laterre, E. and Masson, P. (1982) The concentration of IgM in the cerebrospinal fluid of neurological patients. *J. Neurol. Sci.*, **55**, 339–50.

87. Forsberg, P., Henriksson, A., Link, H. and Ohman, S. (1984) Reference values for CSF-IgM, CSF IgM/S-IgM ratio and IgM index, and its application to patients with multiple sclerosis and aseptic meningoencephalitis. *Scand. J. Clin. Lab. Invest.*, **44**, 7–12.

88. Fagnart, O.C., Sindic, C.M.J. and Laterre, C. (1988) Free kappa and lambda light chain levels in the cerebrospinal fluid of patients with multiple sclerosis and other neurological diseases. *J. Neuroimmunol.* **19**, 119–32.

89. Gallo, P., Piccinno, M., Pagni, S. and Tavolato, B. (1988) Interleukin-2 levels in serum and cerebrospinal fluid of multiple sclerosis patients. *Ann. Neurol.*, **24**, 795–7.

90. Laurenzi, M.A., Mavra, M., Kam-Hansen, S. and Link, H. (1980) Oligoclonal IgG and free light chains in multiple sclerosis demonstrated by thin-layer polycrylamide gel isoelectric focusing and immunofixation. *Ann. Neurol.*, **8**, 241–7.

91. Lolli, F., Siracusa, G., Amato, M.P. *et al.* (1991) Intrathecal synthesis of free immunoglobulin light chains and IgM in initial multiple sclerosis. *Acta Neurol. Scand.*, **83**, 239–43.

92. Rudick, R.A. (1987) Free light chain of immunoglobulins in multiple sclerosis: a putative index of the intrathecal humoral immune response, in *Cellular and Humoral Immunological Components of Cerebrospinal Fluid in Multiple Sclerosis* (eds A. Lowenthal and J. Raus), New York, Plenum, pp. 187–200.

93. Rudick, R.A., French, C.A., Breton, D. and Williams, G.W. (1989) Relative diagnostic value of cerebrospinal fluid kappa chains in MS: comparison with other immunoglobulin tests. *Neurology*, **39**, 946–68.

94. Rudick, R.A., Pallant, A., Bidlack, J.M. and Herndon, R.M. (1986) Free kappa light chains in multiple sclerosis spinal fluid. *Ann. Neurol.*, **20**, 63–9.

95. Stanescu, G.L., Swick, A.R., Tuohy, V.K. and Rudick, R.A. (1991) Sensitive competitive-binding ELISAs for quantifying free kappa and lambda light chains in cerebrospinal fluid. *J. Clin. Lab. Anal.*, **5**, 206–11.

96. Trotter, K. and Brooks, B.R. (1980) Pathophysiology of cerebrospinal fluid immunoglobulins, in *Neurobiology of Cerebrospinal Fluid* (ed J. Wood), New York, Plenum Press, pp. 465–486.

97. Vakaet, A. and Thompson, E.J. (1985) Free light chains in cerebrospinal fluid – an indicator of recent immunological stimulation? *J. Neurol. Neurosurg. Psychiatry*, **48**, 995–8.

98. Esiri, M. (1980) Multiple sclerosis – a quantitative and qualitative study of immunoglobulin-containing cells in the central nervous system. *Neuropathol. Appl. Neurobiol.*, **6**, 9–21.

99. Rudick, R.A. and Whitaker, J.N. (1987) Cerebrospinal fluid tests for multiple sclerosis, in *Neurology and Neurosurgery Update Series* (eds Continuing Professional Education Center, Princeton, NJ), **7**, Lesson 21.

100. Mehta, P., Cook, S., Troiano, R. and Coyle, P. (1991) Increased free light chains in the urine from patients with multiple sclerosis. *Neurology*, **41**, 540–44.

101. Constantinescu, C., Mehta, P. and Rostami, A. (1994) Urinary free kappa light chain levels in chronic progressive multiple sclerosis. *Pathobiology*, **62**, 29–33.

102. Coyle, P.K. and Wolinsky, J.S. (1981) Characterization of immune complexes in progressive rubella panencephalitis. *Ann. Neurol.* **9**, 557–61.

103. Brooks, B.R., Coyle, P.K. and Hirsch, R.L. (1983) Cellular and humoral immune responses in human cerebrospinal fluid, in *The Neurobiology of Cerebrospinal Fluid* (ed. J. Wood), New York, Plenum Press, pp. 263–329.

104. Coyle, P.K. (1985) CSF immune complexes in multiple sclerosis. *Neurology*, **35**, 429–31.

105. Dasgupta, M.K., McPherson, T.A., Catz, I., Warren, K.G. and Dossetor, J.B. (1984) Identification of myelin basic protein (MBP) as an antigenic component of circulating immune complexes (CIC) in MS patients, in *Immunological and Clinical Aspects of Multiple Sclerosis* (eds R. Gonsette and P. Delmotte), Boston, MA, MTP Press pp. 40–6.

106. Procaccia, S., Lanzanova, D., Caputo, D. *et al.* (1988) Circulating immune complexes in serum and in cerebrospinal fluid of patients with multiple sclerosis. *Acta Neurol. Scand.*, **77**, 373–81.

107. Lund, G.A., Arnadottir, T., Hukkanen, V. *et al.* (1983) Detection and characterization of immune complexes in multiple sclerosis patients, in *Actual Problems in Multiple Sclerosis Research* (eds E. Pedersen, J. Clausen and L. Oades), Copenhagen: FADL's Forlag, pp. 277–80.

108. Pedersen, I.R. and Zeeberg, I. (1984) Immunoelectrophoretic characterization of immune complexes from CSF of multiple sclerosis patients, in *Immunological and Clinical Aspects of Multiple Sclerosis* (eds R. Gonsette and P. Delmotte), Boston, MA, MTP Press, pp. 24–7.

109. Jans, H., Heltberg, A., Zeeberg, P. *et al.* (1984) Immune complexes and the complement factors C4 and C3 in cerebrospinal fluid and serum from patients with chronic progressive multiple sclerosis. *Acta Neurol. Scand*, **69**, 34–38.

110. Morgan, B.P., Campbell, A.K. and Compston, D.A.S. (1984) Terminal component of complement (C9) in cerebrospinal fluid of patients with multiple sclerosis. *Lancet*, ii, 251–4.

111. Anonymous (1984) Coming to terms with complement (Editorial). *Lancet*, ii, 264–5.

112. Peter, J., Mc Keown, K. and Agopian, M. (1992) Assessment of different methods to detect increased autochthonous production of immunoglobulin G and oligoclonal immunoglobulins in multiple sclerosis. *Am. J. Clin. Pathol.*, **97**(6), 858–60.

113. Dinarello, C.A. (1991) The proinflammatory cytokines interleukin-1 and tumor necrosis factor and treatment of the septic shock syndrome. *J. Infect. Dis.*, **163**, 1177–84.

114. Hauser, S.L., Doolittle, T.H., Lincoln, R., Brown, R.H. and Dinarello, C.A. (1990) Cytokine accumulations in CSF of multiple sclerosis patients: frequent detection of interleukin-1 and tumor necrosis factor but not interleukin-6. *Neurology*, **40**, 1735–9.

115. Adachi, K., Kumamoto, T. and Araki, S. (1989) Interleukin-2 receptor levels indicating relapse in multiple sclerosis. *Lancet*, **i**, 559–600.

116. Trotter, J., Clifford, D., Andersen, C. *et al.* (1988) Elevated serum interleukin-2 levels in chronic progressive multiple sclerosis [Letter]. *N. Engl. J. Med.*, **318**, 1206.

117. Schindler, R., Mancilla, J., Endres, S. *et al.* (1990) Correlations and interactions in the production of interleukin-6 (IL-6), IL-1, and tumor necrosis factor (TNF) in human blood mononuclear cells: IL-6 suppresses IL-1 and TNF. *Blood*, **75**(1), 40–7.

118. Maimone, D., Gregory, S., Arnason, B.G. and Reder, A.T. (1991) Cytokine levels in the CSF and serum of patients with multiple sclerosis. *J. Neuroimmunol.*, **32**, 67–74.

119. Larrick, J.W. and Wright, S.C. (1990) Cytotoxic mechanism of tumor necrosis factor-α. *FASEB J.*, **4**, 3215–23.

120. Nathan, C.F. (1987) Secretory products of macrophages. *J. Clin. Invest.*, **79**, 319–26.

121. Tracy, K.J., Vlassara, H. and Cerami, A. (1989) Cachectin/tumour necrosis factor. *Lancet*, **1**, 1122–6.

122. Sharief, M.K. and Hentges, R. (1991) Association between tumor necrosis factor-α and disease progression in patients with multiple sclerosis. *N. Engl. J. Med.*, **325**, 467–72.

123. Hirsch, R.L., Panitch, H.S. and Johnson, K.P. (1985) Lymphocytes from multiple sclerosis patients produce elevated levels of gamma interferon in vitro. *J. Clin. Immunol.*, **5/6**, 386–9.

124. Rieckmann, P., Albrecht, M., Kitze, B. *et al.* (1994) Cytokine m RNA levels in mononuclear blood cells from patients with multiple sclerosis. *Neurology*, **44**, 1523.

125. Rieckmann, P., Martin, S., Albrecht, M. *et al.* (1994) Serial analysis of circulating adhesion molecules and TNF receptor in serum from patients with multiple sclerosis. C ICAM-1 is an indicator for relapse. *Neurology*, **44**, 2367–72.

126. Rieckmann, P., Albrecht, M., Kitze, B. *et al.* (1995) Tumor necrosis factor messenger RNA expression in patients with relapsing–remitting multiple sclerosis is associated with disease activity. *Ann. Neurol.*, **37**, 82–8.

127. Sharief, M., Noori, M., Ciardi, M., Cirelli, A. and Thompson, E. (1993) Increased levels of circulation ICAM-1 in serum and cerebrospinal fluid of patients with active multiple sclerosis. Correlation with TNF-α and blood–brain barrier damage. *J. Neuroimmunol.*, **43**, 15–22.

128. Rose, A.S., Kuzma, J.W., Kurtzke, J.F. *et al.* (1970) Cooperative study in the evaluation of therapy in multiple sclerosis: ACTH vs placebo. *Neurology*, **20**, 1–59.

129. Anmarkrud, N. and Slettnes, O. (1989) Uncomplicated retrobulbar neuritis and the development of multiple sclerosis. *Acta Ophthalmol.*, **67**, 306–9.

130. Schipper, H., Neumayer, H. and Poser, S. (1984) Prognostischer Wert der lokalen IgG-Produktion bei monosymptomatischer Optikusneuritis. *Akt. Neurol.*, **11**, 73–6.

131. Stendahl-Brodin, L. and Link, H. (1983) Optic neuritis: oligoclonal bands increase the risk of multiple sclerosis. *Acta Neurol. Scand.*, **67**, 301–4.

132. Frederiksen, J., Larsson, H. and Olessen, J. (1992) Correlation of magnetic resonance imaging and CSF findings in patients with acute monosymptomatic optic neuritis. *Acta Neurol. Scand.*, **86**, 317–22.

133. Sandberg-Wollheim, M. (1975) Optic neuritis: studies on the cerebrospinal fluid in relation to clinical course in 61 patients. *Acta Neurol. Scand.*, **52**, 167–78.

134. Filippini, G., Comi, G., Cosi, V. *et al.* (1994) Sensitivities and predictive values of paraclinical tests for diagnosing multiple sclerosis. *J. Neurol.*, **241**, 132–7.

135. Jacobs, L., Salazar, A.M., Herndon, R. *et al.* (1986) Multicentre double-blind study of effect of intrathecally administered natural human fibroblast interferon on exacerbations of multiple sclerosis. *Lancet*, **ii**, 1411–13.

136. Paty, D.W., Oger, J.J.F., Kastrukoff, L.F. *et al.* (1988) MRI in the diagnosis of MS: a prospective study with comparison of clinical evaluation, evoked potentials, oligoclonal banding, and CT. *Neurology*, **38**, 180–5.

137. Beck, R.W., Cleary, P.A., Anderson Jr, M. *et al.* (1992) A randomized, controlled trial of corticosteroids in the treatment of acute optic neuritis. The Optic Neuritis Study Group. *N. Engl. J. Med.*, **326**(9), 581–8.

138. Baumhefner, R.W., Tourtellotte, W.W., Syndulko, K. and Shapshak, P. (1986) Neuroimmunologic pharmacology of multiple sclerosis. II. Evaluation of immunosuppressive agents, in *Immunotherapies in Multiple Sclerosis* (eds O.R. Hommes, J. Mertin and W.W. Tourtellotte), Suffolk, UK, Stuart Phillips Publications, St Edmundsbury Press, pp. 226–36.

139. Baumhefner, R.W., Tourtellotte, W.W., Syndulko, K. *et al.* (1988) Copolymer I as therapy for multiple sclerosis: the cons. *Neurology*, **38** (Suppl. 2), 69–71.

140. Baumhefner, R.W., Tourtellotte, W.W., Syndulko, K., Staugaitis, A. and Shapshak, P. (1989) Multiple sclerosis intra-blood–brain-barrier IgG synthesis: effect of pulse intravenous and intrathecal corticosteriods. *Ital. J. Neurol. Sci.* **10**, 19–32.

141. Beutler, E., Koziol, J., McMillan, R. *et al.* (1994) Marrow suppression produced by repeated doses of cladribine. *Acta Haematol.*, **91**, 10–15.

142. Jones, H.D., Urquhart, N., Mathias, R.G. and Banerjee, S.N. (1990) An evaluation of oligoclonal banding and CSF IgG index in the diagnosis of neurosyphilis. *Sex. Transm. Dis.*, **17**, 75–9.

143. Tourtellotte, W.W., Haerer, A.F., Heller, G.L. and Somers, J.E. (1964) *Post-Lumbar Puncture Headaches*. Springfield, IL, Charles C. Thomas.

144. Kuntz, K.M., Kokmen, E., Stevens, J.C. *et al.* (1992) Post-lumbar puncture headaches: experience in 501 consecutive procedures. *Neurology*, **42**, 1884–7.

145. Tourtellotte, W.W., Henderson, W.G., Tucker, R.P. *et al.* (1972) A randomized, double-blind clinical trial comparing the 22 versus 26 gauge needle in the production of the post-lumbar puncture syndrome in normal individuals. *Headache*, **12** (2), 73–8.

146. Ellison, G.W., Myers, L.W., Mickey, M.R. *et al.* (1989) A placebo controlled, randomized, double-masked, variable dosage, clinical trial of azathioprine with and without methylprednisolone in multiple sclerosis. *Neurology*, **39**, 1018–26.

147. Hall, W. and Choppin, P. (1981) Measles-virus proteins in the brain tissues of patients with subacute sclerosing panencephalitis. *N. Engl. J. Med.*, **304**, 1152.

6 THE NATURAL HISTORY OF MULTIPLE SCLEROSIS

Brian G. Weinshenker

6.1 Introduction

The natural history of MS refers to the course of MS unaltered by treatment. The natural history of MS must be considered both over the short term (5 years or less), which is relevant to clinical therapeutic trials, and over the long term (more than 5 years), which is ultimately most important to influence favorably by treatment. Given the widespread use of corticosteroid or ACTH treatment for acute exacerbations of MS over the last 20 years, most would accept data from patients treated in this way as natural history data, especially given the best available evidence which suggests that steroids do not significantly alter the ultimate recovery from an attack of MS, merely the rate of recovery[1]. The descriptors of the natural history are both qualitative (disease type and disease state) and quantitative (attack frequency, impairment and disability scores).

The nosology of MS remains uncertain. The diagnosis of MS (Chapter 1), is generally made on clinical grounds based on recurrent or progressive symptoms and signs of central white matter dysfunction, supported by paraclinical studies such as MRI, evoked potentials and CSF studies. However, the ultimate confirmation of multiple sclerosis is based on demonstration of multiple areas of inflammatory demyelinating lesions ('plaques') in the central nervous system. Diagnostic criteria, which are used to define the diagnosis, such as the Poser criteria[2], are clinically valuable but scientifically arbitrary and are generally based on the principle of demonstrating 'lesions disseminated in time and space'. Some diseases, often excluded from the general rubric of MS, differ in distribution, chronicity and severity of white matter inflammation and demyelination. Until they can be distinguished based on etiology and pathophysiology, however, these disorders are best considered under the general rubric 'idiopathic inflammatory demyelinating diseases of the central nervous system', of which MS is the prototype.

The course of MS is difficult to define with a single outcome measure. Early in the course of the prototypic relapsing-remitting form of MS, patients experience exacerbations of impairment reflecting a more or less random distribution of lesions in the neuraxis. Later, a rather typical sequence of deterioration occurs involving, in order, lower extremity and sphincter function, upper extremity function, and bulbar function, although the disease may seemingly 'arrest' after a period of time before the full spectrum of potential impairment is evident. Definition of an optimal and comprehensive scale or set of scales which express the variability in impairments and disabilities encountered in MS patients and adequately measure the evolution of MS both over the short term of clinical trials and over the long term of decades has remained elusive. A task force of the National Multiple Sclerosis Society has been charged with developing such a scale over the next two years. The expanded disability status scale (EDSS) and functional symptoms score (FS) developed by Kurtzke are currently the most widely accepted and officially sanctioned measures of the course of multiple sclerosis.

Survival of MS patients is less than that of the age- and sex-matched general population, but MS rarely causes death in its own right; rather it can result in severe disability which leads to medical complications, which may cause death. Most of the excess deaths in MS patients occur in those with advanced disability. MS can be a 'benign' disease, generally defined by EDSS scores of ≤ 3 after 10 years. The frequency of benign disease has increased, primarily through improved recognition and ascertainment of mild cases in community-based studies.

This chapter will review the nosology of MS and related idiopathic, inflammatory, demyelinating disorders of the central nervous system. The different disease states of multiple sclerosis, and quantitative measures which assess disease progression will be discussed. Predictors of the evolution and outcome of MS will be considered. Finally, the application of knowledge regarding the natural history of MS to the design and interpretation of clinical therapeutic trials will be discussed.

Multiple Sclerosis: Clinical and pathogenetic basis. Edited by Cedric S. Raine, Henry F. McFarland and Wallace W. Tourtellotte. Published in 1997 by Chapman & Hall, London. ISBN 0 412 30890 8.

6.2　The nosology of multiple sclerosis

A number of disorders exist on the fringe of MS, the exact relationship of which to the prototypic disease remains uncertain. These idiopathic inflammatory disorders of the central nervous system are depicted graphically in Figure 6.1.

Optic neuritis and other limited monophasic demyelinating disorders are often indistinguishable from attacks of multiple sclerosis. Acute, incomplete transverse myelitis may more frequently be a harbinger of MS than complete, transverse myelitis [3, 4], but ascertainment and follow-up have not been comparable in examining the natural history of incomplete and complete transverse myelitis studies. Eighty per cent of patients with partial acute transverse myelitis 'convert' to MS within the mean follow-up period of 3 years in one study [3]. Acute transverse myelitis, even when recurrent, may be associated with other discernible and possibly treatable disorders such as herpes simplex virus infection [5] and anticardiolipin antibodies [6]. Therefore, acute transverse myelitis is best regarded as a syndrome, and not always 'an idiopathic' demyelinating disease. Sixty-four per cent of patients followed at the Mayo Clinic with optic neuritis 'converted' to multiple sclerosis by 40 years following the first episode of optic neuritis; 37% had converted to multiple sclerosis within 10 years [7]. The presence of and number of lesions on MRI scan seems to predict conversion from optic neuritis to MS, probably better than any other clinical manifestation [8].

Marburg's variant of MS is an acute severe demyelinating syndrome, generally with multifocal cerebral involvement and often associated with mass effect; a cerebral herniation syndrome, which may be refractory to treatment, has developed and this condition may occasionally be fatal [9]. MS may present as a focal enhancing mass lesion that can be confused with a brain tumor [10]. Acute disseminated encephalomyelitis is generally diagnosed when an acute monophasic demyelinating syndrome with prominent cerebral involvement appears following a viral infection or vaccination. Pathologically and by MRI, acute disseminated encephalomyelitis cannot be reliably distinguished from MS [11] (see Chapter 9).

Devic's syndrome, or neuromyelitis optica, is a syndrome of bilateral optic neuritis and transverse myelopathy, usually occurring in rapid succession (Chapter 2). The course of Devic's syndrome is often severe and recovery from acute episodes is poor. Repeated attacks are common. Pathologically, necrosis and prominent thickening and hyalinization of small vessels are seen. CSF studies are typically negative for oligoclonal bands and elevated immunoglobulin production. MRI scans of the brain are usually negative [12]. A recent review of neuromyelitis optica at the Mayo Clinic reveals that this syndrome is heterogeneous, with some cases being monophasic but an equal number following a relapsing and remitting course with spread beyond the optic nerves and spinal cord. The pathological differences from MS may reflect the severity and chronicity of the inflammatory demyelinating process and not a unique pathogenesis. Recently, it has been suggested that a mitochondrial DNA mutation similar to that associated with a Leber's optic atrophy may account for some cases of a Devic's-like illness [13].

A variant of multiple sclerosis is primary-progressive multiple sclerosis, which most commonly presents as a chronic progressive myelopathy but occasionally as a chronic progressive cerebellar syndrome. There may be cerebral lesions on MRI, but generally there are many fewer lesions than encountered in relapsing-remitting, or relapsing-remitting with secondarily progressive multiple sclerosis [14]. Immunogenetic differences, specifically an excess of individuals with the DR4, DQ8 major histocompatibility haplotype [15], have been reported, although this has not been confirmed in other studies [16] (Chapter 13). There have also been reports that this variant of multiple sclerosis is more refractory to immunosuppressive therapy than those with initially relapsing-remitting disease [17].

For the remainder of the chapter, the discussion will be based on MS as defined by standard criteria, which generally exclude isolated demyelinating syndromes. Devic's syndrome has generally been considered as distinct from MS, although this distinction is not based on an understanding of the etiology of either condition. Primary-progressive MS is generally considered as a variant of MS, and will be included in the discussion that follows.

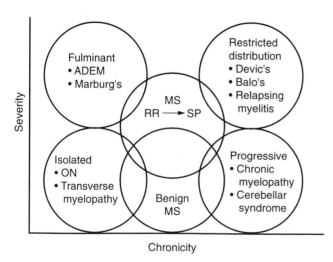

Figure 6.1　The spectrum of idiopathic inflammatory demyelinating diseases of the central nervous system.

6.3 Describing and measuring the outcome of MS

6.3.1 DISEASE STATE

MS has generally been described in terms of a series of disease states – relapsing-remitting (RR), relapsing-progressive (RP), secondary-progressive (SP) and primary-progressive (PP). The definition of these disease states has been subject to controversy and has recently been modified based on a consensus of the Medical Advisory Board of the National MS Society (Figure 6.2). The RR state is encountered in approximately 70% of MS patients, the RP variety in 15% and PP variety in 15% [18]. Of those with RR disease, roughly 50% will have converted to an SP form of MS within 10 years [18, 19]. Relapses tend to affect the central nervous system in a somewhat random fashion and can present as optic neuritis, myelopathy, or oculomotor disturbance, albeit some manifestations such as ascending dorsal column myelopathies are distinctly more common than others; some manifestations, such as, IIIrd nerve palsy, are very rare. However, most individuals who acquire fixed, moderate or greater disability from MS do so in the context of progressive disease and not as a sequel to attacks of relapsing-remitting disease. The long-term outcome and disease burden in most MS patients usually manifests as a progressive paraparesis, followed by upper extremity and then by bulbar impairment, presumably reflecting the frequency and importance of spinal cord disease in MS, and, possibly, the importance of fiber length when axons ultimately undergo degeneration after repeated episodes of inflammatory demyelination [20].

In relapsing-remitting (bout-onset) disease, the major descriptors of the course are the attack frequency and severity. The average attack frequency in the control groups in many prospective clinical trials of patients selected for having active MS is 1–1.5 attacks per year.

In retrospective studies of natural history, the reported attack frequency varies widely from 0.1 to 1 per year. The discrepancy is in large part due to the fact that many mild attacks are overlooked or forgotten in retrospective studies and selection biases are present in prospective studies. There is general agreement that attack frequency declines over time in MS patients. In a prospective follow-up study, Goodkin found that over the short term comparable to the follow-up in a clinical trial, the attack frequency did not decline significantly [21]. However, in clinical trials, decline in attack frequency is almost consistently seen in the placebo groups, likely due to 'regression to the mean', a consequence of selection biases rather than a manifestation of natural history. Individuals selected for a clinical trial because of a high attack frequency are more likely to return to the population average than to sustain a high rate of attacks.

Conversion to a progressive course of MS occurs in 50% of patients with bout-onset MS within 10 years according to a recent Swedish study [19]. This is in accord with a Dutch study which found that conversion to secondarily progressive disease occurred within nine years of onset [22]. 'Progressive MS' is universally accepted as a harbinger of disability. However, prospective clinic-based studies by Goodkin at the Cleveland Clinic [21] and by Ellison et al. at UCLA [23], reveal that a high percentage of patients with 'progressive MS' might be reclassified as being stable within one to two years. The rate of deterioration in terms of EDSS scores once progressive MS has been identified, is approximately 0.5 EDSS points/year for the first five years [18]. The experience in clinical trials of patients with progressive MS shows that 30–50% of the placebo groups deteriorate by 1 EDSS point over 2–3 years follow-up, depending in part on the distribution of baseline EDSS scores at entry [24].

6.3.2 QUANTITATIVE INSTRUMENTS

It is undoubtedly important to quantitate the results of the MS disease process on the function of an individual to address the natural history of MS and to arbitrate the outcome of clinical therapeutic trials. A comprehensive instrument has not yet been universally accepted, nor is it certain that a single clinical instrument can adequately cover the myriad of presentations and combinations of impairments and disabilities that are possible. An optimal instrument, according to a consensus statement from a recent National MS Society-sponsored workshop [25], must be:

1. sensitive to change over the short interval of a clinical trial;
2. reliable, i.e. objective and have high inter- and intra-rater reproducibility;

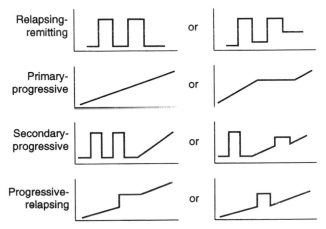

Figure 6.2 The temporal evolution of MS-related impairment in the prototypic disease states of MS based on the new criteria proposed by the National MS Society.

3. able to measure impairment caused by the disease that is clinically important;
4. a measure of components that reflect independent dimensions of disease (cognitive, upper extremity, lower extremity, sphincter etc.);
5. applicable to the range of MS impairments encountered clinically and avoid floor-and-ceiling effects;
6. easy to administer and cost-effective.

Early ordinal scales, such as those devised by McAlpine [26], were heavily oriented to mobility and had a few large steps. These scales were insensitive. While they could broadly classify MS patients in retrospective series for the study of natural history, they were inadequate for use in a clinical trial. Kurtzke developed two sets of scales, the disability status scale (DSS) and the functional scores (FS) for use in a clinical trial of isoniazid. The DSS was later expanded from a 10- to a 20-point scale, the EDSS. Scoring with these scales is determined by examination, except for determination of bladder and bowel function, which is done based on objective elements of the history. The FS, which define system-specific impairment, include pyramidal, cerebellar, sensory, brain stem, bladder and bowel, visual and other systems. Kurtzke points out that some (pyramidal, cerebellar, sensory, brain stem) are more frequently affected than others, and consequently he referred to these FS as major and to the others as minor. Recognizing the ceiling effects of these scores and that a summed score often reaches an unchanging value despite worsening disability, the (E)DSS was retained as a composite impairment score. In the 1.0–4.0 range, the EDSS is determined by the FS. Between 4.0 and 8.0, the scale was designed to reflect the most prominent clinical problem faced by MS patients, namely, ambulation. Beginning at EDSS 6.0, the scale evaluates both distance that can be walked and aids that are necessary to accomplish this task. At EDSS 8.0–9.0, lower extremity function is essentially lost and upper extremity function is the major determinant, whereas at 9.0, bulbar function is the main determinant. The problems with the EDSS include:

1. poor reliability due to imprecision of descriptive terms;
2. limited sensitivity for clinical trials;
3. 'nonlinear' nature and differences in observed staying time and probability of further 1 point worsening at different EDSS levels;
4. emphasis on ambulation in the broad and critical 4.0–8.0 range;
5. inadequate quantitation of mental function.

In parallel with the EDSS, Tourtellotte and others developed a battery of quantitative neuroperformance tests which provide timed measures of functions affected by MS, including cognitive function, finger tapping, foot tapping, tandem walking, and simulated activities of daily living (e.g., dressing, cutting with knife etc.). Syndulko *et al.*, have found that these tests are reproducible and sensitive to change [27]. The quantitative results are more statistically powerful. These tests had not achieved widespread acceptance or interest until recently. Concern has been raised over practice effects. Furthermore, the results of clinical trials expressed in seconds or fractions thereof of timed tests are unconvincing to the clinician as the reason to accept new treatments. None the less, if this approach can be shown to have predictive validity and to be feasible, the neuroperformance battery may become an important and widely used assessment technique.

Cognitive assessment in MS is becoming increasingly important as the frequency of cognitive dysfunction in MS is recognized [28]. However, severe dementia is an uncommon manifestation, affecting fewer than 5% of patients in population-based, cross-sectional studies [29]. The natural history of the neuropsychological test abnormalities in higher order cognitive function tests such as those requiring sustained concentration remains to be clarified, particularly as to whether they are harbingers of dementia.

Other methods of evaluating MS-related impairments, disabilities and handicaps are reviewed elsewhere. A classification of quantitative measures follows.

1. Measures based on scoring of the normal neurologic examination weighted according to the frequency of involvement in MS and role in producing impairment (e.g. Scripps neurological rating scale).
2. Ordinal impairment scales (e.g. EDSS and FS).
3. Disability and handicap scales, which evaluate dysfunction and activities of daily living and social adaptation, which are MS nonspecific (e.g. Functional Independence Measure, Incapacity Status Scale, Environmental Status Scale).
4. Quantitative neuroperformance tests which can be expressed as continuous parametric data, often as a percentage of normal function (e.g. the quantitative evaluation of neurological function of Tourtellotte; the 9-hole peg tests and box and blocks tests of upper extremity function; quantitative neuropsychological test batteries).
5. Global rating scales.
6. Hybrid scales (e.g. Ambulation Index, which is an ordinal scale which includes timed walking).
7. Self-rating scales to assess emotional and functional impact on general health and quality of life; this includes scales to rate fatigue.

It is too early to surmise the outcome of the current deliberations on the clinical outcome measures that will be the basis of measuring the natural history of MS and outcome of clinical trials in the future. Improved ordinal rating scales which provide a readily understandable but more precise picture of overall disease-specific impairment supplemented by quantitative neuroperformance scores to add sensitivity, will likely emerge. Proof of the predictive validity of neuroperformance scores will be crucial.

6.4   Mortality and survival

MS is generally not a fatal disease. The cause of death in MS patients can be classified as:

1. resulting from secondary complications, such as pneumonia, pulmonary embolus, and aspiration;
2. directly due to MS;
3. non-MS related;
4. suicide.

The majority of deaths are due to secondary complications in patients with advanced disability. There are rare exceptions. Marburg's variant of MS (see Chapter 9) has often been reported to be fatal, occasionally as a result of intractable cerebral herniation. Respiratory failure due to progressive upper cervical inflammatory demyelinating disease with diaphragmatic paralysis can occur rarely. Acute neurogenic pulmonary edema due to MS has been reported.

Death due to secondary complications of MS accounts for approximately 50–60% of deaths in patients followed in MS clinics [30]. The mortality ratio (observed to expected) was 4.4 for those with EDSS scores ≥ 7.5 (wheelchair-confined or worse) whereas it was 1.6 for those with mild disability (EDSS ≤ 3.5) and 1.36 if suicides were excluded [31]. The suicide rate has been reported to be increased seven-fold compared to the general population in Canada [30], whereas it was increased two-fold in a large Danish study [32]. The risk of suicide was highest in the first five years following the onset of MS, and the average EDSS scores of patients committing suicide was 4.5 in the Canadian study, a level of impairment compatible with being able to walk approximately two blocks without a walking aid; however, EDSS 4.5 is a level of impairment at which many patients with a relapsing–remitting course enter a secondarily progressive course, and at which MS-related impairments are no longer easily ignored or denied.

Early studies which reported survival in fatal cases give a misleading impression that survival is reduced to a major extent in multiple sclerosis. Prospective studies of survival have been conducted in Olmsted County (Minnesota) at the Mayo Clinic, in Norway, Scotland and Germany. The most complete data are those which emerged from a Danish study. In Denmark, there is a registry of MS with remarkably complete ascertainment [33]. The results from the Danish study are generally similar to those from Olmsted County, Min-

nesota and those of other population-based studies with adequate ascertainment. The Danish study is based on a registry of all patients with MS since 1948 who were classified as having definite, probable or possible MS according to widely accepted criteria. The median survival was 30 years from the onset of MS and 25 years from diagnosis. The 25-year survival probability was 62 ± 1.4% which is marginally lower than the results reported from Olmsted County, Minnesota [34]. Similar to the results obtained from the Mayo Clinic, the mortality ratio was significantly greater in men than women, primarily in those with onset at less than age 29.

The clinical and demographic associations with mortality rate were qualitatively similar in the Danish study to those that have been observed to be associated with probability of reaching advanced disability in a short time in population-based disability studies from London, Ontario [35] and Gothenberg, Sweden [36]. This is not surprising because most of the excess deaths in MS occurred in individuals with advanced disability and not as a result of acute attacks. The excess death rate was 8.6/1000 patient years for those with onset of MS at more than 20 years of age, whereas it was 19.1/1000 patient years for those with onset of MS at over 50 years of age. Purely sensory symptoms in males and optic neuritis in females as a first symptom were associated with 30–40% lower excess death rates than the rates for individuals who had cerebellar involvement at onset. Older age at onset was associated with a higher excess death rate.

While the Mayo Clinic study in Olmsted County, Minnesota, did not find any change in the survival of MS patients over the past seven decades [34], a major improvement in survival was reported from the Danish registry with a decline in the standardized mortality ratio from 4.60 in those with MS onset between 1948 and 1952 to 2.13 for those with onset of MS between 1971 and 1976 [33]. These results are not due to changes in the mortality rate of the general population. What is not clear from this study is whether the improved survival reflects lower rates of advanced disability or better care for the disabled.

6.5   Recovery from attacks

Most MS attacks are rated as mild. In the Betaseron (interferon beta-1b) clinical trial [37], the occurrence of mild attacks in the placebo control group was 0.54/year, whereas the occurrence of moderate and severe attacks occurred at 0.45/year; 20% of attacks were rated as being of unknown severity because patients were not examined at the height of their attack.

Many factors predict the outcome of attacks of MS. The rapidity of onset is strongly associated with recovery: the more rapid the onset, generally the better the recovery. The temporal course of MS is also a critical determinant. Attacks superimposed on a chronically progressive course are much less likely to recover in response to standard courses of steroid therapy. Severity of attacks also seems to be a factor. Kurtzke analyzed recovery from acute attacks in Second World War US Army recruits and found that improvement by ≥ 1 DSS point was equally likely, if not more likely, when an attack produced severe disability. However, he analyzed recovery in terms of improvement by 1 DSS point, and the significance of improvement by 1 DSS point is substantially less when there has been a major attack resulting in a DSS score of ≥ 7. Of 18 soldiers in the US Army during the Second World War who suffered an attack of MS and who had entry EDSS scores of 7–9 (nonambulatory), 39% did not improve at all and 17% improved by a single point. Forty-four per cent improved by 3 or more EDSS points[38]. While recovery from MS attacks can be protracted, in general, the probability of recovery drops markedly after one month following an acute attack[38].

Attacks of demyelination occurring in the context of Devic's syndrome tend to be more severe and are associated with lesser chance of recovery. A poor prognosis might be expected from the histopathology, which is usually encountered in Devic's syndrome, which is characterized by vascular thickening and prominent necrosis of the spinal cord[12].

Rare patients with fulminant presentations of demyelinating disease may die as a result of an acute attack, occasionally as a result of intractable cerebral herniation. In such fulminant syndromes, there may be a single focal cerebral demyelinating lesion producing mass effect or there may be multifocal central nervous system white matter involvement.

6.6   Disabilities and impairments

Most studies which have addressed the accumulation of disabilities and impairments in MS have used the EDSS or other ordinal scales which emphasize ambulation as an endpoint, as this is the most common and perhaps the easiest to quantitate impairment encountered in MS patients. Survival is an insensitive endpoint given the modest reduction in survival in MS patients compared to the general population. Recently, other endpoints, including cognitive dysfunction, have attracted greater interest because of heightened awareness of the impact of cognitive dysfunction, improved neuropsychological test batteries to assess cognitive dysfunction in MS and the strong association between cognitive dysfunction in MRI-determined lesion volume.

Two approaches have been used to evaluate MS-related impairment: cross-sectional analyses and longitudinal studies. Cross-sectional studies provide a 'snapshot' of the burden of disease in a community, while longitudinal studies with two or more serial evaluations provide data on the risk of disability for groups stratified by risk factors in both univariate and multivariate analyses.

Two longitudinal studies employing survival analysis to account for censored data (patients not reaching the endpoint over the follow-up period) are available in the literature. These studies are in whole or in part population-based, with reasonably complete ascertainment; one study is based on an incidence cohort of patients followed for 25 years. [19].

A recent cross-sectional survey from Olmsted County, Minnesota, at the Mayo Clinic reveals that the median EDSS score is 3.5, a level of disability compatible with unrestricted walking ability in 179 patients with definite (n = 162) or probable (n = 17) MS with a median duration of 15.4 years[29]. The distribution of disability scores was bimodal with relative peaks at EDSS 1 (neurological signs only) and 6.5 (bilateral assistance necessary for walking). Fourteen per cent were wheelchair-confined. Severe dementia requiring supervision was found in 4%. Twenty-four per cent had frequent incontinence or need for urinary catheterization. Thirty-three per cent were rated as having a marked para- or hemi-paresis, and 13% had severe cerebellar dysfunction.

Longitudinal studies reveal that 30–40% of patients could be classified as having benign MS, arbitrarily defined as a DSS score ≤ 3 (or equivalent) at 10 years following the first symptoms of MS[39–41]. McAlpine has shown that some patients with benign MS may develop more aggressive MS[39], but Kurtzke has pointed out that those with low DSS scores 5 years from the onset of MS are much more likely to continue to have a benign course than average[42].

Weinshenker *et al.*[18] and Runmarker and Andersen[19], have reported longitudinal studies of MS disability in London, Ontario and Gothenberg, Sweden, respectively. They find that 50% of patients have reached DSS 6 (aids required to walk a distance of one-half block) by 15 years, whereas fewer than 10% had reached DSS 8 (wheelchair-confined) by 15 years.

Cognitive dysfunction, especially in the spheres of recent memory, sustained attention, verbal fluency, conceptual reasoning and visuospatial perception, is encountered in 40% of MS patients[28]. Short-term follow-up over periods of 6 months to 2 years has shown relatively minor change. Whether the frequent cognitive changes in higher order functions encountered in MS patients are harbingers of the dementia encountered in 4% of MS patients in cross-sectional studies[29], awaits the results of longer observation in unbiased cohorts.

6.7 Predicting the outcome of MS

The outcome of MS is notoriously difficult to predict. Some disease inflammatory states are apparently associated with severe attacks and disability, such as Devic's syndrome. For the prototypic relapsing-remitting form of MS, the development of fixed disability generally occurs in the context of a progressive phase of the illness. Increasingly, the distinction between relapsing-remitting and progressive disease has become blurred. In individuals with secondary-progressive MS who have had attacks at some point in their course, it appears as if the MRI changes that are encountered are qualitatively similar when progressive MS supervenes, albeit there is a higher frequency of brain lesions developing per unit time [43]. Recently, it has been suggested that neuronal degeneration may be the end result of repeated inflammatory insults and may be the explanation for the progressive course. This hypothesis is based, in part, on MR spectroscopy studies which reveal a decline in neuronal biochemical markers such as N-acetyl aspartate in individuals with progressive MS [20]. However, in primary-progressive MS, there are many fewer lesions on MRI scans of the head than are encountered in either relapsing-remitting or secondary-progressive disease, despite a progressive course and poor prognosis [14]. Some have speculated that this may reflect the fact that much less inflammation might initiate a progressive neuronal degeneration in individuals with primary-progressive MS.

Since the rate of occurrence of MRI lesions is not routinely determined for individual patients, and since the biological basis for the differences in lesion frequency and pattern of disease (bout-onset versus progressive from onset) is unknown, most predictive studies have addressed clinical and demographic associations with the outcome of MS. A set of associations has emerged from these studies about which there is general, albeit incomplete, consensus. Younger age at onset, female gender, optic neuritis or purely sensory symptoms at onset, low attack frequency, complete symptom remission from a first attack and long first interattack interval are associated with a favorable outcome. Older age at onset (greater than 40 years), male gender, insidious pyramidal tract involvement, prominent cerebellar involvement, frequent attacks and early attainment of moderate fixed disability are generally associated with a poor prognosis [35, 36, 44, 45]. There is some variation in opinion about the influence of gender; however, the disability data suggesting worse outcome in males are supported by a greater reduction in survival in males with MS [33, 34]. Many of the observed associations are consistent with the hypothesis that greater activity of the MS disease process (higher attack frequency, more frequent attacks), and more severe attacks, as well as a tendency to involve systems which prominently affect ambulation are associated with a poor outcome. The association between attack frequency and disability is supported by recent observations that high rates of MRI lesion development early in the disease predicts a worse clinical outcome.

Mathematical models have been developed to predict the time to reach (E)DSS 6 or to develop progressive MS after the onset of symptoms using the associations described above [35, 36]. Accuracy is low for a given individual, and the primary value of such models is to identify subgroups with relatively more homogeneous risk of developing MS-related disability.

6.8 Implications of the natural history for clinical trials

The natural history of MS can be conceived in terms of long-term outcome and short-term outcome. The latter, which refers to the change in MS disabilities over 2–5 years has become particularly relevant given the proliferation of placebo-controlled randomized clinical trials over the past decade. The implications of successfully mollifying the course of MS over the short term on the long-term outcome of MS is uncertain. For practical purposes, however, the behavior of MS over a 2 to 3 year period is all that has been feasible to study in the context of a clinical trial (see also Chapter 19).

The EDSS has been the most widely used instrument to assess impairment in the context of clinical trials. Several difficulties have been encountered resulting from the use of the EDSS as a primary outcome measure [46].

1. The EDSS is open to statistical abuse. Mean change in EDSS, which has been used in several trials, assumes that change at different entry EDSS levels is comparable.
2. There is a relatively low event rate if a treatment failure definition is established requiring a 1 point decline in EDSS scores. In trials using this outcome measure, treatment failure has been encountered in 30–40% of individuals in the placebo group depending on the duration of the trial. A low event rate in the control group seriously compromises the power of a trial.
3. There appears to be substantial difference in the probability of worsening by 1 EDSS point depending on the entry EDSS level. Accordingly, the distribution of EDSS scores in the treatment and control groups may be sufficient to alter the outcome of a clinical trial, especially in a relatively small trial.
4. Inter-rater variability may exceed the definition of treatment failure, particularly at lower ranges of the EDSS where inter-rater variability is higher. The difficulties with inter-rater variation are compounded by the imprecision inherent in the FS, which are used to generate the EDSS at scores less than 4.0.

The low event rate and differences in probability of worsening depending on entry EDSS score may be at least in part circumvented by a modified definition of treatment failure, now widely used in clinical trials, whereby worsening of ≥ 0.5 points is accepted as treatment failure at higher levels of the EDSS (EDSS ≥ 5.5 or 6.0) [47]. At these higher levels, the staying time is longer and the probability of treatment failure is lower [48].

Objectivity may be enhanced by quantitative neuro-performance testing. Recently, a study of oral metho-trexate was shown to be effective in slowing the rate of deterioration in performing quantitative timed upper extremity functional testing (9-hole peg test, box and blocks test), although no other assessment was able to show a benefit [49]. Similar conclusions have been reached for a subset of patients evaluated in the context of the USA cyclosporin study in MS [27].

MRI provides added objectivity and seems to be an excellent short-term screening method for effective therapies which are promising for future phase II and III clinical trials. The addition of quantitative neuro-performance assessments of neurological function as discussed previously may increase sensitivity of clinical trials. However, these endpoints must be shown to have predictive validity, that is, to predict further more important degrees of deterioration.

6.9   Conclusions

The boundaries of MS are not clearly defined. The relationship between the prototypic relapsing-remitting disease with a later secondary-progressive course and other isolated demyelinating syndromes, and between prototypic MS and primary-progressive MS, remains uncertain. Sixty per cent of patients with MS experience the prototypic pattern of relapsing-remitting followed by secondary-progressive multiple sclerosis. Between 20 and 40% of MS patients have benign MS, but there is overlap between the 'benign MS' group of patients and other forms of MS. Approximately 15% of MS patients have a primary-progressive course. The average survival is 30 years from onset and 25 years from diagnosis. Survival is shortened by 15% at 25 years from the onset compared to an age-and-sex matched population. Death occurs primarily in severely disabled patients. Death resulting directly from attacks of MS is uncommon. Ambulation is most commonly impaired as a result of MS and MS-related impairment is usually quantitated by scales which emphasize ambulation. Fifty per cent of MS patients require walking aids to walk a distance of half a block within 15 years. Neuropsychological dysfunction is common, though severe dementia requiring supervision occurs in less than 5% in cross-sectional surveys in completely ascertained populations. A num-ber of clinical and demographic associations with the outcome of MS have been described. While these associations can be used to identify subgroups with greater or lesser risk of severe disability, multivariate regression models are weak in predicting outcome for individuals. Short-term worsening of disability, which is targeted in clinical trials, must be studied to determine its predictive validity for the long-term outcome of MS, particularly with the advent of treatments that can be applied in the early stages of MS with demonstrated short-term benefits on attack rate and on MRI-deter-mined lesion frequency.

ACKNOWLEDGMENTS

Laura Irlbeck and Lori Volkman provided expert assistance in the preparation of the manuscript.

References

1. Myers, L.W. (1992) Treatment of multiple sclerosis with ACTH and corticosteroids, in *Treatment of Multiple Sclerosis* (eds R.A. Rudick and D.E. Goodkin), Springer-Verlag, London, pp. 135–56.
2. Poser, C.M., Paty, D.W., Scheinberg, L. et al. (1983) New diagnostic criteria for multiple sclerosis: guidelines for research protocols. *Ann. Neurol.*, **13**, 227–31.
3. Ford, B., Tampieri, D. and Francis, G. (1992) Long-term follow-up of acute partial transverse myelopathy. *Neurology*, **42**, 250–2.
4. Ropper, A.H. and Poskanzer, D.C. (1978) Prognosis of acute and subacute transverse myelopathy based on early signs and symptoms. *Ann. Neurol.*, **4**, 51–9.
5. Shyu, W.C., Lin, J.C., Chang, B.C. et al. (1993) Recurrent ascending myelitis: an unusual presentation of Herpes simplex virus type I infection. *Ann. Neurol.*, **34**, 625–7.
6. Lavalle, C., Pizarro, S., Drenkard, C. et al. (1990) Transverse myelitis: a manifestation of systemic lupus erythematous strongly associated with antiphospholipid antibodies. *J. Rheumatol.*, **17**, 34–7.
7. Rodriguez, M., Siva, A., Cross, S. et al. (1994) Optic neuritis: a population-based study in Olmsted County, Minnesota. *Neurology*, **44**, A374.
8. Beck, R.W., Cleary, P.A., Trobe, J.D. et al. (1993) The effect of corticosteroids for acute optic neuritis on the subsequent development of multiple sclerosis. *N. Engl. J. Med.*, **329**, 1764–69.
9. Mendez, M.F. and Pogacar, S. (1988) Malignant monophasic multiple sclerosis or 'Marburg's disease', *Neurology*, **38**, 1153–5.
10. Giang, D.W., Poduri, K.R., Eskin, T.A. et al. (1992) Multiple sclerosis masquerading as a mass lesion. *Neuroradiology*, **34**, 150–4.
11. Kesserling, J., Miller, D.H., Robb, S.A. et al. (1990) Acute disseminated encephalomyelitis: MRI findings and the distinction from multiple sclerosis. *Brain*, **113**, 291–302.
12. Mandler, R.N., Davis, L.E., Jeffrey, D.R. et al. (1993) Devic's neuromyelitis optica: a clinicopathological study of 8 patients. *Ann. Neurol.*, **34**, 162–8.
13. Kellar-Wood, H., Robertson, N., Govan, G.G. et al. (1994) Leber's hereditary optic neuropathy mitochondrial DNA mutations in multiple sclerosis. *Ann. Neurol.*, **36**, 109–12.
14. Thompson, A.J., Kermode, A.G., Wicks, D. et al. (1991) Major differences in the dynamics of primary and secondary progressive multiple sclerosis. *Ann. Neurol.*, **29**, 53–62.
15. Olerup, O., Hillert, J., Fredrikson, S. et al. (1989) Primarily chronic progressive and relapsing/remitting multiple sclerosis: two immunogenet-ically distinct disease entities. *Proc. Natl Acad. Sci.*, **86**, 7113–117.
16. Runmarker, B., Martinsson, T., Wahlstrom, J. and Andersen, O. (1994) HLA and prognosis in multiple sclerosis. *J. Neurol.*, **241**, 385–90.
17. Weiner, H.L., Mackin, G.A., Orav, E.J. et al. (1993) Intermittent cyclophos-phamide pulse therapy in progressive multiple sclerosis: final report of the Northeast Cooperative Multiple Sclerosis Treatment Group. *Neurology*, **43**, 910–18.
18. Weinshenker, B.G., Bass, B., Rice, G.P.A. et al. (1989) The natural history of multiple sclerosis: a geographically-based study 1. Clinical course and disability. *Brain*, **112**, 133–46.
19. Runmarker, B. and Andersen, O. (1993) Prognostic factors in a multiple sclerosis incidence cohort with twenty-five years of follow-up. *Brain*, **116**, 117–34.

20. Matthews, P.M., Francis, G., Antel, J. *et al.* (1991) Proton magnetic resonance spectroscopy for metabolic characterization of plaques in multiple sclerosis. *Neurology*, **41**, 1251–6.

21. Goodkin, D.E., Hertsgaard, D. and Rudick, R.A. (1989) Exacerbation rates and adherence to disease type in a prospectively followed-up population with multiple sclerosis. Implications for clinical trials. *Arch. Neurol.*, **46**, 1107–112.

22. Minderhoud, J.M., Van Der Hoeven, J.H. and Prange, A.J.A. (1988) Course and prognosis of chronic progressive multiple sclerosis. Results of an epidemiological study. *Acta Neurol. Scand.*, **78**, 10–15.

23. Ellison, G.W., Myers, L.W. and Leake, G.D. (1993) Defining progression for multiple sclerosis. *Can. J. Neurol. Sci.*, Suppl. 4–S130.

24. Weinshenker, B.G. and Sibley, W.A. (1992) Natural history and treatment of multiple sclerosis. *Curr. Opin. Neurol. Neurosurg.*, **5**, 203–11.

25. Whitaker, J.N., McFarland, H.F., Rudge, P. and Reingold, S.C. (1995) Outcomes assessment in multiple sclerosis clinical trials: a critical analysis. *Multiple Sclerosis*, **1**, 37–47.

26. McAlpine, D. and Compston, N. (1952) Some aspects of the natural history of disseminated sclerosis. *Q. J. Med.*, **21**, 135–67.

27. Syndulko, K., Tourtellotte, W.W., Baumhefner, R.W. *et al.* (1993) Neuro-performance evaluation of multiple sclerosis disease progression in a clinical trial: implications for neurological outcomes. *J. Neurol. Rehab.*, **7**, 153–76.

28. Rao, S.M., Leo, G.J., Bernardin, L. *et al.* (1991) Cognitive dysfunction in multiple sclerosis I. Frequency, patterns, and prediction. *Neurology*, **41**, 685–91.

29. Rodriguez, M., Siva, A., Ward, J. *et al.* (1994) Impairment, disability, and handicap in multiple sclerosis: a population-based study in Olmsted County, Minnesota. *Neurology*, **44**, 28–33.

30. Sadovnick, A.D., Eisen, K., Ebers, G.C. *et al.* (1991) Cause of death in patients attending multiple sclerosis clinics. *Neurology*, **41**, 1193–6.

31. Sadovnick, A.D., Ebers, G.C., Wilson, R.W. *et al.* (1992) Life expectancy in patients attending multiple sclerosis clinics. *Neurology*, **42**, 991–4.

32. Stenager, E.N., Stenager, E., Koch-Henriksen, N. *et al.* (1992) Suicide and multiple sclerosis: an epidemiological investigation. *J. Neurol. Neurosurg. Psychiatry*, **55**, 542–5.

33. Bronnum-Hansen, H., Koch-Henriksen, N. and Hyllested, K. (1994) Survival of patients with multiple sclerosis in Denmark: a nationwide, long-term epidemiologic survey. *Neurology*, **44**, 1901–7.

34. Wynn, D.R., Rodriguez, M., O'Fallon, M. *et al.* (1990) A reappraisal of the epidemiology of multiple sclerosis in Olmsted County, Minnesota. *Neurology*, **40**, 780–6.

35. Weinshenker, B.G., Rice, G.P.A., Noseworthy, J.H. *et al.* (1991) The natural history of multiple sclerosis: a geographically based study 3. Multivariate analysis of predictive factors and models of outcome. *Brain*, **114**, 1045–56.

36. Runmarker, B., Andersson, C., Oden, A. *et al.* (1994) Multivariate analysis of prognostic factors in multiple sclerosis. *J. Neurol.*, **241**, 597–604.

37. The IFNB Multiple Sclerosis Study Group (1993) Interferon beta-1b is effective in relapsing–remitting multiple sclerosis. I. Clinical results of a multicenter, randomized, double-blind, placebo-controlled trial. *Neurology*, **43**, 655–61.

38. Kurtzke, J.F., Beebe, G.W., Nagler, B. *et al.* (1973) Studies on the natural history of multiple sclerosis. 7. Correlates of clinical change in an early bout. *Acta Neurol. Scand.*, **49**, 379–95.

39. McAlpine, D. (1961) The benign form of multiple sclerosis. A study based on 241 cases seen within three years of onset and followed up until the tenth year or more of the disease. *Brain*, **84**, 186–203.

40. Thompson, A.J., Hutchinson, M., Brazil, J. *et al.* (1986) A clinical and laboratory study of benign multiple sclerosis. *Q. J. Med.*, **58**, 69–80.

41. Phadke, J.G. (1990) Clinical aspects of multiple sclerosis in North East Scotland with particular reference to its course and prognosis. *Brain*, **113**, 1597–1628.

42. Kurtzke, J.F., Beebe, G.W., Nagler, B. *et al.* (1977) Studies on the natural history of multiple sclerosis VIII. Early prognostic features of the later course of the illness. *J. Chron. Dis.*, **30**, 819–30.

43. McDonald, W.I., Miller, D.H. and Thompson, A.J. (1994) Are magnetic resonance findings predictive of clinical outcome in therapeutic trials in multiple sclerosis? The dilemma of interferon-beta. *Ann. Neurol.*, **36**, 14–18.

44. Weinshenker, B.G. and Ebers, G.C. (1987) The natural history of multiple sclerosis. *Can. J. Neurol. Sci.*, **14**, 255–61.

45. Weinshenker, B.G. (1995) The natural history of multiple sclerosis. *Neurol. Clin.*, **13**, 119–46.

46. Willoughby, E.W. and Paty, D.W. (1988) Scales for rating impairment in multiple sclerosis: a critique. *Neurology*, **38**, 1793–8.

47. Weinshenker, B. G., Issa, M. and Baskerville, J. (1996) Meta-analysis of the placebo-treated groups in clinical trials of progressive MS. *Neurology*, **46**, 1613–19.

48. Weinshenker, B.G., Rice, G.P.A., Noseworthy, J.H. *et al.* (1991) The natural history of multiple sclerosis: a geographically based study 4. Applications to planning and interpretation of clinical therapeutic trials. *Brain*, **114**, 1057–67.

49. Goodkin, D.E., Rudick, R.A., VanderBrug Medendorp, S. *et al.* (1995) Low-dose (7.5 mg) oral methotrexate reduces the rate of progression in chronic progressive multiple sclerosis. *Ann. Neurol.*, **37**, 30–40.

7 THE EPIDEMIOLOGY OF MULTIPLE SCLEROSIS

John F. Kurtzke

7.1 Epidemiology

For well over a century, multiple sclerosis (MS) has been the subject of study by workers in all the neural sciences. In recent years, especially, these approaches have included epidemiological inquiries. While there are others, one useful definition of this field is that epidemiology is the study of the natural history of disease. Its content and uses are described in Figure 7.1. The epidemiologic unit is a person with a diagnosed disorder. The basic question, after diagnosis, is how common is the disease, and this in turn is delineated by measures of the number of cases (numerator) within defined populations (denominator). These ratios, with the addition of the time factor to which they pertain, are referred to as rates [2, 3].

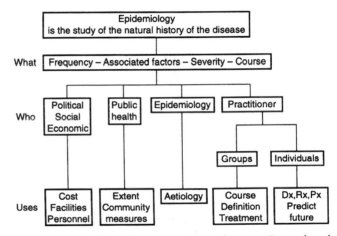

Figure 7.1 Epidemiology: content and uses. (Reproduced from Kurtzke, 1974 [1] with permission.)

7.1.1 RATES

The population-based rates in common use are the incidence rate, the mortality rate, and the prevalence 'rate'. All are ordinarily expressed in unit-population values. For example, 10 cases among a community of 20 000 inhabitants represent a rate of 50 per 100 000 population or 0.5 per 1000 population.

The incidence or attack rate

The incidence or attack rate is defined as the number of new cases of the disease beginning in a unit of time within the specified population. This is usually given as an annual incidence rate in cases per 100 000 population per year. The date of onset of clinical symptoms ordinarily decides the time of accession, though occasionally the date of first diagnosis is used.

The mortality or death rate

The mortality or death rate refers to the number of deaths with this disease as the underlying cause occurring within a unit of time and population, and thus an annual death rate per 100 000 population. The **case fatality ratio** refers to the proportion of the affected who die from the disease. When this is high, as in glioblastoma multiforme, then accurate death rates reflect the disease well. When this is low, as in epilepsy, then death rate data may be strongly biased.

The point prevalence 'rate'

The point prevalence 'rate' is more properly called a ratio, and refers to the number of affected within the community at one point in time, again expressed per unit of population. If over time there is no change in case fatality ratios or annual incidence rates, and no migration, then the average annual incidence rate times the average duration of illness in years equals the point prevalence rate. Both incidence and prevalence rates of diseases are derived from specific surveys within circumscribed populations. Mortality rates come from official published sources. When both numerator and denominator for the rates refer to the entirety of a community, their quotient provides a **crude rate, all ages**. When both terms of the ratio are delimited by age or sex or race or

Multiple Sclerosis: Clinical and pathogenetic basis. Edited by Cedric S. Raine, Henry F. McFarland and Wallace W. Tourtellotte. Published in 1997 by Chapman & Hall, London. ISBN 0 412 30890 8.

other criteria, then we are speaking of **age-specific** or **sex-specific** or similar rates.

Age adjustment

Since different communities will differ in their age distributions, the proper comparisons among communities are those for the age- (and sex-) specific rates. Such comparisons become unwieldy when more than a few surveys are considered, and the proper step then is the calculation of **age-adjusted** rates. One method of age adjustment is to take the age-specific rate for each age group from birth on, and to multiply it by a factor representing that proportion of a standard population that this same age-group contains. The sum of these individual adjusted figures provides an **age-adjusted rate, all ages**, or a **rate all ages, adjusted to a standard population**. One standard population often used is that of the United States for a censal year. This method is especially important when dealing with common disorders that affect primarily either end of the age spectrum.

7.1.2 CASE ASCERTAINMENT

Figure 7.2 indicates how cases of a given disease are ascertained within a community. Within the finite resident population, there will be at any one time a finite number of persons affected with the disease. As is true of almost every illness, some of these will be asymptomatic while a proportion will have symptoms appropriate to the condition. Among the asymptomatic, a

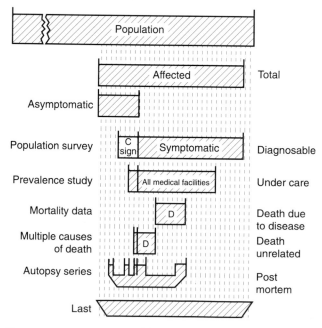

Figure 7.2 Catchment diagram of case ascertainment of disease within a population. (Reproduced from Kurtzke and Kurland, 1973 [4] with permission.)

subset will have abnormalities discoverable by examination or laboratory methods, while the remainder will then be, to all known criteria, free of disease even though affected. By examining the entirety of the population or an appropriate sample thereof, one can discover the symptomatic and abnormal asymptomatic cases. This is called the population survey in Figure 7.2; it has been used for common diseases but is impractical for rare entities. What has generally been done in neurology is the ascertainment of all the affected who have come to medical attention. This I have loosely referred to as the 'prevalence study' rather than a true 'population survey' [2].

One step further removed from complete enumeration of cases is a listing of deaths which the disease has caused. Such data originate in death certificates, and specifically that item written thereon as the 'underlying cause of death'. On the standard certificate there are also places for 'contributory causes of death' and 'associated conditions'. In selected instances they too can be obtained, and provide another (undefined) fraction of the affected. The autopsy series is really a subset of hospital case series, with all the biases implicit in such material [2]. To these are added its own unique biases. Even if all autopsies are collected from all the resources of the community, they will still represent a very fragmentary portion of the affected. In most areas only a small proportion of deaths comes to autopsy (selection bias). Of pertinence to neurology, not all autopsies done include the examination of the brain by neuropathologists, and the spinal cord is seldom examined. Even without these points, we must recognize that the autopsy series contains *some* who die because of the disease, plus *some* who die with the disease known but for other reasons, plus *some* who die with the disease clinically manifest yet undiagnosed, plus *some* in whom the disease would have been impossible to determine during life, and all of these in unknown fractions of those affected within the community.

At every step down the pathway of Figure 7.2, then, a proportion of the diseased will be missed. The further we move away from a true survey of the subject population, the larger and the more undefinable will be this proportion.

7.1.3 METHODS OF ASCERTAINMENT – PREVALENCE

Morbidity data are made available by means of three general kinds of population-based surveys, which I have called the **Assyrian**, the **in-law** and the **spider** [2].

The Assyrian

As Byron put it in *The Destruction of Sennacherib*, 'The Assyrian came down like a wolf on the fold'. This is the type common to most population surveys. It consists of the deployment of a team of workers throughout a community in order to identify the numerator (cases), and to perform whatever examination, laboratory and questionnaire procedures had been planned. All the data required are obtained in a short period, after which the investigators will follow Longfellow and 'Shall fold their tents, like the Arabs, And as silently steal away'. This kind of survey has been directed toward the ascertainment of cases within the population by door-to-door inquiry of its entirety or of a representative sample – what I referred to in Figure 7.2 as the (true) population survey. It has also been directed to the ascertainment of cases known to the medical resources of the community, without investigating the population at large – which I have called the prevalence study.

The in-law

This is a very expensive but important method for carrying out population surveys. The name derives from a perhaps not very complimentary concept of a home visit from one's parents-in-law. The survey team moves into a community, screens the residents and then remains to keep the community under direct surveillance with ongoing or repeated assessments over a prolonged period. In this manner one can directly define incidence as well as prevalence, and can identify risk factors before the event and assess their impact, as well as provide survival estimates and even treatment or prevention comparisons. Such works demand the full and sustained cooperation of both the inhabitants and the medical care providers of the area. They are also limited to regions expected to have little migration, and practicality requires them to be limited to small communities. This last point is important: even after decades the case material will be small.

The spider

Rather than seeking out patients, it would be well to devise studies wherein the patients come to the investigator. When one has an excellent medical facility which serves a defined community as its sole resource, and where the reporting and retrieval systems permit the collection of complete and accurate data, there is then a potential for many excellent epidemiological studies.

7.1.4 METHODS OF ASCERTAINMENT – INCIDENCE AND MORTALITY

Incidence data

If a community survey is carried out for a long enough period, it will afford a direct measure of annual incidence rates as new cases of the disease are encountered. For short-term surveys, incidence can be estimated only by retrospective reconstruction of the appropriate series.

Mortality data

The (underlying) cause of death on the official death certificate is coded according to a three- or four-digit number which represents a specific diagnosis within the International Statistical Classification of Diseases, Injuries and Causes of Death – the ICD, the eighth revision of which was in use for 1968–78 and the ninth until 1994 or 1995 [5, 6]. In the United States a slightly altered version known as the ICDA had been used [7]; this is now ICD9CM (clinical modification). The ICD is revised every 10 years or so, and the changes in both the eighth and the ninth revisions were major ones [8]. Even more striking are those in the new tenth revision with an alphanumeric coding system [9]. Counts of deaths and the death rates for the large number of individual entities so coded are published annually by the governments of many countries. In some lands for many of these disorders the data are also available by age, sex, race or colour, and geographical subdivisions of the country.

The great advantage of these materials is their current availability across time and space for many conditions in which we have an interest. Geographical distributions are especially attractive, since most of the population studies available are of necessity 'spot surveys' which may tell us little about areas that were not investigated. Most often, too, the numbers are larger by magnitudes than prevalence studies can provide. The principal disadvantage is the very real question of diagnostic accuracy. Of secondary importance are questions on coding practices including the choice of the underlying cause of death. There are also the generally minor problems as to demographic errors in both the numerator and denominator (age and residence in particular).

7.1.5 COMMENT

It is well to recall that questions as to diagnosis are not limited to death rates. In virtually all series of MS cases, whether defined for the laboratory or for an epidemiological inquiry, we are dealing with a clinical diagnosis without recourse to a pathognomonic diagnostic test or to pathological verification. A number of schemes for diagnostic criteria have been put forth, none with universal acceptance. In almost all of these, though, there are several grades relating to the degree of confidence in the correctness of the label. If we limit attention to the classes considered the better ones, and discard 'possible MS' and 'uncertain MS', we do in fact have defined groups which are quite similar one to another in time and space. Thus the assessments of morbidity data which follow are based upon series of cases variously labelled **definite, clinically definite** and **probable** MS.

Table 7.1 Schumacher Panel[a] criteria for diagnosis of (clinically definite) multiple sclerosis

1 Neurological examination must reveal objective abnormalities that can be attributed to dysfunction of the central nervous system
2 Examination or case history must supply evidence that two or more parts of the central nervous system are involved
3 Evidence of central nervous system disease must reflect predominant involvement of white matter; that is, long-tract damage
4 Involvement of the neuraxis must have followed one of two time patterns:
  (a) Two or more episodes of worsening, each lasting at least 24 hours and each at least a month apart
  (b) Slow or stepwise progression of signs and symptoms over at least 6 months
[5 At onset the patient must be between 10 and 50 years old][b]
6 A physician competent in clinical neurology should decide that the patient's condition could not better be attributed to another disease

[a] Schumacher et al., 1965 [10].
[b] Should not be obligatory in my view.

Modified from Kurtzke, 1982 [11].

The major clinical criteria in current use for a diagnosis of MS are summarized in Tables 7.1 and 7.2. While this topic is covered extensively elsewhere in this volume, the criteria used are far from irrelevant to measures of frequency. Aside from those cited in these tables, a common earlier categorization that is still used in some MS surveys was that of Allison and Millar [14]: **probable, early probable** or **latent**, and **possible**.

The geographical distribution of MS has been the subject of many mortality and morbidity surveys as well as the topic of several symposia [15–20]. Other major reviews of the epidemiology of MS are those of Acheson [21–24], Alter [25], Dean [26], Detels [27], Gonzales-Scarano et al. [28], Koch-Henriksen [29], Kurland [30], Kurland et al. [31], Kurtzke [2, 32–40], Kurtzke and Kurland [4, 41], Kurtzke et al. [42], Martyn [43], Poskanzer [44, 45], Pryse-Phillips [46], Sadovnick and Ebers [47], Weinshenker and Rodriguez [48], and Wynn et al. [49]. This extensive listing, which still is far from complete, is provided here so that the reader may seek interpretations which may differ – often drastically – from the views to be presented below. Each of these works should be taken in the context of the time in which it was written. Evidence for a number of aspects which earlier authors properly deemed inadequately supported continues to accrue. The most penetrating analyses to 1985 are those of E.D. Acheson [21–24]. His final summation was:

In the summary of the epidemiological chapters in the last edition [of McAlpine's *Multiple Sclerosis*] I concluded that the principal result of work using this approach had been to demonstrate that there are crucial environmental factors which determine

Table 7.2 Diagnostic criteria for MS for research purposes according to Poser et al. [12], compared with Schumacher Panel classification [10]

Category and subclass	No. of attacks	No. of lesions		CSF OCB/IgG	Schumacher classification
		Clinical	Paraclinical		
A Clinically definite					
CDMSA1	2[a]	2[a,b]	n.a.	n.a.	MS
CDMSA2	2[a]	1 *and* 1[c]		n.a.	MS
B Laboratory supported definite					
LSDMSB1	2[a]	1 *or* 1		+	MS or ?MS[d]
LSDMSB2	1	2[a]	n.a.	+	(progr) MS
LSDMSB3	1	1 *and* 1[a]		+	?MS[d]
C Clinically probable					
CPMSC1	2[a]	1[e]	(–)	(–)	MS
CPMSC2	1	2[a]	(–)	(–)	(progr.) MS
CPMSC3	1	1 *and* 1[a]		(–)	?MS[d]
D Laboratory supported probable					
LSPMSD1	2[a]	(–)	(–)	+	Not MS

[a] Separated in time and location of lesion.
[b] One lesion location can be historical only, if 'the information is reliable'.
[c] Separate location of lesion.
[d] Depends on sensitivity, specificity and predictive value of 'paraclinical' evidence of lesions of MS, for which there seem as yet insufficient data; excluding paraclinical evidence for '?MS' gives Schumacher 'not MS'.
[e] Presumably historical evidence is not 'reliable', cf. CDMSA1.

From Kurtzke, 1988 [13].

whether or not an individual acquires multiple sclerosis. Subsequent work has reinforced that conclusion with all the grounds for optimism which stem from it. [24, p. 40].

But what is or are the environmental factor(s) he thought undefined? A worthy update of Acheson's work is that of Christopher Martyn [43]. I *believe* he is trending more toward an interpretation compatible with that presented herein, albeit not by any means consonant in all its aspects. Some of the other recent authors cited seem more impressed with the difficulties inherent in epidemiological works than with the possibilities of integrated inferences. After all, so far every proposed aetiology for this disease has fallen by the wayside. The road to fame for MS investigators has long lain in denying the latest hypothesis, whether from the field or the laboratory.

The reader should be forewarned that my conclusions as to the nature of this disease as derived from its epidemiology are far from being accepted by all neurologists and epidemiologists; conversely, it is fair to state that some, at least, in either category do share my views. Space obviously precludes presentation of most of the data on which my conclusions are based, but I will attempt to provide reference, at least, to most of the principal findings so that the reader may decide the issues.

Despite consultants or laboratory findings, the clinician has to make up his or her own mind as to the diagnosis and treatment of each patient, as theirs alone is this responsibility. They must often so decide with inadequate or incomplete data, but decide they must – realizing that later information may markedly alter that decision. This is my approach to the epidemiology of MS. With all the time and effort, money and people that have gone into its study around the world, can we or can we not at this time come up with some valid conclusions as to the nature of MS? Can we arrive at a diagnosis?

7.2 Mortality data

7.2.1 INTERNATIONAL COMPARISONS

The earliest analysis of MS mortality rates from many countries was made by Limburg [50], who found that death rates were higher in temperate zones than in the tropics or subtropics. He also noted higher rates in northern US and northern Italy than in the southern parts of those countries. Goldberg and Kurland [51] presented death rates for a number of neurological diseases from all countries responding to their request for data. For most countries the deaths were those for five years within the 1951–58 period. All rates were age-adjusted to the 1950 population of the United States, and referred to diseases coded as the underlying

cause of death. These death rates from multiple sclerosis are shown in Figure 7.3. The rates in most of Western Europe were in the order of 2 or more per 100 000 population per year. The northernmost countries of Europe were closer to 1 per 100 000 as too were Canada and US whites, and New Zealand. Deaths from the disease would then appear overall to be notably less common in these groups of countries. The inclusion of Portugal in this 'middle' grouping may be questioned. There are still no good morbidity data for Portugal. In Iceland the rate was only 0.3 per 100 000. This low rate apparently contrasts with the high prevalence of MS in Iceland to be described below, even though the upper 95% confidence limit on this rate is about 0.9. Actually, MS in Iceland appears to have in fact changed in frequency, as will also be discussed later. We shall see that there is support for a rather low death rate in the 1950s. Similar age-adjusted international death rates for 1967–73 were presented by Massey and Schoenberg [52]. Most rates were the same or lower than those in Figure 7.3, but the overall ranking was quite similar. The Portuguese rate was 1.1, in agreement with the earlier rate of 1.2. Iceland, however, then had a rate of 1.0 per 100 000 population, and, again, morbidity data give support for this change.

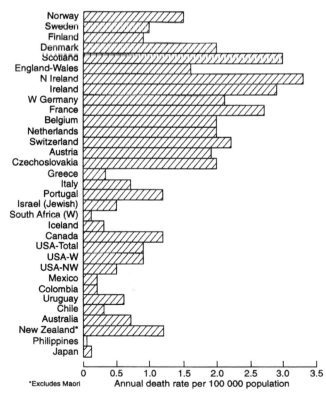

Figure 7.3 Average annual mortality or death rates per 100 000 population for multiple sclerosis from various countries, 1951–8, adjusted for age to the 1950 US population. (Data of Goldberg and Kurland, 1962 [51], reproduced from Kurtzke, 1977 [2] with permission.)

Within Europe there seemed to be a sharp drop between the rates in the north and those for the Mediterranean basin. South American rates were rather low, as were those for US non-whites (of whom more than 90% are African American). The Asian and African rates were clearly the lowest recorded. How accurate all these inferences as to the distribution of MS may be must await consideration of the morbidity data.

7.2.2 UNITED STATES DEATH RATES

The American Public Health Association had sponsored a series of monographs based upon special tabulations of deaths in the US for 1959–61; one of these concerned neurological diseases, including MS [53]. The average annual age-adjusted death rate for MS was 0.8 per 100 000 population, with a slight female and a marked white preponderance. The male:female ratio on the rates was 0.9; the white:non-white ratio was 1.6. Both findings were consistent by geographical (census) region of the US. Crude annual death rates were essentially stable over the 1949–67 period. For 1959–61, among both males and females age-adjusted death rates for MS were nearly three times higher for those who were single or divorced at time of death than rates among the married. Rates for the widowed were intermediate. Males had higher death rates than females among the widowed and divorced. Below age 65, female rates were higher than male for the married and were even more markedly in excess for the single. Geographically, all states south of the 37th parallel of north latitude showed low death rates (mostly 0.3–0.5), while almost all states to the north of this line were well in excess of the national mean (Figure 7.4). This held true for residence at birth as well as at death, and for whites alone as well as for all residents. There was little consistent difference in MS death rates between urban and rural counties within the respective census

Table 7.3 Multiple sclerosis: deaths and average annual death rates per 100 000 population by gender and race, United States, 1959–61[a] and 1979–1981[b]

| | Rate per 100 000 | | | | |
	Total	WM	WF	BM[c]	BF[c]
1959–61					
Crude	0.8	0.7	0.9	0.4	0.5
Age adj.[d]	0.8	0.7	0.9	0.4	0.6
(n)	(4305)	(1756)	(2288)	(106)	(155)
1979–81					
Crude	0.6	0.5	0.8	0.4	0.5
Age adj.[d]	0.6	0.5	0.7	0.5	0.6
(n)	(4287)	(1478)	(2445)	(137)	(216)

[a] From Kurtzke et al., 1973 [42].
[b] From data of NCHS, 1984–86.
[c] Non-whites for 1959–61, almost all black.
[d] Age adjusted to US 1940 population.

regions, though for whites the urban rates tended to be somewhat higher.

When defined by the 506 US state economic areas (SEA), MS death rates for 1965–71 showed a quite similar pattern [55]. For whites, all the significantly high SEAs and almost all SEAs otherwise high were above the 37th parallel. Significantly low SEAs were mostly below 37° north latitude, but again, especially for females, they extended in the east up to 39°. By SEA, the highest (but insignificantly so) rates for the much smaller numbers of non-whites were mostly in the north, and the few significantly low rates in the south.

Rates by sex and colour are shown in Table 7.3 for two periods 20 years apart. There is a clear reduction in that interval, attributable to decreases in white male and female rates. Rates for blacks did not decrease, however.

7.3 Morbidity data: historical geography

The geographic distribution of MS has been studied extensively in prevalence surveys, particularly in the last quarter of a century. However, as far back as 1868, Charcot [56] had commented:

> Après M. Cruveilhier [1835–1842], Carswell, dans l'article *Atrophy* de son Atlas (1838), a fait dessiner des lésions qui se rapportent à la sclérose en plaques. Mais cet auteur, qui a puisé surtout les matériaux de son ouvrage dans les hôpitaux de Paris, ne relate à ce propos aucun fait clinique. Même aujourd'hui [1868], je ne crois pas que la sclérose en plaques soit connue en Angleterre.

Charcot in essence pointed out here that the Englishman Carswell used French material to describe MS in

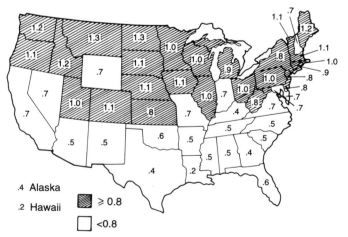

Figure 7.4 Average annual age-adjusted death rates for multiple sclerosis per 100 000 population by state of residence at death: United States, 1959–61. (Reproduced from Kurtzke et al., 1971 [54] with permission.)

his article on Atrophy in his 1838 *Atlas of Neuropathology*, and that even in 1868 there had been no clinical case of MS known (or at least described) in England. The first case report from Britain, indeed, was that of Moxon in 1873 [57], while for most of that century in both France and Germany the disorder had already seemed quite common.

Based on the distribution by state of rates for defects among US Army draftees in the First World War, MS was noted to be especially common among residents of the states bordering the Great Lakes (Illinois, Michigan, Minnesota and Wisconsin), but it was also common in Maine, Pennsylvania, Washington – and Kansas and Missouri [58]. Distribution by race showed the highest rates for Scandinavian and Finnish sections of the country. The distribution was similar when viewed as proportions of MS among injuries and diseases of the nervous system in US troops during that war, as too was the excess for foreign-born, and in particular Scandinavians [59].

7.4   Distribution from prevalence surveys

Prevalence studies provide our best information on the distribution of disease. However, they are expensive in time, people and money. Despite this, there are now well over 300 such surveys for MS. Almost all of them have been performed since the Second World War. Some years ago I tried to collect these studies and to rate them in terms of quality [60, 61]. It is obviously impractical here to list each of them. In the references cited are tables which define for each survey the author, the survey site, its latitude and longitude, the prevalence day, population, number of cases, the prevalence rate and its 95% confidence interval, and my rating as to the quality and hence comparability of the study. Class A studies had published data to indicate that they appeared reasonably complete as to case ascertainment, that they had followed appropriate survey methodology [2], and that they used defined diagnostic criteria. Class B works were generally well done but had some features that might limit comparability – such as a survey performed because the area was thought exceedingly high or low in MS frequency, or lack of detail when this was one part of a broader group (e.g. some from Japan and Italy) that overall seemed acceptable. Class C surveys were clearly not comparable to the others, mostly because of major defects in case ascertainment. Works classified as E provided an *estimate* of MS prevalence from hospital and clinic case series. This estimate was obtained by taking the ratio of cases of MS to cases of amyotrophic lateral sclerosis (ALS) seen in the same interval, and then multiplying this ratio by a rate of 5 per 100 000, which was used as the 'standard' prevalence rate for ALS. The surveys were assigned numbers with or without letter

suffixes so that nos. 1–52 referred to Western Europe, nos. 53–87 to Eastern Europe and Israel; nos. 88–119 to the Americas; nos. 120–135 to Australia–New Zealand; and nos. 136–162 to Asia, the Pacific Islands (including Hawaii), and Africa [60, 61].

7.4.1   PREVALENCE IN EUROPE

Prevalence rates for Europe and the Mediterranean basin as of 1980 are shown in Figure 7.5, correlated with geographical latitude. With so many studies, the confidence intervals were omitted (see below), but when added they served only to emphasize what to me was the best description of MS distribution according to latitude in Europe. It then comprised two clusters, one for prevalence rates of 30 and over, and one for rates below 30 but above 4 per 100 000. Taking only Class A studies, the high prevalence band extended from latitude 44° to 64° N. The medium prevalence zone extended from 32° to 47° N, plus two sites (nos. 11, 12) from the west coast of southern Norway. The only high rate below 44° was that for a small survey of Enna, Sicily (no. 51j), with 15 cases. Except for that one, all surveys from Italy and its islands, Spain, south-eastern France, southern Switzerland, southern Yugoslavia, south-western Romania, probably Bulgaria and Turkey, and Israel, as well as *possibly* Jordan and Tunisia – fell within the medium prevalence band [61]. There was a quite sharp but irregular division in the south between the high and medium frequency zones. From west to east, the dividing line went from the Pyrenees Mountains at 43° N, 2° E, extended upward into Switzerland near 47° N, 8°–9° E, and then dropped down to 45° N, 14° E in north-western Yugoslavia (Figure 7.6). In Romania it curved sharply downward to the Black Sea west of Bucharest. Based largely on relative frequencies from hospitals, the line then went eastward from above the Ukraine and seemed to end at the Ural Mountains at about 60° E longitude.

However, times have changed this interpretation. While the rates in the Shetland–Orkney Islands (no. 6 and 6a in Figure 7.5) were at the time the highest recorded [62–65], Cook *et al.* [66, 67] found both incidence and prevalence to have declined markedly in those islands by 1980 or so. The Outer Hebrides had a rate of 82 per 100 000 population in 1979 [68]. Rates in northeastern Scotland had increased from about 100 to 145 in 1980 [69, 70]. Rates in Wales in 1985 were some 115, including 'possible' MS [71, 72], while the London Borough of Sutton had a prevalence of 104 in the same year [73]. From representative general practices of the United Kingdom, Swingler *et al.* [74] calculated a prevalence rate of 116 for England and Wales in 1991 and 158 for Scotland in 1992.

Later material from Scandinavia indicated a 1979 prevalence of 93 in Vaasa, Finland [75], three times the rate for 1964; in 1972 the rate was 61 (no. 19a of Figure

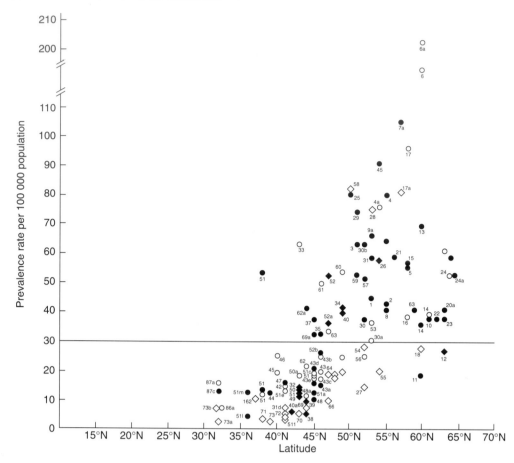

Figure 7.5 Prevalence rates per 100 000 population as of 1980 for probable multiple sclerosis in Europe and the Mediterranean area, correlated with geographical latitude. Numbers identify studies reported by Kurtzke [60,61]. Solid circles represent Class A surveys, open circles Class B, open diamonds Class C and open boxes Class E. Class C studies are listed only if no better quality survey is available for the specific site. (Reproduced from Kurtzke, 1980 [61] with permission.)

7.5). The whole country of Finland averaged 52 in 1979 [76]. Hordaland in western Norway (no.11) also tripled, from 20 in 1963 to 60 in 1983, with a rise in annual incidence from 2 to 4 per 100 000 [77, 78]. Conversely, Troms and Finmark in northern Norway had little change 1973–83; prevalence for probable MS was then 28 [79]. Prevalence in Denmark was stable at 87 for probable MS from 1955 to 1965 [80]. Similar stability at some 60–70 per 100 000 for 1955–85 was reported for Iceland [81, 82].

Other material suggests southwestern France may be of medium prevalence [83, 84], though the Haute-Pyrénées county had a rate of 40 in 1983 [85]. Berne in Switzerland showed 113 per 100 000 in 1986 [86], while (Germanic) Upper Wallis in 1976 had a rate of 38 versus 19 in (Gallic) Lower Wallis [87].

Rates in the 1980s across The Netherlands and Germany ranged from 43 to 68 per 100 000 [88–91]. Prevalence in Flanders, Belgium, was 88 in 1991 [92]. Rates in Hungary were 32 in the south in 1993 [93] and 79 in the west in 1992 [94]. In 1991 several regions of Yugoslavia were between 20 and 40 [95–97]. In an

isolated mountain region, the Gorski Kotar region of Croatia, Sepčić *et al.* [98] reported a 1986 prevalence of 144, and a high familial frequency.

Rates in Czechoslovakia and Poland in 1984 were 71 and 43 per 100 000 respectively [99–101]. In Athens a tentative rate of 10 was offered by Vassilopoulos [102]. For northern Greece Milonas found a 1984 prevalence of 30 [103]. Romania [104, 105] had rates of 27 and 30 in 1979. Bulgaria averaged 21 in 1979 and 1983 [106, 107]. Macedonia's rate was 16 in 1991 [108]; Albania showed 10 in 1988 [109].

Boiko of Moscow University has recently summarized a large literature on the distribution of MS in the former USSR which was previously unavailable in the West [110]. The material for the previous Eastern bloc is largely as stated above. From his Figure 1, much of northwestern Russia down past Kiev and Moscow appears to be of high prevalence (over 30 per 100 000), surrounded to the north, east and south by medium prevalence areas. Overall, the Ukraine and the Caucasus seemed to average in the medium prevalence range. The Asian part of his work will be discussed below.

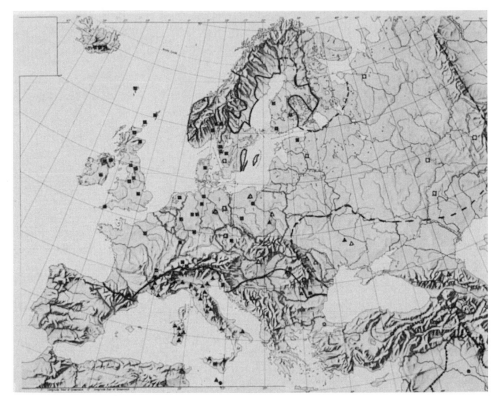

Figure 7.6 MS frequency in Europe and Mediterranean area with survey sites as of 1974. Solid symbols reflect 'good' and open symbols 'poor' studies. High frequency rates are represented by boxes, medium by triangles and low by circles. Solid line separates high from medium frequency zone; dashed line indicates uncertain boundaries. Dotted line outlines a low frequency site in Asia. Scandinavian limits are modified from earlier work by the author [60] to define high vs. medium zones. (Reproduced from Kurtzke, 1980 [61] with permission.)

Geoffrey Dean was the first to question the inclusion of Italy in the medium prevalence zone. In his survey of Enna in Sicily (no. 51j in Fig. 7.5) the rate was 53 per 100 000 [111]. There are now a number of other studies from mainland Italy and its islands to indicate prevalence rates between 30 and 65 per 100 000 in the 1980s [112–120]. Dean has also defined Cyprus as a high risk area with a prevalence of 45 in 1988 [121].

The most recent material has been summarized by Klaus Lauer [122]. Figure 7.7 indicates that there is no longer a high–medium division in Western Europe. The rate of 13 for Portugal was based on records of three neurological services in Lisbon, and the authors themselves thought the 'true' rate for Portugal would equal that of Spain [123]. And much of southeastern Europe may be following a similar course. The principal question is whether this is a change in disease frequency or a change in case ascertainment. For a number of reasons which cannot be detailed here, it is my belief that this is largely a change in the occurrence of MS.

Clustering

When the entirety of a single country is surveyed at a single time by a single team, then it is possible to

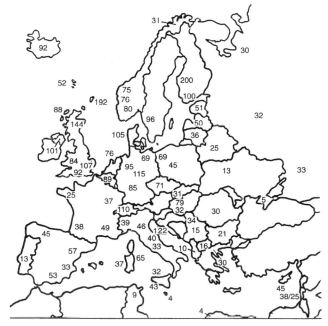

Figure 7.7 MS prevalence rates per 100 000 population in Europe, North Africa and Israel from recent publications for the period since 1980. (Modified from Lauer, 1994 [122] with permission.)

describe in a meaningful way the detailed geographical distribution throughout the land. Such surveys have been accomplished for Norway, Denmark, Switzerland, Northern Ireland, Sweden, northern Scotland, England and Wales, The Netherlands, Iceland, France and Finland. Repeated surveys covering different generations of patients (and doctors) have been accomplished for Norway, Denmark and Switzerland. While the distribution within the small area of Northern Ireland was uniform and that within The Netherlands and Iceland rather equivocal, in all other countries surveyed there were very highly significant deviations from homogeneity, and the high rate areas tended to be contiguous, forming clusters or foci. The differences in the rates between the highest and lowest regions were in the order of six-fold on average, and thus the variations would seem of biological as well as statistical significance [124, 125]. Essentially the same clusters were found when small administrative units rather than large counties were used as the units for testing [126]. In Denmark the clustering was across the middle of the Jutland peninsula on to Fyn, the major island directly east of mid-Jutland; in Switzerland the

concentration was in the north-western part of the country, and in Norway in the central and south-eastern part. Sweden had one southern focus and one in the north-east. The Finnish focus was in the west and south-west. The MS distributions were not related to availability of medical facilities, including hospitals, hospital beds and admissions, all physicians and neural specialists [127].

Not only was there clustering of MS, but in the lands resurveyed a generation apart there was a very strong correlation between the early and the later distributions, with coefficients of correlation of about 0.8 [33, 128]. In Figure 7.8 the rates by county from each survey are correlated for the three countries with such data: Denmark, Switzerland and Norway. Each county rate is expressed as a percentage of its own national (mean) prevalence rate at each survey.

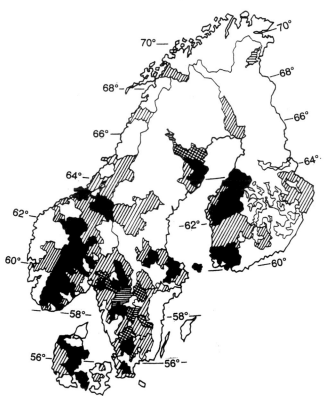

Figure 7.9 Distribution of MS in Fennoscandia. Areas significantly above their respective national means ($\chi^2_a > 4.0$) are in solid black: those high of dubious significance (χ^2_a 2.0–4.0) are cross-hatched: those insignificantly high (χ^2_a < 2.0) are diagonal-lined, those below the national mean are unshaded. Unit boundaries are omitted. Data represent cumulative death rates within 104 small units of Norway (1951–65); prevalence rates from hospital cases within 106 small units of Sweden (1925–34); disability prevalence rates within 20 hospital districts of Finland (1964), and childhood prevalence rates within 23 counties for the national series of Denmark (1949). (Reproduced from Kurtzke, 1974 [128] with permission.)

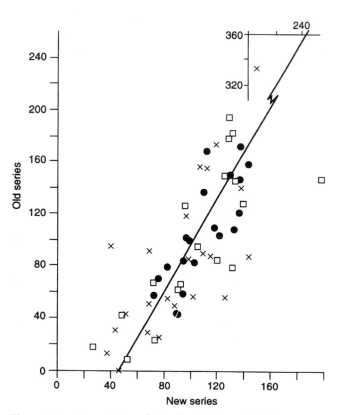

Figure 7.8 Correlation of the distribution of MS by county between old series and new series of prevalence surveys of three countries, each covering different generations of patients: Denmark (solid circles), Switzerland (x), Norway (open squares). Each county rate is expressed as the percentage of its respective national (mean) rate. (Reproduced from Kurtzke, 1974 [128] with permission.)

With this evidence of stability over time, we are able to combine studies from neighbouring countries to determine whether any broader pattern might be apparent. In this fashion, the high frequency MS areas in the north appear to describe one single **Fennoscandian focus** [128, 129]. This focus extended from the waist and south-eastern mountain plains of Norway eastward across the inland lake area of southern Sweden, then across the Bay of Bothnia to south-western Finland, and then back to Sweden in the region of Umeå on the north-eastern shore (Figure 7.9). This clustering, as well as the broader geographical distributions already considered, mean to me that the occurrence of MS is intrinsically related to geography, and therefore that MS can be defined as an acquired, exogenous, environmental disease.

7.4.2 PREVALENCE IN THE AMERICAS

Prevalence surveys from the Americas as of 1974 are denoted in Figure 7.10. Here we see all three risk zones: high frequency from 37° to 52°, medium frequency from 30° to 33°, and low frequency (prevalence less than 5 per 100 000) from 12° to 19° and from 63° to 67° north latitude. The coterminous United States and southern Canada are represented by all the surveys from

nos. 88 to 119a, except for nos. 106 (Greenland), 109 (Jamaica), 113 (Alaska), 117 (Netherland Antilles), and 118 (Mexico City). The Alaskan rate of 0 referred to natives of that state. The prevalence rates for the northern United States and southern Canada then are quite similar to the high frequency rates of Western Europe. Note that there were no studies from South America. More recent data confirmed the North American rates, and there are now several MS/ALS ratio estimates for Argentina and Uruguay, and for Lima, Peru, which indicate these are medium frequency areas. Similar material for Venezuela and Brazil apparently allots these regions to the low frequency zone [61].

In even more recent years a number of well-done surveys have emanated from Canada. Prevalence rates were 68 per 100 000 in Ottawa, Ontario, in 1975 [130] and 94 in London-Middlesex, Ontario, in 1984 [131]. In Saskatoon, Saskatchewan, prevalence was 111 (64 for those resident at onset) in 1977 [132]. On the west coast in the Province of British Columbia the rate was 93 in 1982 [133], while on the east coast the Province of Newfoundland and Labrador had a rate of 55 in 1985 [134]. Four regions of Alberta had rates near 200 in 1989–91 [135–137].

Age-adjusted (US 1950) prevalence rates in Olmsted County (which includes Rochester) and neighboring

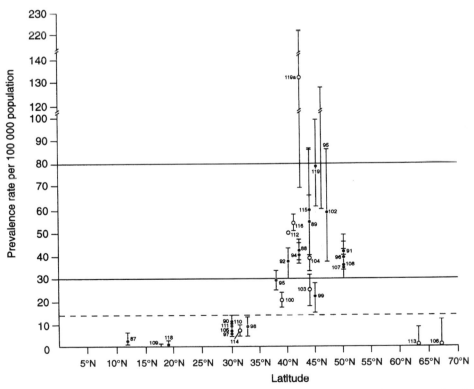

Figure 7.10 Prevalence rates per 100 000 population for probable MS in the Americas as of 1974 correlated with geographical latitude. Numbers identify the surveys as reported by Kurtzke [60]. Solid circles represent Class A studies, open circles Class B, diamonds Class C and squares Class E. Vertical bars define 95% confidence intervals on the rates. (Reproduced from Kurtzke, 1975 [60] with permission.)

Mower County, Minnesota, were respectively 113 and 106 per 100 000 population in 1978 (the crude rates were 102 and 100) [138]. In the northern Colorado counties of Weld and Larimer, the prevalence rate was 65 per 100 000 in 1982 [139]. The question posed by immigration is seen in Los Alamos County, New Mexico [140], where the prevalence rate was 76 per 100 000 (42–128, 95% confidence interval) in what should be a medium risk area; but virtually the entire populace of Los Alamos is migrant.

An 'unusual occurrence' of MS was reported in a letter to *The Lancet* by Sheremata *et al.* [141]. There were stated to be 29 cases of MS ascertained among residents of Key West, Florida, for a prevalence of 110 per 100 000 (74–158 confidence interval). Most patients had symptom onset between 1977 and 1982, and mostly while living in Key West. The State of Florida Department of Health and Rehabilitation Services conducted a case control survey of 22 of these patients with presumed symptom onset in Key West and 76 controls. Its official departmental report states: 'The above findings reveals [sic] that Key West is a high risk area for MS ... [and] health care workers, particularly nurses (representing 41% of the cases), appear to be at a higher risk of acquiring MS than persons not employed in the health care professions' [142]. Helmick *et al.* [143] gave a prevalence rate of 70 with 32 cases; the 25 cases with onset in Monroe County provided a rate of 55. Ingalls [144] discussed seven affected Key West nurses. Helmick *et al.* [143] showed increased risk for nurses but not other health professionals in their own case control study.

US veteran series

The modest number of studies noted in Figure 7.10 and cited above for the United States leaves much of the country undefined as to the distribution of MS. However, our recent history has provided us with a truly unique series. During the Second World War some 16.5 million Americans were in military service, and another 5 million served in the Korean Conflict [145]. US legislation has established multiple sclerosis as a 'service-connected' illness if manifestations of the disease were documented during military service or within seven years after discharge. We have identified 5305 such veterans service-connected for MS. In our diagnostic review of a random sample of these cases 96% met the clinical criteria of the Schumacher Panel [10] for 'definite MS'. Each of the 5305 MS patients was matched to a military peer on the basis of age, date of entry and branch of service, and survival of the war. This provided us with an unbiased, pre-illness case control series of nationwide composition and unprecedented size [146]. Figure 7.11 shows the distribution of MS for white male veterans of the Second World War according to state of residence at entry into

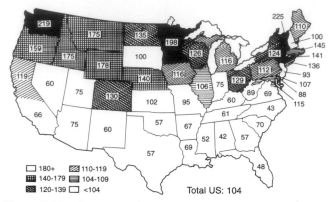

Figure 7.11 Case-control ratios as percentages for US white male Second World War veterans service-connected for MS, according to state of residence at entry into military service. Ratios below 75% are medium frequency. (After Kurtzke, 1978 [145] with permission.)

service, expressed as case-control ratio percentages. From calculations described elsewhere [147], the national case-control ratio of 104% was estimated to be equivalent to a prevalence rate of 41.6 per 100 000. This in turn would define regions of less than 30 prevalence as those of less than 0.75 ratio. As may be seen in Figure 7.11, all states below the 37th parallel of north latitude would then fall within the medium frequency zone. Arizona's ratio was exactly 0.75 but was based on only 9 MS cases and 12 controls. Note the similarity of this nationwide distribution to that from the US death rates in Figure 7.4.

All states (and northern California) above the 37th parallel fall into the high frequency zone, except for Virginia (0.69 for 51 MS vs. 74 controls) and Kentucky (0.60 for 37 vs. 62). In the east, then, the high-to-medium dividing line passes the 39th parallel. The low ration of 0.60 for Nevada in the west can be ignored since it came from only three MS cases and five controls. We therefore have in the United States too a quite sharp division between high and medium frequency bands.

7.4.3 OTHER REGIONS

Australia–New Zealand

In 1974 (Figure 7.12) it seemed that Australia–New Zealand comprised principally a high frequency zone for latitude 44°–34° S, and a medium frequency region for 33°–15° S. The recorded rates which were considered high were toward the lower end of this range. Geographically, this high zone included all of New Zealand as well as south-eastern Australia including Tasmania. The greater part of that continent was of medium frequency. The specific high frequency areas were in New Zealand (nos. 134,135), Tasmania (no. 125) and South Australia (no.127). In all other

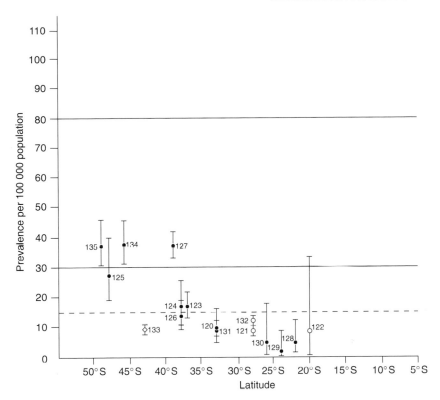

Figure 7.12 Prevalence rates per 100 000 population for probable MS in Australia–New Zealand, as in Figure 7.10. (Reproduced from Kurtzke, 1975 [60] with permission.)

Australian states the rates were essentially of medium frequency, though there was a strong suspicion that Melbourne, Victoria (no. 133), was markedly under-ascertained and should also have been high [60].

The two survey sites of New Zealand were Wellington (no. 134) at the southern tip of North Island and Christchurch (no. 135) at the upper third of South Island. In about 1984 the prevalence in Wellington was 69 per 100 000 [148]. However, in 1981, prevalence in the Waikato region in the middle of North Island was 24 per 100 000 (95% confidence interval 18.2–30.1), while at the same time there was a rate of 69 for the Otago and Southland regions at the lower end of South Island [149]. Both sets of recent authors commented on the rarity of MS among Maoris.

A nationwide prevalence survey of MS in Australia was conducted with 1981 as prevalence day. Compared to an earlier survey (1961), the 1981 crude prevalence rates, including 'possible', were 18 (1961) versus 24 (1981) for Perth, Western Australia; 18 versus 34 for Newcastle, New South Wales; and 29 versus 68 for Hobart, Tasmania [150]. Queensland, which comprises no. 121 and nos. 128–132 in Figure 7.12, had a 1981 rate near 19 per 100 000 [151]. South Australia's rate was near 30; no data were available for Victoria or Northern Territory. The state of Western Australia had a 1981 rate of 25 [152]. In general, then, Australia remains largely as before: mostly of medium prevalence

but with the southeastern quadrant including Tasmania now clearly of high prevalence.

Asia and Africa

Rates from Asia and the Pacific in the northern hemisphere were all low, except that Hawaii (nos. 145, 146) may be in the medium zone (Figure 7.13). No. 147 refers to its occidental immigrants. These study sites extended from latitude 8° to 47° N. Later hospital series in Asia and additional prevalence studies in Japan indicate that there was no site in Asia to 1980 demonstrated to have more than a low frequency for MS [61].

One subtropical locale that may be in the medium range is Las Palmas Province, Canary Islands, which lie at 28° N, 16° W off the southwestern coast of Morocco. Sosa Enriquez *et al.* [153] found 44 cases in the 700 000 (white) population in the 10 years to 1982 for a prevalence of 6 per 100 000. Libya, on the Mediterranean littoral of Africa, could also be within the medium frequency zone, with an age-adjusted (West Germany) prevalence rate of 6 per 100 000 for the 21 patients in Benghazi in 1984 [154]. Immediately west of Libya lies Tunisia. Ben Hamida [155] has reported 100 cases of MS seen in his clinic in Tunis 1974–76, of which 73 were definite and probable MS – and all of whom were native Tunisians. If all these 73 came from

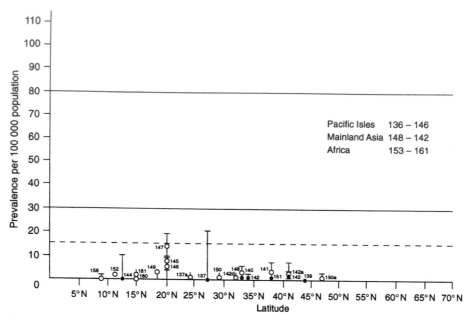

Figure 7.13 Prevalence rates per 100 000 population for probable MS in Asia and Africa (northern hemisphere), as in Figure 7.10. (Reproduced from Kurtzke, 1975 [60] with permission.)

Tunis itself, a prevalence of 10 per 100 000 might be inferred. There is other evidence that MS prevalence is in the medium range for all the quondam colonies of France in North Africa – Tunisia, Algeria and Morocco [Kurtzke and Delasnerie-Lauprêtre, in preparation].

Kurdi et al. [156] have described 32 cases of MS from the King Hussein Medical Center in Amman, Jordan. Of these, 22 were 'urban'. If they all came from Amman itself, a prevalence of 7 per 100 000 might be calculated; the 32 cases would provide a minimum prevalence of 2 per 100 000 for the country as a whole. An age-adjusted (US) rate of 8 per 100 000 was found for Kuwait on the Arabian Gulf in 1984 [157]. As of 1989, its prevalence rate was 13 [158]. An MS:ALS case ratio suggests a prevalence rate of 8 per 100 000 in Riyadh, Saudi Arabia, as of 1986 [159].

The prevalence rate for native-born Israelis, age-adjusted to US 1960 population, was 13 per 100 000 in 1965 [60]. Biton and Abramsky [160] presented in abstract an update of the material to about 1985, and they indicated a crude prevalence rate four times as high in natives with Ashkenazi (European) parents than in those with Sephardic (African-Asian) forebears (43 vs. 11 per 100 000 respectively). However, when the rates as presented were age-adjusted (US 1960), the prevalence rates were identical: 47 and 46 per 100 000 respectively, rates that are now clearly in the high frequency range. Data differed somewhat in the definitive report of Kahana et al. [161]. For all Israel in 1981 the age-adjusted (US 1960) prevalence rate for Israelis born of European parentage was 26 per 100 000; with Afro-Asian parents the rate was 15, and with Israeli-

born parents the rate was 23. For Jerusalem in 1983 the rates in the same order were 43, 36 and 51 per 100 000. I believe the all-Israel rates represent a considerable under-count, and it seems that all Israeli-born residents, regardless of parentage, now show a high prevalence for MS. The Afro-Asian parentage group in Jerusalem did not differ significantly from the others.

Boiko [110], as mentioned above, has summarized prevalence studies from Russia and other parts of the former Soviet Union. In the southern regions of the Ukraine, the Volga area, the Caucasus and into Novosibirsk and Kazakhstan, rates were generally in the medium prevalence range (5–30 per 100 000), while Uzbekistan, Samarkand, Turkistan and Turkmenistan areas overall appeared to be low. In the far east, medium prevalence once again appeared, and rates were indeed in the high range in the central and western parts of the Amur region, which abuts the Pacific ocean above China and includes Vladivostok. In all these areas rates were higher for Russian-born or those of Russian parentage than for the indigenous population. Certainly more detailed information as to methodology (diagnosis and case ascertainment in particular) is required before this material can be properly assessed. One might hope that all the basic papers on which Boiko's presentation is based can now be made available in the West. Boiko himself seems to have made a knowledgeable assessment of the materials, but one is always hesitant to accept findings that cannot be assessed directly.

In China itself, Hou and Zhang [162] summarized their 1986 door-to-door survey in a part of Yunnan Province, which lies in the south central part of the

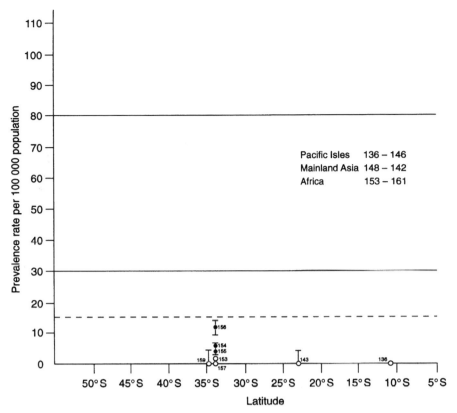

Figure 7.14   Prevalence rates per 100 000 population for probable MS in Asia and Africa (southern hemisphere), as in Figure 7.10. (Reproduced from Kurtzke, 1975 [60] with permission.)

country above Burma. The rate was 2.1 per 100 000 (1.4 age adjusted, US 1970) based on one patient found in a random sample of some 48 000 among the populace of 425 000. In Hong Kong the prevalence was 0.9 per 100 000 with 88 cases in the Chinese population [163].

In the southern hemisphere, with surveys from 30° to 6° S, all rates from Asia and Africa were also low, except for English-speaking native-born whites (no. 156) of South Africa (Figure 7.14). Their rate of 11 contrasted with that of 3 for the Afrikaans-speaking native-born whites (no. 155). Rosman *et al.* [164] found five new cases of MS among Afrikaans-speaking residents of Pretoria for the year ending February 1985; they calculated an incidence rate of 1.6 per 100 000, 'an eight-fold rise' over the annual incidence rate of 0.2 per 100 000 given by Dean [165] for 1958–66. In Cape Town, Kies [166, 167] recorded a prevalence rate in 1986 of 14 per 100 000 for English-speaking and 11 per 100 000 for Afrikaans-speaking native whites. Thus, the ethnic disparity in that country seems to have disappeared; the Afrikaaners have 'caught up' with their English compatriots, and now that nation is an area of medium risk for all whites – but still not for Cape Coloured (prevalence 3), or for blacks, who have virtually no cases known.

7.4.4   WORLDWIDE DISTRIBUTION

In 1966 it appeared that 'the world-wide distribution of MS may be described within three frequency bands: (1) high frequency with prevalence rates of 45 per 100 000 and a range of 30–60 ... ; (2) medium frequency with prevalence of 10 per 100 000 and a range of 5–15 ... ; and (3) low frequency with prevalence of 1 per 100 000 and a range of 0 to 4 ...' [32] Over the years thereafter, the high and medium frequency bands have each provided higher rates, in some areas at least, so that the former is now largely between 50 and 120 and the latter mostly near 25; low frequency, however, remains at less than 5 per 100 000.

I think the general worldwide distribution of MS may still best be described within these three zones of frequency or risk (Figure 7.15). I do not believe a 'super-high' grouping for rates of, say, over 100 is warranted (yet) because of the geographic scatter of such high prevalence figures. It may be necessary in the future to raise the medium-to-high border to (say) 40, but this does not yet seem warranted. The high risk zone, with prevalence rates reported up to 1996 of 30 and above per 100 000 population, includes northern and central Europe into the former Soviet Union, the northern US and almost all of Canada, together with New Zealand

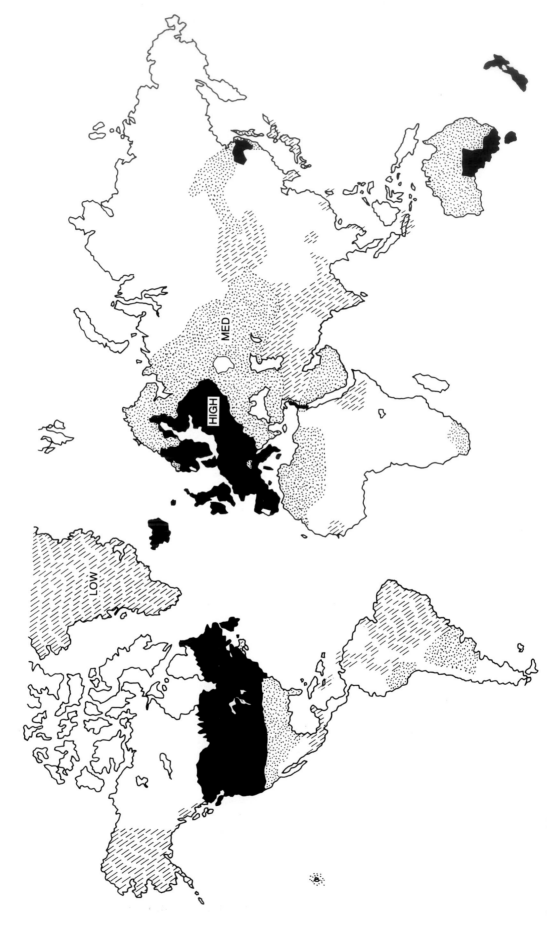

Figure 7.15 World-wide distribution of MS as of 1994. High frequency areas are indicated in black, medium frequency areas with dots and low frequency areas with diagonal dashes. Open areas are regions without data. South American, North African and ex-USSR frequencies are tentative.

and southeastern Australia. Italy, Spain and Cyprus appear to have joined the ranks of high frequency areas. Israel too now appears high, as does part of the Amur region of easternmost Russia. The high zones for southeastern Australia and for more of the Balkan republics have expanded somewhat. Most of the Balkans are midway between high and medium.

All the high risk regions are bounded by areas of medium frequency, with prevalence rates to date between 5 and 29 per 100 000, consisting of the southern US, (less of) southwestern Norway, northernmost Scandinavia, and probably Russia in the southwest and the far east. As stated, most of the northern Mediterranean basin is now high, and much of its southern and eastern margins now appear to be of medium frequency. These seem to be recent changes, in my view (see below).

Most of Australia still falls in the medium zone, as do perhaps Hawaii and the mid-portion of South America. Both ethnic groups of whites of South Africa now share equally in this grouping. Low frequency areas, with prevalence rates below 5 per 100 000, comprise all other known areas of Asia and Africa, Alaska and Greenland, and the Caribbean region to include Mexico and probably northern South America.

The origin and spread of multiple sclerosis

It is clear that MS is a place-related disorder. All the high and medium risk areas are found in Europe or the European colonies: Canada, the United States, Australia, New Zealand, South Africa, and probably central and southern South America and Asiatic Russia. It seems likely therefore that MS originated in northwestern Europe and was brought to these other lands by their European settlers [2]. In Europe itself, although the disease has clearly remained clustered in some countries, there is evidence even within these clusters of a slow diffusion over time. Note in this respect the slope of the regression line in Figure 7.8. There is also the marked change in incidence and prevalence rates found for Hordaland, Norway, discussed above, so that this region is now one of high rather than medium risk (it now joins the Fennoscandian focus of Figure 7.9), as well as the changes seen for Italy and Israel – and likely for Spain.

Following is a *hypothesis* as to the origin and spread of MS which requires much better documentation, but which is a tenable, and partly testable, one. MS may have originated in the south-central Swedish lake region near the centre of the Fennoscandian focus of Figure 7.9, and possibly in about the seventeenth or the beginning of the eighteenth century. It then spread slowly from this nidus to form the focus depicted. Spread into Norway may have been accentuated following the 1815 union with Sweden. From Scandinavia it diffused across the Baltic States, Poland, Russia (?),

Germany and France before the start of the nineteenth century. Further spread into the British Isles took place in the early nineteenth century, and spread to the US (and Canada) primarily by the Scandinavians in the mid and latter part of that century; toward its end came the emplacement in Australia–New Zealand by the British. In this century spread came to South Africa early and Israel, Italy and Spain late, though South Africa is still of only medium prevalence, as are the southern and eastern lands of the Mediterranean basin, also apparently newly established. All of these Mediterranean region changes may well be the consequences of the movements of the military and the populace in the Second World War and its aftermath.

If this hypothesis is correct, then our long-held belief in a latitude gradient for the risk of MS may be an artefact: we may be seeing merely the pattern of spread of MS from Scandinavia outward. And this spread in my view is too rapid to be via genes: epidemiologically MS appears to be an acquired, exogenous, environmental disease, primarily a disease of place rather than person, as noted above. My best guess as to this environmental causative agent is a specific infection; this will be discussed further in a later section.

7.5 Age, gender and race

7.5.1 DEATH RATES

Not only can we contrast death rates for geographical inferences, we can also see whether this terminal part of the illness provides us with useful information as to predilections by gender or race, as well as, of course, the age distributions themselves.

Denmark has long provided the best vital statistics data available. Its death rates for MS for the years 1963–68 are drawn in Figure 7.16. The rates for MS as underlying cause of death are represented by the lower lines with open symbols, while those for all deaths with MS listed on the certificate are defined by the upper lines with solid symbols. The shaded portions are the contributions to the total death rate for MS when this disease was recorded as a contributory cause or associated condition at death. The average annual crude death rate, all ages, was 2.6 per 100 000 for total deaths and 2.0 as underlying cause. By gender the rates respectively were 2.6 and 1.9 for males and 2.6 and 2.0 for females. The age at death showing the maximal rates is the 55–64 age group, regardless of type of cause or gender. The rates below this age were generally somewhat higher in females, and above this age tended to be greater in males.

For the United States age-adjusted death rates by gender and colour were noted in section 7.2.2. Crude death rates for MS, all ages, were 1.3 (total) and 0.9 (underlying) for whites in 1955, as contrasted with 0.5

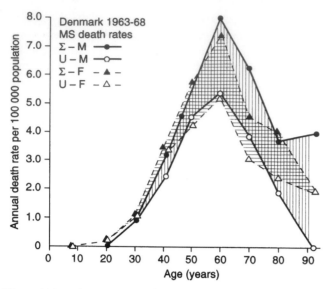

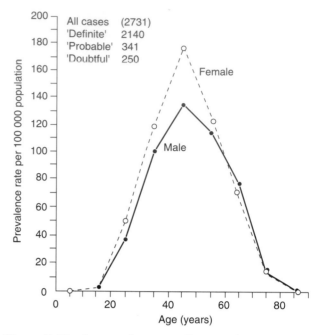

Figure 7.16 Average annual age- and sex-specific mortality rates per 100 000 population for multiple sclerosis in Denmark as the underlying cause of death and as total deaths. Shaded portion represents the contributions from deaths coded as contributory cause or associated conditions. (Reproduced from Kurtzke, 1972 [168] with permission.)

Figure 7.17 Age- and sex-specific prevalence rates per 100 000 population for multiple sclerosis in Denmark, 1949, from data of Hyllested [169]. (Reproduced from Kurtzke and Kurland, 1973 [4] with permission.)

(total) and 0.4 (underlying) for non-whites, of whom some 90% would be black or African American. Similar figures for underlying-cause death rates in 1959–61 were 0.8 white vs. 0.4 non-white [168]. Among the whites, the male rates were 1.3 for total deaths and 0.8 (1955) and 0.7 (1959–61) for underlying-cause deaths, while the female rates were 1.2 total and 1.0 and 0.9 underlying. Non-white rates by gender were about the same as those for both sexes combined, and thus some half the white rates. Note too that the white rates in the US were half those of Denmark.

In contrast to the Danish rates, the age-specific rates for MS as underlying cause in the US were almost plateaued from about age 45 on, with maximum rates near three per 100 000. Adding the 'secondary cause' deaths for white males resulted in a dramatic change in the configuration with a clear maximum at 5 per 100 000 for ages 65–84. This was not seen for white females or for non-whites, whose age-specific death rate curves differed little in configuration with total deaths from those for underlying cause. In both Denmark and the US the proportion of deaths classed as underlying tended to fall with increasing age. The differences in configuration from the curves for Denmark I believe are most likely artefacts of less complete ascertainment and coding for MS as cause of death in the US.

7.5.2 PREVALENCE RATES

The prevalence data for Figure 7.17 are those of the nationwide Danish MS registry of Hyllested [169] as of

October 1949. Note the sharp maximum in the 40–49 age group, where the rate among females was some 180 per 100 000 and that for males was almost 140. With this almost symmetrical and central curve, the differences among age distributions found for native populations of most of the world would have little influence on the rates. Thus for most purposes, age adjustment of MS prevalence rates is unnecessary.

Another well-done nationwide survey of MS, that in Ireland, provides confirmation for the Danish rates. Figure 7.18 shows age- and gender-specific prevalence rates for probable MS in Ireland as of 1971 drawn from the data of Brady *et al.* [170].

7.5.3 INCIDENCE RATES

By taking distributions at onset by age and gender for the Danish prevalent cases of definite and probable MS as of 1949, the population distribution of Denmark for 1940, and the average number of incident cases for 1939–45 (128.86 per year), it was possible to reconstruct age- and gender-specific annual incidence rates for MS [33, 171]. These rates are drawn in Figure 7.19, and demonstrate the female excess in the young and the maximal incidence at age 25–29. The annual incidence rate, all ages, was calculated as 3.35 per 100 000 population (3.00 male and 3.69 female). Here too the configurations do not suggest the need for age-adjustment in the usual material. For no source, mortality or morbidity is there need to separate the data by gender,

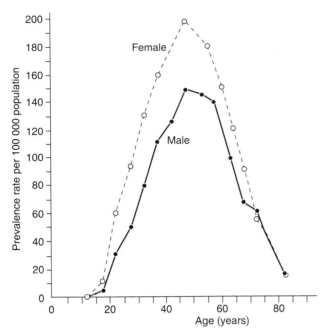

Figure 7.18 Age- and sex-specific prevalence rates per 100 000 population for multiple sclerosis in Ireland, 1971. (Data of Brady *et al.*, 1977 [170]. Reproduced from Kurtzke, 1983 [37] with permission.)

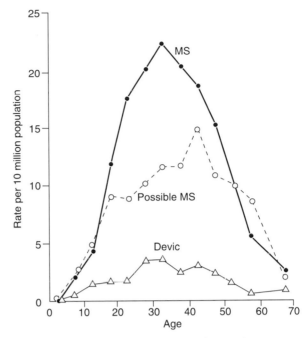

Figure 7.20 Average annual age-specific incidence rates per 10 million population for multiple sclerosis, possible MS and Devic's disease in Japan. (Reproduced from Kurtzke, 1983 [37] with permission.)

even though there is a modest female excess, particularly in the young. However, the female excess is increasing in most recent studies.

We have seen above that Japan is a low-risk area, with a likely overall prevalence rate for probable MS of about 2 per 100 000 population. Shibasaki, Okihiro and Kuroiwa [172] have pointed out the similarities in age at onset, course and duration of MS between Orientals and whites in Hawaii. If duration of illness in Japan is

similar to that in Denmark, then the ratio of the incidence rates in the two lands would equal the ratio of their prevalence rates. In this manner, we could estimate an average annual incidence rate of 11.55 per 10 million

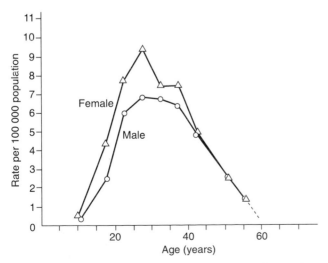

Figure 7.19 Average annual age- and sex-specific incidence rates per 100 000 population for multiple sclerosis in Denmark. (Reproduced from Kurtzke, 1969 [33] with permission.)

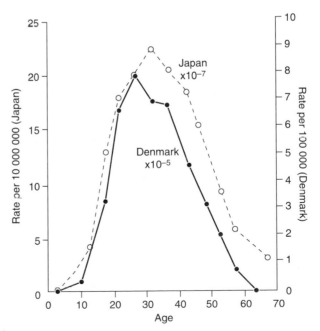

Figure 7.21 Average annual age-specific incidence rates for MS per 100 000 population in Denmark and per 10 million population in Japan. (Reproduced from Kurtzke, 1983 [37] with permission.)

population for MS in Japan. The MS Study Group of Japan [173] reported the age at onset for 497 probable MS, 330 possible MS, and 77 Devic's disease. By adjusting the 1968 population of Japan so that the 497 cases provide a rate of 11.55 per 10 million, age-specific incidence rates for all three conditions can be calculated (Figure 7.20). The annual incidence rate for Devic's disease would be 1.8 per 10 million.

The age-specific incidence rate curve for MS in Japan shows a striking similarity with that for Denmark (Figure 7.21). This is not an artefact of the mode of calculation, since the curve is independent of the absolute rate, all ages. The inference here is that, in so far as these attack rates are concerned, MS in low-risk Japan is the same as in high-risk Denmark.

7.5.4   RACE

We have already pointed out that death rates in the US indicate that non-whites have this disorder recorded as a cause of death only half as often as whites, and both mortality and morbidity data demonstrate low frequencies of the disease in the Orient. In fact, all the high-risk and medium-risk areas for MS have predominantly white populations. Regardless of residence in the US, in our veteran series blacks or African Americans have only half the risk of white males (Table 7.4). Note too that these young white females have nearly twice the risk of MS as do the white males. The group consisting of the 'Other' races suggests a paucity as well in American Indians and in Orientals (Table 7.5). Detels *et*

Table 7.4 US veteran series: case-control ratios by tier of residence at entry into active duty (EAD) for the major gender and race groups, entire series

Gender and race	Tier of residence at EAD			
	North	Middle	South	Total[a]
MS case control ratio				
White male	1.41	1.02	0.58	1.04
White female	2.77	1.71	0.80	1.86
Black male	0.61	0.59	0.31	0.45
Total series[b]	1.41	1.00	0.53	1.00
MS case control				
White male	2195/1544	2059/2022	688/1161	4922/4737
White female	97/35	65/38	20/25	182/98
Black male	28/46	88/150	61/194	177/390
Total series[b]	2323/1647	2213/2219	762/1425	5298/5291

[a] Excludes 1 male case and 11 male controls inducted in foreign countries.
[b] Includes black females and other (non-white, non-black) persons.

Data of Kurtzke *et al.*, 1979 [146].

Table 7.5 US veteran series: case-control ratios for 'other' males by birthplace and race, entire series

Birthplace and race	Ratio	Case/control		
		Total	N[a]	S[a]
Coterminous United States	0.48	11/23[b]	6/12	5/11
Amerindian	0.38	3/8	3/6	0/2
Mexican–Spanish American	0.60	6/10	1/1	5/9
Japanese	0.50	2/4	2/4	0/0
Mexico, Latin America, total	0.29	6/21		
Mexican–Spanish American	0.00	0/5		
Puerto Rican	0.38	6/16		
Hawaii, total	0.00	0/15		
Japanese	0.00	0/10		
Other	0.00	0/5		
Asia, total	0.00	0/14		
Chinese	0.00	0/4		
Filipino	0.00	0/9		
Other	0.00	0/1		
Total	0.23	17/73		

[a] N = Northern and middle tier of birth, S = Southern. For white males the MS/C ratios are 1.2 N and 0.6 S.
[b] Includes 1 Filipino control.

From Kurtzke *et al.*, 1979 [146].

al. [174] in California have presented good evidence for a low prevalence among Japanese-Americans. The apparent deficit we found among Spanish-Americans would seem more a reflection of geography than race. This is borne out when comparisons by race are made among the foreign-born cases in veteran series (Table 7.6). The deficit in the first two groups is equal by race. Japanese and possibly Polynesians in Hawaii are low, as are Filipinos in the Philippines.

MS then is predominantly the white man's burden. However, it is clear that, where there are good data, the

Table 7.6 US veteran series: case-control ratios according to race and birthplace in selected regions, entire series

Region	Ratio	Case/control			
		Total	White	Black	Other
Mexico, Central America	0.14	2/14	1/9	1/0	0/5
Puerto Rico	0.42	14/33	6/14	2/3	6/16
Hawaii	0.06	1/16	1/1	0/0	0/15
Japan, Korea	–	4/0	4/0	0/0	0/0
China	0.00	0/4	0/0	0/0	0/4
Philippines, SE Asia	0.00	0/12	0/2	0/0	0/10

From Kurtzke *et al.*, 1979 [146].

less-susceptible racial groups do share the geographical gradients of the whites, with higher frequencies in high risk areas than in low. This observation differs from that of Alter and Harshe[175], who thought MS rates were similar regardless of race in a given locale; their evidence was primarily for Israel.

7.6 Migration, latency and risk

7.6.1 MIGRATION

The fate of migrants who move into regions of differing risk for MS is critical to our understanding of geography in this disease. Table 7.7 summarizes prevalence rates (all ages) among migrants to and from different MS risk areas. (Specific references are given in my 1993 review[40].) The rates are those regardless of age at immigration and clinical onset. In broad terms, the immigrants do tend to retain much of the MS risk of their birthplace. The evidence for risk retention is better for migrants from high risk areas to low than is the reverse, where data are limited but do suggest an

increase. Rates would be artificially low in Australia because of laws restricting entry of the disabled, but even so, the age-specific rate cited for Perth is twice as high in the immigrants as in the native-born.

Information on low to high area migration remains sparse. Dassel[176] recorded three instances of MS among a probably rather small group of immigrants from Indonesia to Holland. Their onsets were at age 17, 23 and 25 years, and took place respectively 7, 9 and 8 years after their arrival in The Netherlands. Three instances of relapsing-remitting MS have been found among a series of some 3400 persons born in Vietnam of Vietnamese mothers and French fathers, and who came to France under the age of 20[177]. The three MS patients each had clinical onset about 15 years after immigration, which for them had been at under the age of 10. The cumulative risk of MS was 89 per 100 000, with a 95% confidence interval of 18–260. The age-specific prevalence rate was 169 per 100 000 age 20–29 (confidence interval 35–494). Both measures are rather similar to such rates for Denmark and are significantly higher than MS rates for Vietnamese in Vietnam.

Contrary, however, was the conclusion of Detels *et al.*[178]. In their final study of white migrants to northern Washington state and southern California who later developed MS, they found that the northern-born migrants who lived in Washington had an age-adjusted prevalence rate of 55 per 100 000 population age 20 +, while their peers who lived in California had a rate of 30. This reduction is significant and is in accord with the data discussed above for high-to-low migrants. However, their southern-born migrants had adjusted rates of 15 for California and 19 for Washington. The problem here is that this last rate was based on only 17 cases. The 95% confidence interval on this rate would be about 11–30 per 100 000. While this Washington rate is clearly lower than expectations for northern-born, I do not believe it safe to assume that this rate does *not* differ from that for the southern-born who stayed in the south. Their findings and interpretations (and my objection) were the same as they previously reported for MS death rates in the same regions[179]. Northern white migrants to Washington had a death rate of 1.3 per 100 000; those to California a rate of 0.8, both similar to the native-born rates and each significantly different north vs. south. The southern migrants to California had a death rate of 0.4 while those to Washington had a rate of 0.5 – but the 95% confidence interval on this last was 0.3–1.0.

Even more definitive was the conclusion of Dean *et al.*[180] that 'Emigrating to England from low risk parts of the world did not seem to increase the risk of developing MS'. This was based on the frequency of MS among first hospital admissions 1960–72 in Greater London. There were nearly 4000 such cases of MS, including 11% among immigrants. The 'New

Table 7.7 Prevalence rates per 100 000 population for probable multiple sclerosis among native born and immigrants

Immigration site according to its MS risk	Native born	Immigrants from risk areas		
		High	Medium	Low
High				
S. Australia	38	37	4	
Washington State		55	19	
Paris	92[d]			89[d]
Northern US	49		27	
Medium				
Perth, W. Aust.	40[b]	87[b]		
Perth, W. Aust.	14	22		
W. Australia	10	31		
Queensland	9[c]	15		
Israel[a]	9		19[c]	6[c]
Israel	4	33	8	3
Los Angeles		30	15	
Southern US	22	29		
Low				
South Africa	6	48	15	
Neth. Antilles	3	59		
Hawaii[a]	5		35	

[a] May include 'possible' MS.
[b] Age-specific rate, 40–49 years.
[c] Age-adjusted to 1960 US population.
[d] Cumulative risk.

From Kurtzke, 1993 [40].

Commonwealth' immigrants from Asia, Africa and Latin America comprised 33 cases, whereas they calculated 242 were expected.

Dean *et al.*[181] extended this work to the West Midlands for 1967–74, where they found 8 MS vs. 72 expected for New Commonwealth immigrants. They further pointed out that death rates for MS in England and Wales in 1960–72 were equally lacking for such immigrants, and that for ALS, observed and expected cases were equal regardless of origin.

The major problem here is that more than half the New Commonwealth immigrants had been resident in England and Wales only since 1966 or so. For 1960–72, then, even if the immigrants acquired the British risk of MS as soon as they landed in England, even if there is no 'incubation' period after MS acquisition and symptoms begin immediately, and even if the diagnosis is made in the first year of illness, still it seems likely to me that expectations based only on such 'prevalence day' population counts would be grossly inflated when the group at hand is increasing so rapidly. 'The question of risk of MS in migrant populations gets very involved, being dependent not only on a sufficiency of people who change their residence from one risk area to another but also on their ages at immigration, their length of stay in the new land, *and* their age at prevalence day... Another problem further to confound the issue is the apparent racial predilection for MS, regardless of geography...'[182].

'The true population at risk according to age at survey *and* age at migration *and* age at clinical onset can be very difficult to define, and the choice of denominator or the type of rate required (incidence, prevalence, death, cumulative risk) can get very involved. In addition, the desired population denominator is generally not available from routine sources'[36]. There is, however, good evidence for an increased MS risk for low-to-high migrants, aside from the works already discussed in the first part of this section. These data also speak to the influence of age at migration. But one other low-to-high migration needs first be mentioned. This is the paper of Delasnerie-Lauprêtre and Alpérovich[183] for the French Collaborative Group on Multiple Sclerosis, INSERM. From among the some 8000 patients ascertained in a nationwide survey in France in 1986, they identified 246 who had immigrated from North Africa, mostly between 1960 and 1965 consequent to the Algerian war for independence. Of these 246, 86% were of European origin, with the remainder being Arab or Berber. There were 24 patients with MS onset before migration and three at the time of migration, leaving 219 with onset of MS after migration to metropolitan France. There were thus eight times as many patients with onset after migration, in a setting where virtually the entire French population, *les colonnes*, had left North Africa for metropolitan France. In section 7.9.3 below yet another low–high migrant series is considered, namely Faroese who moved to Denmark.

Age of migration

If the risk of MS is defined at or near birth (or the disease is innate), then migrants from low to high regions would demonstrate no increase in the risk of MS, and their MS frequency would be that specified by birthplace alone. In the United States, death rates for MS are distributed so that states to the north of 37° N latitude have twice the rates of those to the south, as described in Figure 7.4. If birthplace is the critical residence, then those who exchange these risk areas would demonstrate the mirror image of Figure 7.4, with MS rates high in the south and low in the north. Actually, as seen in Figure 7.22, for MS deaths 1959–61, those who were born in the north and died in the south, when compared with those born in the south who died in the north, demonstrated an *obliteration* of the north–south difference, and all the death rates were closer to the national mean than were those for the non-migrants[54]. The death rate for US southern-born MS cases who had died in the north (0.68) was significantly higher than southern-born who died in the south (0.46), further supporting an increased risk for low-to-high moves.

Figure 7.11 showed state of residence at entry into military service for the US veteran case control series. In Table 7.4 these residences were allocated within three horizontal tiers for the coterminous United States: a northern tier of states above 41–42° N, a middle tier and a southern tier below 37°, including California from Fresno south. Migrants would be those born in one tier who entered service from another. In Table 7.8 the marginal totals provide the ratios for birthplace and for residence at service entry for white males serving in the Second World War. The major diagonal (north–north, middle–middle, south–south) gives the case-control ratios for non-migrants, and cells off this diagonal define the ratios for the migrants.

All ratios decrease as we go from north to south. The non-migrant ratios are 1.41 north, 1.04 middle and 0.56 south. For the migrants, those born north and entering service from the middle tier have a ratio of 1.26; if they enter from the south their ratio is 0.70, only half that of the non-migrants. Birth in the middle tier is marked by an *increase* in the MS/C ratio for northern entrants to 1.30 and a *decrease* to 0.72 for the southern ones. Migration after birth in the south seems to raise the ratios to 0.62 (middle) and 0.73 (north). The migrant risk ratios are intermediate between those characteristic of their birthplace and their residence at entry.

From the marginal total of Table 7.8, residence at birth has about the same gradient of risk as does

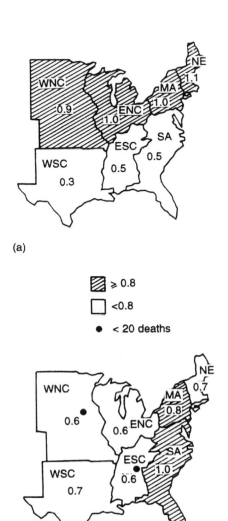

Figure 7.22 Average annual death rates from MS per 100 000 population by residence by census region in the eastern two-thirds of the US, 1959–61: (*a*) region of birth = region of residence at death; (*b*) region of residence at death for those born in opposite tier of states, north or south. NE, New England; MA, Middle Atlantic; SA, South Atlantic; EN/SC, East North/South Central; WN/SC, West North/South Central. (After Kurtzke *et al.*, 1971 [54].)

Table 7.8 MS case-control ratios for white male Second World War veterans[a] by tier of residence at birth and at entry into active duty (EAD): US only

	EAD tier			Birth total
Birth tier	North	Middle	South	
MS/control ratio				
North	1.41	1.26	0.70	1.38
Middle	1.30	1.04	0.72	1.04
South	0.73	0.62	0.56	0.57
EAD total	1.39	1.04	0.58	1.04
Case/control				
North	1611/1140	112/89	32/46	1755/1275
Middle	125/96	1544/1482	68/94	1737/1672
South	16/22	42/68	439/788	497/878
EAD total	1752/1258	1698/1639	539/928	3989/3825

[a] Includes those who also served in the Korean conflict.

From Kurtzke *et al.*, 1985 [184].

groups older at immigration, the prevalence was some 40 to 80 per 100 000, the same as expected from their high-risk homelands. This change was sharp and occurred exactly at age 15 [185, 186]. Two other high-to-low migrant surveys, for Israel [187] and Hawaii [188], also suggest, though with small numbers, that age 15 divides those who retain the risk of their birthplace from those (younger) who acquire a lower risk. On low-to-high migration, Alter, Kahana and Loewenson [189] have suggested that Afro-Asian immigrants arriving in Israel below the age of 5 years have age specific incidence rates similar to such immigrants from Europe, whereas those arriving beyond age of 5 tend to differ: European rates *appear* higher. However, the number of cases, especially for those under age 15 at immigration, would appear too small for meaningful interpretation.

7.6.2   AGE OF ACQUISITION OF MS

The veteran series and the other studies just mentioned also speak to the *age* at which MS may in fact be acquired, as opposed to the age at which symptoms appear. Both sets suggest that an age near puberty might indeed be the critical time wherein geography is most relevant. This is most definitive for the latter studies. The veteran study indicates that changing residence well before onset alters the risk, but does not really give us an upper endpoint by age. Beebe *et al.* [190] reported a similar though smaller group of MS cases. These were some 500 enlisted men whose diagnosis of MS was first made in the US Army and agreed with upon our review in the early 1960s. These men were matched to their military peers by age and date of entry into service. Their residence at birth and at entry into service showed

residence at service entry – and therefore about age 24 for these Second World War veterans. For the migrants there is no clear difference in risk for moves from high to low regions versus low to high.

If the disease is acquired over a short interval, then the point midway between birth and 24 would seem the most reasonable to account for our findings. This would therefore indicate age 10–15, which would be in accord with other data on migrants (see below).

In a study of European immigrants to South Africa, the MS prevalence rate, adjusted to a population of all ages, was 13 per 100 000 for immigration under age 15, which is the same medium prevalence rate as for the native-born English-speaking white South Africans. But for age a strong north–south gradient in the case control ratios, similar to that described above for our much larger veteran series. However, this gradient had totally disappeared when residences during military service but before clinical onset were compared: all ratios, north, middle and south, were then essentially unity.

These data suggest that virtually all the change in risk attributable to change in residence had already taken place well before the third decade of life in this series – and thus well before clinical onset. Other evidence suggesting acquisition of MS between perhaps ages 10 and 15 – based largely on ages of maximal geographical clustering – has been presented elsewhere [2, 33, 34, 191, 192]. Schapira, Poskanzer and Miller [193] came to similar conclusions from the ages of common residence for sibs, both of whom had MS. All these inferences arose from surveys in high-risk areas.

It is premature to state that altered risk ceases by age 20 or so for migrants from low to high MS areas, but the evidence does seem good that for natives of high-risk zones and for migrants from high to low, their risk of MS is by and large determined well before age 20. I have taken this also to mean that the *disease* is acquired well before this age, and that there is in fact an 'incubation' or 'latency' period of some years before clinical symptom onset after disease acquisition; further, that at least part of this 'latent' period is pathologically one of active subclinical disease. In addition, from the European migrants to South Africa discussed above [185, 186], young children in high risk areas are *not* susceptible to this disease. Some idea of an upper limit for age of acquisition of MS may be obtained if we can identify virgin populations into which MS was introduced. To this point the section on MS Epidemics would seem apposite: the suggestion there is that age 45 or so might be the cut-off point. This is also in accord with the North African immigrants to France [40, 183].

7.6.3   RISK OF MS

It was particularly to attack the problems of MS in migrants that I attempted to provide, for one time and area at least, estimates as to the risk of MS by age, sex and interval [194]. Table 7.9 gives a summary of the period risk for MS in Denmark by age at entry for both sexes combined. The cumulative lifetime risk from birth is 201 per 100 000, or one chance in 500. At age 20 the risk of MS beginning within the next five years is 34 per 100 000; after 20 years this figure is 142, and after 30 years 181. For entrance at age 10, the 5-year risk is only 2 per 100 000 and the 20-year risk 92; by 30 years, it reaches 159. For entrants age 50, the lifetime risk of 13 per 100 000 is attained within 10 years.

As we stated above, if we assume that the duration of MS is constant regardless of geography, then the ratios of prevalence rates in different areas are equivalent to the

Table 7.9   Period cumulative risk of multiple sclerosis in Denmark. Approximate number of new cases expected by period per 100 000 population of given age at entry, male and female combined

Age at entry	Period (yr)						
	5	10	15	20	25	30	Lifetime
0	0	2	4	20	52	89	201
5	2	4	21	54	94	128	211
10	2	19	53	92	126	159	210
15	17	51	90	125	158	181	209
20	34	74	109	142	165	181	193
25	40	75	108	131	148	157	160
30	35	69	92	108	118	120	120
35	34	58	74	83	86	86	86
40	24	41	50	53	53	53	53
45	17	27	30	30	30	30	30
50	10	13	13	13	13	13	13
55	3	3	3	3	3	3	3
60	0	0	0	0	0	0	0

Data of Kurtzke 1978 [194].

ratios of incidence rates. Then, too, such ratios can also be applied to these risk estimates. In this case, if 100 000 Japanese were to migrate to Denmark at age 10, they would be expected to provide four MS cases after 20 years if they retained the low risk of their birthplace, but there would be 92 cases if they acquired the high risk of Denmark immediately upon their arrival.

More informative might be a statement as to the number of cases expected to occur within given intervals among a disease-free sample of the general population. In Table 7.10 are such figures derived from the Danish risk estimates and the 1960 US population distribution. In 5 years there will be only 14 cases per 100 000 population – or some 12% of the total anticipated. After

Table 7.10   Number of MS cases per 100 000 population and cumulative percentages expected to develop in given intervals among a disease-free cohort of a high-risk populace[a]

Interval (yr)	Cases per 100 000	Cumulative %
5	14.1	11.6
10	28.8	23.8
15	44.4	36.6
20	61.3	50.6
25	77.9	64.3
30	92.2	76.1
Lifetime	121.2	100.0

[a] Risk estimates for Denmark applied to 1960 US population distribution.

Modified from Kurtzke 1980 [35].

20 years we will have accumulated only *half* the total cases expected. These frequencies understate the absolute risk in high frequency areas, as those affected by age x have been deleted from the calculations. It is this kind of information, however, that must be borne in mind when trying to interpret data for MS among migrants, and it is directly relevant to the immigrants to Britain discussed above [180–182].

7.7 Survival

7.7.1 LIFE TABLE ANALYSIS

One major aspect of epidemiology is the course of illness. At its most basic level, this can be measured by survival. A seemingly esoteric but actually quite simple method is the calculation of survival rates (more properly 'ratios') by means of life table analysis (Table 7.11) [195, 196]. Let us start with 100 patients with parkinsonism whose onset is 1 January 1920, and they all come to our office on that date, whereupon we immediately diagnose them. Suppose we can follow them all until the one-hundredth patient dies. During 1920, 10 die. The annual case fatality ratio in 1920 is 10/100 and the remainder from that fraction is 90/100, so that 90.0% have survived the first year of illness. Let

15 die in 1921, and the annual case fatality ratio is 15/90 or 0.167, the remainder being 0.833. Survival through the second year is (0.833) (0.900) or 75.0%. If 20 die in the third year, the annual fatality ratio is 20/75 or 0.267, survival is (0.733) (0.833) (0.900) or 55.0%, and we start off the fourth year with 55 living patients (Table 7.11, Example A). Note that we have already almost reached the median survival (50%) point, a very useful figure. It is more correct to compute from averages of those at risk of death during the interval in question (see below). Periods, of course, need not be measured in years; one can use decades or months or days – or even hours – when circumstances require, or even unequal intervals.

Example A though provides a quite artificial experience. Closer to usual experience is Example B where, on 31 December 1921, 30 patients emigrated to Nigeria and were thus lost to follow-up. The calculations are the same, but the population at risk in 1922 is limited to those still under observation. A common but potentially misleading method is that of Example B, where all patients are listed from onset regardless of when they first come to attention. But if we first encounter a patient 10 years after onset, that patient will by definition have survived 10 years. One should add the patient to the series only at the time of first observa-

Table 7.11 Hypothetical life table for survival in disease

Sample	Period	Completed year at end of period	No. at start of period	Deaths during period	Withdrawals during period	Added during period	Annual ratio Dead	Annual ratio Alive	Survival %
A	1920	1	100	10	0	0	0.100	0.900	90.0
	1921	2	90	15	0	0	0.167	0.833	75.0
	1922	3	75	20	0	0	0.267	0.733	55.0
	1923	4	55						
B	1920	1	100	10	0	0	0.100	0.900	90.0
	1921	2	90	15	30	0	0.167	0.833	75.0
	1922	3	45	20	0	0	0.444	0.556	41.7
	1923	4	25						
C	1920	1	100	10	0	20	0.100	0.900	90.0
	1921	2	110	15	30	0	0.136	0.864	77.7
	1922	3	65	20	0	10	0.308	0.692	53.8
	1923	4	55						
D	1920	1	100(110)[a]	10	0	20	0.091	0.909	90.9
	1921	2	110(95)	15	30	0	0.158	0.842	76.5
	1922	3	65(70)	20	0	10	0.286	0.714	54.6
	1923	4	55						
E	–	1	100(100)[a]	10	0	(20)	0.100	0.900	90.0
	–	2	110(95)	15	30	0	0.158	0.842	75.8
	–	3	65(65)	20	0	(10)	0.308	0.692	52.5
	–	4	55						

[a] Population at risk during interval.

From Kurtzke, 1992 [196].

tion [197]. Example C in Table 7.11 would then be appropriate if there were in fact 130 patients whose disease started on 1 January 1920, but only 100 of them came to us then. On 31 December 1920 another 20 shuffled into the office, and on 31 December 1922 the last 10 arrived.

Suppose that instead of arriving or departing on 31 December, the additions and departures all took place on 1 July of the cited years. Each such patient would thus contribute one-half a person-year of exposure to the population at risk at the start of that year: departures from 1 January to 30 June; additions from 1 July to 31 December (Table 7.11, Example D). This is, in fact, the standard presumption, that gains and losses are equally distributed over the interval and thus contribute half their numbers to the denominator.

However, in ordinary 'real-life' situations, calendar years are replaced by years from onset (year 1, year 2) for the patients, and results described according to completed years so that '1' represents the first completed year of illness. In this way the entire series starts at 0 (= 1 January 1920 here) and cases are lost by death or withdrawal until the last patient is accounted for. Since, then, the patients are added according to their own time of onset: Example E in Table 7.11 provides the methodology most often used, with denominator adjustment required only for the withdrawals [197].

Survival estimates are important in many neurological disorders. Similar methodology can be used to measure events other than death – for example, the occurrence of a complication or of a second illness. It can also be used to measure the occurrence of an event (such as stroke) in a population at risk (patients with TIA, or hypertension, or diabetes, or carotid surgery). In comparisons of intervention measures in such instances it is the preferred procedure [196].

7.7.2 SURVIVAL IN MS

In studies antedating the Second World War hospital series indicated an average duration of life after onset of MS of about 10 years. The prevalence studies of the early 1950s provided for survival averages of at least 20 years [198]. Survival rates were calculated by life table methods (Figure 7.23) for the patients resident in Rochester, Minnesota [199], and for the US Army male patients hospitalized during the Second World War [200]. Among both Army groups and the Rochester series, the average duration of illness or median survival was estimated to be at least 35 years from onset. About three-quarters of the patients had survived 20 years, and two-thirds 30 years [200]. In the Rochester series, half the survivors were still ambulatory after 20 years of illness.

These findings, considerably in excess of other estimates, probably reflect the more complete ascer-

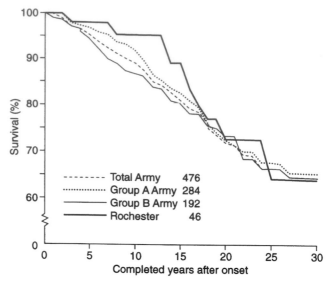

Figure 7.23. Multiple sclerosis: percentage survival by years after clinical onset from life table analyses. Army Second World War series: total, group A (onset bout antedating Army diagnostic bout) and group B (Army diagnosis during onset bout) (data of Kurtzke et al., 1970 [200]); and Rochester, Minnesota, resident series (data of Percy et al., 1971 [199]). (After Kurtzke, 1970 [195].)

tainment (including benign cases) in Rochester and the enumeration of early cases (irrespective of severity) developing in a defined population (Army series), with both cohorts followed over a lengthy period of time. There is, though, additional support for these figures from other population-based series. In Lower Saxony, (West) Germany [201], and the Faroe Islands (Kurtzke, unpublished data), median survival has been calculated

Table 7.12 Percentage survival in population-based series of MS cases from life table analyses

Years post onset	Percentage surviving		
	Rochester, MN[a]	US Army[b]	Saxony, FRG[c]
0	100	100	100
5	98	96	100
10	95	90	93
15	89	83	86
20	73	73	69
25	64	66	63
30	(64)[d]	64	57
35	–	–	50
40	–	–	(50)
N	46	476	224

[a] Percy et al., 1971 [199].
[b] Kurtzke et al., 1970 [200].
[c] Poser et al., 1989 [201].
[d] Rate unstable, small numbers at risk.

Modified from S. Poser et al., 1989 [201].

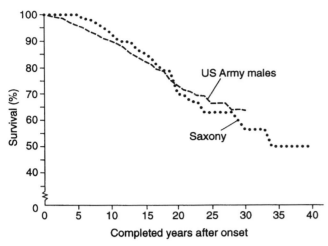

Figure 7.24. Multiple sclerosis: percentage survival by years after clinical onset from life table analyses. Epidemiological series of Lower Saxony, FRG (data of S. Poser *et al.*, 1989[201]) versus Second World War Army males, total series (data of Kurtzke *et al.*, 1970[200]). (After S. Poser *et al.*, 1989[201].)

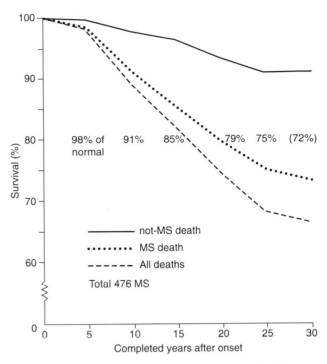

Figure 7.25. Multiple sclerosis: percentage survival by years after clinical onset according to cause of death – MS-related vs. not related to MS – for total US Army Second World War series. (After Kurtzke *et al.*, 1970[200].)

also to be in the order of some 35–40 years from onset. Table 7.12 compares the survival ratios of Saxony with those from the Rochester and the Army series. The German concordance with the Army ratios over the entire study interval is clearly seen in Figure 7.24.

The Rochester experience has recently been updated[202]. It showed an incidence rate of 6 per 100 000 for the decade of 1975–84, a significant increase over prior experience[138, 199]. The 25-year survival ratio was 76% versus 88% expected, the former figure being apparently higher than prior experience (Table 7.12). The Danish National MS Registry data provided a median survival of 30 years from onset[203]. For two Norwegian counties a median survival of 27 years from diagnosis was calculated by Riise *et al.*[204].

Expected survival

While median survival in MS, then, appears to be some 35–40 years after clinical onset, the question remains as to the excess of deaths over those expected for the general population. In the Army series, causes of death were allocated by review of the clinical records and not taken from the death certificates. Those deaths that were not attributable to MS can be taken as the normal expectations of the (selective) population of like age that is reflected by the military.

Figure 7.25 shows the Army survival ratios over time by cause of death, MS or not. The MS-related deaths clearly show a growing discrepancy from the expected (normal) deaths, but even after 25 years of illness, the survival ratio from MS itself was still some three-quarters of normal survival. This held as well for each

subgroup of the Army series, and it was also found for the Rochester series versus population expectations. The similar proportion seems possibly somewhat lower in the Saxony series, but not significantly so (Table 7.13). The excess death rate from onset in Denmark was calculated at 13.0 per 1000 person-years of observation; stated otherwise, there was a standardized mortality ratio of 3.25 for MS in Denmark (the standardized ratio being 1.00)[203].

Table 7.13 Percentage of normal (expected)[a] survival in population-based series of MS cases from life table analyses

Years post onset	Percentage of expected survival		
	Rochester, MN[b]	US Army[c]	Saxony, FRG[d]
0	100	100	100
5	99	98	101
10	98	91	95
15	94	85	88
20	80	79	72
25	74	75	68

[a] expected survival from US whites age 30 for Rochester series; from non-MS deaths among Army series; and from FRG population age 30 for Saxony series.
[b] Percy *et al.*, 1971[199].
[c] Kurtzke *et al.*, 1970[200].
[d] S. Poser *et al.*, 1989[201].

Table 7.14 US Army series: percentage survival in MS according to age at time of Army diagnosis

Years from diagnosis	Age at Army diagnosis			
	20–24	25–29	30–34	35–39
0	100.0	100.0	100.0	100.0
5	96.8	97.9	96.3	94.0
10	91.9	89.4	89.0	90.0
15	87.0	84.4	77.1	82.0
20	75.4	76.2	73.4	75.2
n	(123)	(141)	(109)	(50)

From Kurtzke *et al.*, 1970 [200].

Survival by age and sex

It has often been argued that in MS males have a worse prognosis for life than females, and that old age at onset is also an unfavorable predictor for survival. The first Rochester series was too small to answer these questions. The later one did show worse survival for males. While the Army series could not address sex, there was no difference in survival by age through the first 20 years after diagnosis: whether at age 20–24 or at successive age groups through to age 35–39, the survival ratio at that 20 year point was 75% in every instance (Table 7.14) – but older age onsets (age 40 and beyond) were not represented.

In the Norwegian series, median survival from diagnosis was 23.7 years for males and 'over 30' for females; for onset under age 35 this figure was 34.5 years vs. 21.7 years for older patients [204].

In the survival study of the epidemiological series from Lower Saxony, there was also a significant difference by age at onset, those with clinical onset at age 35 + years faring worse than those with onset under age 35; however, there was no significant variation by sex [201]. Because numbers were small, the same question was investigated with a much larger series of patients diagnosed between 1973 and 1975 in 11 neurological centres throughout West Germany (FRG) and followed for the next nine years or so. Survival was calculated by the same life table (actuarial) method as with the prior studies, with patients entered into the calculations according to time after clinical onset when they were first ascertained [197], and only those under observation for more than 2 years included. While such a (biased towards severity) hospital series cannot give an accurate absolute survival ratio (and in fact the median survival was 29 years), it seems valid to compare the patients *within* that series according to sex and age at onset.

When this was done, there were indeed found significant differences favouring females and young onsets (Figure 7.26). However, when each subgroup was compared with expected survival ratios based upon the

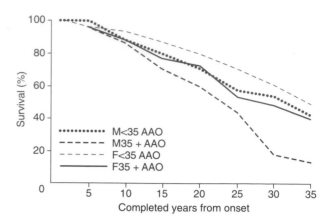

Figure 7.26. Multiple sclerosis: percentage survival by year after 3 years post onset by sex and age at onset (AAO) (< 35, 35 + years of age), West German (FRG) multi-centred hospital series of cases with 2 + years under observation. (Data of S. Poser *et al.*, 1989 [201].)

population of the FRG, there was a striking uniformity among all subgroups (Table 7.15). Regardless of time post onset, the percentage of expected survival in each of the four subgroups varied by, at the most, but a few percentage points from the ratios for the entire series throughout 35 years from onset (Figure 7.27). The conclusion from these data was that differential survival by sex and age at onset in MS is chiefly a reflection of the patterns expected for the entire population of like sex and age. In other words, males fare worse mostly because they are males and not because they have MS, and patients with older onsets die sooner than those with onset at younger years chiefly because they are older. This explanation may not be completely supported in the

Table 7.15 FRG hospital series (revised): percentages of expected survival[a] by gender and age at onset[b] in 1429 patients from 11 neurological centres

Years post onset	Total	M < 35	M 35 +	F < 35	F 35 +
0	100	100	(100)	100	100
5	97	101	99	96	96
10	91	88	93	93	90
15	80	78	77	85	82
20	74	73	71	79	79
25	63	61	67	70	62
30	55	55	(37)	62	69
35	44	(44)	(20)	46	(76)

[a] Expections based on life tables for FRG 1976–78 for entry age 25 (< 35 AAO), age 45 (35 + AAO), age 30 (total), with ratios for both sexes weighted 1:2, M:F.
[b] Age at onset (AAO) under 35 years and 35 + years.
[c] Parentheses indicate less than 10 patients at risk that year.

From S. Poser *et al.*, 1989 [201].

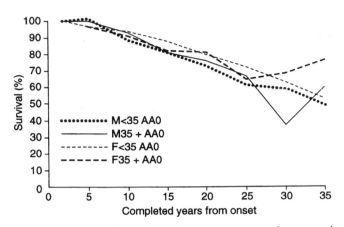

Figure 7.27. Multiple sclerosis: percentage of expected survival by sex and age at onset (AAO) as in Figure 7.26. (Data of S. Poser *et al.*, 1989 [201].)

Danish series, where the standardized mortality ratio was higher for women than men for each age-at-onset group except for those age 20–29 at onset, while the excess death rate was higher for men than women for each group except those age 50 + at onset. However, even there the greater part of the differential survival still appeared to be attributable to the population expectations by sex at least (their Figure 1); survival curves by both age and sex were not provided. I do not believe the Danish work really negates the German findings.

7.8 Demographic risk factors

It is clear from the foregoing that age, sex, race and geography are all important – and independent – risk factors in the expression of MS, but all are quite nonspecific [126]. We clearly need more discriminating characteristics in order to understand this illness. This section will not consider laboratory or familial features of MS, both covered extensively elsewhere in this volume, as well as in prior reviews [37–40].

7.8.1 GEOGRAPHIC CORRELATES

Attempts to identify factors that would explain the unique geographical distribution of MS have been numerous but unsuccessful [21 25, 37–40, 43, 46–49, 205]. Dietary fat [25], trace elements and heavy metals [206–212] have been implicated, but these observations remain largely unsupported. One problem with some studies has been the limited geographical area under investigation with little chance for cases to differ from controls; another has been the question of the representativeness of the patients *or* their controls. It is for these and other reasons that we have paid special attention to the US veteran series of the Second World War and the Korean conflict. Recall that this is a very large, nationwide 'inception cohort' of MS with the availability of unbiased, pre-illness controls *and* with the ability to study factors recorded for both case and control well before the patient became symptomatic.

Table 7.16 US veterans series: case and control (MS/C) pairs by county of birth and latitude of birthplace according to geographic correlates (Factor A) of the birth counties

Factor A	Latitude: case = control pairs w/Factor A			Factor A: case = control pairs w/latitude		
	MS > C	MS < C	P	MS > C	MS < C	P
Mean annual freeze-free period (F-F)	388	359	0.15	501	320	$< 10^{-9}$
Annual solar radiation (SOL)	207	210	0.46	894	530	$< 10^{-21}$
Mean annual hours of sunshine	504	487	0.30	552	307	$< 10^{-16}$
Mean annual days temperature > 90 °F	394	431	0.10	333	222	$< 10^{-5}$
Mean annual days temperature < 32 °F (COLD)	577	537	0.12	170	105	0.00006
Mean July relative humidity	489	486	0.47	616	338	$< 10^{-18}$
Mean annual pan evaporation (PAN)	269	255	0.28	565	359	$< 10^{-10}$
Mean annual days of precipitation (RAIN)	534	517	0.31	504	300	$< 10^{-12}$
Mean annual days forecasted air pollution	653	658	0.46	309	173	$< 10^{-9}$
Ground H_2O minerals	408	392	0.30	821	508	$< 10^{-17}$
Elevation, feet above sea level	553	509	0.09	552	286	$< 10^{-19}$
COLD × RAIN	751	681	0.03	77	39	0.0003
SOL × PAN	376	389	0.33	452	280	$< 10^{-9}$
F-F × RAIN	669	646	0.27	187	139	0.005
COLD × PAN	609	606	0.48	128	81	0.007

Modified from Norman, Kurtzke and Beebe, 1983 [213].

The large data set of the US veterans series was therefore analysed as to geoclimatic correlates of geography for the county of birth of the patients and their controls [213]. Taken singly, all of the characteristics tested were highly significantly related to the risk of MS. However, when adjusted for latitude *per se*, not one of these attributes then showed any significant relationship (Table 7.16). It was concluded that 'an explanation for the [marked] influence of latitude must be sought outside of the realm of conventional meteorologic variables' [213]. Multiple logistic regression analyses confirmed the importance of latitude alone [214, 215].

Population ancestry

In the US veterans series some anomalies in the distribution of MS risk by state (Figure 7.11) indicated that latitude, *per se*, might not be the sole determining factor of risk since at least the northern and middle tiers of latitude contained some states of differing MS risk. In seeking an explanation for such variation, William Page carried out cluster analyses (unpublished) and arrived at a hypothesis that ancestry might be a contributing factor. The lack of ancestry data at that time for the individual MS cases and controls in the cohort required the analysis of population-based information. The US decennial census of 1980 provided these data in tabulated form [216] for some 188 million persons.

Analyses included the ten largest self-reported ancestry groups (English, German, Irish, French, Italian, Scottish, Polish, Dutch, Swedish, and Norwegian) as well as Danish and 'Scandinavian, not otherwise specified'. Data were tabulated separately for respondents who reported 'at least one specific ancestry group' (total response) and for those who reported only 'a single ancestry group' (single response) [217].

Proportions of residents with specific ancestry by state were compared with case-control ratios for white male veterans of the Second World War by state of residence at birth and at entry into active duty (EAD), and correlational and regression analyses carried out with data weighted for state population size.

Table 7.17 shows the correlation coefficients. Most striking are the highly significant positive correlations of Scandinavian ancestry, especially Swedish ancestry, with MS risk; these are statistically significant for all combinations of single or total ancestry and birth or EAD state. Thus, in a given state, the higher the proportion of persons reporting Scandinavian ancestry on the 1980 census, the higher the risk of MS among Second World War white male veterans who were born in or entered military service from that state.

To quantify this association more precisely, weighted stepwise multiple regression models were fit, using all 12 ancestry groups to predict MS risk. Table 7.18 shows the sign of the regression coefficient (indicating positive or negative association) of each significant variable, along with the proportion of variance in MS risk explained, a measure of the strength of association.

Thus ancestry of the state population by itself explains nearly as much of the variation in MS risk (45–60%) as does geography (latitude) *per se* (60–67%). Even when ancestry is combined with geography in a joint model (data not shown), it remains a statistically significant and independent predictor of

Table 7.17 US veterans series: correlation of ancestry (single and total) with MS risk tabulated by birth and EAD state (Pearson correlation coefficients)

Ancestry type	Birth state		EAD state	
	Single ancestry	Total ancestry	Single ancestry	Total ancestry
English	−0.565***	−0.425***	−0.565***	−0.409**
German	0.250	0.276	0.260	0.309*
Irish	−0.136	−0.149	−0.114	−0.066
French	0.152	0.273	0.131	0.294*
Italian	0.212	0.238	0.207	0.228
Scottish	0.156	−0.077	0.107	0.151
Polish	0.296*	0.352*	0.283	0.349*
Dutch	0.077	−0.045	0.101	0.023
Swedish	0.545***	0.545***	0.631***	0.634***
Norwegian	0.401**	0.445**	0.444**	0.497***
Danish	0.306*	0.345*	0.263	0.375**
Scandinavian, n.o.s.	0.489***	0.509***	0.554***	0.566***

*P < 0.05, **P < 0.01, ***P < 0.001.
EAD, entry into active duty; n.o.s., not otherwise specified.

From Page *et al.*, 1993 [217].

Table 7.18 US veterans series: proportion of variance in MS risk explained by ancestry[a] (single and total responses)

Variable and direction of association[b]	Birth state		EAD state	
	Single ancestry (%)	Total ancestry (%)	Single ancestry (%)	Total ancestry (%)
Swedish (positive)	–	29.7	39.8	40.2
Italian (positive)	–	16.2	15.2	17.6
Scandinavian (n.o.s.) (positive)	12.3	–	–	–
Scottish (positive)	16.5	–	–	–
English (negative)	31.9	–	–	–
Total model	60.7	45.9	55.0	57.8

EAD, Entry into active duty; n.o.s., not otherwise specified.

[a] Based on 1980 decennial census data aggregated by state.
[b] Positive means that MS risk increases with increasing values of the variable; negative means that MS risk decreases with increasing values of the variable.

From Page *et al.*, 1993 [217].

MS risk. In this latter analysis, though, the Italian correlation disappears. Although the specific ancestry groups significantly predicting MS risk vary somewhat in the several analyses, Swedish (or, in one case, Scandinavian) ancestry is always a significant positive predictor of MS risk.

Ebers and Bulman [218] had independently done a similar analysis of the published data of our series and concluded that 'the distribution of MS in the United States, at least in part, reflects the distribution of genetic susceptibility factors'. In their full paper Bulman and Ebers [219] found 'the highest correlations between MS prevalence and Scandinavian birth/ancestry (r = 0.73)'. They stated: 'The analysis we report here supports a genetic explanation for the geography of MS in the US' [219].

That these data provide evidence for 'a genetic explanation' seems a premature statement. More appropriate would be that of Page *et al.* [217]: 'These findings provide evidence that ancestry of the resident population – a confounded measure of genetic susceptibility and cultural environment – is part of the complicated picture of MS as a disease of place.'

A link between ancestry and MS risk has older antecedents. Earlier I cited Davenport's presentation of data on drafted men in the First World War [58]. He reported among whites a high rate of MS in the Great Lakes region and the state of Washington. He stated that 'there is some race inhabiting [these regions] that is especially subject to multiple sclerosis... One thinks of the big Swedes that live in this country'. However, he continued that 'whether or not ... multiple sclerosis [is] especially common among Scandinavians cannot be definitely asserted'. Bailey's findings [59] were also cited for MS during service in that war. Geographically, the cases were distributed similar to those of Davenport, and he did note an excess among the foreign-born, and

in particular Scandinavians. Above I presented a conjecture to explain these and other findings as to the distribution of this disease, and below I shall consider ethnicity within the veterans series.

7.8.2 PERSONAL CHARACTERISTICS

Most retrospective case control comparisons by a number of workers have revealed no significant associations, other than the accepted geographical variations [16, 25, 29, 45, 220–227]. Poskanzer [45, 223] reported that patients had tonsillectomy in more instances than had either their spouses or their nearest siblings; but these results have not been replicated. In the Israeli studies there were possible inverse relationships with indices of poor sanitation and a direct relationship to some features of urbanization [220]. Reports implicating canine distemper or dog exposure have been published, but to date these also remain unverified (see [38] for references to 1983; later data, to my mind, do not alter this conclusion).

In Olmsted and Mower counties, Minnesota, small family size was significantly associated with the risk of MS [221]. Whether this reflects socioeconomic status (see below) is uncertain, although urban residence and high educational achievement did have relative risk estimates greater than one. In a small US veteran twin series, Bobowick *et al.* [147] reported a significant excess of prior 'environment events' among affected versus unaffected twins. These 'events' included operations, trauma and infections as the major groups; and differentiating frequencies were mostly within 20 years before clinical onset rather than in early childhood. Operskalski *et al.* [222], in a mailed questionnaire survey, recorded a notably increased risk for a history of infectious mononucleosis, and lesser increases for moves and travel.

Table 7.19 US veterans series: case-control ratios by socioeconomic status (SES)[a] and by urbanization classification of residence at entry into service

Urbanization class	SES scores					
	000–069	*070–109*	*110–149*	*150–200*	*Total*	*No. MS cases*
Metropolitan	2.00	3.67	1.70	3.50	2.40	(48)
Other urban	1.60	1.33	2.17	1.57	1.67	(40)
Mixed	0.63	0.88	1.21	1.52	0.98	(209)
Rural	0.62	0.36	1.09	1.52	0.63	(71)
Total	0.70	0.81	1.33	1.20	1.00	
No. of MS cases	(85)	(96)	(100)	(87)		(368)

[a] Sum of scores for pre-service occupational status (Bureau of Census codes) and codes for educational level, each ranging from 0 to 100; the higher the scores, the higher the SES.

Data of Beebe *et al.*, 1967[190]; from Kurtzke, 1988[39].

Poskanzer *et al.* [65] drew an analogy with poliomyelitis, and suggested that the existence of an infection such as this, if more commonly acquired in early life, protected against MS in low risk areas. This 'subtle hypothesis', as Acheson [21] termed it, is that the cause of MS is much more widespread where MS is rare than where it is common. As was true with polio, early birth order has been reported to increase MS risk [228]; but others have found no relationship to birth order [80, 229, 230].

As noted above, Beebe *et al.* [190] compared MS patients with matched controls from an earlier US Army Second World War series, utilizing data collected *before* multiple sclerosis was diagnosed. Among the characteristics that significantly differentiated patients from controls were geographical location at birth or service entry but not during military service before onset (see section 7.6.2). There was a strong positive correlation with urbanization of residence, high socioeconomic status (SES), and visual defects (refractive errors) at entry into military service. Table 7.19 summarizes the first two of these factors for the Army veterans, indicating each one to be an important variable.

Similar data are still being analysed for the large veteran series, but the findings thus far do include the same factors of high SES, urbanization and refractive errors, all of which appear to hold for white women and black men as well as for white men [231].

That series also provides the first solid evidence for differences in age at clinical onset according to geography [232]. The age at onset for white men in the Second World War series was 26.4 years for service entry from the northern tier, 27.3 years for entry from the middle tier and 28.8 years for entry from the south. Birth tier itself was not a significant variable. Similar were differences for the smaller numbers of black men and white women. Among the white men migrants also increased their age at onset by moving south between birth and service entry.

Individual ethnicity

Above we discussed the relationship of population ancestry of residence at service entry for the veteran series. Thomas Mack of the University of Southern California had developed a computer program to assign subjects to a single ethnic (linguistic) group based upon their surname. He thus categorized the 10 311 males comprising the cases and controls of the Second World War and Korean

Table 7.20 US veterans series: number of MS cases and case-control ratios grouped by surname-derived ethnicity for white males

Ethnicity	No. of cases[a]	Case control ratio
Celtic	556	0.93*
Eastern European	274	1.09
East and SE Asian	4	0.80
English	1567	0.96**
Latino[b]	53	0.79
Middle Eastern	14	0.70
Russian	79	1.34
Scandinavian	180	1.21
Southern European	321	1.35**
Western European	1049	1.15**
Total[a]	4098	1.04

[a] One case, with Hawaiian ethnicity, was not assigned to any ethnic group.
[b] Portuguese/Spanish.

* $P < 0.05$.
** $P < 0.01$.

From Page *et al.*, 1995[233].

Conflict MS series without knowledge of the subject's status as case or control. Details as to methodology may be found in the paper of Page *et al.* [233].

There were 22 ethnicity classes represented. These were combined for further analysis into ten groups (Table 7.20). There were statistically significant deficits (MS/C ratio under 1.0) for Celtic and English ethnicity groups, and significant excesses for Southern European and Western European groups; the case-control ratio of 1.21 for Scandinavians did not achieve statistical significance.

However, when these same ethnic groups were subdivided according to tier of residence at EAD, there was a striking uniformity in the case control gradient of north to middle to south for each ethnicity group (Table 7.21). Within each tier none of the ethnic distributions differed significantly from the others.

Stepwise logistic regression was carried out utilizing latitude of EAD residence; all of the population ancestry groups of the prior study [217] plus Greek ancestry, considering the findings for Southern European ethnicity (only Italian and Greek in this study); and the grouped ethnicity materials of Table 7.20. The result of this analysis indicated that the individual patient's

Table 7.22 US veterans series: effect of state-based ancestry and grouped surname-derived ethnicity on MS risk among white males: odds ratios for significant risk factors in stepwise logistic regression

Risk factor	Odds ratio
Latitude (each additional 5 degrees of northern latitude)	1.382
Swedish ancestry (each additional 5% of the EAD state's population)	1.137
French ancestry (each additional 5% of the EAD state's population)	1.076
Southern European ethnicity (individual yes versus no)	1.245

From Page *et al.* 1995 [233].

ethnicity was subordinate to these other factors in terms of the risk of MS; only Southern European ethnicity showed any independent contribution (Table 7.22). 'In general, we conclude that an individual's ethnicity seems to be of less relative importance in determining MS risk than is the population ancestry of the state of EAD. These findings underscore the fact that MS is a disease of place, with "place" including not only attributes of the locale (e.g., latitude), but also of its populace (e.g., ancestry)' [233].

The evidence for a genetic origin to differing geographic risks of MS, then, becomes quite tenuous. Sex and racial differences need by no means reflect heredity. Some time ago, after considering familial frequency and twin studies [2], I had written: 'My own view has been that a genetic factor is *unnecessary* to consider in seeking an explanation for the cause [of MS] (not that there cannot be one), which cause to me lies in the environment' (p. 132). I have to this date not seen evidence to convince me otherwise.

Table 7.21 US veterans series: cases and case-control ratios grouped by surname-derived ethnicity and EAD latitude tier for white males

Ethnicity	EAD latitude tier		
	Northern	Middle	Southern
Celtic	1.16 (222)	0.94 (241)	0.61 (93)
Eastern European	1.23 (127)	1.03 (139)	[0.57] (8)
English	1.38 (565)	1.00 (677)	0.59 (325)
Latino	1.57 (22)	1.05 (19)	0.74 (12)
Russian	1.45 (45)	1.29 (31)	[0.75] (3)
Scandinavian	1.72 (121)	0.79 (50)	[0.56] (9)
Southern European	1.53 (183)	1.26 (125)	0.72 (13)
Western European	1.41 (523)	1.13 (447)	0.54 (78)
Total	1.38 (1808)	1.04 (1729)	0.58 (541)

Case-control ratios based on 10 or fewer cases are in square brackets []. Numbers of cases are given in round brackets.

From Page *et al.* 1995 [233].

7.9 Epidemics

There has been in the past no reason to consider that MS has occurred in the form of epidemics. All known geographical areas that had been surveyed at repeated intervals up to 1980 provided either stable or increasing prevalence rates, the latter compatible with both better case ascertainment and perhaps improved survival. More recent changes have been considered above (section 7.4.4). Epidemics of MS would serve to define the disease as not only an acquired one, but also a transmissible one. We seem to have encountered separate epidemics of MS, which in fact may have common precipitants, and which have occurred in the ethnically similar lands of the Faroe Islands, the Shetland–Orkney Islands and Iceland.

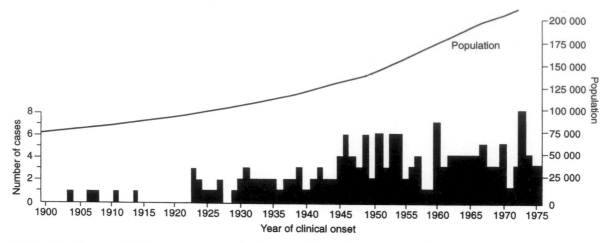

Figure 7.28 Distribution of MS cases among native-born residents of Iceland by calendar year of clinical onset, 1900–75. Icelandic population is recorded. (Data of Kurtzke *et al.*, 1982 [244].)

Recall that an epidemic may be defined as disease occurrence 'clearly in excess of normal expectancy and derived from a common or propagated source' [234, p. 81]. Epidemics are divisible into two types: 'Type 1 epidemics occur in susceptible populations, exposed for the first time to a virulent infectious agent. Type 2 epidemics occur in populations within which the virulent organism is already established' [235, p. 60]. If the entire populace is exposed to a Type 1 epidemic, the ages of those affected clinically will define the age range of susceptibility to the infection. This kind of assessment is how the Faroes previously became medically famous, by Panum having defined the age range of susceptibility to measles (life long) with the 1846 epidemic [236]. Type 2 epidemics will tend to have a young age at onset, as the effective exposure of the patients will then begin when they first reach the age of susceptibility. Epidemics can of course be due to toxins and deficiency states as well as infections, and allegorically may describe any sudden increase in adverse health effects (auto accidents, myocardial infarction). If the causative agent of a 'true' epidemic is persistent in an area, the epidemic will end when the number of susceptibles within the populace is exhausted. Any further cases would then be dependent on the arrival of new susceptibles – by birth, age or immigration. If the agent is transient in occurrence, then new cases can arise after its disappearance only by transmission from those affected to new cohorts of the unaffected, so that successive epidemics in such an instance are limited *de facto* to the action of infectious agents. The occurrence of MS in the Faroe Islands was described as an epidemic in our first presentation of 1975 [237]; the full paper appeared in 1979 [239]. For over 20 years now we have been actively investigating MS on these islands [239–243]. We shall first, though, consider other possibly pertinent materials, starting with another Nordic land.

7.9.1 ICELAND

After our earlier work on the Faroes, an obvious next question was what had happened with MS in Iceland. The same Norse Vikings had settled Iceland at about the same time as the Faroes. Like the Faroes, Iceland had been a county of Denmark, but it had attained semi-independence in 1918. Also like the Faroes, it was occupied in the Second World War – not only by the British, but also by the Canadians and the Americans. Iceland declared its independence as a nation during that war. With Sverrir Bergmann and the late Kjartan Guðmundsson, we had collected between 1974 and 1979 all MS cases known in Iceland with onset from 1900 to 1975 [244]. They numbered 168 among native-born resident Icelanders. In Figure 7.28 are the MS cases by year of onset. There seem to be four chronological phases: a low and sporadic occurrence before the First World War; a sudden rise in 1923 and then a plateau to 1944; then another sudden rise and an irregular plateau

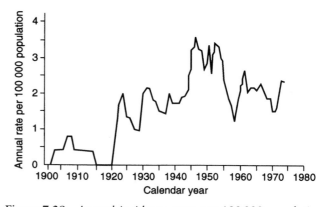

Figure 7.29 Annual incidence rates per 100 000 population for MS in Iceland, calculated as 3-year centred moving averages. (Data of Kurtzke *et al.*, 1982 [244].)

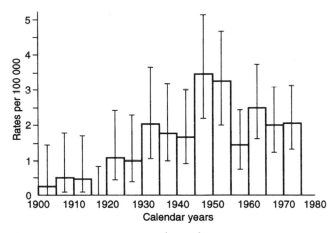

Figure 7.30 Average annual incidence rates per 100 000 population for MS in Iceland; 5-year intervals with 95% confidence limits on the average rates. (Data of Kurtzke *et al.*, 1982 [244].)

from 1945 to 1954; and then a plateau at lower levels thereafter. Annual incidence rates reveal that there does seem to have been at least one definite type 2 epidemic of MS in Iceland beginning in 1945 (Figure 7.29). The average annual incidence rate from 1923 to 1944 was 1.6 per 100 000. For 1945–54 it was significantly higher at 3.2, and then it declined significantly to 1.9 for 1955–74 (Figure 7.30). In fact, most of the individual five-year intervals from 1900 on had incidence rates significantly below those of 1945 to 1949 or 1950 to 1954, and by ten-year intervals all showed the significant difference. Furthermore, age at onset in the 1945 to 1949 interval (23 years) was significantly lower than for any other quinquennium 1900 to 1974. Thus, to us, there did appear to be a postwar epidemic of MS in Iceland. Cook *et al.* [245, 246] had independently come to the same conclusion, and Kjartan Guðmundsson had previously pointed out the significant decline in incidence from 3.1 for 1946–55 to 1.9 for 1956–65 [247]. Conversely, Charles Poser and colleagues have concluded that there was never any significant variation in incidence in Iceland up to 1985, attributing any pre-war deficit to incomplete ascertainment and considering the 1945–54 peak to be not meaningful, since incidence had risen gradually from 1955 to over 4 per 100 000 in the 1980s [81, 82].

7.9.2 OTHER AREAS

The Shetland–Orkney Islands

These islands off northern Scotland were once possessions of Denmark, and in the Viking era had considerable occupations from Norway, as with Iceland and the Faroes. Earlier we had pointed out that the Shetland–Orkneys, taken together, had at the time of study the highest prevalence rates for MS known (nos. 6 and 6a in Figure 7.5). These islands have been formally surveyed as to the occurrence of MS five times. Sutherland in 1954 [62], Allison [63] and Fog and Hyllested in 1961–62 [64], Poskanzer *et al.* in 1970, and Poskanzer *et al.* in 1974 (where the former study is cited) [224] – each group demonstrated progressively increasing prevalence rates so as to attain by the last date rates for probable MS of 258 per 100 000 in the Orkneys and 152 in Shetland. Because of small numbers of cases and population I have tended to combine results for both sets of islands, although Poskanzer [224] pointed out that most of the increase over time was attributable to the Orkneys.

The fifth set of surveys was that of Cook *et al.* In 1985 [66] they observed that MS on the Orkneys seemed to have shown a marked decline in the annual incidence between 1965 and 1973, with few cases thereafter to 1983 when their survey input ended. They concluded that the Orkney experience too was compatible with a post Second World War epidemic, but attributed the increase and decrease in incidence to the occurrence of canine distemper on those islands. A similar decline was found for the Shetland Islands [248] up to 1986 'beginning between 1951 and 1968'. Basic data for the latter work were kindly provided by Dr Cook (personal communication, 9 September 1988), and additional population figures for both island groups by F.G. Thomas of the General Register Office for Scotland (personal communication, 13 March 1987). The onset data of Cook *et al.* for both islands were cited uniformly as one year after those depicted by Poskanzer [224] for the period from 1940; I have accordingly moved Poskanzer's figures as well for the 1930s.

Based on the above, the incidence rates over time for the Shetland–Orkneys are summarized in Table 7.23. The occurrence after 1970 is significantly lower than that for the prior 30 or 35 years. The individual annual incidence rates show considerable fluctuations, and do apparently differ in peaks and troughs somewhat between the islands, but the overall impression of at least one epidemic between 1941 and 1970 seems valid, as does the clear decline after 1970 – at least up to 1983 or 1986. Further assessment is required to consider the possibility of repeated epidemics *within* the 1941–70 interval.

Poskanzer *et al.* [224] were of the opinion that MS in the Shetland–Orkneys had always been of high frequency, citing deaths attributed to disseminated sclerosis as early as 1898 and 1908. 'After that, the [death certificate] diagnoses appeared routinely' [224, p. 232] and averaged 1.6 cases a year, the large majority being, however, 'possible MS'. They thought that previous cases might have been missed by misdiagnosis or by emigration. Still, the available data do indicate a dramatic increase circa 1940 and a dramatic decrease circa 1970 in

Table 7.23 Average annual incidence rates per 100 000 population for probable MS in Shetland and Orkney Islands, 1911–1985

Period	Shetland			Orkney			Both		
	n	Rate	95% CI	n	Rate	95% CI	n	Rate	95% CI
1911–15	1	0.73*	0.02–4.06	0	0*	0–2.89	1	0.38*	0.01–2.10
1916–20	0	0*	0–2.81	0	0*	0–2.99	0	0*	0–1.45
1921–25	2	1.62	0.20–5.84	1	0.84	0.02–4.70	3	1.24*	0.26–3.62
1926–30	0	0*	0–3.26	1	0.88	0.02–4.91	1	0.44*	0.01–2.46
1931–35	3	2.85	0.59–8.32	3	2.66	0.55–7.77	6	2.75	1.01–5.98
1936–40	6	5.94	2.18–12.94	3	2.52	0.52–7.35	9	4.09	1.87–7.76
1941–45	9	9.52*	4.36–18.06	13	10.79*	5.74–18.45	22	10.23*	6.41–15.49
1946–50	11	11.05*	5.51–19.77	10	9.14*	4.39–16.81	21	10.05*	6.22–15.36
1951–55	5	5.27	1.71–12.30	13	12.42*	6.61–21.23	18	9.02*	5.35–14.26
1956–60	11	12.01*	5.99–21.49	8	8.18	3.53–16.12	19	10.03*	6.04–15.67
1961–65	5	5.68	1.84–13.26	10	10.83*	5.20–19.92	15	8.32*	4.66–13.72
1966–70	9	10.48*	4.80–19.90	6	6.84	2.51–14.89	15	8.69*	4.87–14.34
1971–75	2	2.22	0.27–8.00	2	2.31	0.28–8.34	4	2.26	0.62–5.79
1976–80	3	2.85	0.59–8.34	2	2.22	0.27–8.01	5	2.56	0.83–5.98
1981–82	–	–	–	1	2.63	0.07–14.64	–	–	–
1981–85	2	1.66	0.20–5.99	–	–	–	–	–	–
Total	69	4.36	3.39–5.52	73	4.73	3.71–5.95	139	4.69	3.94–5.53
	$\chi^2_{14} = 57.763$			$\chi^2_{14} = 61.539$			$\chi^2_{13} = 100.630$		

$P = 0.00001$ @ $\chi^2_{14} = 48.716$.
*Significantly high or low vs. mean ($\chi^2_a > 4.0$).

Data of Poskanzer *et al.*, 1980 [224] and Cook *et al.*, 1985, 1988 [66, 248]

the occurrence of this disease. Thus there seems clearly to have been at least one wartime–postwar epidemic of MS in the Shetland–Orkney Islands. Martin [249] pointed out that nearly as many cases would have had to be missed in the prewar era as were found later in order to negate the existence of the epidemics. He also raised the question whether this epidemic too was attributable to British troop concentrations there during the war – as was the situation, as we shall see, in the Faroes. But it seems to have persisted after any troop concentrations would have long disappeared and without clearly separate recurrences until the recent decline; the apparent decreases in annual incidence rates do not at first inspection seem to have followed any definable pattern, but further exploration would be in order to see if a patterning other than chance variation can be defined. What is clearly needed, though, is an update of the experience on these islands to cover the most recent 10 or 15 years. Will high rates have returned?

North America

The purported Key West 'epidemic' of Sheremata *et al.* [141] has been discussed previously, as have the later reports of Bigler [142] and Helmick *et al.* [143]. Other MS clusters have been reported in the Americas, such as the six cases occurring in the 500-person population of Mossyrock, Washington [250], and the 13 cases in the 10 000 population of Mansfield, Massachusetts [251]; the 10 cases in the 150 population of a farming area in Colchester County, Nova Scotia [252], seem less well documented. No satisfactory explanation has arisen for these clusters, and no follow-ups have been reported for either the cases or their communities.

Stein *et al.* [253] were contacted in 1982 by an industrial physician of an upstate New York manufacturing plant because of 'an unusual number of cases of MS among the employee population. This industry uses zinc as a principal raw material. Our report of this industry-based MS cluster follows' [253, p. 1672]. After careful review they found 11 cases of MS had occurred in 1970–79 among workers with more than one year of employment before onset, which occurrence they estimated to be significantly in excess of population expectations. No differences in Zn levels or exposure were found in their employee case control study; both sets had Zn levels apparently somewhat higher than local non-plant workers.

Follow-up of this experience was provided by Schiffer *et al.* [254]. There were nine new cases of MS in the

1980–89 decade. No differences in HLA patterns were seen vs. non-plant MS. Transferrin C3 gene frequencies seemed higher in the plant MS patients; C1 and C2 did not differ appreciably between groups (transferrin is an Fe- and Zn-binding protein). The authors state: 'We do not yet have an explanation for the ongoing MS incidence cluster in this manufacturing plant' [254, p. 332].

This New York experience is difficult to evaluate. Only numerator data were provided. The location itself is undefined. While it is understandable that the plant would seek anonymity, there is no way to judge whether these cases are truly a space cluster, since there is no information as to the frequency of MS in the area of the plant – nor the size of the 'area' in view. There is also no information as to characteristics these patients may have had in common aside from their occupation.

7.9.3 THE FAROE ISLANDS

The Faroe Islands comprise a group of 18 major volcanic islands lying in the North Atlantic Ocean at 7° W longitude and 62° N latitude. First settled by Norse Vikings in the ninth century, they had long been a standard county (*amt*) of Denmark. In 1948 the Faroes achieved semi-independence, though remaining part of the Kingdom of Denmark, which is still responsible for their health and welfare services. The population numbered some 48,000 in 1989.

The first hospital in the Faroes opened at Tórshavn, the capital, in 1829. Both Klaksvík Hospital in the north and Tvøroyri Hospital in the south were established in 1904; and there was a tuberculosis hospital near Tórshavn from 1908 to 1962. The State Psychiatric Hospital was opened in 1963 at Tórshavn. Denmark has had nationwide medical coverage provided by the state or the individual counties since 1921. Faroese patients in need of specialized diagnosis and treatment have long been sent to The National [Royal] Hospital (Rigshospitalet) in Copenhagen. Since 1929, this hospital has had a separate Neuromedical Department, although neurological care was under the Medical Departments previously [40, 238–240, 242, 243].

Case ascertainment

Critical to our findings and interpretations is the requirement that we have found *all* cases of MS that have occurred among Faroese in the twentieth century. We are limited by the fact that the person must have been seen medically and neurological symptoms recorded. But two points argue for completeness: MS clinically is a disorder with repeated or progressive symptomatology over time; and medical care for Faroese, not constrained by financial factors, is of high quality and well documented. Further, 'MS' is usually the first consideration for unexplained neurological symptoms in young adults: suspects will be over-reported rather than the reverse.

Ascertainment of potential cases of MS has been ongoing since 1972 utilizing all available resources [238–240, 242, 243]. These include the aforementioned hospital records and death certificates from 1900 on, the National Patient and Death Registries, and the Danish MS Registry. For any patient suspected of MS, all medical records from Denmark and the Faroes were reviewed and the subjects personally examined by us. Diagnostic criteria were those of the Schumacher Panel [10], although most patients also had the appropriate laboratory abnormalities in spinal fluid, evoked responses, and – in some – MR or CT. Clinical features are typical of any series of MS [238–240, 242, 243].

Cases of MS among the Faroese were subdivided according to their residence history, based on criteria first defined in 1974. In order to avoid attributing to the Faroes the occurrence of disease that had in fact been acquired elsewhere, we then decided to exclude from the resident series those we had *a priori* decided had lived 'too long' off the islands before clinical onset: Persons off the Faroes for 3 or more years before onset were thus to be excluded (Group C); those not off (Group A) or off less than 2 years (Group B) were to be included [238–240, 242]. In the recent analysis, requirements for new exclusions (Group C') have been made more stringent because of the potential for exposure to this disease in both Denmark and the Faroes [243]. Validation of the exclusion criteria was provided by the findings for the migrants (next section).

The excluded 'migrant' multiple sclerosis

The patients with foreign residence were not only potential 'rejects' but also comprised two groups of immigrants from a low-risk MS area (Faroes) to a high one (Denmark). Figure 7.31 provides for each patient the ages and durations of foreign residence. For Group C, C', ignoring short childhood visits for one of them, all of the patients had had at least two years of their stay off the Faroes between the ages of 11 and 36, and two years was the minimum period for such stays.

The foreign residences for Group B showed little consistency in time to MS onset. On the other hand, the Group C residences clustered within 10 years or so before clinical onset. Subtracting the 2 years 'exposure' which is common to all from each patient's overseas residence interval gave an 'incubation' period of 7.2 years (range 5–13).

From this we concluded that residence in a high-risk MS area by a susceptible but virgin (as to MS) population for a period of 2 years from age 11 on, could result in clinical MS beginning after a further period of some 7 years. Additionally, residence need not have been maintained in that endemic area for the entire

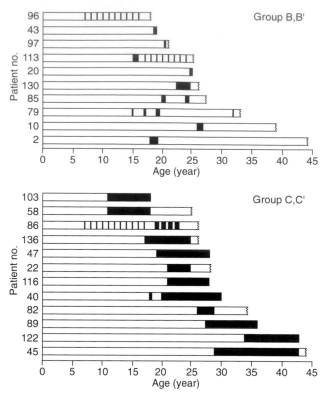

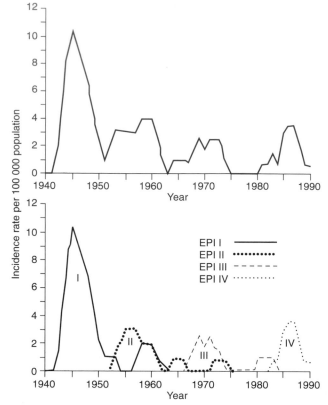

Figure 7.31. Faroese MS. Ages and durations of foreign residences (black segment of bars) for Groups B,B′ and C,C′ patients as of 1991. MS clinical onset is the terminus of each patient's bar with its origin at birth; a straight terminal line indicates symptom onset while overseas, a jagged line, while in the Faroes. Numbers identify the patients in reports by Kurtzke and Hyllested [239]) and Kurtzke *et al.* [243]. (Reproduced from Kurtzke, 1993 [40] with permission.)

Figure 7.32. MS in native resident Faroese. Annual incidence rates per 100 000 population calculated as 3-year centred moving averages as of June 1991. *Upper panel*: total series; *lower panel*: incidence rates by epidemic. (Reproduced from Kurtzke *et al.*, 1993 [243], with permission.)

interval. Thus, 7 years is a true incubation or latent interval between disease acquisition and symptom onset. Further, short periods of residence in the same place and at the same age did not result in MS.

The resident series

By 1991 we had ascertained 42 cases of MS among native-born resident Faroese. We could not find one single resident patient with clinical onset of MS in this century until July 1943. Then there were 16 patients with onset 1943–1949, and another 26 with onset thereafter.

Annual incidence rates per 100 000 population showed an early and dramatic rise and fall, followed by three irregular secondary peaks (Figure 7.32, *top*). The rate exceeded 10 per 100 000 in 1945. The first question was whether this was a single epidemic with a very irregular tail, or whether the incidence rate curve in fact reflected separate epidemics. The migrant series considered above suggested that MS was acquired by Faroese only if they were at least 11 years of age at first exposure, and only if the exposure was then for at least 2 years' duration. Hence, we classified the resident series

according to the calendar time when the patients had attained age 11, whether by 1941 (2 years before first clinical onset) or thereafter. Figure 7.33 shows the results as of 1986; there clearly seemed to be a separation into discrete subsets – or epidemics. The 1991 update of this material provides the annual incidence rates by epidemic shown in Figure 7.32 (*bottom*). Epidemic I then comprised all patients aged 11 + in 1941 plus one (see below) aged 11 by 1943 (*n* = 20). Epidemic I accounted for all cases contributing to the first MS incidence rate peak. Epidemic II comprised the patients aged 11 in 1946–51; they accounted for the second incidence rate peak (*n* = 9). Epidemic III comprised the patients aged 11 in 1956–67; they accounted for the third incidence rate peak (*n* = 6). And Epidemic IV patients achieved age 11 or first effective exposure in 1973–80; hence the fourth incidence rate peak (*n* = 7). Age at clinical onset was similar, near age 21, for epidemics II, III and IV patients, but all were significantly lower than age at onset for epidemic I cases, age 30. Incubation averaged some six years from 1943 or age 13, whichever came later (5, 8, 8, 7 years for epidemics I, II, III, IV) [243].

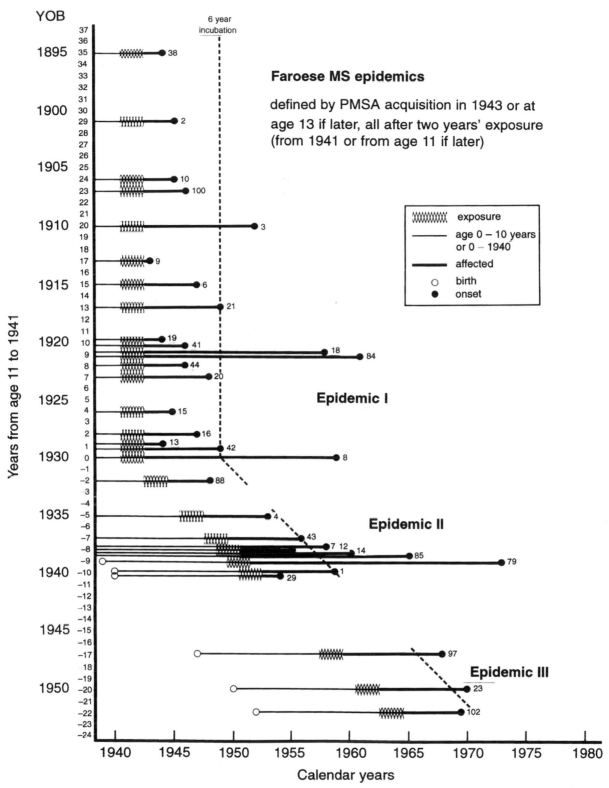

Figure 7.33. MS in native resident Faroese as of 1986. Each patient is represented by a bar with the thin portion the time and ages *before* exposure to PMSA (the primary MS affection; see text) and the 2 years of cross-hatching the period of PMSA exposure, following which (heavy portion of bar) the patient is affected but neurologically asymptomatic (the incubation period). Solid circles at terminus of each bar represent time and age of clinical onset, with the numbers identifying the patient in the report by Kurtzke and Hyllested [240]. Open circles for lower bars define time of birth. Location of each bar on the Y axis is specified by the number of years from 1941 at which time the patient attained age 11; calendar year of birth (YOB) is also identified. Dashed line represents a 6-year incubation period from time of acquisition of PMSA after the 2-year exposure. (Reproduced from Kurtzke and Hyllested, 1987 [240], with permission.)

Table 7.24 Faroese CNMS cases: average annual incidence rates per 100 000 population (with observed and expected MS cases), divided into four epidemic periods of 13 years with each period expected to comprise 7 'high' followed by 6 'low' years

Period	Person-years	MS-O	MS-E	χ^2_a	Rate[a]	95% CI
1943–49	205 033	16	4.888	25.261	7.80	4.46–12.67
1950–55	192 711	4	4.594	0.077	2.08	0.57–5.31
1956–62	239 155	7	5.702	0.295	2.93	1.17–6.03
1963–68	221 324	2	5.276	2.034	0.90	0.11–3.26
1969–75	277 106	5	6.606	0.390	1.80	0.58–4.21
1976–81	257 194	0	6.132	6.132	0.00	0.00–1.43
1982–89[b]	369 205	8	8.802	0.369	2.17	0.93–4.27
Total	1 761 728	42	42.000	34.558	2.38	1.72–3.22

[a] Rate per 100 000 person-years. $\chi^2_6 = 34.556$, $P < 0.00001$.
[b] Results similar for 1982–88.

From Kurtzke *et al.*, 1993 [243].

The existence of the epidemics on the Faroes has been contested by C.M. Poser *et al.* [255] and Poser and Hibberd [256]. The same points were raised again by Benedikz [257] in a symposium supplement edited by Poser [258]. Our detailed response has been published [242].

The median year of symptom onset was 1947 for epidemic I and 1986 for epidemic IV [243]. If this division into four epidemics is valid, there should be an average interval of some 13 years ([1986–1947 = 39]/3) between each epidemic's onset or end. Thus, if there are four epidemics, they should have begun about 1943, 1956, 1969 and 1982 respectively, and the few years before these respective dates should be the 'valleys' or troughs of virtually no cases. Results are given for seven years 'on' (high case expectation) followed by six years 'off' (low) for each epidemic (eight- and five-year division results were quite similar) (Table 7.24).

The hypothesis of three epidemics after the first within *population cohorts*, each defined by the calendar time age 11 occurred, can also be tested with the same *a priori* division of 13-year intervals (seven 'on', six 'off') used above, beginning in 1945. Thus, if this is a valid criterion, age 11 'on' intervals should start near 1945, 1958 and 1971. The denominator for each interval is the number of Faroese aged 11, derived from published data for Faroese aged 10–14 or similar intervals. Even with these very small numbers the findings are still statistically significant (Table 7.25). Consolidating the three 'high' periods and comparing them with the three 'low' gives risk ratios of 1.21 and 0.30 per 1000 respectively, with $\chi^2_c = 6.24$, $0.02 > P > 0.01$. The relative risk is 4.00 for high versus low intervals.

Geographic distribution and British troops

The pertinence of residence location within the Faroes has to do with our assessment of the British occupation in the Second World War. The Faroes were occupied by British troops for five years from April 1940. During

Table 7.25 Faroese series: risk of CNMS per 1 000 population aged 11, for three epidemics after epidemic I divided into periods of 13 years, with each period expected to comprise 7 'high' followed by 6 'low' years

Period	Persons aged 11	Patients aged 11		χ^2_a	Risk[a]	95% CI
		MS-O	MS-E			
1945–51	3 963.6	9	3.112	11.140	2.27	1.04–4.31
1952–57	3 994.5	1	3.137	1.456	0.25	0.01–1.39
1958–64	5 070.5	4	3.981	0.000	0.79	0.21–2.02
1965–70	4 465.5	1	3.506	1.791	0.22	0.01–1.25
1971–77	5 804.4	5	4.558	0.043	0.86	0.28–2.01
1978–83	4 719.1	2	3.706	0.785	0.42	0.05–1.53
Total	28 017.6	22	22.000	15.215	0.79	0.49–1.19

[a] Per 1 000 persons aged 11. $\chi^2_5 = 15.215$, $P < 0.02$.
From Kurtzke *et al.*, 1993 [243].

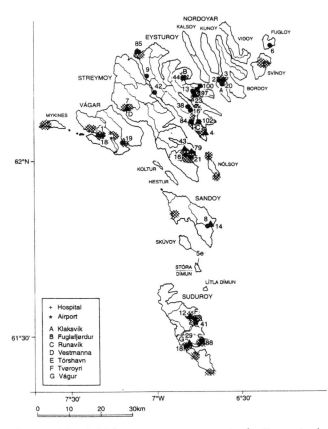

Figure 7.34. British troop encampments in the Faroes in the Second World War (cross-hatched areas), and residence of Faroese MS patients in 1943 or at age 11 if then younger for patients known as of 1986, subdivided by epidemic: I (●), II (▲), III (■). Numbers identify the patients in the report by Kurtzke and Hyllested [240]. (Reproduced from Kurtzke and Hyllested, 1987 [240], with permission.)

1941–44 there were at least 1500 troops stationed on the islands. The most rigid and unbiased criterion for exposure of Faroese to British troops is that Faroese MS patients lived where the troops were billeted (Figure 7.34). It was clear the locations of troop encampments were strongly correlated with the place of residence of all MS patients, regardless of epidemic [239, 240, 243].

Our conclusion was that British troops brought MS to the Faroese in the Faroe Islands during 1941–44 (this was why we included in epidemic I one patient aged 11 in 1943).

It was also clear the disease had *not* spread throughout the islands. There are still the same 21 parishes, containing 25% of the population in 1943, which were free of both MS and British troop occupation.

Parishes of residence for all patients of all four epidemics versus those occupied by British troops during the war are described elsewhere [243]. In formal testing, troop locations versus residence of patients of epidemics I–IV has OR of 20.43 ($P < 0.001$); versus II–IV, OR is 9.00 ($P < 0.01$). There is also a highly significant association between residence of patients of epidemics II–IV and that of epidemic I: OR = 32.63 ($P < 0.001$).

Therefore, this disease has remained geographically stable on the Faroes for half a century, and the MS risk areas remain in essence those defined by the British troop occupation sites of the Second World War.

Transmission of multiple sclerosis in the Faroe Islands

Our principal conclusion from the Faroes work, and one compatible with other epidemiological evidence [38, 40], is that clinical neurological MS (CNMS) is the rare late manifestation of infection with what we call PMSA – the primary MS affection. In this concept PMSA is transmissible; CNMS is not. Evidence as to the characteristics of PMSA derives entirely from the epidemiological features of CNMS. Among Faroese, these indicate that some two years of exposure to PMSA are necessary before its acquisition; Faroese under age 11 are not susceptible; and once PMSA is acquired, those Faroese who develop CNMS do so after an average incubation period of some six or seven years [240, 243]. The proportion of exposed Faroese who acquire PMSA is obviously unknown, but in our models we have taken that value as 100% of the population at risk.

Our transmission models were based on the finding of separate consecutive epidemics of CNMS. To explain this, there must have been separate consecutive cohorts of the population who acquired PMSA. The first cohort (F1) would have acquired PMSA from the British troops during the Second World War occupation. However, since the troops had left the islands by then, the second (F2) cohort must have acquired the disease from the F1 cohort, and then in turn transmitted PMSA to a third (F3) population cohort [240]. If this were true, then the expectation was that the F3 cohort would transmit PMSA to a fourth cohort, and this would be demonstrated by the occurrence of a fourth epidemic of CNMS – which is what has happened [243].

The way in which we were able to construct separate cohorts out of the continuum which is the Faroese population over time was to define an *age* beyond which PMSA would not be transmissible, and we took this age to be the average age of symptom onset of CNMS in general, age 27. Two corollaries are those noted above: susceptibility to PMSA begins at age 11, and 2 years of exposure are required for PMSA to be acquired. All of these numbers – age 11, age 27, 2 years – should be taken as *population averages* about which individuals may well vary appreciably. Each statement of the following should be taken, then, to include 'about' or 'approximately'.

A summation of our concept of PMSA transmission on the Faroes is provided in Figure 7.35, the main part of which represents specified portions of the actual

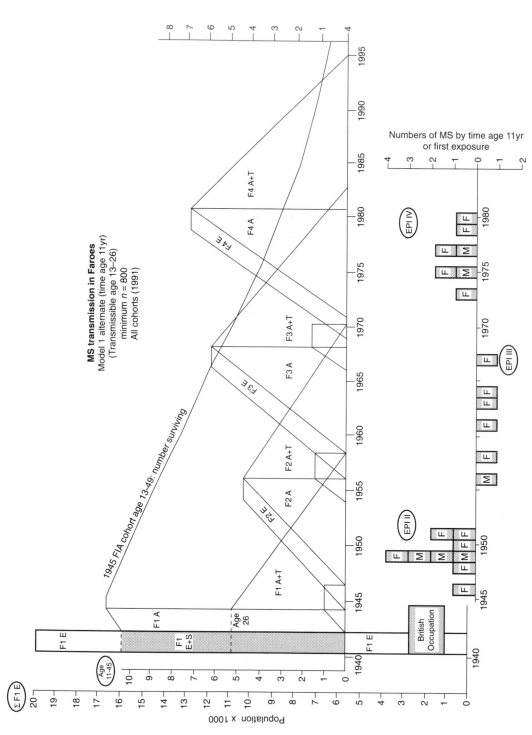

Figure 7.35. Faroese population cohorts exposed to and affected with PMSA. The first Faroese cohort (F1) exposed to PMSA (F1 E) from the British troops (block at lower left) comprises the entire Faroese population, all ages, geographically at risk in 1941 (long bar to left). Only those aged 11–45 in 1941 were susceptible (F1 E + S) to PMSA, based on later occurrence of CNMS (shaded portion of bar). After two years of exposure, F1 E + S becomes the F1 A (affected) cohort. That part of the F1 A cohort under age 27 in 1945 defines the F1 A + T (affected and transmissible) cohort, which declines in number each year as those attaining age 27 are deleted (first decreasing triangle). The F1 A + T cohort transmits PMSA to the second cohort of Faroese (F2), formed from those reaching age 11 each year while F1 A + T is of sufficient size. Their two years of exposure, F2 E (first rising parallelogram), precede the stage of affected (F2 A); when F2 E/F2 A ceases growth it begins its own decline while serving as the F2 A + T cohort for transmission of PMSA to F3 E. Similar is transmission from F3 A + T to F4 E. At the bottom of main figure each patient of epidemics II–IV is identified by time of first exposure to PMSA. The survival curve for the entire F1 A population cohort from 1945 is also drawn in the upper portion. (Reproduced from Kurtzke *et al.*, 1993 [243], with permission.)

population over time. The small block to the lower left represents the British occupation of 1941–44, which is the source of PMSA among the first (F1) cohort of Faroese (long vertical block). Only 0.757 of the total population in 1941 were geographically exposed (see above) to the British and PMSA; thus F1 E (exposed) comprised nearly 20 000 Faroese of all ages. However, only those aged 11–45 in 1941 later developed CNMS; therefore, susceptibility to PMSA is limited to that F1 E + S portion (shaded part of the block). After 2 years of exposure F1 E + S became the F1 A cohort (affected with PMSA). At the time of the British departure, the F1 A cohort numbered nearly 11 000 Faroese aged 13–49. Were this entire cohort able to transmit PMSA throughout its life, there would have been a *steady* input for new cases of CNMS well into the twenty-first century (see 'number surviving' curve in Figure 7.35) and *not* consecutive epidemics. However, the number of persons aged 13–26 in 1945 was some 5300, and *this* was the portion able to transmit (F1 A + T) PMSA. Each year those attaining age 27 ceased to be F1 A + T persons.

The F2 E cohort comprised the geographically appropriate fraction of all Faroese attaining age 11 each year until 2 years before the effective end of F1 A + T input. In Figure 7.35 we have hypothesized 800 Faroese as the minimum number needed to transmit PMSA.

When input to F2 E ceased the F2 A + T cohort began its own decline as its members attained age 27, and until it reached its own effective minimum it was the source of PMSA for the F3 cohort, which again was accrued from those attaining age 11 each year. Similar considerations hold for the F4 E cohort. There is an increasing size to each cohort, the result of both overall population growth and selective movement into our geographical risk areas.

Note that at the time when the magnitude of each cohort is declining, that of its successor is increasing. There will thus be intermittent periods when either cohort, transmitter or transmittee is 'too small', and therefore there will be intermittent periods when PMSA (and thus CNMS) would be less likely to occur. Conversely, when both cohorts are 'adequate' in size – which will also be intermittent – we have more effective PMSA transmission and later CNMS; hence the epidemics [259].

MS in the Faroes: summation

What then can be inferred from the Faroese saga? In outline form I will show the findings from the best evidence available and my interpretations of this material.

1. CNMS did not exist among resident Faroese before 1943.
2. PMSA was introduced into the Faroes by British troops in 1941–44.

3. This introduction led to a point source epidemic of CNMS (epidemic I) within the cohort of Faroese who were affected with PMSA (F1 A) after 2 years' exposure (F1 E).
4. Only Faroese aged 11–45 at onset of exposure were affected with CNMS, and hence PMSA.
5. Those affected Faroese aged 13–26 (F1 A + T) transmitted PMSA to a second cohort of Faroese (F2 E), comprising those attaining age 11 while F1 A + T existed.
6. The F2 A + T cohort included the CNMS of epidemic II and was the source of PMSA in the F3 cohort with its epidemic III of CNMS.
7. The F3 A + T cohort similarly has produced epidemic IV within the F4 cohort with PMSA.

7.9.4 THE NATURE OF MS

I think it is as well established as possible, then, that there have been true epidemics of MS – not only in the Faroes, but also in Shetland–Orkney and Iceland. The dramatic increases in incidence and prevalence noted above for northeastern Scotland, for Turku, Finland, for Hordaland, Norway, for Rochester, Minnesota, for Lower Saxony, Germany, and for several areas of Italy – all these can also be so interpreted. Similarly, the postwar decline in incidence in Denmark is compatible with this thesis, and there was a bactrian-camel curve for annual incidence in Rostock, (East) Germany. In the last, average annual incidence rates were 4.5 per 100 000 for 1963–68; 1.8 for 1969–1973; 3.7 for 1974–78; 1.8 for 1979–83 [260]. And all this is not to mention the apparently recent changes in the entire Mediterranean area discussed above as well.

The best explanation I can offer is that MS is the result of a specific infection transmissible from person to person. This, however, would require a much larger pool of transmissible persons than clinical cases can provide, else the disease would have rapidly died out. The thesis of subclinical disease as such a source of transmissibility, which was raised in 1969 [33], has been elaborated into our current concept of PMSA, the primary MS affection, as a widespread infection that only rarely results in clinical MS. We are hoping to search for a (retro)virus as the PMSA agent. The Faroes are the ideal locus for such a project, since even after 50 years of illness there are *still* areas of the islands where PMSA (as measured by CNMS) has not yet appeared. This gives a dimension to 'controls' that is not possible anywhere else in the world.

I would like to close this chapter with another summary list, this one as to the nature of MS [40].

1. There is a specific, widespread but unidentified infection we call the primary multiple sclerosis affection (PMSA).

2. PMSA is a persistent infection transmitted person to person.
3. A small proportion of persons with PMSA will later develop clinical neurological multiple sclerosis (CNMS).
4. Prolonged exposure (some 2 years virgin; 4 years [?] endemic) is needed to acquire PMSA.
5. PMSA acquisition follows first adequate exposure.
6. Susceptibility to PMSA is limited to about age 11 to 45 at start of exposure.
7. CNMS is *not* transmissible.
8. Therefore, transmissibility of PMSA is limited to a period under usual age of CNMS onset.
9. Existence of PMSA can now be inferred only from existence of CNMS.

7.10   Comment

Epidemiology is the study of the natural history of disease. Measures of disease frequency involve a numerator (cases) and a denominator (population at risk). Incidence and death rates refer to new cases and to deaths per unit time and population; prevalence rates to cases present at one time per unit population. Incidence and prevalence rates arise from specific surveys for the disease within circumscribed populations; death rates come from standard published governmental sources. Selection bias grows as the source of cases departs from a true population survey, and is maximal in autopsy series.

As to multiple sclerosis, the best measures of geographical distribution come from prevalence studies, of which there are now over 300. These works indicate that, geographically, MS is distributed throughout the world within three zones of high, medium and low frequency. High-frequency areas, with prevalence rates of 30 and above per 100 000 population, comprise most of Europe into the former USSR, Israel, Canada and northern United States, New Zealand and south-eastern Australia. These regions are bounded by areas of medium frequency with prevalence rates of 5–29 and mostly 15–25 per 100 000, which then comprise most of Australia, southern US, southwestern Norway and northern Scandinavia, perhaps the southern Mediterranean basin, probably Russia from the Urals into Siberia and the far east as well as the Ukraine, South Africa, and perhaps central South America. All other known areas of Asia and Africa and the Caribbean region, including Mexico and possibly northern South America, are all low, with prevalence rates under 5 per 100 000 population. A number of nationwide prevalence studies in Europe provide evidence for geographical clustering of the disease, which is stable over time, but with evidence of diffusion over time.

All high- and medium-risk areas are among predominantly white populations: MS is the white man's burden. In America, blacks and Orientals, and possibly Native Americans, have much lower rates of MS than do whites, but each group still demonstrates the geographical gradients found for whites.

Migration studies indicate that, on the whole, migrants retain much of the risk of their birthplace. However, this risk is clearly not defined at birth: MS death rates for migrants born in one risk area and dying in another are intermediate between those characteristic of their birthplace and their death residence regardless of the direction of the move. Prevalence studies for migrants from high- to low-risk areas indicate the age of adolescence to be critical for risk retention: those migrating beyond age 15 retain the MS risk of their birthplace; those migrating under 15 acquire the lower risk of their new residence. This also means that young children are *not* susceptible to this disease. Several low-to-high studies show that those migrating in childhood or adolescence do in fact increase their risk of MS. Best data as to migration arise from a nationwide series of MS cases with pre-illness controls from the US military-veteran population. For white male veterans of Second World War military service, case control ratios are clearly decreased by moving from north to south between birth and entry into service, and clearly increased by similar moves in the opposite direction.

The migrant data, plus the geographical distributions and especially the clustering, serve to define MS as an acquired, exogenous, environmental disease. The data fit best the 'simple' or 'prevalence' hypothesis: that the cause of MS will be found where the clinical disease is common. The migrant data also support the idea that MS is ordinarily acquired in early adolescence, with a lengthy 'incubation' or 'latent' period between disease onset and symptom onset, and with young children not susceptible to this illness.

Further migrant studies are required to support (or refute) these interpretations. However, all migrant studies are beset with major difficulties in ascertaining the proper denominator, the true population at risk, since this is a three-fold function of age at migration, duration of residence and age at prevalence day – each aspect of which will have a major influence in defining expected numbers of cases. To obviate those difficulties in some measure, period risk estimates have been calculated for MS in Denmark. They indicate that, after 5 years a disease-free population, all ages, would be likely to provide only some 12% of the MS cases expected over its lifetime, and only half the expected total would be found after 20 years' follow-up.

Recently, epidemics of MS have been defined: one (definite) in the Faroe Islands; the others (probable) in Iceland and the Shetland–Orkneys. To 1991 we have been able to identify on the Faroe Islands 42 cases of multiple sclerosis among native-born resident Faroese.

They comprised four successive epidemics with peaks at 13-year intervals and the first case in 1943. The 20 cases included from the first epidemic met all criteria for a type 1 point-source epidemic. Present evidence as to a source for this epidemic points to the British troops, who occupied the Faroes in large numbers for 5 years from April 1940, and were stationed where the patients lived.

Sverrir Bergmann and the late Kjartan Guðmundsson collected all cases of MS in Iceland from 1900 to 1975, achieving a total of 168. As to their numbers over time, there seem to have been two step-wise increases in the occurrence of new cases of MS: after the First and the Second World Wars, with plateaus following each of these increments. The annual incidence of 3.2 per 100 000 for 1945–54 was twice as high as the rate for 1923–44, and it had returned to 1.9 for 1955–74. Iceland, which shares its origin and history with the Faroes, was also heavily occupied during the Second World War, not only by the British but also by Canadians and Americans.

The Shetland–Orkney Islands, which from the 1950s to the 1970s had the highest prevalence rates in the world, have since then showed marked decreases in incidence, and in retrospect also show a wartime–postwar epidemic.

If these findings are valid, these studies would indicate the definition of MS as not only an acquired disease but also a transmissible one. What we believe is transmissible is a widespread, specific (but unknown) persistent infection of adolescents and young adults, which we call PMSA (the primary multiple sclerosis affection), and which only rarely leads to clinical neurological MS after years of incubation. In this context PMSA is transmissible, CNMS is not. Further, prolonged exposure (at least 2 years) is required to acquire PMSA. Our best guess as to its nature at this time is an undefined (retro)-virus, which we hope to attempt to find in the Faroes, since there is in those islands a unique control group: there are parts of the Faroes which are still free of CNMS, even after 50 years of disease.

Our knowledge as to the epidemiology of MS, then, is not inconsiderable. The underlying goal of all these studies – and of the host of workers who have devoted so much time and effort to their performance – is to define the aetiology of MS. Many clinicians consider this to be an impossibility with the epidemiological approach, and it obviously has not yet been accomplished. But, personally, I think we are getting close. The definitive answer will, I believe, come from the Norse Viking settlements of the North Atlantic islands – the Shetland–Orkneys, Iceland and the Faroes. There is a phrase that came to be one of derision during the Vietnam War, but it is one to which I subscribe in terms of the cause of MS: I think there is light at the end of the tunnel.

ACKNOWLEDGEMENTS

This work was supported by the Department of Veterans Affairs (Neuroepidemiology Research Program, Veterans Affairs Medical Center, Washington, DC) and the National Multiple Sclerosis Society, New York. My thanks to a very large number of colleagues about the world whose thoughts and data over the years have been instrumental in providing the material on which this work has been based. These include not only all of my co-authors, but also the authors of the majority of the papers cited in this chapter.

References

1. Kurtzke, J.F. (1974) Neurologic needs of the community, in *Neuroepidemiology* (ed. J.F. Kurtzke), American Academy of Neurology Special Course. Minneapolis, MN, Education Marketing Corp., pp. 61–5 + tape cassette.
2. Kurtzke, J.F. (1977) Multiple sclerosis from an epidemiological viewpoint, in *Multiple Sclerosis. A Critical Conspectus* (ed. E.J. Field), Lancaster, MTP Press, pp. 83–142.
3. Kurtzke, J.F. (1984) Neuroepidemiology. *Ann. Neurol.*, **16**, 265–77.
4. Kurtzke J.F. and Kurland, L.T. (1973) The epidemiology of neurologic disease, in *Clinical Neurology* (eds A.B. Baker and L.H. Baker), vol. 3, Hagerstown, MD, Harper and Row, 48, pp. 1–80.
5. World Health Organization (1967/1969) *Manual of the International Statistical Classification of Diseases, Injuries, and Causes of Death*, 1965 Revision, Volume I, 2, Geneva, World Health Organization.
6. World Health Organization (1977) *Manual of the International Statistical Classification of Diseases, Injuries, and Causes of Death*, Ninth Revision, Volume I, Geneva, World Health Organization.
7. National Center for Health Statistics (1968) *Eighth Revision International Classification of Diseases, Adopted for Use in the United States*, vol. 1, Tabular List, vol. 2 Alphabetical Index (PHS Publ. No. 1693), Washington, DC, US GPO.
8. Kurtzke, J.F. (1979) ICD 9: a regression. *Am. J. Epidemiol.*, **109**, 383–93.
9. World Health Organization (1992) *International Statistical Classification of Diseases and Related Health Problems*, Tenth Revision, Volume I, Geneva, World Health Organization.
10. Schumacher, G.A., Beebe, G.W., Kibler, R.F. *et al.* (1965) Problems of experimental trials of therapy in multiple sclerosis: report by the panel on the evaluation of experimental trials of therapy in multiple sclerosis. *Ann. NY Acad. Sci.*, **122**, 552–68.
11. Kurtzke, J.F. (1982) Multiple sclerosis: still a clinical diagnosis. *Consultant*, **22**, 359–69.
12. Poser, C.M., Paty, D.W., Scheinberg, L. *et al.* (1983) New diagnostic criteria for multiple sclerosis: guidelines for research protocols. *Ann. Neurol.*, **13**, 227–31.
13. Kurtzke, J.F. (1988) Multiple sclerosis: what's in a name? *Neurology*, **38**, 309–16.
14. Allison, R.S. and Millar, J.H.D. (1954) Prevalence and familial incidence of disseminated sclerosis (a report to the Northern Ireland Hospitals Authority on the results of a three year study). Prevalence of disseminated sclerosis in Northern Ireland. *Ulster Med. J.*, **23** (Suppl. 2), 5–27.
15. Hyllested, K. and Kurland, L.T. (eds) (1966) Studies in multiple sclerosis: VI. Further explorations on the geographic distribution of multiple sclerosis. *Acta Neurol. Scand.*, **42** (Suppl. 19).
16. Alter, M. and Kurtzke, J.F. (eds.) (1968) *The Epidemiology of Multiple Sclerosis*, Springfield, Ill., Charles C. Thomas.
17. Field, E.J., Bell, T.M. and Carnegie, P.R. (eds) (1972) *Multiple Sclerosis: Progress in Research*. Amsterdam, North-Holland.
18. Kranz, J.S. and Kurland, L.T. (1982) General overview of the epidemiology of multiple sclerosis with emphasis on the geographic pattern and long-term trends, in *Multiple Sclerosis: East and West* (eds Y. Kuroiwa and L.T. Kurland), Fukuoka, Japan, Kyushu University Press, pp. 3–29.
19. Kuroiwa, Y. and Kurland, L.T. (eds) (1982) *Multiple Sclerosis East and West*, Fukuoka, Japan, Kyushu University Press.
20. Firnhaber, W. and Lauer, K. (1994) *Multiple Sclerosis in Europe. An Epidemiological Update*, Darmstadt, LTV Press.
21. Acheson, E.D. (1972) The epidemiology of multiple sclerosis, in *Multiple Sclerosis: A Reappraisal* (eds D. McAlpine, C.E. Lumsden and E.D. Acheson), 2nd edn, Edinburgh, E&S Livingstone, pp. 3–80.

22. Acheson, E.D. (1972) Migration prior to onset and the risk of multiple sclerosis: a brief review of the published data, in *Multiple Sclerosis: Progress in Research* (eds E.J. Field, T.M. Bell and P.R. Carnegie), Amsterdam, North-Holland, pp. 204–7.

23. Acheson, E.D. (1977) Epidemiology of multiple sclerosis. *Br. Med. Bull.*, **33**, 9–14.

24. Acheson, E.D. (1985) The epidemiology of multiple sclerosis. 1. The pattern of disease. 2. What does this pattern mean? in *McAlpine's Multiple Sclerosis* (eds W.B. Matthews, E.D. Acheson, J.R. Batchelor and R.O. Weller), Edinburgh, Churchill Livingstone, pp. 3–26, 27–46.

25. Alter, M. (1977) Clues to the cause based upon the epidemiology of multiple sclerosis, in *Multiple Sclerosis A Critical Conspectus* (ed. E.J. Field), Lancaster, MTP Press, pp. 35–82.

26. Dean, G. (1984) Epidemiology of multiple sclerosis. *Neuroepidemiology*, **3**, 58–73.

27. Detels, R. (1978) Epidemiology of multiple sclerosis. *Adv. Neurol.*, **19**, 459–72.

28. Gonzalez-Scarano, F., Spielman, R.S. and Nathanson, N. (1986) Neuro-epidemiology, in *Multiple Sclerosis* (eds W.I. McDonald and D.H. Silberberg), Boston, MA, Butterworths, pp. 37–55.

29. Koch-Henriksen, N. (1989) An epidemiological study of multiple sclerosis. Familial aggregation, social determinants, and exogenic factors. *Acta Neurol. Scand.*, **80** (Suppl. 124), pp. 1–123.

30. Kurland, L.T. (1970) The epidemiologic characteristics of multiple sclerosis, in *Handbook of Clinical Neurology* vol. 9, *Multiple Sclerosis and Other Demyelinating Diseases* (eds P.J. Vinken and G.W. Bruyn), Amsterdam, North-Holland, pp. 63–84.

31. Kurland, L.T., Stazio, A. and Reed, D. (1965) An appraisal of population studies of multiple sclerosis. *Ann. NY Acad. Sci.*, **122**, 520–41.

32. Kurtzke, J.F. (1966) An epidemiologic approach to multiple sclerosis. *Arch. Neurol.*, **14**, 213–22.

33. Kurtzke, J.F. (1969) Some epidemiologic features compatible with an infectious origin for multiple sclerosis. *Int. Arch. Allergy.*, **36**, 59–81.

34. Kurtzke, J.F. (1977) Geography in multiple sclerosis. *J. Neurol.*, **215**, 1–26.

35. Kurtzke, J.F. (1980) Epidemiologic contributions to multiple sclerosis – an overview. *Neurology*, **30** (part 2), 61–79.

36. Kurtzke, J.F. (1980) Multiple sclerosis an overview, in *Clinical Neuroepidemiology* (ed. F.C. Rose), London, Pitman Medical, pp. 170–95.

37. Kurtzke, J.F. (1983) Epidemiology of multiple sclerosis, in *Multiple Sclerosis. Pathology, Diagnosis and Management* (eds J.F. Hallpike, C.W.M. Adams and W.W. Tourtelotte), London, Chapman & Hall, pp. 47–95.

38. Kurtzke, J.F. (1985) Epidemiology of multiple sclerosis, in *Handbook of Clinical Neurology*, vol. 3, revd. ser., *Demyelinating Diseases* (eds P.J. Vinken, G.W. Bruyn and H.L. Klawans), Amsterdam, Elsevier, pp. 259–87.

39. Kurtzke, J.F. (1988) Risk factors, course, and prognosis of multiple sclerosis, in *Virology and Immunology in Multiple Sclerosis: Rationale for Therapy* (eds C.L. Cazzullo, D. Caputo, A. Ghezzi and M. Zaffaroni), Berlin, Springer Verlag, pp. 87–109.

40. Kurtzke, J.F. (1993) Epidemiologic evidence for multiple sclerosis as an infection. *Clin. Microbiol. Rev.*, **6**, pp. 382–427.

41. Kurtzke, J.F. and Kurland, L.T. (1983) The epidemiology of neurologic disease, in *Clinical Neurology*, vol. 4 (eds A.B. Baker and L.H. Baker), Philadelphia, Harper and Row, **66**, 1–143.

42. Kurtzke, J.F., Kurland, L.T., Goldberg, I.D. and Choi, L.T. (1973) Multiple sclerosis, in *Epidemiology of Neurologic and Sense Organ Disorders* (eds L.T. Kurland, J.F. Kurtzke and I.D. Goldberg), Cambridge, MA, Harvard University Press, pp. 64–107.

43. Martyn, C. (1991) The epidemiology of multiple sclerosis, in *McAlpine's Multiple Sclerosis* (eds W.B. Matthews, A. Compston, I.V. Allen and C.N. Martyn), 2nd edn, Edinburgh, Churchill Livingstone, pp. 3–40.

44. Poskanzer, D.C. (1967) Neurological disorders, in *Preventive Medicine* (eds D.W. Clark and B. McMahon), Boston, MA, Little, Brown, pp. 373–402.

45. Poskanzer, D.C. (1968) Etiology of multiple sclerosis: Analogy suggesting infection in early life, in *The Epidemiology of Multiple Sclerosis* (eds M. Alter and J.F. Kurtzke), Springfield, IL, Charles C. Thomas, pp. 62–82.

46. Pryse-Phillips, W. (1990) The epidemiology of multiple sclerosis, in *Handbook of Multiple Sclerosis* (ed. S.D. Cook), New York, Marcel Dekker, pp. 1–24.

47. Sadovnick, A.D. and Ebers, G.C. (1993) Epidemiology of multiple sclerosis: a review and critique of the epidemiological literature. *Can. J. Neurol. Sci.*, **20**, 17–29.

48. Weinshenker, B.G. and Rodriguez, M. (1994) Epidemiology of multiple sclerosis, in *Handbook of Neuroepidemiology* (eds P.B. Gorelick and M. Alter), New York, Marcel Dekker, 533–64.

49. Wynn, D.R., Rodriguez, M., O'Fallon, W.M. and Kurland, L.T. (1989) Update on the epidemiology of multiple sclerosis. *Mayo Clin. Proc.*, **64**, 808–17.

50. Limburg, C.C. (1950) The geographic distribution of multiple sclerosis and its estimated prevalence in the United States. *Proc. Assoc. Res. Nerv. Ment. Dis.*, **28**, 15–24.

51. Goldberg, I.D. and Kurland, L.T. (1962) Mortality in 33 countries from disease of the nervous system. *World Neurol.*, **3**, 444–65.

52. Massey, E.W. and Schoenberg, B.S. (1982) International patterns of mortality from multiple sclerosis. *Neuroepidemiology*, **1**, 189–96.

53. Kurland, L.T., Kurtzke, J.F. and Goldberg, I.D. (1973) *Epidemiology of Neurologic and Sense Organ Disorders*, Cambridge, MA, Harvard University Press.

54. Kurtzke, J.F., Kurland, L.T. and Goldberg, I.D. (1971) Mortality and migration in multiple sclerosis. *Neurology*, **21**, 1186–97.

55. Mason, T.J., Fraumeni, J.F. Jr, Hoover, R. and Blot, W.J. (1981) *An Atlas of Mortality from Selected Diseases*, NIH Publication No. 81–2397. USDHS, PHS, NIH, Washington DC, US GPO.

56. Charcot, J.-M. (1877) *Leçons sur les maladies du système nerveux fautes a la salpêtrière: recuellies et publiées par Bourneville*, tome premier, troisième édition, Paris, V. Adrien Delahaye et Cie, pp. 189–417.

57. Moxon (1873) Case of insular sclerosis of brain and spinal cord. *Lancet*, i, 236.

58. Davenport, C.B. (1922) Multiple sclerosis from the standpoint of geographic distribution and race. *Proc. Assoc. Res. Nerv. Ment. Dis.*, **2**, 8–19.

59. Bailey, P. (1922) Incidence of multiple sclerosis in United States troops. *Proc. Assoc. Res. Nerv. Ment. Dis.*, **2**, 19–22.

60. Kurtzke, J.F. (1975) A reassessment of the distribution of multiple sclerosis. *Acta Neurol. Scand.*, **51**, 110–36; 137–57.

61. Kurtzke, J.F. (1980) The geographic distribution of multiple sclerosis: an update with special reference to Europe and the Mediterranean region. *Acta Neurol. Scand.*, **62**, 65–80.

62. Sutherland, J.M. (1956) Observations on the prevalence of multiple sclerosis in northern Scotland. *Brain*, **79**, 635–54.

63. Allison, R.S. (1963) Some neurological aspects of medical geography. *Proc. R. Soc. Med.*, **56**, 71–6.

64. Fog, M. and Hyllested, K. (1966) Prevalence of disseminated sclerosis in the Faroes, the Orkneys and Shetland. *Acta Neurol. Scand.*, **42** (Suppl. 19), 9–11.

65. Poskanzer, D.C., Schapira, K. and Miller, H. (1963) Multiple sclerosis and poliomyelitis. *Lancet*, ii, 917–21.

66. Cook, S.D., Cromarty, J.I., Tapp, W., Poskanjer, D.C. *et al.* (1985) Declining incidence of multiple sclerosis in the Orkney Islands. *Neurology*, **35**, 545–51.

67. Cook, S.D., MacDonald, J., Tapp, W., Poskanzer, D. and Dowling, P.C. (1988) Multiple sclerosis in the Shetland Islands: an update. *Acta Neurol. Scand.*, **77**, 148–51.

68. Dean, G., Goodall, J. and Downie, A. (1981) The prevalence of multiple sclerosis in the Outer Hebrides compared with north-east Scotland and the Orkney and Shetland Islands. *J. Epidemiol. Commun. Hlth*, **35**, 110–13.

69. Phadke, J.G. and Downie, A.W. (1987) Epidemiology of multiple sclerosis in the north-east (Grampian Region) of Scotland – an update. *J. Epidemiol. Commun. Hlth*, **41**, 5–13.

70. Shepherd, D.I. and Downie, A.W. (1978) Prevalence of multiple sclerosis in northeast Scotland. *Br. Med. J.*, **2**, 314–16.

71. Swingler, R.J. and Compston, D.A.S. (1986) The distribution of multiple sclerosis in the United Kingdom. *J. Neurol. Neurosurg. Psychiatry*, **49**, 1115–24.

72. Swingler, R.J. and Compston, D.A.S. (1988) The prevalence of multiple sclerosis in South East Wales. *J. Neurol. Neurosurg. Psychiatry*, **51**, 1520–4.

73. Williams, E.S. and McKeran, R.O. (1986) Prevalence of multiple sclerosis in a south London borough. *Br. Med. J.*, **293**, 237–9.

74. Swingler, R.J., Rothwell, P., Taylor, M.W. and Hall, G.C. (1994) Prevalence of multiple sclerosis in 604 general practices in the United Kingdom. *Ann. Neurol.*, **36**, 303 (abstract).

75. Kinnunen, E. (1984) Multiple sclerosis in Finland: evidence of increasing frequency and uneven geographic distribution. *Neurology*, **34**, 457–61.

76. Wikström, J., Kinnunen, E. and Palo, J. (1983) The epidemiology of multiple sclerosis in Finland, in *Actual Problems in Multiple Sclerosis Research* (eds E. Pedersen, J. Clausen and L. Oades), Copenhagen, FADL's Forlag, p. 223.

77. Larsen, J.P., Aarli, J.A., Nyland, H. and Riise, T. (1984) Western Norway, a high-risk area for multiple sclerosis: a prevalence/incidence study in the country of Hordaland. *Neurology*, **34**, 1202–7.

78. Larsen, J.P., Kvalle, R., Riise, T., Nyland, H. and Aarli, J.A. (1984) An increase in the incidence of multiple sclerosis in Western Norway. *Acta Neurol. Scand.*, **69**, 96–103.

79. Grønning, M. and Mellgren, S.I. (1985) Multiple sclerosis in the two northernmost counties of Norway. *Acta Neurol. Scand.*, **72**, 321–7.

80. Koch-Henriksen, N. and Hyllested, K. (1988) Epidemiology of multiple sclerosis: incidence and prevalence rates in Denmark 1948–64 based on the Danish Multiple Sclerosis Registry. *Acta Neurol. Scand.*, **78**, 369–80.

81. Benedikz, J.E.G., Magnússon, H., Poser, C.M. *et al.* (1991) Multiple sclerosis in Iceland 1900–1985. *J. Trop. Geogr. Neurol.*, **1**, 16–22.

82. Poser, C.M., Benedikz, J. and Hibberd, P.L. (1992) The epidemiology of multiple sclerosis: the Iceland model. Onset-adjusted prevalence rates and other methodological considerations. *J. Neurol. Sci.*, **111**, 143–52.

83. Alperovitch, A. and Bouvier, M.-H. (1982) Geographical pattern of death rates from multiple sclerosis in France. An analysis of 4912 deaths. *Acta Neurol. Scand.*, **66**, 454–61.

84. Gallou, M., Madigand, M., Masse, L. *et al.* (1983) Epidémiologie de la sclérose en plaques en Bretagne. *Presse Méd.*, **12**, 995–9.

85. Blanc, M., Clanet, M., Berr, C. *et al.* (1986) Immunoglobulin allotypes and susceptibility to multiple sclerosis. An epidemiological and genetic study in the Hautes-Pyrénées county of France. *J. Neurol. Sci.*, **75**, 1–5.

86. Kesselring, J. (1987) High prevalence of multiple sclerosis in Switzerland. *Neurology* **37** (Suppl. 1), 151 (abstract).

87. Bärtschi-Rochaux, W. (1980) MS in Switzerland – canton Wallis, in *Progress in Multiple Sclerosis Research* (eds H.J. Bauer, S. Poser and G. Ritter), Berlin, Springer-Verlag, pp. 535–8.

88. Meyer-Rienecker, H.J. and Buddenhagen, F. (1983) Grundlagen and Problematik der Epidemiologie der Multiplen Sklerose. *Psychiat. Neurol. Med. Psychol.*, **35**, 697–707.

89. Prange, A.J.A., Lauer, K., Poser, S. *et al.* (1986) Epidemiological aspects of multiple sclerosis: a comparative study of four cities in Europe. *Neuroepidemiology*, **5**, 71–9.

90. Schmidt, R.M., Kissing, B., Kuppe, G. and Neumann, V. (1985) Frequency and distribution of MS in the district of Halle. Presented at IFMSS Symposium: MS in Europe, Hamburg, 7 September 1985.

91. Wikström, J., Ritter, G., Poser, S., Firnhaber, W. and Bauer, H.J. (1977) Das Vorkommen von Multipler Sklerose in Südniedersachsen. Ergebnisse einer Feldstudie über 12 Jahre. *Nervenarzt*, **48**, 494–9.

92. Van Ooteghem, P., D'Hooghe, M.B., Vlietinck, R. and Carton, H. (1994) Prevalence of multiple sclerosis in Flanders, Belgium. *Neuroepidemiology*, **13**, 220–5.

93. Pálffy, G., Czopf, J., Kuntár, L. and Gyodi, E. (1994) Multiple sclerosis in Hungarians and in Gipsies, in *Multiple Sclerosis in Europe. An Epidemiological Update* (eds W. Firnhaber and K. Lauer), Darmstadt, LTV Press, pp. 274–8.

94. Guseo, A. Jofejü, E. and Kocsis, A. (1994) Epidemiology of multiple sclerosis in Western Hungary 1957–1992, in *Multiple Sclerosis in Europe. An Epidemiological Update.* (eds W. Firnhaber and K. Lauer), Darmstadt, LTV Press, pp. 279–86.

95. Buddenhagen, F. and Pantovič, M.M. (1985) Vergleichende epidemiologische Analyse der Multiplen Sklerose in Gebieten des mittleren und südlichen Europas. *Psychiat. Neurol. Med. Psychol.*, **37**, 565–72.

96. Lević, Z., Pantović, M. and Sepčić, J. (1985) Epidemiologic studies of multiple sclerosis in Yugoslavia. *Neurologija*, **34**, 89–96.

97. Materljan, E., Sepčić, J, Antonelli, L. and Šepčić-Grahovac, D. (1989) Multiple sclerosis in Istria, Yugoslavia. *Neurologija*, **38**, 201–12.

98. Sepčić, J., Antonelli, L., Materljan, E. and Šepčić-Grahovac, D. (1989) Multiple sclerosis cluster in Gorski Kotar, Croatia, Yugoslavia, in *Multiple Sclerosis Research* (ed. M.A. Battaglia), Amsterdam, Elsevier, pp. 165–9.

99. Jedlička, P. (1985) Epidemiology of MS in CSSR. Presented at IFMSS Symposium: MS in Europe, Hamburg, 7 September 1985.

100. Wender, M., Pruchnik-Grabowska, D., Hertmanowska, H. *et al.* (1985) Epidemiology of multiple sclerosis in Western Poland – a comparison between prevalence rates in 1965 and 1981. *Acta Neurol. Scand.*, **72**, 210–17.

101. Wender, M., Kowal, P., Pruchnik-Grabowska, D. *et al.* (1985) The clustering of multiple sclerosis in various administrative units of Western Poland. *J. Neurol.*, **232**, 240–5.

102. Vassilopoulos, D. (1984) Epidemiological data for multiple sclerosis in Greece. *Neuroepidemiology*, **3**, 52–6.

103. Milonas, I. (1994) Epidemiological data of multiple sclerosis in northern Greece, in *Multiple Sclerosis in Europe. An Epidemiological Update* (eds W. Firnhaber and K. Lauer), Darmstadt, LTV Press, pp. 332–3.

104. Petrescu, A. and Verdes, F. (1989) Epidemiology of multiple sclerosis in Romania. *Rev. Roum. Méd. Neurol. Psychiat.*, **27**, 261–71.

105. Popescu, D. and Popescu, V.G. (1981) Contributii la studiul factorilor de risc în scleroza multiplă – cercetři epidemiologice în judetul Arges. [Contributions to the study of risk factors in multiple sclerosis – epidemiologic investigations in the Arges region.] *Neurol. Psihiat. Neurochir.*, **26**, 23–31.

106. Kalafatova, O.I. (1987) Epidemiology of multiple sclerosis in Bulgaria. *Acta Neurol. Scand.*, **75**, 186–9.

107. Yordanov, B.I. (1985) Multiple sclerosis in Bulgaria. Presented at IFMSS Symposium: MS in Europe, Hamburg, 7 September 1985.

108. Ljapchev, R. and Daskalovska, V. (1994) Epidemiological studies of multiple sclerosis in the Republic of Macedonia, in *Multiple Sclerosis in Europe An Epidemiological Update* (eds W. Firnhaber and K. Lauer), Darmstadt, LTV Press, pp. 301–8.

109. Kruja, J. (1994) Multiple sclerosis in Albania, in *Multiple Sclerosis in Europe. An Epidemiological Update* (eds W. Firnhaber and K. Lauer), Darmstadt, LTV Press, pp. 309–15.

110. Boiko, A.N. (1994) Multiple sclerosis prevalence in Russia and other countries of the USSR, in *Multiple Sclerosis in Europe. An Epidemiological Update* (eds W. Firnhaber and K. Lauer), Darmstadt, LTV Press, pp. 219–30.

111. Dean, G., Grimaldi, G., Kelly, R. and Karhausen, L. (1975) Multiple sclerosis in southern Europe. I: prevalence in Sicily 1975. *J. Epidemiol. Commun. Hlth*, **33**, 107–10.

112. Granieri, E. and Rosati, G. (1982) Italy: a medium- or high-risk area for multiple sclerosis? An epidemiologic study in Barbagia, Sardinia, southern Italy. *Neurology*, **32**, 466–72.

113. Granieri, E., Rosati, G., Tola, R. *et al.* (1983) The frequency of multiple sclerosis in Mediterranean Europe. An incidence and prevalence study in Barbagia, Sardinia, insular Italy. *Acta Neurol. Scand.*, **68**, 84–9.

114. Granieri, E., Tola, R., Paolina, E. *et al.* (1985) The frequency of multiple sclerosis in Italy: a descriptive study in Ferrara. *Ann. Neurol.*, **17**, 80–4.

115. Morganti, G., Naccarato, M., Elian, P. *et al.* (1984) Multiple sclerosis in the Republic of San Marino. *J. Epidemiol Commun. Hlth*, **38**, 23–8.

116. Rosati, G., Aiello, I., Granieri, E. *et al.* (1986) Incidence of multiple sclerosis in Macomer, Sardinia, 1912–1981: onset of the disease after 1950. *Neurology*, **36**, 14–19.

117. Rosati, G., Aiello, I., Pirastru, M.I. *et al.* (1987) Sardinia, a high-risk area for multiple sclerosis: a prevalence and incidence study in the district of Alghero. *Ann. Neurol.*, **21**, 190–4.

118. Rosati, G., Aiello, I., Pirastru, M.I. *et al.* (1988) Incidence of multiple sclerosis in the town of Sassari, Sardinia, 1965–1985: evidence for increasing occurrence of the disease. *Neurology*, **38**, 384–8.

119. Rosati, G., Granieri, E., Carreras, M. *et al.* (1981) Multiple sclerosis in northern Italy. Prevalence in the province of Ferrara in 1978. *Ital. J. Neurol. Sci.*, **2**, 17–23.

120. Savettieri, G., Elian, M., Giordano, D. *et al.* (1986) A further study on the prevalence of multiple sclerosis in Sicily: Caltanissetta city. *Acta Neurol. Scand.*, **73**, 71–5.

121. Middleton, L.T. and Dean, G. (1991) Multiple sclerosis in Cyprus. *J. Neurol. Sci.*, **103**, 29–36.

122. Lauer, K. (1994) Multiple sclerosis in the old world: the new old map, in *Multiple Sclerosis in Europe. An Epidemiological Update* (eds W. Firnhaber and K. Lauer), Darmstadt, LTV Press, pp. 14–27.

123. de Sá, J. and Magalhaes, A. (1994) Epidemiology of multiple sclerosis in Portugal, in *Multiple Sclerosis in Europe. An Epidemiological Update* (eds W. Firnhaber and K. Lauer), Darmstadt LTV Press, pp. 192–4.

124. Kurtzke, J.F. (1966) An evaluation of the geographic distrubution of multiple sclerosis. *Acta Neurol. Scand.*, **42** (Suppl. 19), pp. 91–117.

125. Kurtzke, J.F. (1967) Further considerations on the geographic distribution of multiple sclerosis. *Acta Neurol. Scand.*, **43**, 283–97.

126. Kurtzke, J.F. (1967) On the fine structure of the distribution of multiple sclerosis. *Acta Neurol. Scand.*, **43**, 257–82.

127. Kurtzke, J.F. (1965) Medical facilities and the prevalence of multiple sclerosis. *Acta Neurol. Scand.*, **41**, 561–79.

128. Kurtzke, J.F. (1974) Further features of the Fennoscandian focus of multiple sclerosis. *Acta Neurol. Scand.*, **50**, 478–502.

129. Kurtzke, J.F. (1968) A Fennoscandian focus of multiple sclerosis. *Neurology*, **18**, 16–20.

130. Bennett, L., Hamilton, R., Neutel, C.I. *et al.* (1976) Survey of persons with multiple sclerosis in Ottawa 1974–1975. *Can. J. Publ. Hlth*, **60**, 141–7.

131. Hader, W.J., Elliott, M. and Ebers, G.C. (1988) Epidemiology of multiple sclerosis in London and Middlesex County, Ontario, Canada. *Neurology*, **38**, 617–21.

132. Hader, W.J. (1982) Prevalence of multiple sclerosis in Saskatoon. *Can. Med. Assoc. J.*, **127**, 295–7.

133. Sweeney, V.P., Sadovnick, A.D. and Brandejs, V. (1986) Prevalence of multiple sclerosis in British Columbia. *Can. J. Neurol. Sci.*, **13**, 47–51.

134. Pryse-Phillips, W.E.M. (1986) The incidence of multiple sclerosis in Newfoundland and Labrador, 1960–1984. *Ann. Neurol.*, **20**, 323–8.

135. Warren, S., Warren, K.G. (1992) Prevalence of multiple sclerosis in Barrhead County, Alberta, Canada. *Can. J. Neurol. Sci.*, **19**, 72–5.

136. Warren, S. and Warren, K.G. (1993) Prevalence, incidence and characteristics of multiple sclerosis in Westlock County, Alberta, Canada. *Neurology*, **43**, 1760–3.

137. Klein, G.M., Rose, M.S. and Seland, T.P. (1994) A prevalence study of multiple sclerosis in the Crowsnest Pass region of Southern Alberta. *Can. J. Neurol. Sci.*, **21**, 262–5.

138. Scarlett Kranz, J.M., Kurland, L.T., Schuman, L.M. and Layton, D. (1983) Multiple sclerosis in Olmsted and Mower Counties, Minnesota. *Neuroepidemiology*, **2**, 206–18.

139. Nelson, L.M., Hamman, R.F., Thompson, D.S. *et al.* (1986) Higher than expected prevalence of multiple sclerosis (MS) in northern Colorado: dependence on methodologic issues. *Neuroepidemiology*, **5**, 17–28.

140. Hoffman, R.E., Zack, M.M., Davis, L.E. and Burchfiel, C.M. (1981) Increased incidence and prevalence of multiple sclerosis in Los Alamos County, New Mexico. *Neurology*, **31**, 1489–92.

141. Sheremata, W.A., Poskanzer, D.C., Withum, D.G., MacLeod, C.L. and Whiteside, M.E. (1985) Unusual occurrence on a tropical island of multiple sclerosis. *Lancet*, **2**, 618 (Letter).

142. Bigler, W.J. (1986) An epidemiological investigation of multiple sclerosis in Key West, Florida. A preliminary report. State of Florida HRS Department Report, 17 February 1986.

143. Helmick, C.G., Wrigley, J.M., Zack, M.M. *et al.* (1989) Multiple sclerosis in Key West, Florida. *Am. J. Epidemiol.*, **130**, 935–49.

144. Ingalls, T.H. (1986) Endemic clustering of multiple sclerosis in time and place, 1934–1984. Confirmation of a hypothesis. *Am. J. Forensic Med. Pathol.*, **7**, 3–8.

145. Kurtzke, J.F. (1978) Data registries on selected segments of the population: Veterans, in *Neurological Epidemiology: Principles and Clinical Applications* (ed. B.S. Schoenberg), New York, Raven Press, pp. 55–67.

146. Kurtzke, J.F., Beebe, G.W., Norman, J.E. Jr (1979) Epidemiology of multiple sclerosis in US veterans: 1. Race, sex, and geographic distribution. *Neurology*, 29, 1228–35.

147. Bobowick, A.R., Kurtzke, J.F., Brody, J.A. *et al.* (1978) Twin study of multiple sclerosis: an epidemiologic inquiry. *Neurology*, 28, 978–87.

148. Miller, D.H., Hornabrook, R.W., Dagger, J. and Fong, R. (1986) Ethnic and HLA patterns related to multiple sclerosis in Wellington, New Zealand. *J. Neurol. Neurosurg. Psychiatry*, 49, 43–6.

149. Skegg, D.C.G., Corwin, P.A., Craven, R.S., Malloch, J.A. and Pollock, M. (1987) Occurrence of multiple sclerosis in the north and south of New Zealand. *J. Neurol. Neurosurg. Psychiatry*, 50, 134–9.

150. Hammond, S.R., McLeod, J.G., Millingen, K.S. *et al.* (1988) The epidemiology of multiple sclerosis in three Australian cities: Perth, Newcastle and Hobart. *Brain*, 111, 1–25.

151. Hammond, S.R., de Wytt, C., Maxwell, I.C. *et al.* (1987) The epidemiology of multiple sclerosis in Queensland, Australia. *J. Neurol. Sci.*, 80, 185–204.

152. Hammond, S.R., McLeod, J.G., Stewart-Wynne, E.G., McCall, M.G. and English, D. (1988) The epidemiology of multiple sclerosis in Western Australia. *Aust. NZ J. Med.*, 18, 102–10.

153. Sosa Enriquez, M., Leon Betancor, P., Rosas, C. and Navarro, M.C. (1983) La esclerosis múltiple en la provincia de Las Palmas. *Arch. Neurobiol.*, 46, 161–6.

154. Radhakrishnan, K., Ashok, P.P., Sridharan, R. and Mousa, M.E. (1985) Prevalence and pattern of multiple sclerosis in Benghazi, north-eastern Libya. *J. Neurol. Sci.*, 70, 39–46.

155. Ben Hamida, M. (1977) La sclérose en plaques en Tunisie. Étude clinique de 100 observations. *Rev. Neurol.*, 133, 109–17.

156. Kurdi, A., Ayesh, I., Abdallat, A. and McDonald, W.I. (1977) Multiple sclerosis and IA-like antigens. Presented 11th World Congress of Neurology, Amsterdam, 11–16 September, 1977.

157. Al-Din, A.S.N. (1986) Multiple sclerosis in Kuwait: clinical and epidemiological study. *J. Neurol. Neurosurg. Psychiatry*, 49 928–31.

158. Al-Din, A.S.N., Shakir, R.A., Poser, C.M. and Khogali, M. (1992) Multiple sclerosis in Arabs. *J. Trop. Geogr. Neurol.*, 2, 57–62.

159. Yaqub, B.A. and Daif, A.K. (1988) Multiple sclerosis in Saudi Arabia. *Neurology*, 38, 621–3.

160. Biton, V. and Abramsky, O. (1986) Newer study fails to support environmental factors in etiology of MS. *Neurology*, 36 (Suppl. 1), 184 (abstract).

161. Kahana, E., Zilber, N., Abramson, J.H. *et al.* (1994) Multiple sclerosis: genetic versus environmental aetiology: epidemiology in Israel updated. *J. Neurol.*, 241, 341–6.

162. Hou, J.B. and Zhang, Z.X. (1992) Prevalence of multiple sclerosis: a door-to-door survey in Lan Cang La Hu Zu Autonomous County, Yunnan Province of China. *Neuroepidemiology*, 11, 52.

163. Yu, Y.L., Woo, E., Hawkins, B.R., Ho, H.C. and Huang, C.Y. (1989) Multiple sclerosis amongst Chinese in Hong Kong. *Brain*, 112, 1445–67.

164. Rosman, K.D., Jacobs, H.A. and Van der Merwe, C.A. (1985) A new multiple sclerosis epidemic? A pilot survey. *S. Afr. Med. J.*, 68, 162–3.

165. Dean, G. (1967) Annual incidence, prevalence and mortality of multiple sclerosis in White South-African-born and in White immigrants to South Africa. *Br. Med. J.*, 2, 724–30.

166. Kies, B.M. (1989) An epidemiological study of multiple sclerosis in Cape Town, South Africa. Abstracts, XIVth World Congress of Neurology, New Delhi, India, 22–27 October 1989 (abstract 612B05), p. 287.

167. Kies, B.M. (1990) An epidemiological study of multiple sclerosis in Cape Town, South Africa, 1990 (unpublished manuscript).

168. Kurtzke, J.F. (1972) Multiple sclerosis death rates from underlying cause and total deaths. *Acta Neurol. Scand.*, 48, 148–62.

169. Hyllested, K. (1956) *Disseminated Sclerosis in Denmark. Prevalence and Geographical Distribution.* Copenhagen, J Jørgensen.

170. Brady, R., Dean, G., Secerbegovic, S. and Secerbegovic, A-M. (1977) Multiple sclerosis in the Republic of Ireland. *J. Irish Med. Assoc.*, 70, 500–6.

171. Kurtzke, J.F. and Hamtoft, H. (1976) Multiple sclerosis and Hodgkin's disease in Denmark. *Acta Neurol. Scand.*, 53, 358–75.

172. Shibasaki, H., Okihiro, M.M. and Kuroiwa, Y. (1978) Multiple sclerosis among Orientals and Caucasians in Hawaii: a reappraisal. *Neurology*, 28, 113–8.

173. Kuroiwa, Y. (1973) Multiple sclerosis case reports from all Japan (2nd report). Special Report by MS Study Group. Health and Welfare Department of Japan, 1–19.

174. Detels, R., Visscher, B., Malmgren, R.M. *et al.* (1977) Evidence for lower susceptibility to multiple sclerosis in Japanese-Americans. *Am. J. Epidemiol.*, 105, 303–10.

175. Alter, M. and Harshe, M. (1975) Racial predilection in multiple sclerosis. *J. Neurol.*, 210, 1–20.

176. Dassel, H. (1972) Discussion of the epidemiology of MS, in *Multiple Sclerosis – Progress in Research* (eds E.J. Field, T.M. Bell and P.R. Carnegie) Amsterdam, North-Holland, pp. 241–2.

177. Kurtzke, J.F. and Bui, Q.H. (1980) Multiple sclerosis in a migrant population. 2. Half-Orientals immigrating in childhood. *Ann. Neurol.*, 8, 256–60.

178. Detels, R., Visscher, B.R., Haile, R.W. *et al.* (1978) Multiple sclerosis and age at migration. *Am. J. Epidemiol.*, 108, 386–93.

179. Detels, R., Brody, J.A. and Edgar, A.H. (1972) Multiple sclerosis among American, Japanese and Chinese migrants to California and Washington. *J. Chron. Dis.*, 25, 3–10.

180. Dean, G., McLoughlin, H., Brady, R., Adelstein, A.M. and Tallett-Williams, J. (1976) Multiple sclerosis among immigrants in Greater London. *Br. Med. J.*, 1, 861–4.

181. Dean, G., Brady, R., McLoughlin, H., Eliam, M. and Adelstein, A.M. (1977) Motor neurone disease and multiple sclerosis among immigrants to Britain. *Br. J. Prevent. Soc. Med.*, 31, 141–7.

182. Kurtzke, J.F. (1976) Multiple sclerosis among immigrants. *Br. Med. J.*, 1, 1527–8.

183. Delasnerie-Lauprêtre, N. and Alpérovitch, A. (1992) Migration and age at onset of multiple sclerosis: some pitfalls of migrant studies. *Acta Neurol. Scand.*, 85, 408–11.

184. Kurtzke, J.F., Beebe, G.W. and Norman, J.E. Jr (1985) Epidemiology of multiple sclerosis in US veterans: III. Migration and the risk of MS. *Neurology*, 35, 672–8.

185. Dean, G. and Kurtzke, J.F. (1971) On the risk of multiple sclerosis according to age at immigration to South Africa. *Br. Med. J.*, 3, 725–9.

186. Kurtzke, J.F., Dean, G. and Botha, D.P.J. (1970) A method of estimating the age at immigration of white immigrants to South Africa, with an example of its importance. *S. Afr. Med. J.*, 44, 663–9.

187. Alter, M., Leibowitz, U. and Speer, J. (1966) Risk of multiple sclerosis related to age at immigration to Israel. *Arch. Neurol.*, 15, 234–7.

188. Alter, M. and Okihiro, M. (1971) When is multiple sclerosis acquired? *Neurology*, 21, 1030–6.

189. Alter, M., Kahana, E. and Loewenson, R. (1978) Migration and risk of multiple sclerosis. *Neurology*, 28, 1089–93.

190. Beebe, G.W., Kurtzke, J.F., Kurland, L.T., Auth, T.L. and Nagler, B. (1967) Studies on the natural history of multiple sclerosis. 3. Epidemiologic analysis of the Army experience in World War II. *Neurology*, 17, 1–17.

191. Kurtzke, J.F. (1965) On the time of onset in multiple sclerosis. *Acta Neurol. Scand.*, 41, 140–58.

192. Kurtzke, J.F. (1972) Migration and latency in multiple sclerosis, in *Multiple Sclerosis. Progress in Research* (eds E.J. Field, T.M. Bell and P.R. Carnegie), Amsterdam, North-Holland, pp. 208–28.

193. Schapira, K., Poskanzer, D.C. and Miller, H. (1963) Familial and conjugal multiple sclerosis. *Brain*, 86, 315–32.

194. Kurtzke, J.F. (1978) The risk of multiple sclerosis in Denmark. *Acta Neurol. Scand.*, 57, 141–50.

195. Kurtzke, J.F. (1970) Clinical manifestations of multiple sclerosis, in *Handbook of Clinical Neurology*, vol. 9. *Multiple Sclerosis and Other Demyelinating Diseases* (eds P.J. Vinken and G.W. Bruyn), Amsterdam, North-Holland, pp. 161–216.

196. Kurtzke, J.F. (1992) Neuroepidemiology, in *Clinical Neurology* (ed. R.J. Joynt); rev. edn, vol. 4, Philadelphia, Lippincott, ch. 66A, pp. 1–29.

197. Kurtzke, J.F. (1989) On estimating survival; a tale of two censors. *J. Clin. Epidemiol.*, 42, 169–75.

198. Kurland, L.T. and Westlund, K.B. (1954) Epidemiologic factors in the etiology and prognosis of multiple sclerosis. *Ann. NY Acad. Sci.*, 58, 682–701.

199. Percy, A.K., Nobrega, F.T., Okazaki, H., Glattre, E. and Kurland, L.T. (1971) Multiple sclerosis in Rochester, Minnesota – a 60 year appraisal. *Arch. Neurol.*, 25, 105–11.

200. Kurtzke, J.F., Beebe, G.W., Nagler, B. *et al.* (1970) Studies on the natural history of multiple sclerosis: V. Long-term survival in young men. *Arch. Neurol.*, 22, 215–25.

201. Poser, S., Kurtzke, J.F., Poser, W. and Schlaf, G. (1989) Survival in multiple sclerosis. *J. Clin. Epidemiol.*, 42, 159–68.

202. Wynn, D.R., Rodriguez, M., O'Fallon, W.M. and Kurland, L.T. (1990) A reappraisal of the epidemiology of multiple sclerosis in Olmsted County, Minnesota. *Neurology*, 40, 780–6.

203. Brønnum-Hansen, H., Koch-Henriksen, N. and Hyllested, K. (1994) Survival of patients with multiple sclerosis in Denmark: a nationwide, long-term epidemiologic survey. *Neurology*, 44, 1901–7.

204. Riise, T., Grønning, M., Aarli, J.A. *et al.* (1988) Prognostic factors for life expectancy in multiple sclerosis analyzed by Cox-models. *J. Clin. Epidemiol.*, 41, 1031–6.

205. Barlow, J.S. (1960) Correlation of geographic distribution of multiple sclerosis with cosmic-ray intensities. *Acta Psychiat. Neurol. Scand.*, 35 (Suppl. 147), pp. 108–30.

206. Campbell, A.M.G., Herdan, G., Tatlow, W.F.T. and Whittie, E.G. (1950) Lead in relation to disseminated sclerosis. *Brain*, 73, 52–70.

207. Ho, S-Y., Catalanotto, F.A., Lisak, R.P. and Dore-Duffy, P. (1986) Zinc in multiple sclerosis. II. Correlation with disease activity and elevated plasma membrane-bound zinc in erythrocytes from patients with multiple sclerosis. *Ann. Neurol.*, 20, 712–15.

208. Ryan, D.E., Holtbecher, J. and Stuart, D.C. (1978) Trace elements in scalp-hair of persons with multiple sclerosis and of normal individuals. *Clin. Chem.*, **24**, 1996–2000.

209. Warren, H.V., Delavault, R.E. and Cross, C.H. (1967) Possible correlations between geology and some disease patterns. *Ann. NY Acad. Sci.*, **136**, 657–710.

210. Wikström, J., Westermarck, T. and Palo, J. (1976) Selenium, vitamin E and copper in multiple sclerosis. *Acta Neurol. Scand.*, **54**, 287–90.

211. Stein, E.C., Schiffer, R.B., Hall, W.J. and Young, N. (1987) Multiple sclerosis and the workplace: report of an industry-based cluster. *Neurology*, **37**, 1672–7.

212. Schiffer, R.B., Weitkamp, L.R., Ford, C. and Hall, W.J. (1994) A genetic marker and family history study of the upstate New York multiple sclerosis cluster. *Neurology*, **44**, 329–33.

213. Norman, J.E. Jr, Kurtzke, J.F. and Beebe, G.W. (1983) Epidemiology of multiple sclerosis in US veterans: 2. Latitude, climate and the risk of multiple sclerosis. *J. Chron. Dis.*, **36**, 551–9.

214. Norman, J.E. Jr, Kurtzke, J.F. and Beebe, G.W. (1983) Latitude, climate and the risk of multiple sclerosis. Authors' reply. *J. Chron. Dis.*, **36**, 565–7.

215. Norman, J.E. Jr (1984) Logistic regression and multiple sclerosis. Response. *J. Chron. Dis.*, **37**, 676.

216. Bureau of the Census (1983) *1980 Census of Population. Ancestry of the Population by State: 1980*. Supplementary Report. PC80-S1-10. Washington, DC: US Government Printing Office.

217. Page, W.F., Kurtzke, J.F., Murphy, F.M. and Norman, J.E. Jr (1993) Epidemiology of multiple sclerosis in US veterans. V: Ancestry and the risk of MS. *Ann. Neurol.*, **33**, 632–9.

218. Ebers, G.C. and Bulman, D. (1986) The geography of MS reflects a genetic susceptibility. *Neurology*, **36** (Suppl.), 108 (abstract).

219. Bulman, D.E. and Ebers, G.C. (1992) The geography of MS reflects genetic susceptibility. *J. Trop. Geogr. Neurol.*, **2**, 66–72.

220. Antonovsky, A., Leibowitz, U., Medalie, J.M. *et al.* (1967) Epidemiological study of multiple sclerosis in Israel. Part III. Multiple sclerosis and socio-economic status. *J. Neurol. Neurosurg. Psychiatry*, **30**, 1–6.

221. Kranz, J.S. (1983) A multiple sclerosis case-control study in Olmsted and Mower Counties, Minnesota. PhD Thesis, University of Minnesota.

222. Operskalski, E.A., Visscher, B.R., Malmgren, R.M. and Detels, R. (1989) A case-control study of multiple sclerosis. *Neurology*, **39**, 825–9.

223. Poskanzer, D.C. (1965) Tonsillectomy and multiple sclerosis. *Lancet*, ii, 1264–6.

224. Poskanzer, D.C., Prenney, L.B., Sheridan, J.L. and Yonkondy, J. (1980) Multiple sclerosis in the Orkney and Shetland Islands. I. Epidemiology, clinical factors and methodology. *J. Epidemiol. Commun. Hlth*, **34**, 229–39.

225. Poskanzer, D.C., Schapira, K. and Miller, H. (1963) Epidemiology of multiple sclerosis in the counties of Northumberland and Durham. *J. Neurol. Neurosurg. Psychiatry*, **26**, 368–76.

226. Poskanzer, D.C., Sheridan, J.L. and Prenney, L.B. (1980) Multiple sclerosis in the Orkney and Shetland Islands. II. The search for an exogenous aetiology. *J. Epidemiol. Commun. Hlth.*, **34**, 240–52.

227. Westlund, K.B. and Kurland, L.T. (1953) Studies on multiple sclerosis in Winnipeg, Manitoba, and New Orleans, Louisiana. I. Prevalence. Comparison between the patient groups in Winnipeg and New Orleans. *Am. J. Hyg.*, **57**, 380–96.

228. Isager, H., Anderson, E. and Hyllested, K. (1980) Risk of multiple sclerosis inversely associated with birth order position. *Acta Neurol. Scand.*, **61**, 393–6.

229. Alperovitch, A., Le Canuet, P. and Marteau, R. (1981) Birth order and risk of multiple sclerosis: are they associated and how? *Acta Neurol. Scand.*, **63**, 136–8.

230. Visscher, B.R., Liu, K.-S., Sullivan, C.B., Valdiviezo, N.L. and Detels, R. (1982) Birth order and multiple sclerosis. *Acta Neurol. Scand.*, **66**, 209–15.

231. Kurtzke, J.F., Page, W.F., Murphy, F.M. and Norman, J.E. Jr (1994) Epidemiology of multiple sclerosis in U.S. veterans: risk factors for multiple sclerosis. *Ann. Neurol.*, **36**, 302 (abstract).

232. Kurtzke, J.F., Page, W.F., Murphy, F.M. and Norman, J.E. Jr (1992) Epidemiology of multiple sclerosis in US veterans. 4. Age at onset. *Neuroepidemiology*, **11**, 226–35.

233. Page, W.F., Mack, T.M., Kurtzke, J.F., Murphy, F.M. and Norman, J.E. Jr (1995) Epidemiology of multiple sclerosis in US veterans. 6: Population ancestry and surname ethnicity as risk factors for multiple sclerosis. *Neuroepidemiology*, **14**, 286–96.

234. MacMahon, B. (1967) Epidemiological methods, in *Preventive Medicine* (eds D.W. Clark and B. MacMahon), Boston, Little Brown, pp. 81–104.

235. Paul, J.R. (1966) *Clinical Epidemiology*, rev. edn. Chicago: University of Chicago.

236. Panum, P.L. (1940) Observations made during the epidemic of measles on the Faroe Islands in the year 1846 (translated A.S. Hatcher), in *Panum on Measles*, New York, Delta Omega Society (distributed by American Public Health Association).

237. Kurtzke, J.F. and Hyllested, K. (1975) Multiple sclerosis: an epidemic disease in the Faeroes. *Trans. Am. Neurol. Assoc.*, **100**, 213–15.

238. Kurtzke, J.F. and Hyllested, K. (1979) Multiple sclerosis in the Faroe Islands: I. Clinical and epidemiological features. *Ann. Neurol.*, **5**, 6–21.

239. Kurtzke, J.F. and Hyllested, K. (1986) Multiple sclerosis in the Faroe Islands. II. Clinical update, transmission, and the nature of MS. *Neurology*, **36**, 307–28.

240. Kurtzke, J.F. and Hyllested, K. (1987) Multiple sclerosis in the Faroe Islands. III. An alternative assessment of the three epidemics. *Acta Neurol. Scand.*, **76**, 317–39.

241. Kurtzke, J.F. and Hyllested, K. (1987) MS epidemiology in Faroe Islands. *Rivista Neurol.*, **57**, 77–87.

242. Kurtzke, J.F. and Hyllested, K. (1988) Validity of the epidemics of multiple sclerosis in the Faroe Islands. *Neuroepidemiology*, **7**, 190–227.

243. Kurtzke, J.F., Hyllested, K., Heltberg, A. and Olsen, Á. (1993) Multiple sclerosis in the Faroe Islands. 5. The occurrence of the fourth epidemic as validation of transmission. *Acta Neurol. Scand.*, **88**, 161–73.

244. Kurtzke, J.F., Guðmundsson, K.R. and Bergmann, S. (1982) Multiple sclerosis in Iceland: I. Evidence of a postwar epidemic. *Neurology*, **32**, 143–50.

245. Cook, S.D., Dowling, P.C., Norman, J. *et al.* (1979) Multiple sclerosis and canine distemper in Iceland. *Lancet*, **1**, 380–1.

246. Cook, S.D., Gudmundsson, G., Benedikz, J. and Dowling, P.C. (1986) Multiple sclerosis and distemper in Iceland, 1966–1978. *Acta Neurol. Scand.*, **61**, 244–51.

247. Guðmundsson, K.R., Bergmann, S., Björnsson, O.J. and Ellertsson, A.B. (1974) Further studies on multiple sclerosis in Iceland. *J. Neurol. Sci.*, **21**, 47–58.

248. Cook, S.D., MacDonald, J., Tapp, W., Poskanzer, D. and Dowling, P.C. (1988) Multiple sclerosis in Shetland Islands: an update. *Acta Neurol. Scand.*, **77**, 148–51.

249. Martin, J.R. (1987) Troop-related multiple sclerosis outbreak in the Orkneys? *J. Epidemiol. Commun. Hlth.*, **41**, 183–4.

250. Koch, M.J., Reed, D., Stern, R. and Brody, J.A. (1974) Multiple sclerosis: a cluster in a small northwestern United States community. *J. Am. Med. Assoc.*, **228**, 1555–7.

251. Eastman, R., Sheridan, J. and Poskanzer, D.C. (1977) Multiple sclerosis clustering in a small Massachusetts community, with possible common exposure 23 years before onset. *N. Engl. J. Med.*, **389**, 793–4.

252. Murray, T.J. (1976) An unusual occurrence of multiple sclerosis in a small rural community. *Can. J. Neurol. Sci.*, **3**, 163–6.

253. Stein, E.C., Schiffer, R.B., Hall, W.J. and Young, N. (1987) Multiple sclerosis and the workplace: report of an industry-based cluster. *Neurology*, **37**, 1672–7.

254. Schiffer, R.B., Weitkamp, L.R., Ford, C. and Hall, W.J. (1994) A genetic marker and family history study of the upstate New York multiple sclerosis cluster. *Neurology*, **44**, 329–33.

255. Poser, C.M., Hibberd, P.L., Benedikz, J. *et al.* (1988) Analysis of the 'epidemic' of multiple sclerosis in the Faroe Islands. I. Clinical and epidemiological aspects. *Neuroepidemiology*, **7**, 168–80.

256. Poser, C.M. and Hibberd, P.L. (1988) Analysis of the 'epidemic' of multiple sclerosis in the Faroe Islands. II. Biostatistical aspects. *Neuroepidemiology*, **7**, 181–9.

257. Benedikz, J.E.G., Magnússon, H. and Guðmundsson, G. (1994) Multiple sclerosis in Iceland, with observations on the alleged epidemic in the Faroe Islands. *Ann. Neurol.*, **36** (S2), S175–S179.

258. Poser, C.M. (ed.) (1994) Multiple sclerosis: epidemiology and genetics. Reviews and recommendations of a workshop by the Alghero Group organized and directed by Charles M. Poser, MD . . . and Giulio Rosati, MD . . . *Ann. Neurol.*, **36** (S2), S163–S247.

259. Kurtzke, J.F., Hyllested, K. and Heltberg, A. (1995) Multiple sclerosis in the Faroe Islands: transmission across four epidemics. *Acta Neurol. Scand.*, **91**, 321–5.

260. Meyer-Rienecker, H. and Buddenhagen, F. (1988) Incidence of multiple sclerosis: a periodic or stable phenomenon. *J. Neurol.*, **235**, 241–4.

8 RISK FACTORS IN MULTIPLE SCLEROSIS

William A. Sibley

8.1 Introduction

Although there is a strong genetic influence determining the occurrence of multiple sclerosis (MS), it is probable that some environmental factors play a role, either in causation or in triggering of exacerbations. Thus, while there is a high degree of concordance of MS in identical twins, this never exceeds about 40% – suggesting that non-genetic factors are also important. Clusters such as that affecting the Faroe Islands after the Second World War are one example of many reported clusters of MS cases which are not easily explained. These experiences, and the data regarding a changing risk of MS with migration, have prompted Kurtzke to define MS as an 'acquired exogenous environmental disease' [1].

Environmental factors that might be responsible for causation have seldom been sought in an organized systematic way in a prospective study of the populations at main risk – chiefly caucasians of northern European origin. It is impossible to identify people who are destined to develop MS, and follow this group closely to settle the matter, because the occurrence of MS is unpredictable. One would have to mount a detailed study of hundreds of thousands of individuals, and the logistics and expense of such a study make it unlikely that it will ever be done.

An interesting alternative method of investigation, available to certain large clinics supervising almost all of the care of certain populations, and having accessible records for many past decades, is to identify a historical cohort of patients hypothetically at risk, and 'prospectively' follow this cohort for the possible development of MS. This method has been used productively by the Mayo Clinic in Rochester, Minnesota. Almost all of the population of Olmsted County receives all of their medical care from Mayo Clinic facilities [2].

Another way of potentially gaining information about the environmental origins of MS consists of making a systematic study of factors that influence exacerbation and disability progression rates in established cases. Most studies of this in the past have been retrospective, often involving medical chart reviews, or questioning of patients and their relatives. Medical charts are often sketchy and very selective in the information recorded: for example, an attack of retrobulbar neuritis following 'flu would probably be recorded as such, but an episode of 'flu not followed by a change in the disease might not be mentioned. Similarly with episodes of physical trauma and episodes of psychological stress. Selective medical recording and selective memory recording make it difficult to use information derived in this way to establish any of the putative factors as true risk factors.

Dr Harry Weaver, former Director of Research at the National Multiple Sclerosis Society, USA, recognizing this problem, took a leading role in establishing a center at the University of Arizona whose task over the ensuing 8 years was to focus on environmental risk factors, by careful systematic long-term recording of these in patients with known MS followed closely to determine exacerbations and the rate of progression of disability.

8.2 Methodology

8.2.1 PATIENTS

Gradually, beginning in 1976, 170 patients with clinically probable or definite MS by the Schumacher Criteria [3] entered the program. All patients were eligible who were able to come to the clinic periodically, who were willing to complete a monthly questionaire, and who were not taking prophylactic immunosuppressive drugs. Our patients received only symptomatic treatment during the program, although many received corticotropin or prednisone, in declining dosage, for 10–14 days after acute exacerbations.

The mean age at entry was 43 years and the F:M ratio was 1.6:1. Almost half of the patients (83) were mildly affected by MS at entry, with a Disability Status Scale (DSS) [4] of 0–4, 12 were DSS 5, 32 were DSS 6 and 28 were DSS 7. Only 15 patients were chair- or bed-confined, 9 being DSS 8 and 6 being DSS 9. The study

Multiple Sclerosis: Clinical and pathogenetic basis. Edited by Cedric S. Raine, Henry F. McFarland and Wallace W. Tourtellotte. Published in 1997 by Chapman & Hall, London. ISBN 0 412 30890 8.

Table 8.1 Exacerbation and progression during a prospective 5.2 year study in 170 symptomatically[a] treated patients

Entry DSS	No. of patients	Mean exac./yr	Exit DSS	Mean increase DSS/yr
0	10	0.16	0.6	0.12
1	22	0.50	2.3	0.22
2	19	0.50	3.4	0.31
3	18	0.39	4.1	0.24
4	14	0.30	5.2	0.24
5	12	0.30	5.7	0.12
6	32	0.16	6.5	0.09
7	28	0.17	7.7	0.12
8	9	0.03	8.3	0.05
9	6	0.02	9.1	0.05

[a]Treated occasionally with 10–14 days of steroids for acute exacerbations.

was conducted over a period of 8 years, but some patients spent less time in the study due to entering late, or to relocation. Four left to start prophylactic immuno-therapy, and 5 because of advanced disability. The mean time in the program per patient was 5.2 years.

Table 8.1 shows the yearly exacerbation rates and rate of progression in these patients during the 5 years. Note that the clinical exacerbation rate was 0.3–0.5 per year for patients in the earlier stages of the illness. For patients with a DSS of 6–9 the mean annual exacerbation rate was only 0.02–0.16. Likewise for DSS ratings greater than 4 at entry the mean annual increase in DSS was very low, ranging from 0.05 to 0.12. Thus, while cranial MRI scanning shows that patients with chronic progressive disease may have as many as four to six new lesions per year on serial scans [5], it is apparent that patients with a DSS rating of over 5 (those requiring assistance to walk) were poor clinical indicators of disease activity. This has obvious implications, not only for a prospective study of risk factors, but also for long-term trials of treatment.

8.2.2   CONTROLS

Controls were included in the study primarily to compare the frequency of various environmental factors in the two groups. There were 134 controls, mostly women (F:M ratio 1.7:1), and the mean age at study entry was 40 years. The majority were healthy and working, although they acquired an assortment of illnesses during the program.

8.2.3   EXACERBATION

This was rather strictly defined, as a new symptom, or worsening of an old symptom, associated with a

confirmatory change on neurological examination, all lasting at least 48 hours in the absence of fever. Magnetic resonance imaging (MRI) scans were not available during the early years of the study, and were not used routinely to confirm localization. However, the term 'exacerbation', in our usage, implied a new lesion or enlargement of an old lesion. New symptoms suggesting exacerbation required the patient to attend clinic again, as soon as possible, for re-examination and confirmation.

8.2.4   PROCEDURAL DETAILS

All patients and controls completed a questionaire monthly, answering a wide variety of questions about changes during the previous month. Included were questions about physical and emotional trauma, infections, immunizations and changes in either dietary habits, medication or exercise patterns. If the answers were not returned promptly, they were obtained by telephone by the clinic nurse.

At entry, and routinely every 3 months, and in the event of symptoms suggesting an exacerbation, all patients had a complete neurological examination, interval history and a new Kurtzke functional symptoms (FS) score and disability status scale (DSS) rating.

8.2.5   DATA ANALSYSIS: PERIODS AT RISK (AR) AND NOT AT RISK (NAR)

In order to establish any factor as a risk factor in MS it is necessary to show that exacerbation or worsening of the disease occurs statistically more frequently when at risk (AR) for that factor than when not at risk (NAR). Exacerbation rates can be determined during the cumulative time AR and during cumulative time NAR for the same group of patients, for any given factor.

Deciding what period AR to use was not always easy because we know so little about the cause of MS lesions. In the intercurrent viral infection portion of the study, we chose a period AR of 7 weeks: 2 weeks prior to clinical symptoms (because prior mass culture studies had sometimes shown viral shedding as early as 14 days prior to clinical symptoms) [6], and 5 weeks after the infection: the latter period was chosen because it is at the upper end of the incubation range of post-rabies vaccination encephalomyelitis in man [7]. We reasoned that if the viral infection is a trigger similar to this known myelin antigen, perhaps by molecular mimicry, this should be an appropriate time period.

In the analysis of stressful life events the AR period was the actual duration of the perceived stress as reported by the patient plus 3 months: thus in some cases of marital discord ending in divorce the AR period might be 15 months or longer.

In the trauma study we arbitrarily used an AR period of 6 months in a preliminary report [8]. Recently, in a report of our completed prospective study of trauma in MS we employed both a 3-month and 6-month analysis [9]. We included the 3-months AR period because it was one used by McAlpine *et al.* [10, 11], and some had objected that the 6-month period might be unreasonably long. In the trauma study, whether using a 3-month or 6-month period, the AR period ceased either in 3 or 6 months, or at the time of the next traumatic event: AR periods were not allowed to overlap. With simultaneous traumas, the AR period was arbitrarily assigned to the most serious injury: for example, it would be assigned to a head injury rather than to an abraded knee, if both occurred at the same time.

The change in Kurtzke DSS score during the study provided a method of measuring the influence of all these factors on progression of disability, for example, if stressful life events are a risk factor, one might expect a statistically significant more rapid progression of the disease in patients experiencing many of these, in comparison to patients leading more tranquil lives.

8.2.6 STATISTICAL METHODS

We assumed the null hypothesis, that if a factor was not a risk factor in MS, exacerbations would distribute themselves randomly during AR and NAR periods. This hypothesis was tested using a simple chi-square analysis on the occurrences (exacerbations) during cumulative AR and NAR periods, using 1 degree of freedom. The critical value for chi-square in most of the tables in this chapter is 3.84, for $P = 0.05$.

The not-at-risk (NAR) periods were all times in the study when the patients were not at risk for any given factor. The cumulative NAR periods were calculated for the same group of patients as had been determined to be at risk.

8.3 Results

8.3.1 VIRUS-LIKE INFECTIONS

Logistical problems and expense did not allow us to do viral cultures in all patients, and the infections were identified simply as a 'clinical viral infection' because the clinical description matched what one usually associates with such infections. Most were upper respiratory tract infections ranging from frank influenza to colds; some were gastrointestinal with low grade fever and diarrhea or sore throat. Often other family members were sick with similar symptoms at the same times. The details are given in the primary publication [12].

The higher annual exacerbation rates in our study, when at risk for such infections, is illustrated in Figure 8.1: note that the much higher rate of exacerbation when at risk for viral infections was equally evident in

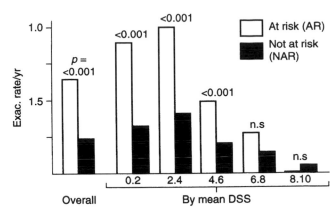

Figure 8.1 Relationship between MS exacerbations and 779 viral infections in 170 patients in 5.3 years.

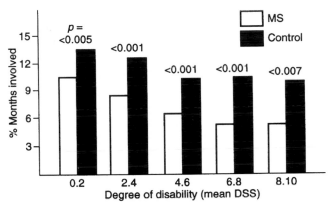

Figure 8.2 Comparison of frequency of common viral infections in MS patients with varying degrees of disability and age matched controls. Mean DSS = average of entry and exit DSS scores: mean follow-up 5.3 years.

ambulatory patients and in patients with more advanced physical impairment.

Another major finding in this portion of our study was that patients with MS experience 25–60% fewer symptomatic viral infections than controls (Figure 8.2). One might expect that this was due to sheltering with fewer infectious contacts, but the best evidence that this was not the entire explanation is contained in the first column of Figure 8.2 – even patients with minimal disability, who were working daily, and had the same number of young children at home as controls, had 25% fewer clinically apparent infections.

8.3.2 THE EFFECT OF STRESSFUL LIFE EVENTS

This is perhaps the most difficult of the putative risk factors to study. Not only is stress difficult to quantify, the problem is compounded by the fact that patients with multiple cerebral lesions complain more of stress than those equivalently disabled by lesions confined to the spinal cord, suggesting that the MS cerebral lesions themselves enhance perception of stress, as noted by

Table 8.2   *Types of stressful life events*

1   Bereavement – spouse or immediate family
2   Death of other close family member
3   Marital stress
4   Job loss or severe work stress
5   Job loss – spouse
6   Personal illness (not MS), trauma, surgery
7   Illness, serious, in family member
8   Interpersonal conflict (includes financial problems)
9   Miscellaneous: friend or pet death etc.

Rabins *et al.* [13]. The greater frequency of conversion reactions [14], depression [15–17], and cognitive disorders almost certainly has a similar explanation. Some have found the greater frequency of depression to be correlated with cognitive disorders [17], but others have not [15]. Even early MS patients have a higher frequency of depression, however, and the rate of suicide in MS patients is 7.5 times that of the general population [16].

In our study, because of difficulties in measuring the severity of stress, we chose rather to count episodes of stressful life events, but only if they were perceived as stressful by the patient. Those chosen are indicated in Table 8.2, which is modified from our publication on this topic [18].

Table 8.3 presents data on the effects of stress on exacerbation rates in the 95 patients who had exacerbations in the study. The types of stress are grouped into only four categories, corresponding to Types 1–2, 3–5, 6–7 and 8–9 in Table 8.2.

In our original publication [18], the data for each type of stress were analyzed separately, and none of the rows showed a statistically significant difference between the proportion of exacerbations AR and NAR, although there was a trend to a positive association with marital and job stress. In Table 8.3 one sees that the combined marital and job stress category shows a significant positive relationship to exacerbation when only the 95 patients who had exacerbations are analyzed, although this association is not seen in any of the other categories. Scrutiny of the data showed that this positive association could be due, at least partly, to several instances in which there was concurrent reporting of both a stressful work or marital situation and the exacerbation; in the

case of 16 exacerbations, both the new exacerbation and a stressful event were reported at the same time. For example, one patient had 4 exacerbations and on each occasion attributed it to a stressful situation at work during the same month.

We analyzed the data to see if there was a relationship between the frequency of stressful life events and the progression of the disease. We grouped patients entering the study with a DSS score of 0–5 into two groups: those with more than 5 stressful life events during the study and those with less than 5. Thirty-four patients had a mean of 7 such events during the program and 61 patients had a mean of only 2.1 events: none the less, both groups advanced in their disability by the same mean 1.1 DSS points. We concluded that we had no evidence that life stress accelerated the disability imposed by MS.

8.3.3   THE EFFECT OF PHYSICAL TRAUMA

A detailed account of our completed analysis of the effect of trauma during the entire prospective study has been presented elsewhere, and the reader is referred to this publication and a related editorial [9, 19].

All physical traumas were divided into the following categories: dental procedures, major surgery, minor surgery, burns, sprains, head injuries, fractures, and abrasions/lacerations/contusions (ab/lac/con). The frequency of these events, and the number of patients involved with each, is presented in Table 8.4, which is an analysis of the data using a 6-month AR period. Note that there is no significant difference in the proportion of exacerbations occurring AR and NAR in any row, although a trend toward a negative correlation is seen in the case of surgical procedures and fractures. In the primary publication on this subject [9], we repeated the analysis using only the 95 patients having one or more exacerbations during the study; here the tendency for a negative correlation was more striking, and when surgical procedures and fractures were grouped and compared to other types of trauma, there was a statistically significant negative correlation between surgical procedures and fractures and new activity of the illness. We saw no logical reason to group the categories this way, except as a way to illustrate the primary source

Table 8.3   Stressful life events and exacerbations of MS in 95 patients with exacerbations during the program

Type stress	No. of patients	No. episodes	No. exac. AR	Yr AR	No. exac. NAR	Yr AR	Exac./yr AR (mean)	Exac./yr NAR (mean)	χ^2	
Bereavement	21	26	1	6.5	38	98.6	0.15	0.38	1.1	
Marital and job	44	81	24	25.0	101	182.7	0.96	0.55	6.1	$P < .02$
Personal and family illness	61	152	20	37.9	135	266.7	0.53	0.50	0.0	
Interpersonal, miscellaneous	57	256	10	33.3	130	268.8	0.30	0.48	2.3	n.s.

Table 8.4 Annual exacerbation rates following various types of trauma, compared to rates in the same patients when not at risk for any trauma, using a 6-month at-risk period

Type trauma	No. of patients	No. episodes	No. exac. AR	Time AR (mth)	No. exac. NAR	Time NAR (mth)	Exac./yr AR (mean)	Exac./yr NAR (mean)
Dental	78	162	16	613	56	2642	0.31	0.25
Minor surgery	83	147	5	557	55	2816	0.11	0.23
Major surgery	42	73	5	320	36	1264	0.19	0.34
Burns	71	157	12	618	62	1969	0.23	0.37
Sprains	61	93	10	331	46	1510	0.36	0.37
Fractures	32	55	1	231	15	968	0.05	0.19
Head injuries	67	140	16	534	63	2071	0.35	0.36
Ab/lac/con	137	580	50	2071	109	4050	0.28	0.32
Totals		1407	115	5275	*	*		

*These columns cannot be totalled since many patients are represented several times in the various subcategories when NAR for any trauma. Ab/lac/con, abrasions, lacerations, contusions.

of the negative correlation. There is no ready explanation for this phenomenon. However there is some precedent: Ridley and Schapira reported no exacerbations in 57 surgical cases in the first postoperative month [20].

Analysis of the data using a 3-month AR period, in the same way, resulted in no different interpretations, with one exception: the subcategory of electric shock was statistically significantly related to exacerbation using the 3-month AR category, but not using the 6-month period AR [9]. All of the electrical injuries were mild, not producing significant burns, and almost all were due to contact with a cooking device using 110 volt alternating current. In most cases the current flow was hand to hand or hand-to-foot. In the case of one man shocked while repairing a television set, we could not be sure of the direction of current flow; we could not ascertain whether his head was grounded since it may have been positioned inside the rear of the television cabinet. Five days later this patient had an acute exacerbation with ataxia and facial pain. The history of another of our patients with a very short time between electric shock and exacerbation was included in a previous report [8].

However, one of the patients reporting an electric shock had an exacerbation during the AR period, 2 months after reporting a shock from a transcutaneous stimulator. Since low voltage currents of the type involved in these devices are not known to produce biological injury [21, 22], it might be argued that it was inappropriate to include this patient. Therefore in Table 8.5 we have re-analyzed the data excluding this case, and the association no longer reaches significance. Table 8.5 probably gives a more accurate analysis of electrical shock and risk of MS exacerbation than that published in our earlier reports [8, 9].

A short interval between the time of trauma and exacerbation has been stressed as convincing evidence of a causative relationship between trauma and exacerbation by several authors. In our 3-month AR analysis of 1407 traumas, 86 exacerbations occurred during a 3-month period after trauma; 15 of these cases happened during the first 15 days after a trauma, only one more than would be expected by chance. The most important results of the study, however, are that exacerbations occurred no more commonly after various types of trauma than they occurred in the same patients when no trauma had occurred.

8.3.4 THE EFFECT OF PREGNANCY

Too few pregnancies occurred in our prospective study to draw conclusions. However, Dr Donald Paty and I previously [23] investigated the effect of pregnancy retrospectively, by asking 72 women patients in our MS

Table 8.5 Electrical injury and MS exacerbations[a]

Period AR	No. of patients	No. episodes	No. exac. AR	Time AR (yr)	No. exac. NAR	Time NAR (yr)	Exac./yr AR (mean)	Exac./yr NAR (mean)	χ^2
3 months	16	18	3	3.6	20	65.5	0.83	0.30	2.9 n.s.
6 months	16	18	4	6.2	18	49.9	0.64	0.36	1.1 n.s.

[a]In this analysis, one patient having an exacerbation 2 months after a reported shock from a transcutaneous stimulator was eliminated for reasons cited in the text. The critical value for χ^2 is 3.84 ($P < 0.05$).

Clinic in Arizona and 82 patients in the MS Clinic at the University of Western Ontario, London, Ontario, two questions: 'Did your first MS symptoms begin during the nine months of a pregnancy, or during the 9 months following a pregnancy?' and 'Did any subsequent relapses occur during a pregnancy, or during 9-month periods following a pregnancy?' In Arizona 2/74 patients (2%) and in Canada 8/82 patients (9%) reported onset of MS during a pregnancy, while the corresponding figures for onset during a 9-month post-partum period were 9/67 (13%) in Arizona and 15/82 (18%) in Canada. Subsequent relapse occurred during a pregnancy in 1.4% of Arizona patients and in 9.7% of Canadian patients, while figures for later relapse during a 9-month post-partum period were 15% in Arizona and 14% in Canada.

The fact that relatively fewer exacerbations occur during pregnancy is the consensus of most who have investigated this area. The subject was recently reviewed by Abramsky [24]. Most authors have noted that the ratio of exacerbations in the puerperium to those during pregnancy varies from 2:1 to 6:1 Possible reasons include the immunosuppressive effects of corticosteroids, progesterone, interferon beta and transforming growth factor beta (TGFβ), which are increased during pregnancy.

8.4   Discussion and conclusions

8.4.1   RELATIVE IMPORTANCE OF PUTATIVE ENVIRONMENTAL FACTORS

In the majority of acute relapses in MS patients there is no history of recent trauma, no history of preceding infection and no history of preceding unusual stress. If it were otherwise, the associations would have been recognized by most experienced neurologists, and there would be no controversy. Less obvious precipitants might easily be missed, however. Now that we have analyzed data relating to all of the major putative risk factors, it has become clear that clinical viral infections are the most important risk factor uncovered in this study. While only about 8% of 779 such infections were

followed by clinical MS exacerbation, 27% of MS attacks were preceded by such infections. Table 8.6 is a summary showing the relative importance of those studied prospectively and concurrently, all of which have been favored candidates as possible precipitants over the years. Note that the chi-square value for the significance of viral infection far overshadows the relatively weak positive relationship with stressful life events, and that we were unable, overall, to confirm a relationship with trauma.

Confirmation of our data about the triggering of MS exacerbations by viral infections first came from the University of Ottawa. Narod and associates, in a small series, found that 32% of exacerbations were preceded by viral infections, a figure very similar to ours [25]. Later Andersen et al. made similar observations, finding a significant increased risk of exacerbation during viral infection AR periods. They also found a significant correlation between the number of AR relapses and the number of virus-like infections among 60 patients with benign MS [26]. Still more recently, Panitch reported a strong correlation between upper respiratory infections and MS relapses in patients: nearly two-thirds of relapses occurred in AR periods [27]. In this study, interferon beta-1b prevented relapses, but did not reduce the frequency of symptomatic infections.

The finding of many fewer viral infections in MS patients than in controls is also a matter of interest. We interpret this to mean that MS patients have fewer *clinically apparent infections*, not fewer infections. It seems unlikely that, as a group, they have fewer viral infections, because antibody titers to most common viruses are as high or higher than controls, including titers to several strains of influenza [28, 29]. We believe, furthermore, that the lower numbers of apparent viral infections is not entirely due to sheltering or sequestration of the patients, since even active working patients, with the same average number of young children in the household, had 25% fewer infections than controls. The reduction in numbers of viral infections, in comparison to controls, progressively escalated with increasing disability. While this may have been due to sheltering, one must also consider the possibility that increased immune capability may have

Table 8.6   Prospective and concurrent study of risk factors in MS (170 patients, 887 patient-years)

	No. episodes	No. exac. AR	Time AR (mth)	No. exac. NAR	Time NAR (mth)	Exac./yr AR (mean)	Exac./yr NAR (mean)	χ^2
Viral infection	779	67	1246	179	9401	0.64	0.23	56.3
Stress	576	55	1819	191	8828	0.36	0.26	4.8
Trauma	1407	115	5274	131	5373	0.26	0.29	0.8

Note: The AR period following traumatic episodes is 6 months in this table; the 0.8 χ^2 is not significant; the χ^2 for stress is significant at $P < 0.05$ (see text for possible caveats).

determined both fewer apparent infections and the severity of disability from MS.

When one considers this evidence that MS patients experience inapparent infections more often than controls, and that probably as many as 50% of viral infections are inapparent[6], it seems probable that viral infection is the major triggering factor for most new MS bouts.

In view of the fact that the frequency of stress did not influence the progression of disability, and since none of the categories of stressful life events had a significant influence on exacerbations individually, it seems unlikely that stress is an important risk factor in MS. This conclusion is similar to that of the only other prospective study of this factor, by Rabins *et al.*[13], and with the recent study of the influence of the acute stress of daily missile attacks on the frequency of exacerbation in MS patients in Tel Aviv during the Persian Gulf war[30]. It is a conclusion also in accord with an earlier retrospective study by Pratt[31]. While marital and job stresses, when combined, bore a significant relationship to exacerbation, bereavement and other stressful life events showed no such trend. While a number of explanations could be considered, we suspect that shaky marriages and insecure job situations, stressed further by chronic illness, were blamed unrealistically for worsening during periods when concurrent reporting of stress and exacerbation was possible. It seems likely that concurrent reporting in studies of this kind is less reliable, since it allows expression of patient bias. A patient survey by Rabins *et al.*[13] found that MS patients were biased in the belief that stress resulted in exacerbation, even though stressful life event scores, in their study, were no higher in the month before exacerbations than at other times. At least 16 exacerbations were reported concurrently with a life stress in this portion of our study, and one patient, as already noted, consistently blamed work stress for each of four concurrently reported exacerbations.

A number of retrospective investigations of emotional stress and its relationship either to the onset or exacerbation of MS have been reported, suggesting that stress may play a role[32–36]. All potentially suffer from the major problem with such studies: fallible memories, possible failure to record all stresses, especially those not associated with exacerbation, and a tendency to recall selectively those stresses followed by worsening of MS. These studies also do not take into account the more frequent reporting of stress by MS patients, noted in the study of Rabins *et al.*[13].

Our study, considered in combination with a study from the Mayo Clinic[2], suggests that physical trauma should no longer be seriously considered as a precipitant of MS worsening. Our data clearly indicate that there is no linkage between disability progression in MS

patients and the frequency with which they suffer physical trauma, nor is there any correlation between common traumas and exacerbation of MS. Certainly the results of the study provide no support for the notion that minor head injuries or peripheral trauma to the limbs are risk factors. The data do not, however, provide definite information about the effects of severe or penetrating trauma to the head or spine, since we had no such cases. Two of our patients with steady and fairly rapid progression of disability during the previous two years continued to progress at about the same rate after thalamotomy. We agree with Kelly[37] who noted that all of his patients having this procedure did badly afterwards; this has been our experience too, but we have been equally impressed with the rapidity and severity of the preoperative course in most such cases.

The prospective portion of the confirmatory study on MS and trauma from the Mayo Clinic found that exacerbations occurred no more commonly in the 6 months after trauma, than in the 6 months prior to trauma[2, 38]. This study also included prospective follow-up of a historically identified cohort of 819 non-MS patients with moderate or severe head injuries living in Olmsted County, Minnesota. Follow-up over a period of up to 30 years indicated that only two patients developed MS – one 2 years and one 30 years after injury. These lengthy intervals made a relationship to trauma unlikely, and the frequency of development of MS was no higher than modern estimates of its expected prevalence.

Poser[39] has hypothesized that even relatively minor injuries to the head or spine may cause increased permeability of the blood–brain barrier and precipitate MS lesions; his case reports are highly selected ones, and his publications do not include MS population studies indicating that more exacerbations *actually occur* after trauma than at other times, and prove nothing in a disease normally so variable and active as MS. We have had an opportunity to comment on this problem in greater detail in a recent editorial[19].

8.4.2 ETIOLOGIC IMPLICATIONS

If trauma and stress are not impressive risk factors, we are left with the conclusion best supported by the data: that MS is probably a post-infectious phenomenon. There is precedent for demyelination occurring after infection – in the peripheral nerves in the Guillain–Barré syndrome, and in the central white matter in the post-infectious perivenous encephalomyelitides. The common post-infectious demyelinating disorders, such as those following the childhood exanthemata, are almost always uniphasic, one-time conditions. This may be because the responsible viruses usually establish solid immunity in the host. Re-infection is common, however, with many other common viruses, especially those producing upper respiratory symptoms. Some of these are therefore candidate viruses which may trigger the recurrent lesions of MS.

The mechanism of such triggering by viruses is still conjectural. However, the phenomenon of molecular mimicry, whereby amino acid homologies exist between certain viruses and certain myelin proteins, provides one possible explanation [40]. This possibility has recently received support from the study of Wucherpfennig and Strominger [41], showing that T lymphocytes from MS patients reactive to myelin basic protein also react strongly against peptides from a number of common viruses. Another possibility is that persistent sensitized clones of lymphocytes, directed against white matter of the CNS, are resident in the blood and brain of MS patients at all times, but attack only when the target cells (possibly oligodendrocytes) display class II histocompatibility antigens on their surface. Interferon gamma, produced by sensitized T cells in response to antigenic stimulation, including that produced by viral infection, promotes the expression of such antigens on cell surfaces. Panitch *et al.* have reported that gamma interferon, used in treatment efforts, increased the frequency of MS exacerbation [42].

It is an intriguing possibility that immune systems efficient in defeating common viral infection have had special survival value in cold climates over the millions of years of human existence. This could account for the increased frequency of DR2 and related genes in northern European populations and their descendants. It is possible that the immune systems in some individuals, destined to develop MS, have become overly aggressive and mistake peptide sequences in certain brain proteins for virus, and attack them.

References

1. Kurtzke, J.F. (1983) The epidemiology of multiple sclerosis, in *Multiple Sclerosis* (eds J.F. Hallpike, C.W.M. Adams and W.W. Tourtellotte), Baltimore, MD, Williams and Wilkins.
2. Siva, A., Radhakrishnan, K., Kurland, L.T. *et al.* (1993) Trauma and multiple sclerosis: a population-based cohort study from Olmsted County, Minnesota. *Neurology*, 43, 1878–82.
3. Schumacher, G.A., Beebe, G., Kibler, R.F. *et al.* (1965) Problems of experimental trials of therapy in multiple sclerosis: report by the panel on evaluation of experimental trials of therapy in multiple sclerosis. *Ann. NY Acad. Sci.*, 122, 552–68.
4. Kurtzke, J.F. (1961) On the evaluation of disability in multiple sclerosis. *Neurology*, 11, 686–94.
5. Koopmans, R.A., Li, D.K.B., Oger, J.J.F. *et al.* (1989) Chronic progressive multiple sclerosis: serial magnetic resonance brain imaging over six months. *Ann. Neurol.*, 26, 248–56.
6. Fox, J.P. and Hall, C.E. (1980) *Viruses in Families*. Littleton, MA, PSG.
7. Shiraki, H. and Otani, S. (1959) Clinical and pathological features of rabies post-vaccinal encephalomyelitis in man, in '*Allergic*' *Encephalomyelitis* (eds M.W. Kies and E.C. Alvord), Springfield, IL, Charles C. Thomas.
8. Bamford, C.R., Sibley W.A., Thies, C. *et al.* (1981) Trauma as an etiologic and aggravating factor in multiple sclerosis. *Neurology*, 31, 1229–34.
9. Sibley, W.A., Bamford, C.R., Clark, K.P., Smith, M.S. and Laguna, J.F. (1991) A prospective study of physical trauma and multiple sclerosis. *J. Neurol. Neurosurg. Psychiatry*, 54, 584–9.
10. McAlpine, D. and Compston, N. (1952) Some aspects of the natural history of disseminated sclerosis. *Q. J. Med.*, 21, 135–67.
11. McAlpine, D., Lumsden, C.E. and Acheson, E.D.S. (1972) *Multiple Sclerosis. A Reappraisal*, Edinburgh and London, Churchill Livingstone.
12. Sibley, W.A., Bamford, C.R. and Clark, K. (1985) Clinical viral infections and multiple sclerosis. *Lancet*, i, 1313–15.
13. Rabins, P.V., Brooks, B.R., O'Donnell, P. *et al.* (1986) Structural brain correlates of emotional disorder in multiple sclerosis. *Brain*, 109, 585–97.
14. Caplan, L.R. and Nadelson, T. (1980) Multiple sclerosis and hysteria. *J. Am. Med. Assoc.*, 243, 2418–20.
15. Jouvent, R., Montreuil, M., Benoit, N. *et al.* (1989) Cognitive impairment, emotional disturbances and duration of multiple sclerosis, in *Mental Disorders and Cognitive Deficits in Multiple Sclerosis* (eds K. Jensen, L. Knudsen, E. Stenager and I. Grant), London and Paris, John Libbey.
16. Sadovnick, A.D., Eisen, K., Ebers, G.C. and Paty, D.W. (1991) Cause of death in patients attending multiple sclerosis clinics. *Neurology*, 41, 1193–6.
17. Stenager, E., Knudsen, L. and Jensen, K. (1989) Correlation of Beck depression inventory score, Kurtzke disability status scale, and cognitive functioning in multiple sclerosis, in *Mental Disorders and Cognitive Deficits in Multiple Sclerosis* (eds K. Jensen, L. Knudsen, E. Stenager and I. Grant), London and Paris, John Libbey.
18. Sibley, W.A. (1988) Risk factors in multiple sclerosis – implication for pathogenesis, in *A Multidisciplinary Approach to Myelin Diseases* (ed. G. Serlupi Crescenzi) New York, Plenum Press, pp. 227–32.
19. Sibley, W.A. (1993) Physical trauma and multiple sclerosis (Editorial). *Neurology*, 43, 1871–4.
20. Ridley, A. and Schapira, K. (1961) Influence of surgical procedures on the course of multiple sclerosis. *Neurology*, 11, 81–92.
21. Shealy, C.N. (1974) Transcutaneous electrical stimulation for control of pain. *Clin. Neurosurg.*, 21, 269–77.
22. Panse, F. (1974) Electrical trauma, in *Handbook of Clinical Neurology*, vol. 23, (eds P.J. Vinken and G.W. Bruyn) Amsterdam, North Holland, p. 686.
23. Sibley, W.A. and Paty, D.W. (1981) A comparison of multiple sclerosis in Arizona (USA) and Ontario (Canada). *Acta Neurol. Scand.*, 64 (Suppl. 87), 60–5.
24. Abramsky, O (1994) Pregnancy and multiple sclerosis. *Ann. Neurol.*, 36, S38–S41.
25. Narod, S. Johnson-Lussemburg C.M., Zheng, Q. and Nelson, R. (1985) Viral infections and MS (Letter). *Lancet*, 2, 165.
26. Andersen, O., Lygner, P., Bergstrom, T. *et al.* (1993) Viral infections trigger multiple sclerosis relapses: a prospective seroepidemiological study. *J. Neurol.*, 240, 417–22.
27. Panitch, H.S. (1994) Influence of infection on exacerbations of multiple sclerosis. *Ann. Neurol.*, 36, S25–S28.
28. Sibley, W.A. and Foley, J.M. (1965) Infection and immunity in multiple sclerosis. *Ann. NY Acad. Sci.*, 122, 457–68.
29. Johnson, R.T. (1994) The virology of demyelinating diseases. *Ann. Neurol.*, 36, S54–S60.
30. Nisipeanu, P. and Korczyn, A.D. (1993) Psychological stress as a risk factor for exacerbations in multiple sclerosis. *Neurology*, 43, 1311–12.
31. Pratt, R.T.C. (1951) An investigation of the psychiatric aspects of disseminated sclerosis. *J. Neurol. Neurosurg. Psychiatry*, 14, 326–36.
32. Langworthy, O.R. (1948) Relation of personality problems to onset and progress of multiple sclerosis. *Arch. Neurol. Psychiatry*, 59, 13–28.
33. Philippopoulos, G.S., Wittkower, E.D. and Cousineau, M.A. (1958) The etiologic significance of emotional factors in onset and exacerbations of multiple sclerosis. *Psychosom. Med.*, 20, 458–73.
34. Warren, S., Greenhill, S. and Warren, K.G. (1982) Emotional stress and the development of multiple sclerosis: case-control evidence of a relationship. *J. Chron. Dis.*, 35, 821–31.
35. Grant, I., Brown, G.W., Harris, T. *et al.* (1989) Severely threatening events and marked life difficulties preceding onset or exacerbation of multiple sclerosis. *J. Neurol., Neurosurg. Psychiatry*, 52, 8–13.
36. Franklin, G.M., Nelson, L.M., Heaton, R.K. *et al.* (1988) Stress and its relationship to acute exacerbations in multiple sclerosis. *J. Neurol. Rehab.*, 2, 7–11.
37. Kelly, R. (1985) Clinical aspects of multiple sclerosis, in *Handbook of Clinical Neurology* (ed. J.C. Koetsier), Amsterdam, Elsevier, p. 64.
38. Kurland, L.T. (1994) Trauma and multiple sclerosis. *Ann. Neurol.*, 36, S33–S37.
39. Poser. C. (1987) Trauma and multiple sclerosis. An hypothesis. *J. Neurol.*, 234, 155–9.
40. Jahnke, U., Fischer, E.H. and Alvord, E.C. (1985) Sequence homology between certain viral proteins and proteins related to encephalomyelitis and neuritis. *Science*, 229, 282.
41. Wucherpfennig, K.W. and Strominger, J.L. (1995) Molecular mimicry in T cell-mediated autoimmunity: viral peptides activate human T cell clones specific for myelin basic protein. *Cell*, 80, 695–705.
42. Panitch, H.S., Haley, A.S. and Hirsch, R.L. (1986) A trial of gamma interferon in multiple sclerosis. *Neurology*, 36, 285.

PART TWO

NEUROPATHOLOGY AND ETIOPATHOGENESIS

9 THE NEUROPATHOLOGY OF MULTIPLE SCLEROSIS

Cedric S. Raine

9.1 Introduction

In comparison to a period of relative stagnation of about 100 years following the perceptive clinicopathological analyses of multiple sclerosis of Charcot in the late 1860s and others at the beginning of the twentieth century, the past two decades have seen a veritable explosion of activity in the field, as high resolution morphology, histochemistry, immunology and molecular biology have become established and applied to human central nervous system tissue. Similarly, for the clinical neurologist, the great advances seen in imaging technology (Chapter 3) have provided more precise monitoring of disease progression and have allowed for more meaningful clinicopathological correlation, thus promising advances key to the evaluation of future therapeutic strategies (Chapters 17 and 18).

Multiple sclerosis (MS) is the paradigmatic demyelinating disease. The term 'demyelination', or more precisely 'primary demyelination', has been much abused in the literature. Its definition, underscored by a number of seminal chapters on the subject, concerns the loss of myelin from areas of white matter (central and peripheral) with relative sparing of axons [e.g. 1–6]. 'Relative' sparing because in most MS lesions there is some proclivity for an appreciable percentage of axons to be lost during the early phases of plaque formation and, with time, considerable axonal attrition is not unusual as lesions become established and fibrotic. The above definitive accounts notwithstanding, one can still find the term (albeit with decreasing frequency) applied to conditions in which there is widespread loss of both myelin and axons, namely the hereditary metabolic disorders of myelin (see below). 'Myelinoclasis', a term sometimes applied to the demyelinating diseases and encountered mainly in older texts, is still promulgated by some authors who choose it over the more traditional term 'demyelinating' in order to emphasize the differences between the MS type of disease and the dysmyelinating diseases. However, such emphasis is redundant since the latter group of conditions is entirely different from MS and displays marked axonal pathology. The conditions therefore do not even qualify as demyelinating diseases. The historical nosology of the subject is given in greater detail elsewhere [6].

9.2 Classification

In order to set the stage for the neuropathology of MS, the following perspective is presented in the form of a schema to show how myelin and/or myelination abnormalities have been used to segregate several families of diseases.

9.2.1 DISORDERS OF MYELIN

Group 1 Acquired, inflammatory or infectious demyelinating conditions

Examples: chronic MS; MS variants; acute disseminated encephalomyelitis; acute hemorrhagic leukoencephalopathy; progressive multifocal leukoencephalopathy; and Guillain–Barré syndrome and variants. These conditions typically display primary demyelination, usually developing against a background of inflammation. Many have a suspected or proven viral etiology.

Group 2 Hereditary metabolic disorders of myelin

Examples: (a) metachromatic leukodystrophy; Krabbe's (globoid) leukodystrophy; adrenoleukodystrophy. These examples display massive white matter lesions, often symmetrical, and loss of both myelin and axons, with onset occurring *after* myelin has formed. (b) Pelizaeus–Merzbacher disease; Canavan's disease; Alexander's disease. These conditions also show diffuse involvement of white matter with both axons and myelin affected, but are of the hypomyelinating type in that they have their onset *before* myelination is complete.

Multiple Sclerosis: Clinical and pathogenetic basis. Edited by Cedric S. Raine, Henry F. McFarland and Wallace W. Tourtellotte. Published in 1997 by Chapman & Hall, London. ISBN 0 412 30890 8.

Group 3 Acquired toxic-metabolic disorders of myelin

Examples: central pontine myelinolysis; Machiafava–Bignami disease; vitamin B_{12} deficiency. Each of these diseases has an unusual or unique lesion topography and is associated either with electrolyte imbalances or the lack of intrinsic factors.

Group 4 Traumatic disorders of myelin

Examples: compression adjacent to a tumor; trauma.

The above four groups are unified by the common incidence of large areas of myelin loss such as would show up in any routine myelin-stained preparation (Luxol fast-blue; Heidenhain, Kultschitzky etc.). However, only those diseases listed under the first group (the acquired, inflammatory or infectious conditions) constitute the true demyelinating disorders. As stated above, Groups 2, 3 and 4 display, in addition to myelin depletion, massive loss of axons. The demyelinating diseases proper (Group 1) can be further subdivided as shown below.

9.2.2 ACQUIRED DEMYELINATING DISEASES

- **Central nervous system (CNS)**

1. Chronic MS
2. Variants of MS
   Acute MS (Marburg type)
   Neuromyelitis optica (Devic's)
   Concentric sclerosis (Balo's)
3. Acute disseminated encephalomyelitis
   Post-infectious encephalomyelitis
   Post-vaccination encephalomyelitis
   Post-immunization encephalomyelitis
4. Acute hemorrhagic leukoencephalopathy
5. Progressive multifocal leukoencephalopathy

- **Peripheral nervous system (PNS)**

6. Idiopathic polyneuritis
7. Diphtheric neuropathy

Multiple sclerosis, the archetypical demyelinating disease, is the most prevalent of the group. It has enormous socioeconomic ramifications, afflicting young adults in their prime, with a duration commonly spanning several decades (Chapter 1). In its most encountered forms, MS displays a chronic relapsing-remitting or chronic progressive course although it is not unknown for the disease to manifest itself for a relatively short period and then remit for many years or completely. The so-called variants of MS (Marburg type, Devic's and Balo's) are acute, much rarer and usually characterized by a more severe fulminant course of shorter duration, often with an early, fatal outcome. Diagnosis of the latter is often difficult in life and confirmed only at autopsy. The varied clinical picture of MS is presented elsewhere in this volume (Chapter 1). Suffice it to say at this juncture that MS is probably a collection of diseases of varied etiology (probably infectious) but sharing the same lesion, the demyelinated plaque, a lesion with a common inflammatory (immune-mediated) pathogenesis.

9.3 The battlefield – white matter

9.3.1 MYELIN

White matter is white because it is made up of millions of nerve fibers, each of which is insulated and separated from its neighbors by multiple lengths (internodes) of a lipid (fat)-rich membrane, myelin. Each myelin sheath is formed from layers of compacted cell membrane (myelin) unusually high in lipids (70% lipid, 30% protein) that serve to isolate the axon functionally and expedite impulses along its length by saltatory conduction [7]. The cell responsible for the elaboration and maintenance of myelin in the CNS is the oligodendrocyte, and in the peripheral nervous system its counterpart is the Schwann cell. In normal white matter myelin is the major structural component and accounts for about 25% of the dry weight of the brain. Each myelin sheath is elaborated around a segment of axon by the flattening and spiral wrapping of a single cell process from an oligodendrocyte. This forms an internode of myelin and each end is demarcated by a node of Ranvier. The onset and cessation of myelination are believed to be orchestrated by neuronal signals [8].

Myelin possesses a number of unique constituents which are potent and unique antigens. The possession of such antigens – e.g. myelin basic protein (MBP), proteolipid protein (PLP) – renders the CNS potentially vulnerable to autoimmune-mediated processes. For example, there is the distinct possibility that whenever the blood–brain barrier is breached (e.g. by trauma), its so-called immunologic privilege might be compromised and cells of the immune system might enter, fail to recognize as self certain constitutive components of the CNS (from which they have been previously sequestered) and mount an immunologic attack. The ability of the investigator to induce in animals a pattern of myelin pathology similar to that observed in MS by sensitization against a number of myelin antigens or fragments thereof (or by the intravenous transfer of syngeneic lymphocytes activated by the same antigens or their encephalitogenic epitopes), has led to suggestions that in its complex montage, MS may have an autoimmune component (Chapter 15). However, the nature of the putative antigen(s) in MS remains to be elucidated and whether autoimmunity is involved is still highly controversial.

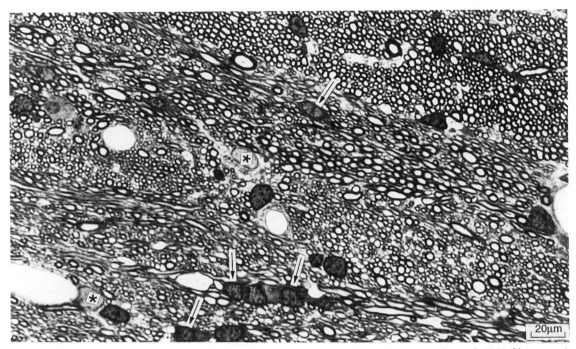

Figure 9.1 Normal white matter from a paraventricular region of a rat brain shows myelinated CNS fibers cut in various planes. Note the densely staining, rounded interfascicular oligodendrocytes (*arrows*), sometimes arranged in rows (*below*), and the occasional astrocyte (*). The blood vessels appear as clear empty spaces and display no perivascular cellularity. (Toluidine-blue stained; 1 μm epoxy section.)

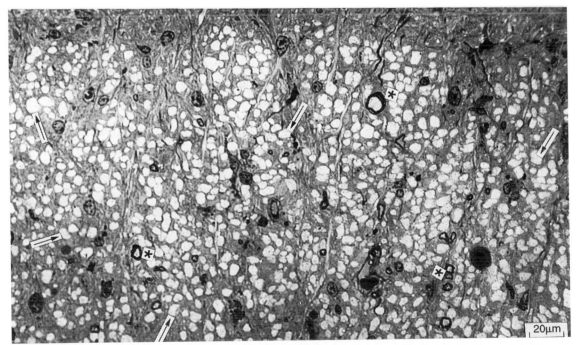

Figure 9.2 Demyelinated spinal cord white matter from a chronic MS plaque for comparison with Figure 9.1. Note the spared, naked axons (*arrows*) and the fibrous astrogliotic matrix of the plaque. An occasional preserved myelin sheath(*) is present but no surviving oligodendrocytes are in evidence.

9.3.2 GLIAL CELLS

Aligned often in rows among bundles of myelinated axons are interfascicular oligodendrocytes, the cells responsible for CNS myelination (Figure 9.1). Oligodendrocytes are heavily outnumbered by the myelin sheaths they produce, and it has been estimated that each is capable of elaborating and maintaining between 30 and 50 internodes (segments). This 1:30 to 1:50 ratio means that throughout its lifespan, the oligodendrocyte must make and support 1000–3000 times its own cell membrane at considerable distances from the cell soma [9]. Most myelin-specific molecules also occur in oligodendrocytes, albeit transiently in some cases and in lower concentrations. Thus, the cell body is also a potential target for immunologic attack. The oligodendrocyte does not respond actively (e.g. by mitosis) after injury and frequently degenerates – a key feature in the formation of the MS plaque. Separating and penetrating the bundles of myelinated nerve fibers in the CNS are astrocytes, the second macroglial cell type and the major supporting and structural elements of gray and white matter. Like oligodendrocytes, astrocytes are of ectodermal origin but unlike oligodendrocytes, they respond readily to injury by proliferating and synthesizing glial fibrils. This fibrillary astrogliosis leads to a state of sclerosis (scarring), a major hallmark of the MS plaque. Astrocytes in gray matter (so-called protoplasmic astrocytes) and white matter (fibrous astrocytes) closely surround the perivascular space (forming a *glia limitans*) and provide a second barrier (after the endothelial cell layer of the blood vessel) to molecules passing from the bloodstream or meninges into the CNS parenchyma. Completing the components that make up white matter are microglia, the resident macrophages of the CNS which are of mesodermal (hematogenous) origin, ciliated ependymal cells lining the ventricles, and blood vessels. The manner in which these structural components (oligodendrocytes, astrocytes, microglia and blood vessels) interact with the cells of the immune system heavily influences the pathogenesis of the demyelinated lesion, which characteristically is ultimately reduced to scar tissue containing bundles of naked axons (Figure 9.2).

9.4 Multiple sclerosis lesions

9.4.1. HISTORY

Multiple sclerosis has been estimated to account for 1 in every 1000 adult deaths around the world. While it may have been described as early as 1433 in a 53-year-old woman [10], the first seriously considered, reported case involved a grandson of George III whose clinical manifestations began in 1822 with a bout of optic neuritis which was the beginning of a 25-year clinical history [11]. Although credit for the first clinical descriptions and accounts of the pathology of spinal cord lesions go separately to Cruveilhier and Carswell in 1835 [6, 11], it was Charcot [12] who provided the first complete clinicopathologic accounts of typical chronic MS – dubbing the condition 'sclérose en plaques' – and who also recognized other forms of MS affecting the spinal cord. The cardinal observations that MS lesions were chronic and inflammatory in nature and were often centered on veins had been noted earlier by Rindfleisch [13], but it was Charcot who identified the white matter problem as being related to selective primary demyelination. Other pioneers who made seminal contributions include Moxon (1875), who was the first to recognize MS as widespread in England, and Hammond (1871), the first to describe MS in the United States – reviewed by Raine [6]. The nosologic origin of 'multiple sclerosis' is difficult to trace except to say that the term was already in use in an article by Schule in 1870 in which the term 'multiple sklerose' is found [6]. Dejong [11], in his review of the history of MS, attributes the first use of the term 'multiple sclerosis' to Hammond in the USA in 1871. For the British school, the preferred terminology until relatively recently was 'disseminated sclerosis'. From the pathogenetic standpoint, in his doctoral thesis in 1916 Dawson [14] provides us with one of the most comprehensive accounts on the pathology of MS and of the thinking on the disease mechanism(s) at the turn of the twentieth century. He places clear emphasis on the perivascular nature of the lesions and postulates their being causally related to autotoxins emanating from the circulation. The reader interested in the early history of MS would be well advised to consult Dawson's treatise.

9.4.2 GROSS PATHOLOGY AND LESION DISTRIBUTION

Classic accounts of the gross pathology of the CNS in MS refer to the disease process as being purely white-matter related with a tendency for lesions to display a predilection for hemispheric paraventricular zones (Figures 9.3–9.7) and subpial areas in the brain stem and spinal cord (Figure 9.8). The proclivity for outwardly extending lesions to follow the course of blood vessels has been long recognized (Figure 9.7), and such finger-like projections of lesions have long been termed 'Dawson's fingers', after Dawson [14] (Figures 9.9, 9.10). The brain weight is usually within the normal range and externally displays no abnormalities except for a mild degree of cortical atrophy on rare occasions. The optic nerves and chiasm frequently display gray (demyelinated) zones, are unusually firm (due to fibrous astrogliosis) and often atrophic. Moving distally, the brain stem might reveal gray islands on the surface of the basis pontis (Figure 9.8), around the IVth ventricle, the cerebellar peduncles and the pial surface of the

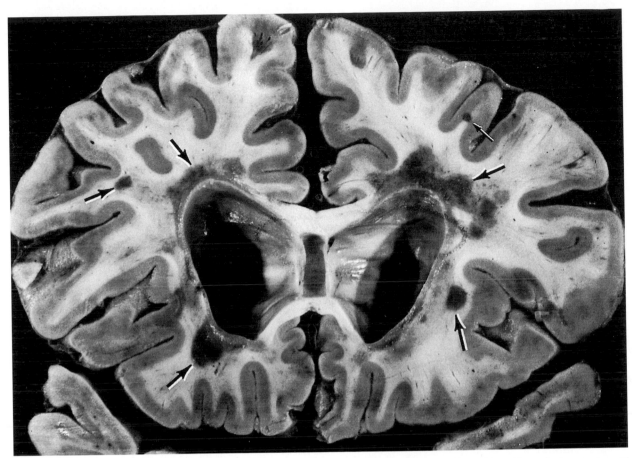

Figure 9.3 Coronal section, chronic MS. The disseminated nature of old, intensely sclerotic, demyelinated plaques is evident (*large arrows*), particularly in periventricular areas. The ventricles are enlarged due to loss of white matter parenchyma and a small lesion at the tip of a gyrus (*small arrow*), spills over into adjacent gray matter.

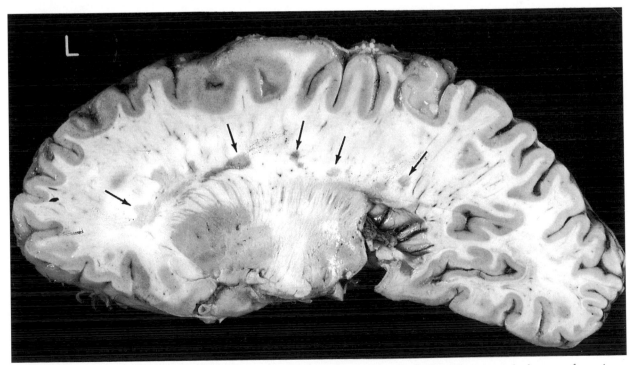

Figure 9.4 A central sagittal section through a cerebral hemisphere shows multiple, disseminated plaques of varying ages (*arrows*) in periventricular locations. (Courtesy of Professor C.W.M. Adams.)

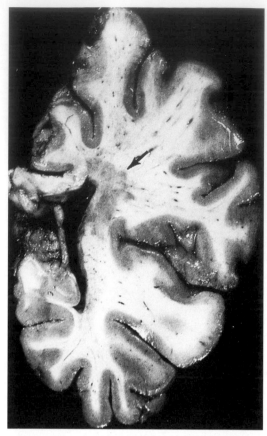

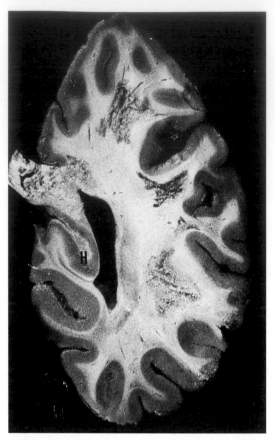

Figure 9.5 A coronal section through a single hemisphere in the region of ventricular trigone shows a single large demyelinated plaque (*arrow*) at the angle of the lateral ventricle. Note that the lesion is less chronic than those in Figure 9.3 and the irregular margins may be formed by the coalescence of smaller lesions.

Figure 9.6 A hemispheric section more rostral to Figure 9.8 (note the posterior hippocampus at **H**), from another case of chronic MS, contains several large white matter plaques which show cystic degeneration.

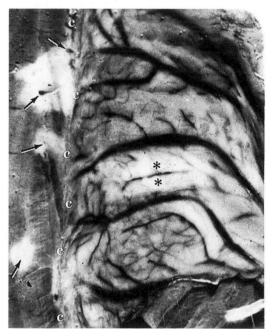

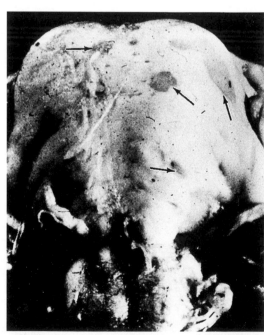

Figure 9.7 A gross specimen shows the surface of the lateral ventricle with its parallel veins extending away from the paraventricular white matter which is sectioned perpendicularly, the cut edge indicated by (**c**). In the cut surface of the paraventricular white matter, sleeves of demyelination appear to follow the course of subependymal venules (*arrows*). Note also the myelin pallor (*) flanking some of the parallel veins on the ventricle wall. (Nile blue staining.) (Courtesy of Professor C.W.M. Adams.)

Figure 9.8 A gross specimen from the inverted pons of a case of chronic MS. Note the multiple small gray, demyelinated plaques (*arrows*) which have broken through the surface from deeper areas.

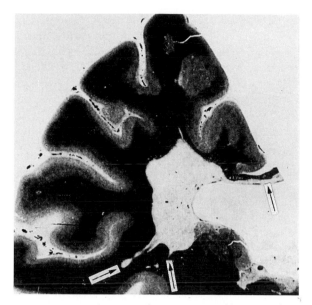

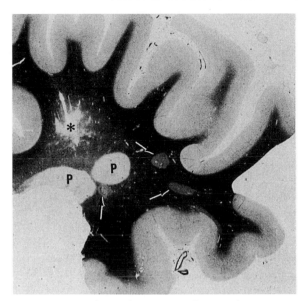

Figure 9.9   A myelin-stained preparation depicts a chronic silent periventricular plaque from which radiate several Dawson's fingers (*arrows, left*) – sleeves of demyelination which follow blood vessels. The plaque also extends periventricularly along the corpus callosum (*arrow, right*).

Figure 9.10   Two deep white matter chronic plaques (**P**) and several shadow plaques (*arrows*) are seen in this Luxol fast blue-stained section. An evolving chronic lesion (*) with an irregular margin and several Dawson's fingers is also seen. (Reproduced from Adams, 1989 [5], with permission.)

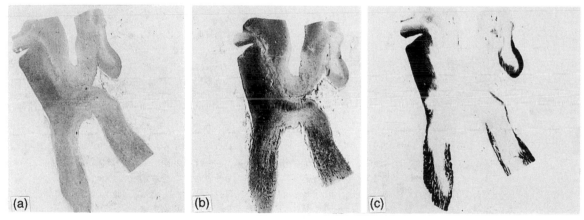

Figure 9.11   A series of paraffin sections across the optic chiasm shows: (a) the general histology (H & E); (b) axonal sparing (Bodian); (c) widespread loss of myelin (Heidenhain).

medulla oblongata. These are lesions that have either arisen in superficial areas or have broken through from deeper levels. The spinal cord, like the optic nerves, can be severely atrophic, displaying disseminated depressed demyelinated superficial plaques along its entire length. No predilection for any particular level or tract is apparent. One technique used by the author in the localization of lesions in the undissected spinal cord is to run a gloved finger gently along its length – plaques can often be detected by their firmer texture and they will feel like small knots. Proximal regions of cranial nerves and spinal nerve roots are sometimes atrophic, an alteration usually attributed to the loss of CNS myelin in

such areas or to the proximity of lesions in the CNS proper. Macroscopically, the PNS appears normal.

Dissection of the brain reveals in coronal section large demyelinated lesions (plaques), varying in appearance and texture depending upon age and activity (Figure 9.3). Plaques also differ in size, shape, number and topography. Pink soft plaques indicate recent activity (acute or active lesions), while older lesions are gray, somewhat translucent (hyaline, glassy), gelatinous and firm. Chronic lesions are difficult to slice thinly since they possess the consistency of soft rubber and shrink away from the adjacent normal white matter upon contact with air. Recently active chronic plaques may display whitish rings or margins – zones which are seen by microscopy to comprise large populations of lipid-laden macrophages. Even in patients succumbing after relatively short clinical histories (3–5 years), lesions in the spinal cord and optic nerve are almost invariably older, firmer and more brittle than hemispheric lesions. Optic nerve chiasm and tract lesions can be deep or superficially located, focal or widespread and might traverse the entire nerve for considerable lengths (Figure 9.11). Visual system white matter lesions usually correlate well with clinical history although a few anecdotal reports do exist to the contrary.

Within the cerebral hemispheres, white matter lesions vary from less than one millimeter to several centimeters in diameter and display a tendency to coalesce and arborize via Dawson's fingers (Figures 9.9 and 9.10). The location of plaques usually defies clinical and anatomical correlation, and prior to the days of magnetic resonance imaging (MRI) (Chapter 3) the degree of involvement revealed at autopsy exceeded by far that which might have been predicted by the clinical history. There are also numerous reports indicating autopsy diagnosis of MS in the total absence of a previous clinical history (benign MS). Although the entire central neuraxis appears to be equally vulnerable, the heaviest concentration of changes is almost invariably in paraventricular locations but no pattern is pathognomonic. Indeed, what is typical of MS is the complete unpredictability of plaque topography and the massive extent to which central white matter can be involved in a totally disseminated fashion. One commonly involved area is the angle between the caudate nucleus and the corpus callosum – the so-called 'Wetterwinkel' zone or 'storm center' of Steiner [15] (Figures

9.3, 9.5, and 9.9). Discrete white matter lesions at gray/white matter junctional areas often spill over into adjacent gray matter parenchyma since such areas of gray matter also contain myelinated fibers, e.g. at the tips of gyri (Figure 9.3). All brain white matter regions are vulnerable to attack – striatum, pallidum, thalamus, around the IIIrd ventricle (Figure 9.12), the cerebral peduncles, folia and deeper regions, and the roof and floor of the IVth ventricle. On occasion, old white

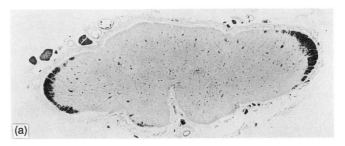

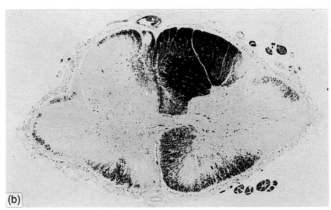

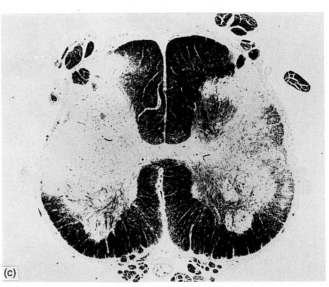

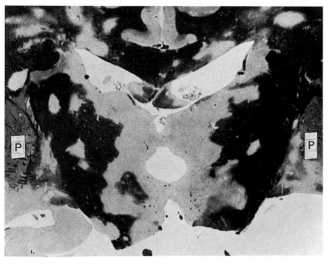

Figure 9.12   Note the symmetrical, extensive involvement of white matter around the IIIrd ventricle at the level of the mass intermedia. Scattered old plaques are seen throughout in this Luxol fast blue-stained preparation. The putamen (P) lies to the left and right.

Figure 9.13   Three different levels of spinal cord from a case of chronic MS demonstrate variation in degree of involvement. Note the almost total loss of myelin in (a) (cervical), where axons are well preserved, the asymmetrical, large lesions in (b) (midthoracic) and the disseminated involvement in (c) (lumbar). (Heidenhain stain.)

matter lesions can display cystic changes [6], a feature presumed to be the result of earlier, highly inflammatory, activity having led to parenchymal necrosis (Figure 9.6).

The brain stem is another commonly affected region, with lesions developing around the aqueduct of Sylvius and the periphery of the basis pontis. Well-defined plaques often extend down into the medulla and upper cervical cord. Brain stem lesions sometimes correlate with recent clinical events like coma or respiratory failure. Spinal cord lesions show no regularity in distribution and display total disregard for anatomical and functional boundaries. It is not unusual to find one level (frequently cervical) completely devoid of myelin and atrophic in transverse section and other, more distal, levels uninvolved or involved incompletely, with patchy, disseminated lesions criss-crossing sensory and motor, ascending and descending tracts (Figure 9.13). In the vast majority of cases there is spinal cord involvement, and for a complete diagnosis the neuropathologist should sample the spinal cord. Many a report on

equivocal cases of MS would probably have been more definitive had spinal cord been sampled. It is generally accepted that optic nerve and spinal cord lesions frequently occur concomitantly. According to the literature, both optic nerve and spinal cord lesions can sometimes be traced initially to changes around the pial vasculature. While a subpial distribution is the common pattern in animal models (Chapter 15), this pattern is not typical in MS. In most cases, optic nerve and spinal cord lesions usually display the most chronic changes, even in patients with ostensibly short clinical acute histories (weeks to months prior to death).

9.4.3 HISTOPATHOLOGY OF THE MS PLAQUE

Incredible though it may seem, relatively little new (emphasis on 'new') has been added to the list of histologic features characterizing the MS plaque from other types of white matter pathology since the seminal works of Charcot and Dawson. Based largely on the extent of scarring and inflammatory activity, MS

Table 9.1 Anatomical distribution and % frequency of MS plaques[a]

Anatomical site	No.	%	Anatomical site	No.	%
Cerebral cortex	37/168	22.0	Pons, tegmentum	56/104	53.8
Subcortical WM	77/168	45.8	Pons, decussation	56/104	53.8
Central WM	145/168	86.3	Inferior cerebellar peduncle	10/29	34.5
Frontal lobe	77/168	45.8	Medulla		
Parietal lobe	60/168	35.7	Dorsal nuclei	28/92	30.4
Temporal lobe	65/168	38.7	Reticular	33/92	35.9
Occipital lobe	17/168	10.1	Olives	22/92	23.9
Periventricular			Pyramids	12/92	13.0
IIIrd	14/126	11.1	Cerebellum		
Lateral	98/126	77.7	Cortex	1/102	1.0
Corpus callosum	20/36	55.6	Dentate nucleus	2/102	2.0
Hippocampus	8/37	21.6	Digital WM	8/102	7.8
Caudate nucleus	6/63	9.5	Central WM	31/102	30.4
Thalamus	10/63	15.9	Optic nerve[b]	11/20	55.0
Putamen	6/63	9.5	Optic chiasm	7/20	35.0
Globus pallidus	8/63	12.7	Optic tract	4/17	21.0
Internal capsule	16/63	25.4	Spinal cord[c]	35/59	59.3
Fornix	2/41	4.9	Lateral column	30/59	50.8
Hypothalamus	3/46	6.5	Ventral column	11/59	18.5
Insula/claustrum	4/26	15.4	Gray	2/59	3.4
Tectum	16/34	47.1	Cord thoracic, post. column	17/59	28.8
Tegmentum	16/34	47.1	Lateral column	16/59	27.1
Periaqueductal	19/34	55.9	Ventral column	6/59	10.2
Red nucleus	10/34	29.4	Gray	2/59	3.4
Substantia nigra	10/34	29.4	Cord lumbar, post. column	5/59	8.5
Basis pedunculi	12/34	35.3	Lateral column	5/59	8.5
Brachium pontis	50/104	48.1	Ventral column	5/59	8.5
Periventricular IVth	56/104	53.8	Gray	1/59	1.7

[a] Based on a study by C.W.M. Adams (unpublished) of 2138 plaques in about 2850 sections taken from 180 cases of MS.

[b] Total optic pathology = 14/25 (56.0%).

[c] Total spinal cord = 48/59 (81.4%).

plaques fall into four broad categories – chronic, chronic active, acute/recent and shadow plaques. The types are arranged in this sequence based upon the frequency with which they are encountered at autopsy. It is possible that as other, more molecular, criteria are incorporated into our determination of the age of lesions (e.g. cytokines, adhesion molecules, lymphocyte subsets, T cell receptors etc.), this traditional morphologic categorization might have to be amended (see Cannella and Raine [16]).

The chronic MS plaque

Supporting the old adage that the diagnosis of MS depends upon the existence of lesions separated in time and space, chronic MS lesions are the most common type encountered at autopsy and they usually occur at multiple levels of the neuraxis (see Table 9.1). Myelin staining will reveal them as areas of white matter devoid of myelin and demarcated from adjacent myelinated parenchyma by a sharp edge, imparting upon the lesion a punched-out appearance (Figures 9.9, 9.10 and 9.12). Staining of parallel sections for glial fibrils (Holzer) will show that the areas of myelin depletion correspond to areas of intense fibrillary astrogliosis (Figure 9.14) and

indeed, the majority of the demyelinated plaque parenchyma is replaced by a network of astroglial scar tissue. Axon stains (e.g. the Palmgren or Bodian silver methods), will reveal a moderate decrease in the number of axons at the periphery of the lesion while deeper regions will be more depleted. Microdensitometric estimation of lesions of different ages [5] showed an approximate 68% loss of staining for myelin lipids in both acute (n = 4) and chronic (n = 12) plaques, whereas axonal staining was reduced by 7% in acute plaques but by 48% in chronic plaques. A small amount of Wallerian degeneration and a few axonal spheroids are occasionally seen at lesion edges. Long-term demyelinated axons display a marked decrease in axonal diameter [6].

Astrocytes display a robust, proliferative and hypertrophic response during the active stages of lesion formation (see below), but by the time the chronic plaque has developed, the cells are well separated, rigid-appearing, enlarged, full of GFAP+ fibrils, often multinucleated, display increased oxidative and hydrolytic enzyme activity by histochemistry, and sharply demarcate the lesion area from normal white matter (Figure 9.15). About the rim of the chronic lesion (which almost invariably displays some smoldering activity), astrocytes are frequently reactive and display evidence of prolifera-

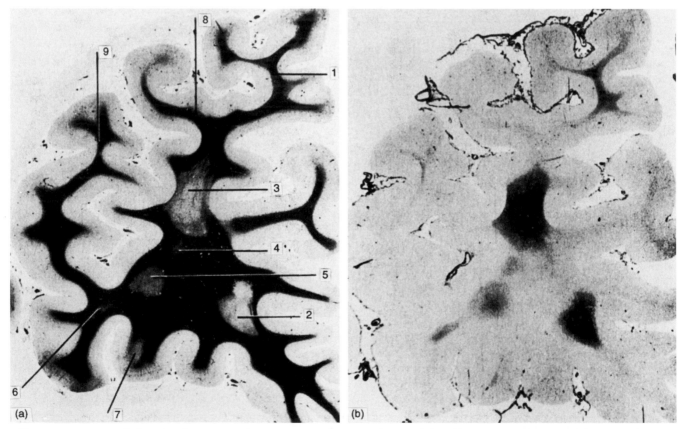

Figure 9.14 Several chronic plaques are shown in a myelin-stained (Luxol fast blue) preparation (a) and in an adjacent gliofibril-stained (Holzer) preparation (b). Note the different degrees of demyelination in (a) evidenced by the variation in fibrillary gliosis (b).

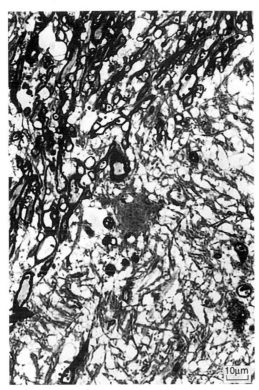

Figure 9.15 The edge of a chronic lesion shows the abrupt change from the fibrous astrogliotic plaque (*right*) to the adjacent myelinated white matter (*left*). A hypertrophic astrocyte is seen in the center. (Toluidine blue-stained; 1 μm epoxy section.)

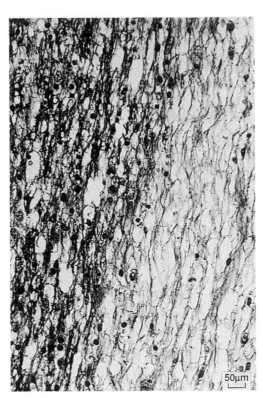

Figure 9.16 Isomorphic gliosis is seen at the margin of a chronic, burnt-out plaque. Note the sharp edge to the lesion and the apparently normal adjacent white matter (*left*). (Phosphotungstic acid-hematoxylin) (Reproduced from Adams, 1989 [5], with permission.)

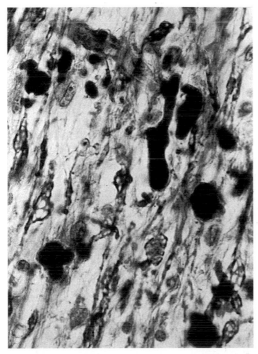

Figure 9.17 Rosenthal fibers are shown at the margin of a chronic plaque. (Heidenhain stain) (Reproduced from Adams, 1989 [5], with permission.)

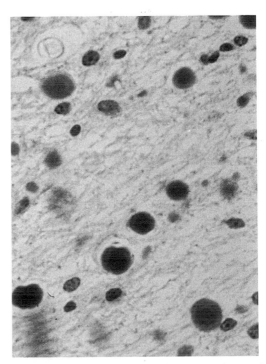

Figure 9.18 Corpora amylacea are shown in a chronic lesion. (Phosphotungstic acid-hematoxylin.) (Reproduced from Adams, 1989 [5], with permission.)

tion. This is in agreement with observations from acute lesions that show the astrocyte to be one of the first CNS elements to respond and it does so by proliferating and undergoing hypertrophy. In the most chronically demyelinated plaques, fibrous astrogliosis is intense, with glial processes forming parallel rows, a phenomenon known in the older literature as 'isomorphic gliosis' (Figure 9.16). Astrocyte degeneration is not a feature of the MS lesion. Some chronic lesions may display the formation of Rosenthal fibers (Figure 9.17) and around the perimeter of old lesions, particularly within the spinal cord, corpora amylacea produced by fibrous astrocytes (a nonspecific consequence of aging and gliosis), occur in high numbers (Figure 9.18).

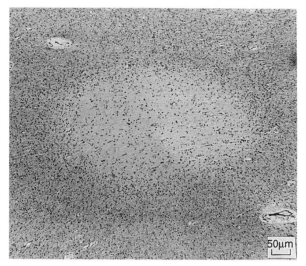

Figure 9.19 An H&E stained section shows a pale-staining small, rounded chronic plaque around the margin of which a zone of oligodendroglial hyperplasia is apparent.

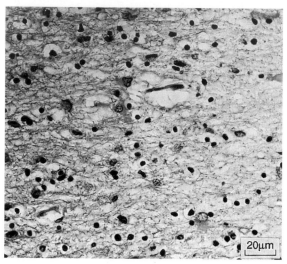

Figure 9.20 The same lesion at higher magnification to show the hypercellular margin. The small, rounded nuclei are typical of oligodendroglial cells.

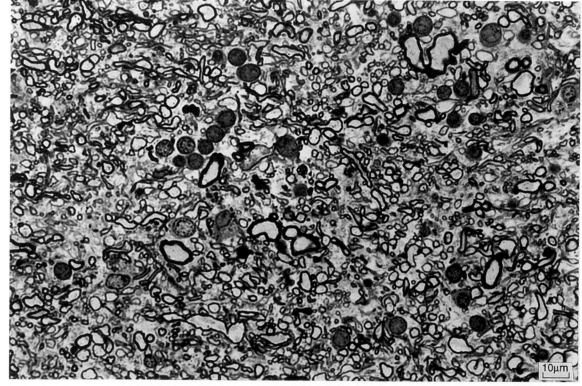

Figure 9.21 At the perimeter of a chronic plaque, the white matter contains an unusually large number of oligodendrocytes (small rounded cells with narrow rims of cytoplasm) among many thinly myelinated (remyelinated) CNS nerve fibers. (Toluidine blue-stained; 1 μm epoxy section.

Oligodendrocyte depletion is readily apparent throughout the center of the chronic MS plaque. However, it is not unusual to find a rim of proliferated oligodendrocytes around the lesion edge (Figures 9.19 and 9.20), sometimes in association with CNS remyelination (Figure 9.21). These topics are discussed in more detail in Chapter 15.

Some evidence of inflammatory activity is a common finding, albeit at a low grade and affecting a few vessels only, even in silent-appearing MS lesions (Figure 9.22). Such activity comprises a few small lymphocytes, numerous plasma cells, large mononuclear cells and the occasional mast cell. Polymorphonuclear leukocytes have never been described in MS lesions. Sometimes, inflammatory activity in old lesions can be correlated with ante-mortem systemic infection. Residual macrophage activity is not an uncommon finding in the chronic MS lesion, particularly towards the lesion margin where smoldering demyelination can sometimes be encountered (Figure 9.23), but concentrations of cells laden with myelin debris and oil-red-O positive lipid, indicative of recent demyelinative activity, are rare to absent. Foamy macrophages containing neutral lipid droplets may be scattered randomly throughout the lesion and adjacent white matter, or may occur in small clusters around blood vessels (Figure 9.24). Typical rod-shaped microglia (the resident macrophage of the CNS, of mesodermal origin) are relatively rare within the lesion proper. It is widely held that many of the rounded, foamy macrophages in the chronic lesion are

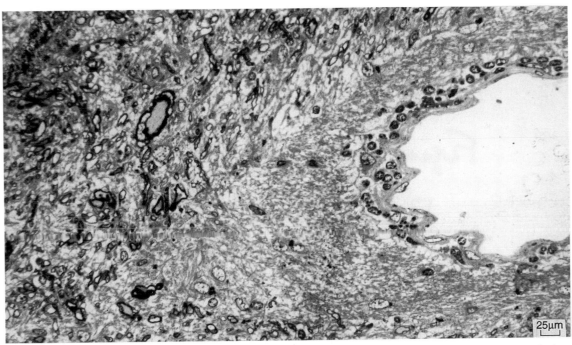

Figure 9.22 At the edge of a chronic plaque, a venule displays some inflammatory activity (probably recent) and a broad sleeve of fibrous astrogliosis – evidence of more chronic activity. (Toluidine blue-stained, 1 μm epoxy section.)

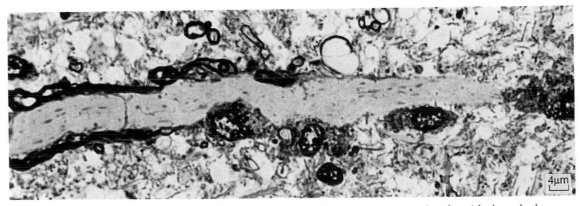

Figure 9.23 A myelinated nerve fiber enters a chronic MS plaque and is seen to lose its sheath, with the naked segment (*right*) flanked by macrophages. (Toluidine blue-stained; 1 μm epoxy section.)

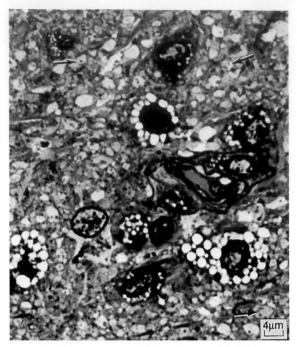

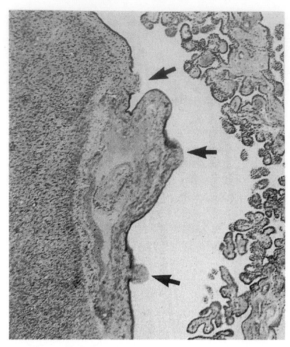

Figure 9.24 Within the center of a chronically demyelinated spinal cord plaque, foamy macrophages (probably reactive microglia) are seen near a small blood vessel. Note the many demyelinated axons (*arrows*). (Toluidine blue-stained; 1 µm epoxy section.)

Figure 9.25 Along the wall of a lateral ventricle in a case of chronic MS, granular ependymitis is apparent by virtue of the focal areas of deficient ependyma and their replacement by glial nodules (*arrows*). (Van Gieson) (Reproduced from Adams, 1989[5] with permission.)

derived from ramified microglia. However, what percentage of the foamy macrophages derive from cells of recent monocytic origin and what percentage might have differentiated from resident microglial cells is an age-old question, insoluble with autopsy tissue. From the examination of many inflammatory lesions and the knowledge that foamy macrophages in MS can persist for months to years within chronic lesions, it is this author's opinion that the foamy macrophage in the MS lesion is derived from a cell of microglial lineage rather than from a 'conventional' monocyte. In cases where infiltrating monocytes are known to be involved in CNS damage (e.g. during trauma or in experimental situations in animals), monocytes enter the CNS, become engaged in phagocytosis and then leave the tissue within days to weeks. This is not the case with foamy macrophages in chronic MS, where such cells persist for indefinite periods.

In some chronic MS lesions which encroach upon the ventricular system, there is some ventricular dilatation (related sometimes to hydrocephalus *ex vacuo*, occurring secondarily to loss of white matter parenchyma; Figure 9.3), which in turn may be associated with a granular ependymitis[17] (Figure 9.25). This has been claimed to lead to attenuation of the ependymal lining resulting in discontinuities which might be repaired locally by accumulations of fibrous astroglial cells and their processes. Whether such microanatomical impedi-

ments might contribute to the abnormal CNS permeability in MS is yet to be proven.

Another change common to the chronic MS plaque relates to the walls of small veins which can display extensive deposition of collagen, some duplication of basement membrane material and a few macrophages within an enlarged Virchow–Robin space, particularly within deeper lesions. These features are consistent with widespread persistent damage to the blood–brain barrier in chronic MS[18, 19]. Sometimes veins display perivascular sleeves of glial scarring, probably the result of previous inflammation (Figure 9.22). While the immunopathology of the vascular lesion in MS is well covered in Chapter 10, the histologic findings point collectively to increased vascular permeability as a major precipitating feature of the developing, growing and established MS lesion, a feature supported by MRI patterns with gadolinium enhancement (Chapter 3). Like the age-old debate on the origin of microglial cell, the role of blood vessels in the pathogenesis of the MS plaque (more of an issue in acute MS, see below) has also been the basis of much speculation. That the vascular change may be the primary lesion *per se* (e.g. due to a nonspecific focal inflammatory venulitis resulting in damage to the vessel wall), is unlikely. The latter statement is based on evidence from studies from many disciplines (namely epidemiologic, immunologic, genetic, pathologic, virologic), but it does address an issue regularly reincarnated in the literature. More acceptable to most workers is the concept that in genetically predisposed individuals, periodic fluctuations in the circulating immune system (e.g. changes in the levels of different phenotypic subpopulations of lymphocytes and/or their soluble products, cytokines), lead to increased permeability of previously damaged and undamaged vessels which renders them accessible to waves of inflammatory activity. This, in turn, leads to the selective perivascular white matter pathology. One presumes that since the vascular damage is confined to white matter, some degree of CNS specificity must be attributed to the inflammation. However, attempts to demonstrate, for example, specific reactivity to CNS myelin antigens by the cells of the perivascular infiltrates and their by-products have thus far been unsuccessful, but remain an area of intense research.

Most speculations in this area have derived from the well-established, myelin-specific, T cell-mediated laboratory model for MS, experimental allergic encephalomyelitis (EAE), and extrapolations to MS should be interpreted with caution (Chapter 15). Interestingly, even in EAE where etiology is known, only a very small percentage of the CNS infiltrating cells (about 1–3%) are reactive to the disease-inducing antigen, MBP[20, 21]. This probably means that the vast majority of the infiltrating cells in inflammatory demyelinating lesions are non-CNS antigen specific and that the selective myelin damage is most likely related to a cascade of events associated with non-CNS specific cells and their soluble mediators, rather than to any cell or factor specifically anti-myelinic in nature. Finally, in favor of perivascular inflammation in MS being pathogenetically significant are the many other instances in neuropathology in which extensive perivascular infiltration occurs but in which there is little or no accompanying effect upon adjacent myelinated white matter (e.g. herpes simplex encephalitis). Perhaps in addition to antigen- or cytokine-related specificities, future studies on the inflammatory cells will have to take into consideration T cell receptor usage, currently a controversial subject in the analysis of the neuroimmunology of MS[22] (Chapter 13).

The chronic active MS plaque

This lesion is histologically midway between the established chronic plaque (see above) and the acute or recent MS lesion (see below). The fine structural aspects of chronic active plaques are covered in Chapter 15. The major features distinguishing this type of lesion from silent lesions is the superimposition of a prominent inflammatory component upon a previously demyelinated, fibrous astrogliotic plaque (Figure 9.26). In addition, there is astroglial hypertrophy, oligodendrocyte hyperplasia and ongoing demyelination, evi-

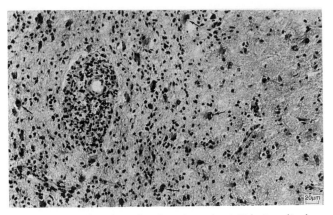

Figure 9.26   The edge of a chronic active MS lesion displays extensive perivascular and parenchymal infiltration by hematogenous cells. Hypertrophic astrocytes (*arrows*) are common. The lesion center is to the left and the margin of the plaque abuts gray matter (*right*). (H&E stain.)

denced histologically by Marchi or oil-red-O positive debris in macrophages and immunocytochemically by widespread class II MHC reactivity[23]. Perivascular cuffing is seen around previously involved and uninvolved venules and the lesion edge is relatively sharp. This type of lesion differs from the smaller, acute MS lesion by lacking an indistinct margin and being less edematous. Lipid-laden macrophages occur in great numbers, sometimes visible grossly as concentric white rings or layers around vessels or along the lesion edge. The plaque margin is broad and markedly hypercellular due to parenchymal infiltrates, oligodendroglial hyperplasia, hypertrophic astrocytes and abundant macrophages. The center of the plaque can be identical to that of the chronic silent plaque but sometimes, in the case of smaller lesions, the entire lesion might be infiltrated and only distinguishable from acute lesions by prominent fibrillary gliosis.

Chronic active lesions frequently correlate with a history of chronic progressive MS of short duration (5–10 years) and a downhill course. On occasion, when they affect clinically strategic sites (e.g. brain stem), such lesions can be matched with recent symptoms. Correlation between lesion activity and MRI-detected activity has been presented[24] and it is worth repeating that the most striking features of these lesions were recent inflammatory infiltrates, ongoing myelin degradation, oligodendroglial survival and increase in number, remyelination and hypertrophic astrocytes[25, 26]. One interesting, recent development arising from the study of chronic active MS lesions emerged from a report by Selmaj *et al.* in 1991[27] which showed that the centers of chronic active lesions sometimes contained an unusual population of T cells bearing γδ T cell receptors (TCR), as opposed to the more commonly encountered T cells bearing αβ chains. TCRγδ T cells are as yet of unknown function, are usually CD4⁻C8⁻ and are believed by some to be cytolytic. These T cells are known to be stimulated by families of proteins expressed by cells under stress, generically termed heat shock proteins (HSP). In keeping with this dogma and of potential significance to our understanding of the chronic active MS lesion, was the colocalization of cytoplasmic HSP-65 on proliferated, MBP⁺ immature oligodendrocytes around the edges of chronic lesions containing TCRγδ T cells. It was speculated that this colocalization might be indicative of impending oligodendroglial cell damage. The presence of this hitherto undescribed population of T cells in the center of chronic lesions may be related to the perpetuation of the disease process in MS and the later destruction of oligodendrocytes. It has since been shown that HSP positivity on oligodendrocytes is not a specific feature of MS, being encountered in a wide range of neurodegenerative states, although it is not normally seen in the cytoplasm of oligodendrocytes in normal CNS tissue [28, 29a].

The paradoxical (almost inappropriate) coexistence of myelin destruction and oligodendroglial hyperplasia and remyelination [25], also a feature of the acute MS lesion (see below), appears to underscore a reparatory attempt (albeit abortive) on the part of the CNS in MS in the face of lesion progression. CNS remyelination in MS can usually be found to some degree around lesions of all ages and it occurs extensively around chronic active plaques.

The acute MS lesion

What constitutes an acute MS lesion is an area of controversy among some neuropathologists. Invariably difficult to identify with certainty in the absence of histology and special staining, acute MS lesions in the gross specimen are fresh, pink, indistinct and sometimes punctate. They share a similar topography to chronic MS lesions and tend to be more common in hemispheric sites. Although usually associated with cases of acute MS, acute MS lesions also occur in severe cases of chronic progressive MS. In such cases, lesion activity in previously uninvolved CNS tissue is often identical to the fresh lesion of acute MS.

The margin of the acute lesion is indistinct due to ongoing demyelinative activity (Figure 9.27), and the entire area is frequently infiltrated by perivascular and parenchymal hematogenous cells (Figure 9.28), the immunocytochemical phenotyping of which has been reported elsewhere [29]. Oil-red-O positive, myelin debris-laden and foamy, lipid-laden macrophages occur throughout the lesion (Figure 9.29). The lesion center is highly edematous with an extensive extracellular space (Figure 9.30). Hypertrophic astrocytes are common, many of them associated with proliferated oligo-

dendrocytes (see below). Demyelinated axons are present but somewhat depleted in number. Intense fibrous astrogliosis is not prominent and most astrocytes are hypertrophic, globoid, and display a diffuse positivity for GFAP, rather than the intensely GFAP⁺ twig-like profiles which are a major feature of older lesions. One of the most striking histologic appearances of the acute MS lesion is the intense inflammatory response and the clear association of lesion activity with small venules (Figure 9.27). In the presence of such an intense inflammatory event, it becomes difficult to arrange chronologically the immunologic events with the concomitant myelin damage and CNS response. Suffice it to say that accompanying the breakdown of the blood–brain barrier in these areas there occurs perivenous fibrin deposition, complement deposition, some hemorrhage and disruption and duplication of vessel basement membrane material [5, 30, 31] (Chapter 10). The mechanism of demyelination in MS is covered in Chapter 15 and demonstrates similarities with models of immune-mediated demyelination.

The demyelinated center of the acute MS lesion displays a depletion of axons. Some axonal spheroids can be seen among the hypertrophic astrocytes and foamy macrophages. Around the central zone, there is frequently a broad band of macrophages containing recognizable myelin debris. It is also not unusual to encounter zones of cells with glial cell features but nothing definitive of astrocytes or oligodendrocytes – these may represent an early reparatory event. Along the interphase of the lesion with myelinated white matter, the hypertrophic astrocytes and scattered macrophages containing recognizable myelin debris are prominent features. Remyelination is not a feature of the margin of the acute MS lesion but remyelination (probably abortive) has been described in the center of the acute MS lesion [32, 33].

Hypertrophic astrocytes in MS lesions frequently display associations with oligodendrocytes, particularly common in the centers of acute and chronic active MS lesions [34]. This phenomenon, described originally in MS by Ghatak and colleagues [35, 36] and Prineas *et al.* [37], involves the close apposition and internalization of immunocytochemically and ultrastructurally identifiable oligodendrocytes by hypertrophic astrocytes, a process known as emperipolesis in the immunologic literature (Figures 9.30–9.32). The phenomenon was considered by Ghatak [35] not to be representative of phagocytosis and possibly not specific for MS, while Prineas *et al.* [37] alluded to its being indicative of phagocytosis and unusual to MS. A later study on a large number of lesions from MS and non-MS cases revealed that, in contrast to previous workers who linked the phenomenon to resolving MS lesions, these oligodendrocyte/astrocyte associations were most common in chronic active and acute MS lesions and, more impor-

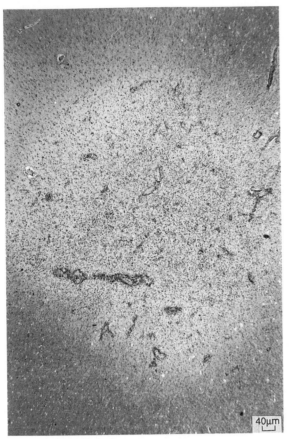

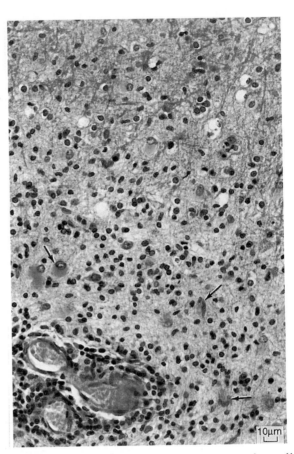

Figure 9.27 An acute MS lesion is shown in an H&E section. Note the indistinct margin and the extensive perivascular and parenchymal infiltration throughout the entire lesion.

Figure 9.28 Detail from Figure 9.27. A perivascular cuff of small mononuclear cells (*lower left*) abuts a lesion area infiltrated by inflammatory cells. Note the edematous nature of the tissue, the many hypertrophic astrocytes (*arrows*) and the adjacent less affected white matter (*above*).

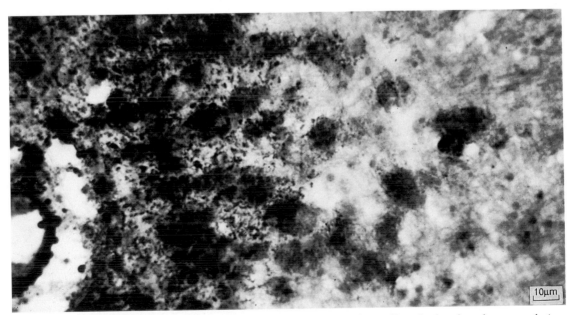

Figure 9.29 Oil-red-O positive macrophages extend away from a perivascular cuff at the border of an acute lesion.

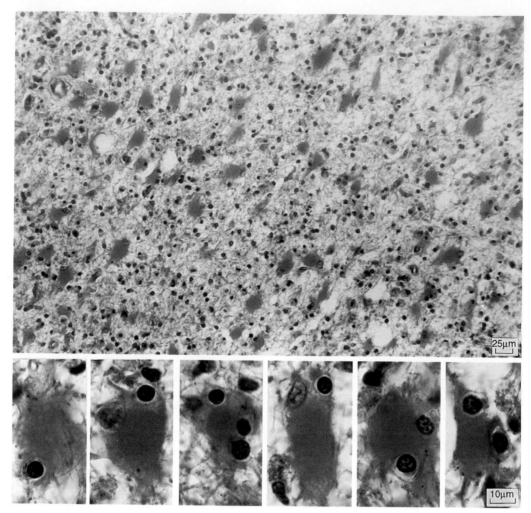

Figure 9.30 The center of an acute MS lesion displays hypertrophic astrocytes amid a background containing small mononuclear cells, many associated with the astrocytes. The six high magnification images below are hypertrophic astrocytes taken from the above field. Note the various interactions of small rounded oligodendrocytes with each astrocyte, from superficial contact to total investment. (H&E stained paraffin section.)

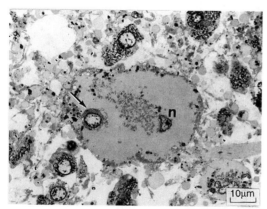

Figure 9.31 An hypertrophic astrocyte (nucleus at **n**) from the center of an acute MS lesion contains an internalized oligodendrocyte (*arrow*). (Toluidine blue stained; 1 μm epoxy section.)

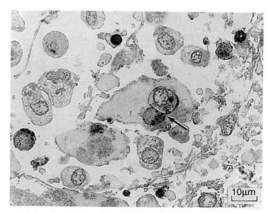

Figure 9.32 A 1 μm epoxy section is double-stained with antibodies against HNK-1 (for oligodendrocytes) and GFAP (for astrocytes). Note the two HNK-1⁺ oligodendrocytes (*arrow*) inside the GFAP⁺ hypertrophic astrocyte in the center of this acute MS lesion. Other HNK-1⁺ oligodendrocytes are present in the surrounding edematous parenchyma. Many unstained foamy macrophages are also seen.

tantly perhaps, they also occurred in a wide variety of etiologically unrelated, non-MS conditions [34]. Interestingly, the glial associations were almost invariably related to areas of inflammation, namely in association with CNS infarcts, adrenoleukodystrophy, globoid leukodystrophy, bacterial and viral encephalitis, AIDS and tumors. The conclusions of the latter study were that as a result of an ongoing inflammatory response, oligodendrocyte proliferation had occurred and that local hypertrophic astrocytes associated with these cells perhaps to protect them from complement- or cytokine-mediated lysis. The phenomenon did not appear to be a phagocytic event since oligodendrocyte necrosis was not apparent (Figures 9.31, 9.32). This postulated protection of oligodendrocytes by hypertrophic astrocytes is probably short term, inasmuch as oligodendrocyte depletion occurs eventually in MS [29a]. It is likely that cytokines produced by the nonspecific inflammatory response in these varied conditions figure prominently in the phenomenon.

The shadow plaque

A lesion unique to MS, the shadow plaque, has had a controversial history since its first description at the beginning of the twentieth century [6]. It is seen most frequently as a diffusely staining pale myelinated area, lying either adjacent to older, demyelinated lesions or in isolated locations, particularly in the spinal cord (Figures 9.33, 9.34). H&E and myelin staining shows it to comprise thinly myelinated fibers – hence the consensus today that such a lesion represents an area of CNS remyelination. Shadow plaques are probably single-hit lesions, regions of CNS white matter that have been afflicted on a single occasion by the disease process and then been left to remyelinate. Earlier descriptions, like those of Alzheimer (1910) and Zimmerman and Netsky (1950) (reviewed by Raine [6]), regarded shadow plaques as lesions in the early stages of development, i.e. incompletely demyelinated. However, the lack of ongoing inflammatory or demyelinative activity and ultra-

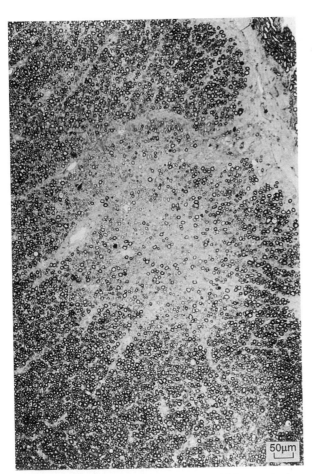

Figure 9.33   A shadow plaque is seen within a spinal cord anterior column. Note the myelin pallor and lack of ongoing disease activity. (Toluidine blue-stained; 1 μm epoxy section.)

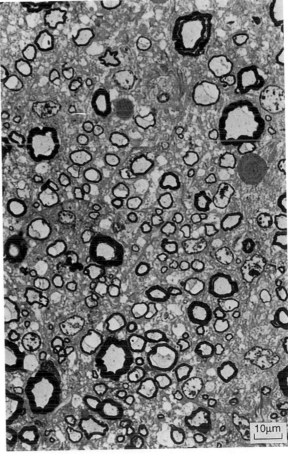

Figure 9.34   Detail from Figure 9.33. Note how many nerve fibers have disproportionately thin myelin sheaths, a morphologic hallmark of remyelination. Mild background gliosis and a few corpora amylacea are also apparent.

structural features of remyelination cause most modern neuropathologists to regard them as areas of repair.

9.5   Conclusions

The above brief account emphasizes the more classical aspects of the neuropathology of MS, other aspects being covered in Chapters 10 and 15, and is intended to provide the reader with an updated, broad overview of the major macro- and microscopical features of the condition. It is not difficult to distinguish the unique features of the MS lesion inasmuch as no other condition displays such a degree of selectivity for CNS myelin, while at the same time sparing previously invested axons. When interpreted against the histologic picture being centered on the CNS vasculature and the observation that lesion enlargement occurs in the presence of recent infiltrates of hematogenous cells, the involvement in MS lesion pathogenesis of a specific immunologic response (against as yet unidentified antigens), is difficult to discount. However, conclusive proof of this still escapes the investigator although immunogenetic and neuroimmunologic findings continue to support the concept. Thus, the analysis of the cells and molecules of the immune system present (and perhaps involved) in the MS plaque continue to provide a major focus of research. Should these research avenues lead to the understanding of the progressive destruction of myelin in MS, the therapeutic implications will be enormous, to say the least.

ACKNOWLEDGMENTS

The author thanks his many colleagues at the Albert Einstein College of Medicine, Bronx, NY, for their advice and collaboration over the years; in particular, Drs Robert D. Terry, Celia F. Brosnan, Krzysztof Selmaj, Herbert H. Schaumburg, Dennis W. Dickson, Anne H. Cross, Barbara Cannella, G.R. Wayne Moore, Dikran S. Horoupian and the late Murray B. Bornstein. Close collaboration with colleagues at NIH (Drs Henry McFarland, David Katz and the late Dale E. McFarlin) is also acknowledged. The technical assistance of Everett Swanson, Miriam Pakingan and Howard Finch has been a key feature in the continuity of this work.

Supported in part by USPHS grants NS 08952; NS 11920 and NS 07098; and National MS Society grant, RG 1001-I-9.

Figures 9.1, 9.3–9.6, 9.9, 9.11, 9.14, 9.21, 9.23, 9.26, 9.33 and 9.34 are reproduced in modified form from Raine, C.S. (1990) Demyelinating diseases, in *Textbook of Neuropathology* (eds R.L. Davis and D.M. Robertson), Baltimore, MD, Williams and Wilkins, pp. 535–620, with permission.

References

1. Adams, R.D. and Sidman, R.L. (1968) *Introduction to Neuropathology*. McGraw-Hill, New York, pp. 149–70.
2. Lumsden, C.E. (1970) The neuropathology of multiple sclerosis, in *Handbook of Clinical Neurology* (eds P.J. Vinken and G.W. Bruyn), Amsterdam, North-Holland, vol. 9, pp. 217–309.
3. Greenfield, J.G. and Norman, R.M. (1971) Demyelinating diseases, in *Greenfield's Neuropathology* (eds W. Blackwood, W.H. McMenemey, M. Meyer, R.M. Norman and D.S. Russell), London, Arnold pp. 474–519.
4. Allen, I.V. (1984) Demyelinating diseases, in *Greenfield's Neuropathology* (eds J.H. Adams, J.A.N. Corsellis and L.W. Duchen), New York, Wiley pp. 338–84.
5. Adams, C.W.M. (1989) *Color Atlas of Multiple Sclerosis and Other Myelin Disorders*, New York, Sheridan House, pp. 1–231.
6. Raine, C.S. (1990) Demyelinating diseases, in *Textbook of Neuropathology* (eds P.L. Davis and D.M. Robertson), Baltimore, MD, Williams and Wilkins, pp. 535–620.
7. Ritchie, J.M. (1984) Physiological basis of conduction in myelinated nerve fibers, in *Myelin* (ed. P. Morell), New York, Plenum, pp. 117–46.
8. Raine, C.S. (1984) The morphology of myelin and myelination, in *Myelin* (ed. P Morell), New York, Plenum, pp. 1–50.
9. Raine, C.S. (1990) Oligodendrocytes and central nerous system myelin, in *Textbook of Neuropathology* (eds, R.L. Davis and D.M. Robertson), Baltimore, MD, Williams and Wilkins, pp. 115–40.
10. Medaer, R. (1979) Does the history of MS go back as far as the 14th century? *Acta Neurol. Scand.*, **60**, 189–92.
11. Dejong, R.N. (1970) Multiple sclerosis: history, definition and general considerations, in *Handbook of Clinical Neurology* (eds P.J. Vinken and G.W. Bruyn), Amsterdam, North-Holland, vol. 9, pp. 45–62.
12. Charcot, J.M. (1868) Histologie de la sclérose en plaques. *Gaz. Hôp. (Paris)*, **41**, 554–66.
13. Rindfleisch, E. (1863) Histologisches Detail zu der grauen Degeneration von Gehirn und Rückenmark. *Virchows Arch. Pathol. Anat.*, **26**, 474–83.
14. Dawson, J.W. (1916) The histology of disseminated sclerosis. *Trans. R. Soc. Edinb.*, **50**, 517–740.
15. Steiner, G. (1931) *Krankheitserreger und Gewebsbefund bei Multiple Sklerose*, Berlin, Springer.
16. Cannella, B., Raine, C.S. (1995) The adhesion molecule/cytokine profile of multiple sclerosis lesions. *Ann. Neurol.*, **37**, 424–35.
17. Adams, C.W.M., Abdulla, Y.H., Torres, E.M. and Poston, R.N. (1987) Periventricular plaques in multiple sclerosis: their perivenous origin and relationship to granular ependymitis. *Neuropathol. Appl. Neurobiol.*, **13**, 141–52.
18. Kwon, E.E. and Prineas, J.W. (1994) Blood–brain barrier abnormalities in longstanding multiple sclerosis lesions. An immunohistochemical study. *J. Neuropathol. Exp. Neurol.*, **53**, 625–36.
19. Claudio, L., Raine, C.S. and Brosnan, C.E. (1995) Evidence of generalized blood–brain barrier abnormalities in chronic-progressive multiple sclerosis. *Acta Neuropathol. (Berlin)*, **90**, 228–38.
20. Cross, A.H., Cannella, B., Brosnan, C.F. and Raine, C.S. (1990) Homing to central nervous system vasculature by antigen specific lymphocytes. I. Localization of ^{14}C-labeled cells during acute, chronic and relapsing experimental allergic encephalomyelitis. *Lab. Invest.*, **63**, 162–70.
21. Raine, C.S., Cannella, B., Duijvestijn, A.M. and Cross, A.H. (1990) Homing to central nervous system vasculature by antigen-specific lymphocytes. II. Lymphocyte/endothelial cell adhesion during the initial stages of autoimmune demyelination. *Lab. Invest.*, **63**, 476–89.
22. Martin, R. and McFarland, H.F. (1992) T cell receptor usage in neurological disease: the case for multiple sclerosis. *Semin. Neurosci.*, **4**, 243–8.
23. Raine, C.S. (1994) The Dale E. McFarlin Memorial Lecture: the immunology of the multiple sclerosis lesion. *Ann. Neurol.*, **36**, 561–72.
24. Katz, D., Taubenberger, J.K., Cannella, B. *et al.* (1993) Correlation between MRI findings and lesion development in chronic active multiple sclerosis. *Ann. Neurol.*, **34**, 661–9.
25. Raine, C.S., Scheinberg, L.C. and Waltz, J.M. (1981) Multiple sclerosis: oligodendrocyte survival and proliferation in an active, established lesion. *Lab. Invest.*, **45**, 534–46.
26. Prineas, J.W., Kwon, E.E., Goldenberg, P.Z. *et al.* (1989) Multiple sclerosis: oligodendrocyte proliferation and differentiation in fresh lesions. *Lab. Invest.*, **61**, 489–503.
27. Selmaj, K., Brosnan, C.F. and Raine, C.S. (1991) Colocalization of TCR-γδ lymphocytes and hsp 65$^+$ oligodendrocytes in multiple sclerosis. *Proc. Natl. Acad. Sci. (USA)*, **88**, 6452–56.
28. Raine, C.S., Wu, E. and Brosnan, C.F. (1994) The immunologic response of the oligodendrocyte in the active multiple sclerosis lesion, in *A Multidisciplinary Approach to Myelin Diseases* (ed. S. Salvati), New York, Plenum, pp. 143–51.
29. Raine, C.S. and Scheinberg, L.C. (1988) On the immunopathology of plaque development and repair in multiple sclerosis. *J. Neuroimmunol.*, **20**, 189–201.

29a. Raine, C.S., Wu, E., Iranyi, J., Katz, D. and Brosnan, C. F. (1996) Multiple sclerosis: a protective or pathogenic role for heat shock protein 60 in the central nervous system? *Lab. Invest.*, **75**, 109–20.

30. Compston, D.A.S., Morgan, B.P., Campbell, A.K. *et al.* (1989) Immunocytochemical localization of the terminal complement complex in multiple sclerosis. *Neuropathol. Appl. Neurobiol.*, **15**, 307–16.

31. Gay, D. and Esiri, M.M. (1991) Blood–brain barrier damage in acute multiple sclerosis plaques. An immunocytological study. *Brain*, **114**, 557–72.

32. Prineas, J.W., Barnard, R.O., Kwon, E.E., Sharer, L.R. and Cho, E.S. (1993) Multiple sclerosis: remyelination of nascent lesions. *Ann. Neurol.*, **33**, 137–51.

33. Raine, C.S. and Wu, E. (1993) Multiple sclerosis: remyelination in acute lesions. *J. Neuropathol. Exp. Neurol.*, **52**, 199–205.

34. Wu, E. and Raine, C.S. (1992) Multiple sclerosis: interactions between oligodendrocytes and hypertrophic astrocytes and their occurrence in other, non-demyelinating conditions. *Lab. Invest.*, **67**, 88–99.

35. Ghatak, N.R. (1992) Occurrence of oligodendrocytes within astrocytes in demyelinating lesions. *J. Neuropathol. Exp. Neurol.*, **51**, 40–6.

36. Ghatak, N.R., Leshner, R.T., Price, A.C. and Felten, W.L. (1989) Remyelination in the human central nervous system. *J. Neuropathol. Exp. Neurol.*, **48**, 507–18.

37. Prineas, J.W., Kwon, E.E., Goldenberg, P.Z., Cho, E.S. and Sharer, L.R. (1990) Interaction of astrocytes and newly formed oligodendrocytes in resolving multiple sclerosis lesions. *Lab. Invest.*, **63**, 624–36.

10 THE IMMUNOCYTOCHEMISTRY OF MULTIPLE SCLEROSIS PLAQUES

Margaret M. Esiri and Derek Gay

10.1 Introduction

Classical histological techniques and histochemical reactions have been used for many years to characterize the cellular components of multiple sclerosis (MS) plaques (Chapter 9). Various recognizable inflammatory cells – lymphocytes, plasma cells, macrophages, microglial cells and mast cells – have been shown to accumulate, particularly during the relatively early stages of development of the plaque. Yet the factors that influence the appearance of these cells in discrete foci in the central nervous system (CNS) and the respective roles they play in destroying myelin and interfering with neurological function in MS, remain elusive. To some extent this reflects the difficulty of understanding a generally long-lasting disease that can, for the most part, only be studied morphologically, with rare exceptions, after death; and one that only occasionally results in death at an acute stage. Recent developments in immunocytochemistry and *in situ* hybridization, applied to the inflammatory cells and related proteins in MS lesions, have raised hopes of throwing light on the pathogenesis of this baffling disease. This chapter reviews the findings of immunocytochemical and *in situ* hybridization studies of MS plaques that have been published during the past 15 years or so. At the end of this review an attempt is made to present a synthesis of current views. Reviews of some of the studies surveyed here have already been published [1–3].

Some of the studies reviewed have made use of monoclonal antibodies to cellular antigens that identify subpopulations of lymphocytes, macrophages and immunologically significant surface molecules such as those of the Class I and Class II major histocompatibility complex (MHC). Others provide information on the localization of locally synthesized, membrane-bound or secreted proteins such as immunoglobulins, complement, adhesion molecules and cytokines. What such studies might be expected to provide is a description of the cellular components of the immune system and of

their bound or ingested soluble products that are present at sequential stages of plaque formation and maturation. The functional significance of immunocytochemical findings in MS must, however, be interpreted with caution and supplemented with information derived from *in situ* hybridization studies. These enable the sites of production of secreted molecules to be identified and distinguished from sites of uptake. Likewise, we need information on the distribution of receptors for secreted molecules since this gives clues to the likely site of influence of the proteins they bind. Information gained from studies that have been published so far is limited by the need for fresh frozen cryostat sections in order to make use of many of the relevant antibodies and nucleic acid probes. This requirement restricts material that can be studied mainly to cases dying in the recent past and also means that histological definition in the sections that can be used is less satisfactory than in formalin-fixed paraffin sections. The lack of a generally accepted method of determining the age of plaques, particularly in frozen sections, hampers comparison between different studies and probably accounts for some discrepant findings in the literature. Likewise, the use of different immunological reagents and techniques can lead to differing findings between research groups. The use of autopsy material fortunately does not appear to impair detection of antigens and mRNA sequences of interest [4, 5]. The review of published findings that follows is divided for convenience into sections that deal separately with the following:

1. Adhesion molecules
2. T lymphocytes and MHC Class I antigens
3. Macrophages, microglial cells and MHC Class II antigens
4. B lymphocytes and plasma cells
5. Cytokines
6. Immunoglobulins and complement
7. Oligodendrocytes.

Multiple Sclerosis: Clinical and pathogenetic basis. Edited by Cedric S. Raine, Henry F. McFarland and Wallace W. Tourtellotte. Published in 1997 by Chapman & Hall, London. ISBN 0 412 30890 8.

10.2   Adhesion molecules

The mononuclear inflammatory cells that appear in MS plaque parenchyma and perivascular spaces have been derived from the blood. Before considering the nature of the cells in detail it is logical first to pay some attention to the mechanisms that have allowed their egress across the blood–brain barrier. Vessels outside the nervous system allow leucocytes to enter tissues as an aid to immune surveillance. The vessels in the CNS, by contrast, allow very few if any such cells to enter the brain and spinal cord under normal conditions, though activated leucocytes may be capable of entry. In order for leucocytes to enter the brain they must undergo a sequence of carefully regulated events, commencing with their contact with endothelial cells. This is followed by slowing of their movement in the blood, rolling against the endothelium, adhering to it, taking on a flattened shape and then migrating between or directly through endothelial cells into the perivascular space. Most such migration of leucocytes occurs at post-capillary venules. A cascade of molecular reactions is thought to underlie this process, involving four sequential steps:

1. **tethering**, mediated by interaction between selectins found on endothelium and leucocytes, which provokes slowing and rolling;
2. **triggering**, principally by cytokines, of activation of previously inactive integrins, strongly adherent leucocyte surface molecules that have receptors (cell adhesion molecules) on endothelial cells; binding of integrins to endothelial cells mediates –
3. **strong adhesion**, and this is followed by –
4. **motility**, stimulated by chemotactic factors, principally some of the cytokines (see reviews by Adams and Shaw [6] and Fabry et al. [7].

Control of leucocyte migration is individually tailored to each cell type.

In normal brain there is low expression of one integrin receptor, intercellular cell adhesion molecule (ICAM)-1 [8, 9]. In MS plaques and surrounding white matter ICAM-1 is expressed more strongly and, in addition, in chronic plaques there is expression of another integrin receptor – vascular cell adhesion molecule (VCAM)-1 (Figure 10.1) [9–11]. E-selectin, which promotes slowing and rolling of leucocytes, is also expressed in some, but not all, plaques [9]. ICAM-1 binds the integrins LFA-1, found on lymphocytes, and Mac-1 found on neutrophils and monocytes, while VCAM-1 binds the integrin VLA-4, found on lymphocytes and monocytes. Upregulation of ICAM-1 and expression of VCAM-1 and E-selectin are common features of inflammation generally. They are, in fact, found also in non-inflammatory CNS conditions such as neurodegeneration [10]. They are therefore likely to be

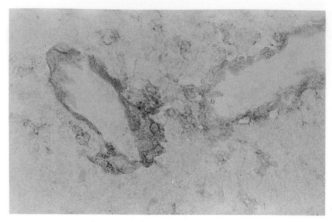

Figure 10.1   A frozen section from a chronic active MS lesion displaying moderate reactivity by endothelial cells and macrophages for VCAM-1. (Courtesy of Dr C.S. Raine and *Annals of Neurology.*)

necessary but not sufficient in themselves to provoke leucocyte entry. The key additional factor is probably the local presence of cytokines in plaques (see below), which can trigger activation of the leucocyte integrins.

10.3   T lymphocytes and MHC class I antigens

The chief findings in the major published reports on the number and distribution of T lymphocytes in and around plaques are summarized in Table 10.1. As can be seen from this table, there is an accumulation of T lymphocytes in plaques, particularly those associated with active demyelination (acute plaques and chronic active ones, i.e. those with evidence of continuing demyelination at their margins). There is some controversy regarding the relative preponderance of CD4 helper/inducer and CD8 cytoxic/suppressor cells in plaques at different stages of their formation and maturation. Overall, most studies find that CD8 cells outnumber CD4 cells in plaques, particularly in the parenchyma and particularly in quiescent lesions. CD4 cells outnumber CD8 cells in the most acute lesions and show rather more tendency than CD8 cells to remain confined to the perivascular Virchow–Robin spaces which usually contain a marked predominance of CD4 cells (Figure 10.2). Some T cells, particularly in acute lesions, express a marker of activation, the receptor for interleukin 2 (IL-2). Some of the CD8 cells may express the natural killer cell marker NKH1 [15], though this marker was not detected in a later study [20]. A subset of CD4 cells expressing a marker of T cells that have, as yet, failed to encounter antigen to which they are responsive [24], 2H4 (CD45R), was found to be decreased in MS plaques [19]. A decrease in 2H4+ cells was found also in the blood in MS [25] as well as in

Table 10.1 Studies of T lymphocytes in multiple sclerosis lesions

Reference	Findings
Nyland et al., 1982 [12]	Many CD8 and fewer CD4 cells in plaque parenchyma. Many CD4 and fewer CD8 cells in perivascular spaces in plaques
Traugott et al., 1983 [13]	Many CD4 and CD8 cells in acute plaques; approx equal numbers of each in chronic active plaques but CD4 cells predominating in surrounding white matter. Few T cells in chronic silent plaques
Booss et al., 1983 [14]	Lymphocytes sparse in plaque parenchyma with CD8 cells predominating. Approx. equal numbers of CD8 and CD4 cells in perivascular spaces. No clear relationship between extent of demyelinating activity and number or proportion of T lymphocytes. Fewer cells expressed the pan-T CD3 marker than CD8 and CD4 markers
Traugott et al., 1984 [15]	NK/Leu 7-positive natural killer cells and cytotoxic CD4 cells in acute and chronic active plaques
Hauser et al., 1986 [4]	T lymphocytes most numerous in the acute and chronic active plaques. Most situated in perivascular spaces with relatively few in parenchyma. CD8 T cells predominated overall with ratios of CD8:CD4 cells varying from 1:1 to 50:1. Surrounding white matter contained few lymphocytes, most of them CD8
Woodroofe et al., 1986 [16]	Findings similar to Hauser et al. [4]. Additionally observed T cells bearing the activation marker IL-2 receptor only in acute plaques, in perivascular spaces
Hofman et al., 1986 [17]	Studied chronic active plaques and found low numbers of T cells, CD4 cells outnumbering CD8 cells. Many cells expressed the IL-2 receptor
McCallum et al., 1987 [18]	Quantitative study of 17 plaques (active, chronic active and chronic silent). CD8 cells slightly exceeded CD4 cells overall and both were maximal at the borders and more numerous in active than silent lesions. CD4 cells in particular were focused near the margins of active plaques
Sobel et al., 1988 [19]	Found abundant T cells in viral encephalitis and fewer in MS. CD4 cells slightly outnumbered CD8 cells in MS but not in viral encephalitis. CD4 cells with 2H4 (CD45R) marker were decreased in MS compared with viral encephalitis
Hayashi et al., 1988 [20]	Studied 9 active plaques, each from differing subjects. Found CD8 cells predominated. No cells were detected with the natural killer cell marker NKH-1 and most T cells did not express the IL-2 receptor
Selmaj et al., 1991 [21]	Studied the minority population of T cells that bear γ/δ cell receptor chains that are thought to be CD8− and CD4−. In chronic plaques these cells formed the majority of T cells in parenchyma. They were less common or absent in other plaques. They were not prominent in other inflammatory conditions
Wucherpfennig et al., 1992 [22]	Extracted RNA from frozen sections of MS plaques and amplifed cDNAs by PCR using primers for TCR Vα and Vβ genes. Showed broad TCR Vα and β repertoire in active lesions with variation between plaques
Hvas et al., 1993 [23]	Found γ/δ T cells in MS lesions. Using PCR studies with primers to Vγ and Vδ regions it was found that the γ/δ T cell response involved a number of different clones possibly in response to several inflammatory antigenic stimuli

other immune-mediated diseases such as rheumatoid arthritis. The decrease may reflect the chronicity of such diseases and is thought likely to be a consequence rather than a cause of the disease.

Most recent of the studies of T cells are those that analyse the proportions of T cells in MS lesions that bear the γ/δ T cell receptor chains [22, 23, 26, 27]. These cells are thought to represent a lineage of T cells distinct from the better known CD4+ or CD8+ T cells which bear α/β T cell receptor chains. Thus γ/δ T cells are usually CD8− and CD4− and they form a small minority of T cells in normal spleen and peripheral blood. γ/δ T cells are remarkably prominent in the immune response provoked by the exceptionally immunogenic, evolutionarily highly conserved, heat shock proteins (HSP). HSP are constitutively expressed in bacteria as well as animal cells and their production is increased in response to stress, including heat shock. A major component of the immune response of animals to infective organisms is directed against HSP (see [28]). HSP in mammalian cells that have been damaged by pathogens such as viruses and bacteria may in turn have the capacity to provoke an autoimmune

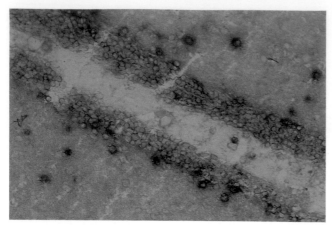

Figure 10.2 Frozen section from an acute MS plaque double-stained to show CD4+ (pink) and CD8+ (navy blue) T cells. CD4+ cells make up the majority of the cells in this perivascular cuff and are not seen in the nearby parenchyma. In contrast, CD8+ cells are present in the cuff and in neighbouring parenchyma.

reaction. Alternatively, immune reactions in response to HSP of infective organisms may inadvertently damage host cells containing HSP or other cell proteins with shared antigenic epitopes. Thus HSP and γ/δ T cells that respond so prominently to them are of considerable interest in relation to the pathogenesis of immune mediated diseases. In MS γ/δ T cells were found in the plaque parenchyma, most commonly in chronically demyelinated plaques, where they comprise the majority of T cells [26]. Oligodendrocytes at the margins of plaques that contained substantial numbers of γ/δ T cells were found to express one of the HSP, HSP-65 [29]. The significance of the γ/δ subset of T cells in MS remains unclear, but a direct cytolytic effect of these cells, isolated from blood, on cultured oligodendrocytes has been shown [30], raising the possibility that they may have a similar role *in vivo*. However, more recent studies have indicated that HSP-65 is also expressed in astrocytes, microglia and endothelial cells, in addition to oligodendrocytes in acute MS lesions, and is expressed in oligodendrocytes and astrocytes in a wide range of other CNS diseases so that expression of this protein is in no way specific for MS [31].

MHC Class I antigens are normally detectable in the CNS only on endothelial cells [32]. These antigens must be present on the surface of cells that form targets for damage by most cytotoxic T cells. Therefore, if the CD8 cells that have been found in MS plaques are active in a cytotoxic capacity, it would be necessary for MHC Class I antigens to be present on their targets. In acute MS plaques MHC Class I antigens have been described as being diffusely expressed, probably on the surface of macrophages and lymphocytes infiltrating the plaques as well as in blood vessel walls [16, 20]. No comment was made on particular localization on myelin sheaths

at the margins of plaques or on oligodendrocytes, and further studies are needed to confirm and clarify the localization of any abnormal MHC Class I antigen expression in the CNS in MS.

10.4   Macrophages, microglial cells and MHC class II antigens

Histochemical reactions for acid phosphatase and non-specific esterase, and the oil-red-O and Sudan black reactions for neutral fat have been used in the past to detect macrophages in MS plaques. These reactions reflect the phagocytic and digestive capabilities of the cells.

Some of the first reports on the immunocytochemistry of MS plaques utilized antibodies to MHC Class II antigens to detect macrophages. At the time there were no antibodies available that reliably identified tissue macrophages in the CNS. The first available mono-clonal antibodies to human macrophage lineage cells reacted with monocytes in peripheral blood and with some tissue macrophages, but their reactions with CNS tissue macrophages (microglial cells) were weak and inconstant. MHC Class II antigens were known to be expressed predominantly on macrophages, though B lymphocytes and activated T cells were also reactive. However, the latter could be distinguished from macrophages using separate antibodies to T and B lymphocytes. Detection of MHC Class II antigens has intrinsic interest in relation to MS because their expression on the surface of macrophages is essential for an important immunological function of macrophages – that of presenting antigen to helper/inducer T lymphocytes, and thereby fuelling immune responses. Recently several monoclonal antibodies have been described which react with certain classes of macrophages and in some cases with microglial cells [33]. Thus, the macrophage populations can now be studied directly in CNS lesions.

Classical histological studies of MS have emphasized not only the presence of large numbers of foamy macrophages in active lesions, but also the presence of numerous activated microglial cells at and beyond the margins of acute and chronic active plaques. Activated, process-bearing microglial cells are generally acknowledged to be derived from blood monocytes [34] and to represent a specialized form of tissue macrophage. Though the origin of resting microglial cells is more controversial, there is now good evidence from recent immunocytochemical studies that they also belong to the mononuclear phagocyte lineage of cells [34, 35]. Activated microglial cells, and a small proportion of resting microglial cells (more weakly), express MHC Class II antigens [32, 35, 36]. One may, therefore, expect them to be detectable with the MHC Class II antibodies used to study MS plaques.

Numerous immunocytochemical studies of macrophages and MHC Class II antigens in MS have been published (Table 10.2). These studies all agree that there are numerous MHC Class II-positive macrophages in established, acutely demyelinated, plaques (Figure 10.3). These cells are much more numerous than T cells in such plaque parenchyma but T cells usually predominate in perivascular spaces. Beyond the borders of acute and chronic active plaques there are numerous activated microglial cells reactive with macrophage antibodies, their numbers falling off fairly abruptly within a short distance of the border (Figure 10.3c). All these cells are strongly reactive for MHC Class II antigens, making them potentially antigen-presenting cells. Other sites of MHC Class II antigen expression in plaques, particularly acute and chronic active ones, are endothelial cells and, according to some studies though not others, astrocytes.

Table 10.2 Studies of T lymphocytes in multiple sclerosis lesions

Reference	Findings
Traugott et al., 1983 [13]	Many MHC Class II-positive macrophages in acute plaques and at the margins of chronic active plaques. Few macrophages in chronic silent plaques, only some of which were MHC Class II-positive
Traugott and Raine, 1985 [37]	Many MHC Class II-positive macrophages and a smaller number of MHC Class II-positive astrocytes found in MS plaques. Endothelial cells in acute plaques were also reactive for MHC Class II antigens
Nyland et al., 1985 [38]	Identified receptors for the FC portion of immunoglobulin on macrophages in actively demyelinating plaques in parenchyma and perivascular spaces. Some endothelial cells were also reactive for this receptor
Hauser et al., 1986 [4]	MHC Class II-positive macrophages much more abundant than T cells in the centre and at margins of actively demyelinating plaques
Hofman et al., 1986 [17]	Many MHC Class II-positive macrophages in actively demyelinating plaques and many MHC Class II-positive astrocytes present also. Macrophages were concentrated mainly at plaque margins
Woodroofe et al., 1986 [16]	Numerous macrophages found in acute plaque parenchyma and perivascular spaces and at plaque borders. Beyond the plaque margins were many activated microglia reactive with the macrophage antibodies used (UCHM1). Both macrophages and microglia reacted for MHC Class II antigens, as did a few astrocytes, which represented about 1% of the MHC Class II-positive cells
Esiri and Reading, 1987 [36]	Numerous macrophages in acute and chronic active plaques in parenchyma and perivascular spaces. In the latter compartment they were less numerous than T cells. Macrophage antibodies used (EBM11, UCHM1) also reacted with many reactive microglial cells beyond plaque margins. All macrophages and microglial cells were reactive for MHC Class II. Acute plaques only contained some macrophages reactive with a further macrophage antibody used (RFD7). Chronic silent plaques contained few macrophages, only some of which reacted for MHC Class II
Hayashi et al., 1988 [20]	Double-labelling experiments showed that most MHC Class II-expressing cells in acute MS plaques were endothelial cells or macrophages and not astrocytes
Adams et al., 1989 [39]	Perivascular macrophages in acute MS were reactive for lysozyme and Mac387. Few parenchymal macrophages reacted for these markers
Lee et al., 1990 [40]	Many MHC Class II-expressing macrophages and a few MHC Class II-expressing astrocytes found in MS plaques
Sanders et al., 1993 [41]	Intensity and severity of MHC Class II expression on macrophages in MS plaques was correlated with extent of demyelinating activity
Washington et al. 1994 Ref [9]	Vessels isolated from MS plaques and surrounding white matter showed expression of MHC Class II antigens
Ulvestad et al., 1994 [42]	Perivascular macrophages of haematogenous origin reacted for non-specific esterase, myeloperoxidase, L1, lysozyme, C14 and RFD7 in chronic active MS lesions. Parenchymal microglia were positive for CD11c and CD68
Bö et al., 1994 [43]	MHC Class II abundant on microglia, phagocytic and perivascular macrophages. Astrocytes and endothelial cells MHC Class II-negative

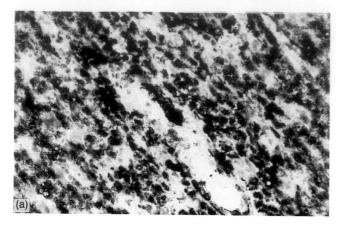

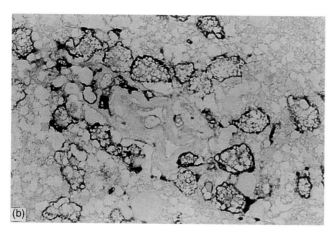

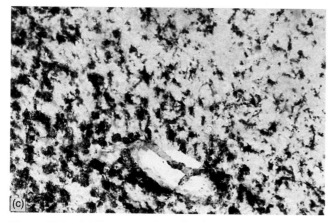

10.5   B cells and plasma cells

Antibodies to B lymphocytes have been used in a few studies of MS plaques and findings have been generally consistent. B cells make up only a very small proportion of the lymphocytes in most perivascular infiltrates in active plaques, though occasional infiltrates may contain up to 40% of B cells [16]. B cells are not found, in the authors' experience, in plaque or non-plaque parenchyma but only in perivascular spaces, mainly in acute plaques. Chronic active plaques may show rare B cells in perivascular spaces but they are generally absent from chronic silent plaques. Plasma cells, into which B cells mature under the influence of B cell growth and maturation factors, produced by activated T helper/ inducer (CD4) cells, can be detected in active MS plaques significantly more commonly than in inactive ones [44, 45] (Figure 10.4). Immunoglobulin-containing cells were located chiefly in perivascular spaces, but were also found in acute plaque parenchyma, often close to vessels which were surrounded by immunoglobulin-containing perivascular cells with the same light or heavy chain content. Normal-appearing white matter around plaques did not show infiltration of the parenchyma by immunoglobulin-containing cells but occasionally contained a few plasma cells in perivascular spaces, and plasma cells were frequently seen in the meninges along with some lymphocytes and macrophages.

In contrast to the above studies in which plasma cells were correlated with active demyelination, Prineas and Wright [46], in a light and electron microscopic study, considered that chronic silent plaques contained more

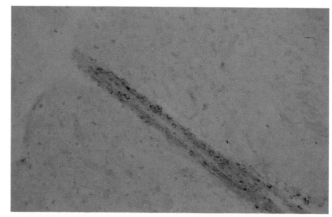

Figure 10.3   (a) Frozen section of a chronic active MS plaque immunostained with the macrophage-specific monoclonal antibody EBM11. Numerous macrophages occupy the plaque parenchyma. (b) 1 μm epoxy section from a chronic active MS lesion immunostained for MHC Class II antigens. Many foamy macrophages in this perivascular field are intensely stained. (Courtesy of Dr C.S. Raine and *Annals of Neurology*.) (c) Frozen section of the edge of an acute multiple sclerosis plaque treated with monoclonal antibody RFDR1 to MHC Class II determinants. Reactive cells with macrophage morphology are seen bottom left within the plaque, while at the top right reactive cells have microglial cell morphology in surrounding white matter. (Counterstained with haematoxylin.) (Reproduced from Esiri and Reading, 1987 [36], courtesy of the Editor and publisher of *Neuropathology and Applied Neurobiology*.)

Figure 10.4   Frozen section of the same perivascular cuff of cells shown in Figure 10.2 from a case of acute MS. The section has been treated with an antibody to IgG and shows numerous perivascular plasma cells (red cytoplasm) and occasional parenchymal plasma cells. The section was photographed under polarized light and shows largely intact myelin at top right with degenerate myelin to left and below the vessel.

Figure 10.5 Cytokine expression in MS: confocal microscopy at the edge of a chronic active lesion. TNFα-positive macrophages (red) are visible alongside IL-10-positive astrocyte processes (green). (Courtesy of Dr C.S. Raine and *Annals of Neurology*.)

plasma cells than active ones. In a recent study based on immunocytochemical techniques Lassmann *et al.* [47] came to the same conclusion.

10.6 Cytokines (Figure 10.5)

The role of cytokines in MS is poorly understood at present, but it is recognized that it is likely to be important. Further studies are needed to provide a full picture of known cytokine expression and the likely effect of cytokines at different stages of MS plaque development. Immunocytochemistry alone is an imprecise technique for assessing cytokine expression since cytokines are secreted proteins that are released from the cells synthesizing them and act on these and other cells in the same vicinity or more distantly, that have receptors for them. Thus, information is needed not only on their distribution (using immunocytochemistry) but also on their sites of synthesis (using *in situ* hybridization) and on the distribution of their receptors (using immunocytochemistry or ligand studies), together with an analysis of their local concentrations, for a comprehensive understanding of their potential roles in MS. Information available at present, fragmentary at best, is summarized in Table 10.3.

Cytokines, including those that have been detected in MS plaques, can be broadly divided into those that are generally pro- and anti-inflammatory. The former include tumour necrosis factor alpha (TNFα) (Figure 10.5), interleukin 1 and interleukin 2 (IL-1, IL-2) interferon γ (IFN-γ) and certain chemokines, small molecular weight cytokines with chemotactic properties. Anti-inflammatory cytokines include interferons alpha and beta (IFN-α, IFN-β), transforming growth factor beta (TGF β) and interleukin 4 (IL-4). Some cytokines have mixed pro- and anti-inflammatory activity, for example interleukin 6 (IL-6), which promotes B cell stimulation and induction of acute phase responses [50], but is also likely to have a restraining influence on the inflammatory and demyelinating process in MS by inducing production of tissue inhibitors of metalloproteinases, enzymes produced by macrophages known to be capable of breaking down myelin [3, 51, 52]. Most of the cytokines detected in MS

Table 10.3 Cytokine expression in MS lesions

Reference	Method	Findings
Hofman *et al.*, 1986 [17]	ICC	Detected TNF in macrophages and astrocytes and IL-1 and IL-2 in MS plaques
Traugott and Lebon, 1988 [48]	ICC	Detected IFNγ in astrocytes and endothelial cells in MS plaques
Hofman *et al.*, 1989 [49]	ICC	Detected TNF in MS plaques
Selmaj *et al.*, 1991 [21, 26]	ICC	Detected TNFα and TNFβ (lymphotoxin) in MS plaques. TNFα was found in astrocytes at the edge of plaques and in microglia within plaques and TNFβ in microglial cells at plaque margins
Woodroofe and Cuzner, 1993 [5]	ISH	Detected mRNA for IL-1α, IL-2, IL-4, IL-6, IL-10, IFNγ, TNFα, TGFβ-1 and 2 in MS plaques. IL-6, IFNγ and TNFα predominated in cells in perivascular spaces; other cytokines were more weakly expressed
Cannella and Raine 1995 [10]	ICC	Detected high levels of IL-1, IL-2, IL-4, IL-10, TNFα, TGFβ and IFNγ in MS lesions, particularly chronic active ones. Localized to microglial cells and astrocytes

plaques are known to be produced by macrophages (IL-1, IL-6, TGFβ, TNFα) and lymphocytes (IL-2, IL-4 IFN-γ, TNFα, TNFβ, IL-6). These are the cells (particularly in perivascular spaces) in which mRNA directing their synthesis was detectable in the study by Woodroofe and Cuzner [5]. However, TNFα, IFN-γ and IL-4 have also been localized to astrocytes either as a result of uptake from the extracellular space or possibly because these cells are also capable of synthesizing them. Cytokines that were particularly associated with demyelinating activity were IL-6, IL-4, TNFα and IFN-γ [5].

The distribution of cytokine receptors in MS lesions has not yet been reported. However, some of the likely effects of local cytokine production in MS can be inferred from their known properties in other inflammatory conditions and from *in vitro* studies of the effects of cytokines. These effects and the possible factors stimulating cytokine production in MS plaques are discussed in section 10.9.

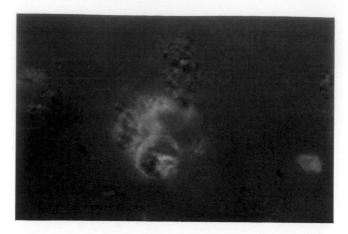

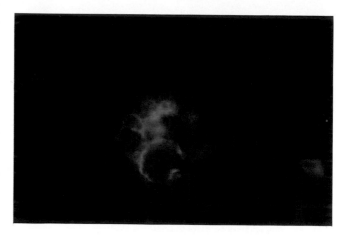

10.7 Immunoglobulin and complement

Several studies have described IgG deposits on myelin sheaths at the borders of demyelinated plaques [53–56], but the significance of this finding has been in doubt because IgG in normal serum can bind to myelin basic protein non-specifically through the Fc part of the molecule [57–59], and such IgG deposits found in multiple sclerosis are readily washed away, suggesting that they are not tightly bound [54, 55]. For the IgG deposits to be significant in immunologically mediated breakdown of myelin, they should be accompanied by other bound molecules, particularly complement components, at the same site. This has not been shown to occur, though there is some evidence that suggests the formation of membrane attack complexes of complement in the CNS and consumption of the terminal C9 complement component in MS [60]. Although complement components have not been located on myelin sheaths in MS, C9 has recently been located in the adventitia of blood vessels [61] and vascular basement membranes, some of which were disrupted [62]. There is also co-localization of C3d and IgM or IgG on macrophage membranes only in acute plaques and associated with ingestion of myelin fragments (Figure 10.6), a feature particularly well demonstrated using antibodies to C3d [53]. These findings suggest that complement-fixing immune complexes may be formed in close association with the demyelinating process, though not, apparently, on myelin sheaths. Further evidence that immune complexes form locally at the site of demyelination was provided by Prineas and Graham [54], who observed capping of IgG on the surface of macrophages in the vicinity of active demyelination – an occurrence that implies combination of

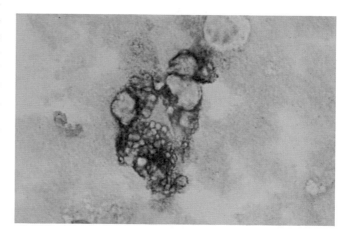

Figure 10.6 Oil-immersion photographs of a frozen section from an acute MS plaque which had been double-stained to show C3d (*a*, green) and IgG (*b*, red). In this field is a macrophage containing ingested myelin fragments, seen with polarized light in (*a*) occupying two of the cytoplasmic vacuoles which contain IgG and C3d co-localized in the surrounding cytoplasmic rims. In a similar cell in which C3d is localized with peroxidase (*c*, brown) the reaction product can be seen in the membrane lining the vacuoles.

immunoglobulin with antigens as complexes or with anti-IgG antibody on the surface of macrophages.

10.8   Oligodendrocytes

On the basis of observations on the light microscopy and ultrastructure of MS lesions it was established that oligodendrocytes disappear from chronic lesions but that they are increased in numbers at the margins of some active plaques (Chapter 15). Immunocytochemical observations using antibodies that specifically attach to oligodendrocytes have now added to information about the fate of oligodendrocytes in MS. Reactions on active MS lesions using antibodies to galactocerebroside, carbonic anhydrase II, 2′, 3′-cyclic nucleotide 3′-phosphodiesterase and myelin basic protein show more intense staining for these myelin-associated proteins and enzymes involved in myelin synthesis than in normal, mature oligodendrocytes [21, 63–65]. They also show increased numbers of oligodendroctyes in active plaques, some of them in pairs or small clusters (Figure 10.7), though some loss of oligodendrocytes in the very early stage (first month) of plaque formation was detected by Prineas et al. [66]. The reactive oligodendrocytes in most actively demyelinating lesions are interpreted by some authors as relatively immature, based on their expression of the HNK-1 antigen [64], and their presence strengthens the evidence for oligodendrocyte replenishment in MS, though the source of this replenishment is not clear at present. They do suggest that there is considerable potential for myelin regeneration in MS, at least in the initial stages. Unusual interactions of oligodendrocytes

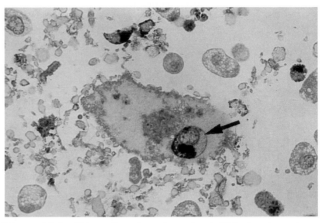

Figure 10.8   Edge of a chronic active MS lesion in a 1 μm section reacted for HNK-1 and glial fibrillary acidic protein. The cell in the centre is a GFAP-stained hypertrophic astrocyte which has engulfed an HNK-1⁺ oligodendrocyte (*arrow*). (Courtesy of Dr C.S. Raine and *Annals of Neurology.*)

with hypertrophic astrocytes which engulf them have been described in some studies [67], possibly as a protective mechanism [68] (Figure 10.8). The expression of HSP by oligodendrocytes in MS and other conditions has already been referred to above.

In chronic silent MS plaques there is a marked loss of immunocytochemically detectable oligodendrocytes similar to the more diffuse loss of such cells found in other chronic demyelinating conditions such as leucodystrophies [65]. This suggests that in the face of prolonged or repeated demyelinating disease oligodendrocyte numbers diminish as their reserve capacity is exhausted.

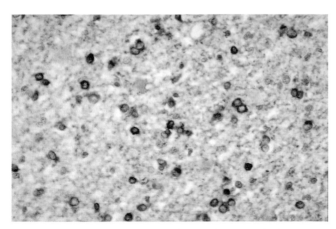

Figure 10.7   Immunostaining for carbonic anhydrase isoenzyme II on a formalin-fixed, paraffin-embedded section of a chronic active MS plaque. There are increased numbers of oligodendrocytes and an increased intensity of immunostaining of their cytoplasm compared with normal white matter. Some of the immunostained oligodendrocytes are lying in pairs. (Section prepared by Dr C.S. Morris.)

10.9   A synthesis of the evidence on the immunocytochemistry of MS plaques

In light of evidence so far presented, it seems that MS plaques can be regarded as foci of inflammation and demyelination in which the inflammatory cells occupy both the perivascular spaces and the plaque parenchyma. It may be helpful to consider these two as different compartments in which immunological events can occur [69]. Perivascular infiltrates are found in the Virchow–Robin spaces around veins and venules; inflammatory cells at this site are a rich source of cytokines that act locally and diffuse into the neighbouring parenchyma, where they facilitate myelin damage, and to endothelium where they promote disruption of the blood–brain barrier and migration of leucocytes. Inflammatory cells reach the parenchyma mainly from these spaces.

In acute plaques the perivascular infiltrates are composed principally of T lymphocytes, including many that are activated, possessing IL-2 receptors. Macrophages account for most of the rest of the cells present. Overall, there are smaller numbers of B cells and plasma cells, although a few infiltrates contain a predominance of these antibody-producing cells. Both CD8 and CD4 cells are abundant in perivascular spaces. Differences in ratios between CD4 and CD8 cells can be attributed in part to variable maturity of plaques studied [19]. CD8 cells frequently migrate into acute plaque parenchyma but CD4 cells, in the authors' experience, and that of Nyland et al. [12], tend to remain in perivascular spaces, where they have a greater opportunity to interact with the relatively scarce B cells. Whether the T cells recruited into plaques are antigen-specific remains largely unknown. B cells appear to mature to plasma cells in the perivascular spaces, following which some of them move into the parenchyma. The heterogeneity of acute plaques with respect to their immunoglobulin-containing cells would be consistent with these cells being derived locally from a relatively small number of B cells. The precise role of humoral, locally produced, antibody in the demyelinating process is at present unclear. Most IgG deposits in plaques seem to be readily washed away, implying that they are not bound to tissues. Complement (C3d) deposits can be unequivocally demonstrated on vascular basement membranes at the margins of acute plaques and complexed with immunoglobulin on macrophages, but their role in the production of demyelination is obscure.

We have seen from this review of the cellular and cytokine studies that there are all the components of both cell-mediated and humoral immune responses in MS plaques. Thus, lymphocytes, macrophages and cytokines of the type associated with cell-mediated immunity, now recognized to be particularly promoted by a subset of activated CD4 T cells known as TH1 cells – TNFβ, IFN-γ, IL-2 – are present, together with B cells, plasma cells, complement and cytokines associated with activity of a second subgroup of CD4 cells known as TH2 – IL-4, IL-5, IL-6, IL-10, IL-13 – which promote antibody responses and in some circumstances eosinophilia [70].

There has been a recent tendency to emphasize the role of cell-mediated immunity in MS, largely based on the predominance of this type of immunity in experimental allergic encephalomyelitis (EAE), widely promoted as a model for MS. However, it is perhaps premature to downplay the potential importance of humoral mechanisms in MS. Even in EAE myelin damage can be much more convincingly demonstrated when humoral as well as cell-mediated mechanisms are brought to bear [71, 72]. There are some features of EAE that differ from MS, cautioning against assumptions of their near-identity. For example, disease-promoting and disease-limiting cytokines seem to be different in the two diseases [3], and whereas EAE is clearly an artificially induced autoimmune disease there is no direct evidence of an autoimmune aetiology in MS. The greatest enigma in MS is the nature of the antigenic stimulus provoking the formation of multiple foci of immune reaction in the CNS. Clues to the nature of such an inciting stimulus may be derivable from a close examination of the nature of the immune response generated. Thus, cell-mediated immunity is particularly provoked by cellular infection by viruses, whilst humoral responses and responses of γ/δ T cells are prominently induced by bacteria and their products. The long-recognized occurrence of oligoclonal immunoglobulin in CSF, the recent evidence of γ/δ T cells in plaques and in CSF, many of the latter responsive to mycobacterial antigens [73], and the presence of plasma cells and complement in acute lesions in MS, all point to the need not to dismiss the possibility of a bacterial trigger for the disease.

Certain Gram-positive and Gram-negative bacterial cell wall molecules and exotoxins are potent T and B cell mitogens [74]. These 'superantigens' activate large numbers of T and B lymphocytes without regard to antigenic specificity and this has led to the speculation that they may amplify and render pathogenic autoreactive clones. The ability of staphylococcal enterotoxins to activate human T lymphocytes reactive with myelin autoantigens [75] adds credence to these ideas in relation to MS. The induction of relapsing EAE with similar enterotoxins [76] provides a model in which these types of reaction may be further investigated. Bacterial products are a direct and potent stimulus to local cytokine production which, in turn, provokes alterations in endothelium that encourage entry of inflammatory cells to the focus of cytokine production. These in turn produce more cytokines that amplify the inflammatory response which generates secreted molecules well capable of damaging local myelin and eventually, through the production of immunoregulatory cytokines, control of the response. The possibility also exists that myelin peptide products resulting from the action of secreted proteinases could provide an antigenic stimulation for a super-added autoimmune reaction [3].

Studies of oligodendrocytes in vitro indicate that they are susceptible to a whole range of leucocyte products known or likely to be present in MS plaques: complement, TNFα, perforins produced by T cells, leucotrienes, proteases, nitric oxide and oxygen radicals produced by macrophages. They are also susceptible to attack by activated macrophages in the presence or absence of opsonizing anti-oligodendrocyte antibodies by CD4 T cells, and to γ/δ T cells, the T cell damage occurring in the absence of an MHC-restricted mechanism [30, 77–79]. Oligodendrocyte proliferation and myelin regeneration may also be influenced to some extent by products of inflammatory cells in MS plaques. Some cytokines (e.g. IL-2) may simulate their proliferation and developing oligodendrocytes have receptors on their surface for another cytokine, platelet-derived growth factor [80].

In chronic silent and chronic active plaques the inflammation is absent or much reduced and there is a markedly greater overall excess of CD8 cells over CD4 cells than in active plaques. As the relative lengths of survival of different T cell subsets in plaques are not known it is uncertain whether this CD8 cell excess represents longer-surviving cells left over from an earlier, active stage of inflammation, or whether CD8 cells migrate into established plaques to a greater extent than CD4 cells. However, taking all the evidence together it is reasonable to suggest that formation and extension of the plaque is associated with a relative excess of CD4 cells in and immediately around the plaques, whether this is detectable as an absolute excess of CD4 cells [13, 19], as a reduced excess of CD8 over CD4 cells, or as a reduced absolute number of CD8 cells [18]. Conversely, arrest of demyelination is associated with an extra preponderance of CD8 cells. It is tempting to speculate that the balance in the populations of these classes of T cells controls the state of the plaque, with each subset acting in an opposing fashion. Because CD8 cells are particularly dominant in the less active lesions it is easier to envisage them as suppressor rather than cytoxic in function. CD8 cells have the capacity to regulate TH1 and TH2 CD4 T cells, probably through their capacity to secrete cytokines such as IL-4 and IFN-γ [81]. There are many CD8 cells present in active plaques, in parenchyma as well as perivascular spaces, but it is difficult to envisage a cytotoxic role for these cells in the absence of demonstrable MHC Class I molecules on targets in and around MS plaques. In contrast, activated CD4 cells can well be envisaged to provoke damage in MS plaques through their capacity to produce IFN-γ, which enhances MHC Class II antigen expression on macrophages and in turn amplifies helper/inducer cell activation by macrophages. Activated CD4 cells also produce cytokines that promote humoral responses. There would seem to be ample opportunity for such interactions to occur between CD4 cells, macrophages and B cells, particularly in the perivascular spaces of acute plaques where T cells, macrophages and B cells are found intermingled.

Present evidence on the involvement of CD8 cells in MS plaques suggests that measures designed to increase their suppressor capacity and decrease their cytotoxic capacity should be beneficial to the patient. Similarly, measures designed to reduce the local CD4 population, or their capacity to respond to immune stimulation, would also be expected to be beneficial.

10.10 Is there a unique inflammatory cell profile in the CNS in MS?

It may be asked to what extent the profile of immunologically competent cells in MS plaques resembles that of cells drawn into the CNS by a known antigenic stimulus. It could be that features seen in MS simply reflect aspects of the general behaviour of inflammatory cells in the CNS. On the other hand, there may be atypical aspects to the MS infiltrate that reflect faulty immunoregulation [82]. In this context, it is worthwhile to refer briefly to immunocytochemical studies of other inflammatory disorders of the CNS (Table 10.4) in order to compare them with MS.

Comparison between T cell studies in MS and other CNS inflammatory conditions shows that total numbers of T cells are lower in MS plaques than in viral encephalitis and the CD8 subset predominates to a greater extent in viral encephalitis than in MS [19]. The 2H4+ CD4 cells are selectively reduced in MS lesions compared with viral encephalitis [19] and the γ/δ T cells are not found in viral encephalitis as they are in MS [26, 30]. The presence of numerous MHC Class II-positive macrophages and microglial cells is also found in viral encephalitis and in many non-inflammatory CNS diseases as well as in MS. The extent of parenchymal macrophage accumulation is largely dependent on the degree of necrosis or demyelination. B cells are relatively uncommon in the perivascular infiltrates in all forms of encephalitis as well as in MS, and the immunoglobulin-containing plasma cells occur in a similar distribution, but in greater abundance in most forms of encephalitis than in MS, though they are notably scarce in perivenous encephalitis. Studies of complement deposition in SSPE [62, 96] and perivenous encephalitis [62] show deposits of complement in vessel walls, but none of the destructive changes in vessel and basement membrane components found in MS. Studies of cytokine detection in SSPE indicate that a similar spectrum of cytokines is present here as in MS.

Thus, we have to conclude that with the possible exceptions of the shortage of 2H4+ cells, the increased numbers of γ/δ T cell receptor-bearing cells, and the deposits of immunoglobulin and complement on macrophages as illustrated in Figure 10.7, the evidence available at present suggests that the inflammatory response in the CNS, regardless of the cause, is relatively stereotyped and that any differences between MS and encephalitis seem as likely to be explicable on the basis of a differing tempo in the responses in the various diseases and/or subtle variation in the nature of the antigenic stimulus as to be due to any fundamental difference in the nature of the response. In particular, there is no evidence so far from studies of MS lesions to suggest that the immune response in this disease, in so far as it is assessable from an examination of the

Table 10.4 Some *in situ* studies of CNS inflammatory disorders other than MS

Reference	Condition	Findings
Johnson *et al.*, 1985 [83]	Japanese B encephalitis	Preponderance of T cells in perivascular cuffs, only a minority of which were CD8 cells. T cells sparse in brain parenchyma, where they were greatly outnumbered by macrophages. B cells uncommon and confined to perivascular spaces
Sobel *et al.*, 1986 [84]	Herpes simplex encephalitis	Parenchymal and meningeal infiltrates consisted chiefly of T cells with variable numbers of macrophages and few B cells and natural killer cells. MHC Class I and II detected on parenchymal cells including neurons. Many T cells were activated, expressing IL-2 receptor
Esiri *et al.*, 1981 [85]	Subacute sclerosing pan-encephalitis (SSPE)	Many IgG-containing plasma cells in the inflammatory infiltrate in perivascular cuffs and brain parenchyma
Kreth *et al.*, 1982 [86]	SSPE	Many T cells in perivascular spaces in SSPE
Hofman *et al.*, 1991 [87]	SSPE	Immunocytochemical study of cytokines and inflammatory cells showed both CD4 and CD8 cells in brain parenchyma. Positive cellular staining obtained for TNFα and IFN-γ
Nagano *et al.* 1994 [88]	SSPE	Immunocytochemical study that detected in SSPE: IL-1β, IL-2, IL-6, TNF, lymphotoxin and IFN-γ; in lymphocytes, (IL-2, IL-6 (rare), lymphotoxin), macrophages/microglia (IL-1β, IFN-γ, IL-6, TNF, lymphotoxin), astrocytes (IL-1β, IL-6, TNF, IFN-γ) and endothelial cells (IL-1β, TNF, IFN-γ)
Griffin *et al.*, 1985 [89]	Adrenoleukodystrophy	Immunocytochemical study of perivascular cuffs, showing 59% were T cells (34% CD4, 16% CD8), 24% B cells and 11% macrophages
Sobel *et al.*, 1988 [5]	Herpes simplex encephalitis and SSPE	Found plentiful 2H4+ (CD45R) cells, in contrast to MS where this subset of CD4 cells was selectively decreased. Rather more CD8 cells found than in MS
Esiri *et al.*, 1989 [90]	Various	Lymphocytic infiltrate consisted chiefly of T cells with CD8 cells predominating. CD4 cells more numerous in acute than chronic cases. B cells sparse
Esiri *et al.*, 1980 [91]	Poliomyelitis	Many immunoglobulin-containing cells in acute phase in damaged areas of CNS: fewer in chronic lesions. Many plasma cells contained IgA. Perivascular cuffs and CNS parenchyma contained plasma cells
Esiri, 1983 [92]	Herpes simplex encephalitis	Inflammation peaked at 3–4 weeks from onset. Many immunoglobulin-containing cells present in perivascular spaces and brain parenchyma. Most of the immunoglobulin was IgG
Nagano *et al.*, 1994 [88]	Progressive multifocal leucoencephalopathy	Rare cells contained IL-1β, IL-2 and lymphotoxin. IL-6 detectable in some microglial cells. Scattered TNF+ macrophages, endothelial cells and oligodendrocytes with enlarged nuclei. IFN-γ detected in some macrophages and astrocytes
Tyor *et al.*, 1992 [93]	HIV infection	Majority of infiltrating CNS cells were macrophages, and reactive microglia, reactive for MHC Class I and II, IL-1 and TNFα
Glass *et al.*, 1993 [94]	HIV infection	High levels of mRNA for TNFα in frontal white matter correlated with clinical evidence of dementia
Stanley *et al.*, 1994 [95]	HIV infection	Many activated microglia were reactive for IL-1α, and astrocytes for S100β
Ulvestad *et al.*, 1994 [42]	Encephalitis (type not specified)	Haematogenously derived macrophages reactive for non-specific esterase myeloperoxidase, L1, lysozyme, RFD7 and CD14 infiltrate parenchyma to a greater extent than in MS

immunocytochemistry of plaques, is at all intrinsically atypical. Immunocytochemical studies on MS demonstrate an immune response of conventional type, but with a most distinctive distribution, localized to the plaques and their immediate environs. What is still lacking is knowledge of the provoking antigen.

10.11   Conclusion

MS plaques are inflammatory lesions about which a wealth of information has now been collected regarding the types of cells that are present and many of their secreted molecules. Even so, the picture is not complete, for more information is needed about expression of receptors for secreted cytokines and growth factors if understanding about their complex effects is to be gained. Amongst the molecules detected are several that are known to be myelinotoxic, such as tumour necrosis factor and complement, while others are capable of damping down the immune response and promoting repair. Likewise, among the cellular constituents of plaques are some cells that are likely to exert destructive effects on myelin – the activated macrophages, for example – and others that may moderate these effects. Knowledge of the key immune players in the disease, and how they interact, offers undoubted therapeutic opportunities but efforts to intervene can be more confidently made when we gain insight into what provokes this myelin-damaging process in the first place.

References

1. Ffrench-Constant, C. (1994) Pathogenesis of multiple sclerosis. *Lancet*, **343**, 271–5.
2. Raine, C.S. (1994) Multiple sclerosis: immune system molecule expression in the central nervous system. *J. Neuropathol. Exp. Neurol.*, **53**, 328–37.
3. Opdenakker, G. and Van Damme, J. (1994) Cytokine-regulated proteases in autoimmune disease. *Immunol. Today*, **15**, 103–10.
4. Hauser, S.L., Bhan, A.K., Gilles, F. *et al.* (1986) Immunohistochemical analysis of the cellular infiltrate in multiple sclerosis lesions. *Ann. Neurol.*, **19**, 578–87.
5. Woodroofe, M.N. and Cuzner, M.L. (1993) Cytokine mRNA expression in inflammatory multiple sclerosis lesions: detection by non-radioactive *in situ* hybridisation. *Cytokine*, **5**, 583–8.
6. Adams, D.H. and Shaw, S. (1994) Leucocyte–endothelial interactions and regulation of leucocyte migration. *Lancet*, **343**, 831–6.
7. Fabry, Z., Raine, C.S. and Hart, M.N. (1994) Nervous tissue as an immune compartment: the dialect of the immune response in the CNS. *Immunol. Today*, **15**, 218–24.
8. Sobel, R.A., Mitchell, M. and Fondren, G. (1990) Intercellular adhesion molecule-1 (ICAM-1) in cellular immune reactions in the human central nervous system. *Am. J. Pathol.*, **136**, 1309–16.
9. Washington, R., Burton, J. Tood, R.F. *et al.* (1994) Expression of immunologically relevant endothelial cell activation antigens on isolated CNS microvessels from patients with multiple sclerosis. *Ann. Neurol.* **35**, 89–97.
10. Cannella, B. and Raine, C.S. (1995) The adhesion molecule and cytokine profile of multiple sclerosis lesions. *Ann. Neurol.*, **37**, 424–35.
11. Raine, C.S. (1994) The Dale E. McFarlin Memorial Lecture: The immunology of multiple sclerosis lesions. *Ann. Neurol.*, **36**, 561–72.
12. Nyland, H., Matre, R., Mork, S. *et al.* (1982) T-lymphocyte subpopulations in multiple sclerosis lesions. *N. Engl. J. Med.*, **307**, 1643–4.
13. Traugott, U., Reinherz, E.L. and Raine, C.S. (1983) Multiple sclerosis: distribution of T cells, T cell subsets and Ia-positive macrophages in lesions of different ages. *J. Neuroimmunol.*, **4**, 201–21.
14. Booss, J., Esiri, M.M., Tourtellotte, W.W. and Mason, D.Y. (1983) Immunohistological analysis of T-lymphocyte subjects in the central nervous system in chronic progressive multiple sclerosis. *J. Neurol. Sci.*, **62**, 219–32.
15. Traugott, U. (1984) Characterisation and distribution of lymphocyte subpopulations in multiple sclerosis plaques versus autoimmune demyelinating lesions. *Springer Semin. Immunopathol.*, **8**, 71–95.
16. Woodroofe, M.N., Bellamy, A.S., Feldman, M. *et al.* (1986) Immunocytochemical characterisation of the immune reaction in the central nervous system in multiple sclerosis: possible role for microglia in lesion growth. *J. Neurol. Sci.*, **74**, 135–52.
17. Hofman, F.M., von Hanwehr, R.I., Dinarello, C.A. *et al.* (1986) Immunoregulatory molecules and IL2 receptors identified in multiple sclerosis brain. *J. Immunol.* **136**, 3239–45.
18. McCallum, K., Esiri, M.M., Tourtellotte, W.W. and Booss, J. (1987) T cell subsets in multiple sclerosis: gradients at plaque borders and differences in non-plaque regions. *Brain*, **110**, 1297–308.
19. Sobel, R.A., Hafler, D.A., Castro, E.E., Morimoto, C. and Weiner, H.L. (1988) The 2H4 (CD45R) antigen is selectively decreased in multiple sclerosis lesions. *J. Immunol.*, **140**, 2210–14.
20. Hayashi, T., Morimoto, C., Burks, J.S., Kerr, C. and Hauser, S.L. (1988) Dual-label immunocytochemistry of the active multiple sclerosis lesion: major histocompatibility complex and activation antigens. *Ann. Neurol.*, **24**, 523–31.
21. Selmaj, K., Raine, C.S., Cannella, B. and Brosnan, C.F. (1991) Identification of lymphotoxin and tumour necrosis factor in multiple sclerosis lesions. *J. Clin. Invest.*, **87**, 949–54.
22. Wucherpfennig, K., Newcombe, J., Li, H. *et al.* (1992) Gamma/delta T cell receptor repertoire in acute multiple sclerosis lesions. *Proc. Natl Acad. Sci. (USA)*, **89**, 4588–92.
23. Hvas, J., Oksenberg, J.R., Fernando, R., Steinman, L. and Bernard, C.C.A. (1993) T cell receptor repertoire in brain lesions of patients with multiple sclerosis. *J. Neuroimmunol.*, **46**, 225–34.
24. Sanders, M.E., Malegapuru, N.M. and Shaw, S. (1988) Alterations in T cell subsets in multiple sclerosis and other autoimmune diseases. *Lancet*, **ii**, 1021.
25. Morimoto, C., Hafler, D.A., Weiner, H.L. *et al.* (1987) Selective loss of the suppressor-inducer T cell subset in progressive multiple sclerosis. *N. Engl. J. Med.*, **316**, 67–72.
26. Selmaj, K., Brosnan, C.F. and Raine, C.S. (1991) Colonisation of TCR gamma/delta lymphocytes and hsp⁺ oligodendrocytes in multiple sclerosis. *Proc. Natl Acad. Sci. (USA)*, **88**, 6452–6.
27. Shimonkevitz, R., Colburn, C., Burnham, J.A., Murray, R.S. and Kotzin, B.L. (1993) Clonal expansion of active gamma/delta T cells in recent onset multiple sclerosis. *Proc. Natl Acad. Sci. (USA)*, **90**, 923–7.
28. Ransohoff, R.M. and Rudick, R.A. (1993) Heat shock proteins and autoimmunity: implications for multiple sclerosis. *Ann. Neurol.*, **34**: 5–7.
29. Selmaj, K., Brosnan, C.F. and Raine, C.S. (1992) Expression of heat-shock protein-65 by oligodendrocytes *in vivo* and *in vitro*: implications for multiple sclerosis. *Neurology*, **42**, 795–800.
30. Freedman, M.S., Ruijs, T.C.G., Selin, L.K. and Antel, J.P. (1991) Peripheral blood γ/δ T cells lyse fresh human brain-derived oligodendrocytes. *Ann. Neurol.*, **30**, 794–800.
31. Raine, C.S. (1994) The immunology of multiple sclerosis lesions. *Ann. Neurol.*, **36**, 561–72.
32. Lampson, L.A. and Hickey, W.F. (1986) Monoclonal antibody analysis of the MHC expression in human brain biopsies: tissue ranging from 'histologically normal' to that showing different levels of glial tumour involvement. *J. Immunol.*, **136**, 4045–62.
33. Esiri, M.M. (1993) Role of the macrophage in HIV encephalitis, in *The Neuropathology of HIV Infection* (ed. F. Scaravilli), London, Springer, pp. 235–50.
34. Perry, V.H. and Gordon, S. (1988) Macrophages and microglia in the nervous system. *Trends Neurosci.*, **11**, 273–7.
35. Hayes, G.M., Woodroofe, M.N. and Cuzner, M.L. (1987) Microglia are the major cell type expressing MHC Class II in human white matter. *J. Neurol. Sci.*, **80**, 25–37.
36. Esiri, M.M. and Reading, M.C. (1987) Macrophage populations associated with multiple sclerosis plaques. *Neuropathol. Appl. Neurobiol.*, **13**, 451–65.
37. Traugott, U. and Raine, C.S. (1985) Multiple Sclerosis. Evidence for antigen presentation in situ by endothelial cells and astrocytes. *J. Neurol. Sci.*, **69**, 365–70.
38. Nyland, H., Mork, S. and Matre, R. (1985) Fc and receptors in multiple sclerosis brains. *Ann. NY Acad. Sci. (USA)*, **436**, 476–9.
39. Adams, C.W.M., Poston, R.N. and Buk, S.J. (1989) Pathology, histochemistry and immunocytochemistry of lesions in acute multiple sclerosis. *J. Neurol. Sci.*, **92**, 291–306.
40. Lee, S.C., Moore, G.R., Golenwsky, G. and Raine, C.S. (1990) Multiple sclerosis: a role for astroglia in active demyelination suggested by Class II MHC expression and ultrastructural study. *J. Neuropathol. Exp. Neurol.*, **49**, 123–36.
41. Sanders, V., Conrad, A.J. and Tourtellotte, W.W. (1993) On classification of post-mortem multiple sclerosis plaques for neuroscientists. *J. Neuroimmunol.*, **46**, 207–16.

42. Ulvestad, E., Williams, K., Mork, S., Antel, J. and Nyland, H. (1994) Phenotypic differences between human monocytes/macrophages and microglial cells studied in situ and in vitro. *J. Neuropathol. Exp. Neurol.*, 53, 492–501.

43. Bö, L., Mörk, S., Kong, P.A. *et al.* (1986) Detection of MHC class II antigens on macrophages and microglia but not on astrocytes and endothelia in active multiple sclerosis lesions. *J. Neuroimmunol.*, 51, 135–46.

44. Esiri, M.M. (1977) Immunoglobulin-containing cells in multiple sclerosis plaques. *Lancet*, ii, 478–80.

45. Esiri, M.M. (1980) Multiple sclerosis: a quantitative and qualitative study of immunoglobulin-containing cells in the central nervous system. *Neuropathol. Appl. Neurobiol*, 6, 9–21.

46. Prineas, J.W. and Wright, R.G. (1978) Macrophages, lymphocytes and plasma cells in the perivascular compartment in chronic multiple sclerosis. *Lab. Invest.*, 38, 409–21.

47. Lassmann, H., Suchanek, G. and Ozawa, K. (1994) Histopathology and blood-cerebrospinal fluid barrier in MS. *Ann. Neurol.*, 36, 542–6.

48. Traugott, U. and Lebon, P. (1988) Interferon-gamma and 1a antigen are present on astrocytes in multiple sclerosis lesions. *J. Neurol. Sci.*, 84, 257–64.

49. Hofman, F.M., Hinton, D.R., Johnson, K. and Merrill, J.E. (1989) Tumor necrosis factor identified in multiple sclerosis brain. *J. Exp. Med.*, 170, 607–12.

50. Parekh, R.B., Swek, R.A., Rademacher, T.W., Opdenakker, G. and Van Damme, J. (1992) Glycosylation of interleukin-6 purified from normal human blood mononuclear cells. *Eur. J. Biochem.*, 203, 135–41.

51. Lotz, M. and Guerne, P.-A. (1990) Interleukin-6 induces the synthesis of tissue inhibitor of metalloproteinases (TIMP-1/EPA). *J. Biol. Chem.*, 266, 2017–20.

52. Chantry, A. and Glynn, P. (1990) A novel metalloproteinase originally isolated from brain myelin membranes is present in many tissues. *Biochem. J.*, 268, 245–8.

53. Lumsden, C.E. (1971) The immunogenesis of the multiple sclerosis plaque. *Brain Res.*, 28, 365–90.

53a. Hays, A.P., Lee, S.S.L. and Latov, N. (1988) Immune reactive C3d on the surface of myelin sheaths in neuropathy. *J. Neuroimmunol.*, 18, 231–44.

54. Tavolato, B.F. (1975) Immunoglobulin G distribution in multiple sclerosis brain. An immunofluorescence study. *J. Neurol. Sci.*, 24, 1–11.

54a. Prineas, J.W. and Graham, J.S. (1981) Multiple sclerosis: capping of surface immunoglobulin G on macrophages engaged in myelin breakdown. *Ann. Neurol.*, 10, 149–58.

55. Mehta, P.D. *et al.* (1981) Bound antibody in multiple sclerosis brains. *J. Neurol. Sci.*, 49, 91–8.

56. Ma, B.I., Joseph, B.S., Walsh, M.J. *et al.* (1981) Immunoglobulin binding of multiple sclerosis serum and cerebrospinal fluid to Fc receptors of oligodendrocytes. *Ann. Neurol.*, 9, 371–81.

57. Aarli, J.A., Aparicio, S.R., Lumsden, C.E. and Tonder, O. (1975) Binding of normal human IgG to myelin sheaths, glia and neurons. *Immunology*, 28, 171–85.

58. Sindic, C.J., Cambiaso, C.L., Masson, P.L. and Laterre, E.C. (1980) The binding of myelin basic protein to the Fc region of aggregated IgG and to immune complexes. *Clin. Exp. Immunol.*, 41, 1–7.

59. Poston, R.N. (1984) Basic proteins bind immunoglobulin G; a mechanism for demyelinating disease? *Lancet*, i, 1268–71.

60. Morgan, B.P., Campbell, A.K. and Compston, D.A.S. (1984) Terminal component of complement (C9) in cerebrospinal fluid of patients with multiple sclerosis. *Lancet*, ii, 251–4.

61. Compston, D.A.S., Morgan, B.P., Campbell, A.K. *et al.* (1989) Immunocytochemical localisation of the terminal complement complex in multiple sclerosis. *Neuropathol. Appl. Neurobiol.*, 15, 307–16.

62. Gay, D. and Esiri, M.M. (1991) Blood–brain barrier damage in acute multiple sclerosis plaques. An immunocytochemical study. *Brain*, 114, 557–72.

63. Lee, S.C. and Raine, C.S. (1989) Multiple sclerosis: oligodendrocytes do not express Class II major histocompatibility molecules in active lesions. *J. Neuroimmunol.*, 25, 261–6.

64. Prineas, J.W., Kwon, E.E., Goldenberg, P.Z. *et al.* (1989) Multiple sclerosis: oligodendrocyte proliferation and differentiation in fresh lesions. *Lab. Invest.*, 61, 489–503.

65. Morris, C.S., Esiri, M.M., Sprinkle, T.J. and Gregson, N. (1994) Oligodendrocyte reactions and cell proliferation markers in human demyelinating diseases. *Neuropathol. Appl. Neurobiol.*, 20, 272–81.

66. Prineas, J.W., Barnard, R.O., Kwon, E.E., Sharer, L.R. and Cho, E.-S. (1993) Multiple sclerosis: remyelination of nascent lesions. *Ann. Neurol.*, 33, 137–51.

67. Wu, E. and Raine, C.S. (1992) Multiple sclerosis: interactions between oligodendrocytes and hypertrophic astrocytes and their occurrence in other non-demyelinating conditions. *Lab. Invest.*, 67, 88–99.

68. Wu, E., Brosnan, C.F. and Raine, C.S. (1993) SP-40, 40 immunoreactivity in inflammatory CNS lesions displaying astrocyte/oligodendrocyte interactions. *J. Neuropathol. Exp. Neurol.*, 52, 129–34.

69. Esiri, M.M. and Gay, D. (1990) Annotation: immunological and neuropathological significance of the Virchow–Robin space. *J. Neurol. Sci.*, 100, 3–8.

70. Clerici, M. and Shearer, G.M. (1994) The Th$_1$-Th$_2$ hypothesis of HIV infection. *Immunol. Today*, 15, 575–81.

71. Brosnan, C.F., Traugott, U. and Raine, C.S. (1983) Analysis of humoral and cellular events and the role of lipid haptens during CNS demyelination. *Acta Neuropathol. (Berlin)*, Suppl. 9, 59–70.

72. Linington, C., Berger, T., Perry, L. *et al.* (1993) T cells specific for the myelin oligodendrocyte glycoprotein mediate an unusual autoimmune inflammatory response in the central nervous system. *Eur. J. Immunol.*, 23, 1364–72.

73. Birnbaum, G., Kotilinek, L. and Albrecht, L. (1993) Spinal fluid lymphocytes from a subgroup of multiple sclerosis patients respond to mycobacterial antigens. *Ann. Neurol.*, 34, 18–24.

74. Smith, H. (1995) The revival of interest in mechanisms of bacterial pathogenicity. *Biol. Rev.*, 70, 277–316.

75. Burns, J., Littlefield, K., Gill, B.S. and Trotter, J.L. (1992) Bacterial toxin superantigens activate human T lymphocytes reactive with myelin autoantigens. *Ann. Neurol.*, 32, 352–7.

76. Brocke, S., Gaur, A., Plercy, C. *et al.* (1993) Induction of relapsing paralysis in experimental autoimmune encephalomyelitis by bacterial superantigen. *Nature*, 365, 642–4.

77. Scolding, N.J. and Compston, D.A.S. (1991) Oligodendrocyte-macrophage interactions *in vitro* triggered by specific antibodies. *Immunology*, 72, 127–32.

78. Merrill, J.E. and Zimmerman, R.P. (1991) Natural and induced cytotoxicity of oligodendrocytes by microglia is inhibitable by TGFβ. *Glia*, 4, 327–31.

79. Antel, J.P., Williams, K., Blain, M., McRea, E. and McLaurian, J.A. (1994) Oligodendrocyte lysis by CD4 + T cells independent of tumour necrosis factor. *Ann. Neurol.*, 35, 341–8.

80. Pringle, N.P., Mudhar, H.S., Collarini, E.J. and Richardson, W.D. (1992) PDGF receptors in the rat CNS: during late neurogenesis PDGF alpha receptor expression appears to be restricted to glial cells of the oligodendrocyte lineage. *Development*, 115, 535–51.

81. Kememy, D.M., Noble, A., Holmes, B.J. and Diaz-Sanchez, D. (1994) Immune regulation: a new role for the CD8 + T cell. *Immunol. Today*, 15, 107–10.

82. Raine, C.S. and Scheinberg, L.C. (1988) On the immunopathology of plaque development and repair in multiple sclerosis. *J. Neuroimmunol.*, 120, 189–201.

83. Johnson, R.T., Burke, D.S., Elwell, M. *et al.* (1985) Japanese encephalitis: immunocytochemical studies of viral antigen and inflammatory cells in fatal cases. *Ann. Neurol.*, 18, 567–73.

84. Sobel, R.A., Collins, A.B., Colvin, R.B. and Bhan, A.K. (1986) The in situ cellular immune response in acute herpes simplex encephalitis. *Am. J. Pathol.*, 125, 332–8.

85. Esiri, M.M., Oppenheimer, D.R., Brownell, B. and Haire, M. (1981) Distribution of measles antigen and immunoglobulin-containing cells in the CNS in subacute sclerosing panencephalitis (SSPE) and atypical measles encephalitis. *J. Neurol. Sci.*, 53, 29–43.

86. Kreth, H.W., Dunker, R., Rodt, H. and Meyermann, R. (1982) Immunohistochemical identification of T-lymphocytes in the central nervous system of patients with multiple sclerosis and subacute sclerosing panencephalitis. *J. Neuroimmunol.*, 2, 177–83.

87. Hofman, F.M., Hinton, D.R., Baemayr, J., Weil, M. and Merrill, J.E. (1991) Lymphokines and immunoregulatory molecules in subacute sclerosing panencephalitis. *Clin. Immunol. Immunopathol.*, 58, 331–42.

88. Nagano, I., Nakamura, S., Yoshioka, M. *et al.* (1994) Expression of cytokines in brain lesions in subacute sclerosing panencephalitis. *Neurology*, 44, 710–15.

89. Griffin, D.E., Moser, H.W., Mendoza, Q. *et al.* (1985) Identification of the inflammatory cells in the central nervous system of patients with adrenoleukodystrophy. *Ann. Neurol.*, 18, 660–4.

90. Esiri, M.M., Reading, M.C., Squier, M.V. and Hughes, J.T. (1989) Immunocytochemical characterisation of the macrophage and lymphocyte infiltrate in the brains of 6 cases of human encephalitis of varied aetiology. *Neuropathol. Appl. Neurobiol.*, 15, 289–305.

91. Esiri, M.M. (1980) Poliomyelitis: immunoglobulin-containing cells in the central nervous system in acute and convalescent phases of the human disease. *Clin. Exp. Immunol.*, 40, 42–8.

92. Esiri, M.M. (1983) Immunohistological studies of immunoglobulin-containing cells and viral antigen in some inflammatory diseases of the nervous system, in *Immunology of Nervous System-Infections* (eds P.O. Behan, V. ter Meulen and F. Clifford Rose), *Progress in Brain Research*, 59, pp. 209–19.

93. Tyor, W.R., Glass, J.D., Griffin, J.W. *et al.* (1992) Cytokine expression in the brain during the acquired immunodeficiency syndrome. *Ann. Neurol.* 31, 349–60.

94. Glass, J.D. Wesselingh, S.L., Selnes, O.A. and McArthur, J.C. (1993) Clinical-neuropathologic correlation in HIV-associated dementia. *Neurology* 43, 2230–7.

95. Stanley, L.G., Mrak, R.E., Woody, R.C. *et al.* (1994) Glial cytokines as neuropathogenic factors in HIV infection: pathogenic similarities to Alzheimer's disease. *J. Neuropathol. Exp. Neurol.* 53, 231–8.

96. Sottel, A., Ronthal, M. and Ross, D.B. (1983) Subacute sclerosing panencephalitis: an immune complex disease? *Neurology*, 33, 885–90.

11 GENES AND DEVELOPMENT OF MYELIN-FORMING CELLS

Greg Lemke

11.1 Introduction

The debilitating nature of multiple sclerosis (MS) starkly highlights the importance of myelin-forming cells. These are, by number and function, among the most significant cellular constituents of higher nervous systems. Until recently, however, little was known with regard to the details of their lineage, development and differentiation. This situation is now rapidly changing – thanks to molecular investigations centered on myelin structure, myelin protein biochemistry, and more recently, myelin molecular genetics. As a consequence, the development of oligodendrocytes in the central nervous system (CNS) and Schwann cells in the peripheral nervous system (PNS) is currently the focus of considerable attention.

This attention and interest is in part due to the fact that oligodendrocytes and Schwann cells can be purified in bulk, using immunoselection and other techniques, from the brains and peripheral nerves of mice, rats, sheep, fish and humans (among others), and cultured as homogeneous populations *in vitro*. Under appropriate conditions, these cultured cells are capable of playing out their full program of differentiation, including the myelination of axons, a feature that has made myelination a useful general model for studying developmental interactions in the nervous system.

In addition, many of the genes unique to myelinating cells, whose protein products are used specifically for myelination, have now been cloned. Some of these proteins are essential structural elements of the myelin sheath itself; others appear to be involved in myelin assembly. Some act at early stages in the development of myelinating cells, and may be critical regulators of myelin gene expression; others function in fully differentiated cells. Together with recent studies of the molecular genetics of inherited hypomyelinating and demyelinating diseases, the molecular analysis of myelination has provided a number of important general insights into outstanding problems in neurobiology, such as the structure and function of cell adhesion molecules, and the regulation of neural cell development and differentiation. In this chapter, I will consider a number of illustrative examples of the structural and regulatory molecules involved in myelination, and of the ways in which these molecules mark and mediate the development of Schwann cells and oligodendrocytes.

11.2 Myelinating cell types and their organelles

The two cell types charged with the task of myelin formation, oligodendrocytes and Schwann cells, have distinct developmental origins in the neural tube and neural crest, respectively. The myelin organelles that these cell types elaborate are also morphologically and molecularly distinct, although their structure and function are, to a first approximation, similar. In the electron microscope, both CNS and PNS myelin in cross-section appear as highly regular, tightly wrapped spirals of membrane that are contiguous with the plasma membranes of oligodendrocytes and Schwann cells, and that ensheathe and insulate large diameter axons. Topologically, the repeatedly wrapped lamellae of myelin are often analogized to a rolled-up sleeping bag, in that when a sleeping bag is rolled, two distinct surface appositions are created – one resulting from the interface between the inner surfaces of the sleeping bag, and another from the interface between its outer surfaces. In a myelin-forming cell, the inner interface corresponds to the association of apposed cytoplasmic membrane surfaces (often referred to by microscopists as the 'major dense line'), while the outer interface corresponds to apposed extracellular membrane surfaces (the 'intraperiod line'). A key feature of myelin is the compaction of the sheath that occurs at these two membrane interfaces – the total cross-sectional 'repeat period' from one point in the myelin sheath to the next topologically equivalent point (e.g. from one major dense line to the next) is only of the order of 150Å.

Multiple Sclerosis: Clinical and pathogenetic basis. Edited by Cedric S. Raine, Henry F. McFarland and Wallace W. Tourtellotte. Published in 1997 by Chapman & Hall, London. ISBN 0 412 30890 8.

To arrive at this compacted spiral organelle – whose appearance marks the end-stage of oligodendrocyte and Schwann cell differentiation – myelinating glia must undergo a spectacular topological reorganization. The initial wrap of the sheath about the axonal membrane is always constrained in the same fashion – tucked under, between the myelinating cell body and the axon. This initial tuck results in a final structure in which the myelin sheath is always interposed between the axon and the cell body (cytoplasm and nucleus) of the myelinating cell. As a result of the enormous amount of membrane synthesized during myelination, the total membrane surface area of a myelinating cell may increase several thousand-fold during the process.

While the overall appearance of CNS and PNS myelin sheaths is similar, there are none the less important differences in the repertoire of myelin structural proteins contained in these sheaths (summarized below), and in the number of myelin organelles that Schwann cells and oligodendrocytes elaborate. A given Schwann cell forms a single myelin sheath around a single axon. In contrast, oligodendrocytes have the remarkable capacity to elaborate independent myelin sheaths, individually, around multiple axons. This means that damage to a single oligodendrocyte, as occurs in CNS demyelinating diseases, may have the devastating effect of demyelination of a relatively large number of axons.

11.3   Myelin-specific genes and their protein products

The myelin proteins that have received the greatest attention thus far are structural components of the sheath. The most abundant in terms of their representation in myelin – often referred to as the 'major myelin proteins' – are protein zero (P_0), proteolipid protein (PLP) and myelin basic protein (MBP). Other myelin-specific or myelin-restricted proteins of demonstrated or presumed importance to the development or mature function of myelin-forming cells include peripheral myelin protein 22 (PMP22), myelin-associated glycoprotein (MAG), oligodendrocyte-myelin glycoprotein (OMgp)[1], $2'3'$ cyclic nucleotide $3'$ phosphodiesterase (CNP)[2–4], myelin oligodendrocyte glycoprotein (MOG)[5], P_2[6] and several additional proteins recently identified through differential cDNA cloning[7]. With the exception of CNP and P_2 all of these proteins are structural components of the myelin sheath.

11.3.1   PROTEIN ZERO (P_0)

Protein zero (P_0) is the most abundant protein of peripheral myelin[8]. Its expression in higher (but not lower) vertebrates is absolutely restricted to PNS myelin[9], where it accounts for >50% of the protein in

the organelle. Neither P_0 protein nor RNA has been detected in any cell type other than Schwann cells. The structure of P_0 is reminiscent of other simple transmembrane glycoproteins – it contains an amino-terminal signal sequence, followed by a relatively hydrophobic and glycosylated immunoglobulin (Ig)-related extracellular domain, a single transmembrane domain bounded by charged residues, and a highly basic carboxy-terminal intracellular domain [10, 11]. This structure and orientation places the P_0 extracellular domain at the intraperiod line of the myelin sheath, and the intracellular domain at the major dense line. Like many proteins that contain Ig domains, the P_0 extracellular domain has the ability to serve as a homophilic recognition molecule that binds to itself in a calcium-independent manner.

P_0 is the main protein responsible for intraperiod line compaction in peripheral myelin. This conclusion has been drawn from cell adhesion experiments using P_0-negative (P_0^-) cell lines that have been stably transfected with the rat P_0 cDNA [12, 13], and more definitively, from the observed ultrastructural phenotype of myelin in mice that lack P_0 (generated through homologous recombination in embryonic stem cells)[14]. These mice fail to achieve normal myelination as a result of a failure of intraperiod line compaction. Although they exhibit a striking neurological phenotype manifested by poor motor coordination, tremors and occasional convulsions that develop after the third postnatal week, P_0-deficient mice are none the less viable for many months under laboratory conditions. The failure of intraperiod line compaction in P_0-deficient mice corroborates the structural and biochemical evidence that P_0 functions as a homophilic adhesion molecule responsible for intraperiod line compaction. In addition, evidence from single and double-mutants at the P_0 and *shiverer* (MBP deletion) loci (see below), suggest that P_0 and MBP may cooperate to bring about compaction at the major dense line as well. These demonstrations of the importance of P_0 to peripheral myelination in mouse mutants have been reinforced by the finding that the inherited demyelinating neuropathy Charcot–Marie–Tooth disease 1B (CMT1B) results from mutations in the P_0 gene (see below). In addition to its dramatic effect on peripheral myelination, loss of P_0 appears to result in secondary effects on Schwann cell gene expression, such as the failure to down-regulate expression of certain (but not all) genes that normally mark early Schwann cell progenitors and non-myelinating Schwann cells (see below)[14].

11.3.2   PROTEOLIPID PROTEIN

Proteolipid protein is the major structural component of CNS myelin, accounting for ~50% of its protein[15]. It appears to have been one of the last neural-specific proteins to have arisen during the course of vertebrate evolution. The product of a single copy gene on the X chromosome, from which two alternatively spliced mRNAs are produced, PLP exists as an ~ 30 kD protein and as a smaller 26 kD protein designated DM-20[16]. Both oligodendrocytes and Schwann cells express PLP, although Schwann cells express very much less; the protein is not detectable in other cell types, although neurons express structurally related proteins designated M6a and M6b[17,18]. PLP is predicted to span the myelin membrane multiple times (four or five, in differing models), in a manner reminiscent of gap junction subunits[15,19,20]. It is therefore likely to display non-membrane domains at both the major dense and intraperiod lines.

The sequence conservation of PLP between different species is striking – there are no amino acid differences between the mouse, rat and human proteins. This conservation, together with the genetic data discussed below, suggests a rigorous structure–function relation for PLP that is not well understood. In spite of the lack of detailed knowledge as to PLP function, it is clear that the protein is critically involved in at least two different stages of oligodendrocyte development – first during normal oligodendrocyte differentiation, when absence of PLP results in premature cell death and subsequent hypomyelination, and secondly during myelination, when PLP may help to mediate myelin compaction at the intraperiod line in the CNS. These conclusions have been drawn almost exclusively from studies on the myriad of naturally occurring mutations in the *PLP* gene, which have been identified in a variety of vertebrate species[21–27].

With only a few exceptions (the well-known *jimpy* mouse being an important one), these mutations involve single base missense changes that alter single amino acids within the PLP protein. Most affect the putative membrane-spanning regions of the protein, and a number account for a set of lethal X-linked myelination disorders in humans, known collectively as Pelizaeus–Merzbacher disease (PMD)[28–31]. Manifested by nystagmus and head tremor in the neonatal period, followed by ataxia and myoclonic seizures, the connatal form of PMD generally results in death by the age of 3. The CNS of a patient with PMD is essentially devoid of myelin, although the PNS is to a first approximation normal.

Mutations in the mouse *PLP* gene typically result in CNS demyelination or hypomyelination, but also lead to an earlier developmental phenotype – the widespread degeneration and death of oligodendrocytes. For example, the *jimpy* mouse exhibits premature oligodendrocyte cell death during postnatal CNS development prior to the onset of myelination, yielding a markedly reduced number of oligodendrocytes in the mature animal relative to wild-type. These observations have been interpreted to suggest a role for PLP/DM-20 in oligodendrocyte development prior to the elaboration and final compaction of CNS myelin. DM-20, in particular, has been cast in this role, since it is abundant relative to full-length PLP during CNS embryogenesis[32]. An important exception to the dual effects of PLP mutations is seen in the mouse mutant *rumpshaker*[33]. Phenotypically, this mouse possesses dramatically reduced levels of CNS myelin, yet exhibits a nearly normal life span. *Rumpshaker* oligodendrocytes do not exhibit the early degeneration and cell death seen in *jimpy* and other PLP mutants, but remain compromised in their ability to elaborate CNS myelin. This mutant also results from a single base pair change (in exon 4 of the PLP gene, within sequence encoding a putative transmembrane domain). It has been speculated that the *rumpshaker* mutation may spare the 'early' developmental function of PLP/DM-20, while compromising its 'late' function in intraperiod line compaction of CNS myelin[27]. A clear mechanistic appreciation of the late versus early functions of PLP remains lacking.

11.3.3 MYELIN BASIC PROTEIN

Myelin basic protein (MBP) is the second most prominent component of both CNS and PNS myelin. MBP actually represents a family of small, very basic proteins (most < 20 kD) that arise from alternative splicing of a single elemental gene containing seven exons[34], which is in turn part of a much larger transcription unit. This larger gene – designated *golli-MBP* – contains transcribed sequences from several exons upstream of the elemental gene, and is capable of generating a myriad of distinct transcripts, some of which are likely to encode additional proteins[35]. Although the importance of MBP to myelination is undisputed (see below), the functional significance of the large variety of different MBP isoforms remains unclear, and they are generally referred to collectively as 'MBP'.

Unlike the other major myelin proteins, MBP is not a transmembrane protein but an exclusively cytoplasmic, extrinsic membrane protein that is localized to the major dense line of myelin. Multiple lines of evidence indicate that MBP acts at the major dense line to compact the myelin sheath. Perhaps the strongest of these comes from studies on two naturally occurring MBP mouse mutants, the best known of which is *shiverer*. The phenotype of *shiverer* homozygotes includes an early generalized intention tremor, followed by progressively increasing convulsions, and death 50–100 days after birth. These mice essentially lack CNS myelin. Where present, it appears as dysmorphic whorls of membrane that are tightly compacted at the intraperiod line, but uncompacted at what would normally be the major dense line.

No MBP mRNA or protein is detectable in *shiverer* homozygotes, and molecular analysis of the mutation reveals an ~20 kb deletion that removes most of the *MBP* gene [36, 37]; re-introduction of the wild-type *MBP* gene into *shiverer* mice rescues the mutant phenotype [38, 39]. The mechanism by which MBP promotes membrane compaction at the major dense line is unknown. Both homophilic interactions between apposed MBP molecules and electrostatic interactions between MBP and apposed acidic lipids have been advanced as possibilities [40]. The lack of a strong ultrastructural or behavioral phenotype associated with the PNS myelin of *shiverer* homozygotes has led to the suggestion that a PNS-specific myelin protein is capable of substituting for MBP in its absence, and the basic cytoplasmic domain of P_0 has been put forward as a candidate molecule for this function [10]. Recent double mutant analyses, involving the generation of $MBP^{-/-}/P_0^{-/-}$ mice, support this hypothesis [41].

11.3.4 MYELIN-ASSOCIATED GLYCOPROTEIN

The myelin-associated glycoprotein (MAG) is a myelin-specific protein that accounts for roughly 1% of myelin protein in the CNS, and somewhat less in the PNS. Two different isoforms exist, which represent alternatively spliced products from a single copy gene, and contain cytoplasmic domains encoded by either of two exons [42–44]. Like P_0, MAG is a member of the Ig superfamily, although its significantly larger size and overall configuration are closer to prototypical members of the superfamily, such as N-CAM and L-1 [45]. The protein contains a small cytoplasmic domain, a single transmembrane domain and a large extracellular domain composed of five homologous and tandemly configured Ig repeats. In marked contrast to the major myelin proteins, MAG is present in the non-compacted regions of myelin. These regions include the innermost layer of the sheath (immediately adjacent to the axon, and known as the inner mesaxon), the outermost layer (the outer mesaxon), and other non-compacted regions such as the paranodal loops and Schmidt–Lanterman incisures. Given its localization to the inner mesaxon and its early expression prior to the onset of overt myelination, MAG has been hypothesized to act as an adhesion molecule that might mediate axon–glial recognition events that precede myelination in both the CNS and PNS. Experiments with MAG knock-out mice, however, have called this possibility, as well as the overall importance of MAG to myelination, into question (46, 47). Mice that lack MAG develop normally, and have, at least to a first approximation, normally myelinated axons in both the CNS and PNS, although subtle abnormalities in CNS myelination have been noted by some workers. The possibility that other Ig-related recognition proteins might compensate for MAG in its absence remains a viable one.

11.3.5 PERIPHERAL MYELIN PROTEIN 22

Unlike the myelin-specific proteins mentioned above, peripheral myelin protein 22 (PMP22) was first identified as a gene induced in NIH3T3 fibroblasts upon growth arrest in culture, and was therefore designated gas3, for growth arrest specific gene 3 [48]. Two groups later identified this same gene when using techniques to clone mRNAs (cDNAs) that are induced or downregulated in Schwann cells following peripheral nerve transection or crush injury [49, 50]. cDNAs for PMP22 predict a protein of ~17 kD that does not exhibit significant primary structure homology to previously described proteins, except for weak homology to a variety of membrane proteins. In its secondary structure, however, PMP22 is predicted to span the membrane four times, in a manner analogous to that of gap junction subunits, and not dissimilar to that of PLP [48]. Although not a myelin-specific protein *per se*, PMP22 is abundantly expressed by myelinating Schwann cells, which are probably the predominant site of synthesis in adult mammals [51]. Detailed mechanistic insights into PMP22 function are lacking, but much speculation has centered on its potential as a gap-junction-like ion channel or pore.

As for PLP, MBP and P_0, studies of naturally occurring mutations have provided what is perhaps the most satisfying demonstration of the importance of PMP22 to peripheral myelination [52]. Prominent among these has been the *Trembler* mutation in the mouse, and Charcot–Marie–Tooth disease (CMT), the most common inherited peripheral neuropathy in humans. *Trembler (Tr)* is an autosomal semi-dominant mutation that maps to mouse chromosome 11, and presents as a Schwann cell autonomous defect characterized by dramatic peripheral nerve hypomyelination and continuous Schwann cell proliferation into adulthood [53–56]. *Trembler* mice carry a point mutation in the PMP22 gene [57]. Like most of the characterized PLP mutations, this PMP22 mutation is a single base missense mutation within a putative membrane-spanning domain, in this case the fourth such domain; a distinct allele of *Trembler*, known as *Trembler^J* carries an independent point mutation in the *PMP22* gene, a missense mutation within the first membrane-spanning domain [58].

The region of mouse chromosome 11 that contains the *Trembler* mutations is syntenic with a region on the short arm of human chromosome 17 that contains the locus for Charcot–Marie–Tooth disease Type 1A (CMT1A) [59, 60]. Patients with this disease present with progressive distal muscle weakness and atrophy, distal sensory impairment and tremor. Their peripheral nerves show markedly decreased conduction velocities, and nerve biopsies reveal segmental demyelination, partial remyelination and Schwann cell proliferation [61]. The most common CMT1A mutation is not a point mutation, but instead a relatively large (> 1 megabase) interstitial duplication of the chromosomal region that contains the *PMP22* gene [62–64]. This represents the first known example of a dominantly inherited human disorder that arises from a large scale DNA duplication. The phenotype of CMT1A is believed to result from increased dosage (1.5 × normal) of the normal PMP22 protein. Interestingly, a related but milder inherited peripheral neuropathy – hereditary neuropathy with liability to pressure palsies (HNPP) – results from the corresponding meiotic recombination event that results in *decreased* dosage (0.5 × normal) of the *PMP22* gene [65]. Thus, either increased or diminished expression of PMP22 appears to result in dysmyelinating neuropathies. Interestingly, point mutations (and an in-frame 3-base deletion) within sequences encoding the Ig domain of P_0 have been implicated in the related disorder CMT1B [66].

11.4 Cellular origins, development and differentiation

11.4.1 SCHWANN CELL DIFFERENTIATION

To a significant extent, analysis of the developmental regulation of the myelin-related genes discussed above has motivated the molecular study of Schwann cell and oligodendrocyte lineages. Like the majority of cell types that eventually make up the PNS, Schwann cells originate in the embryonic neural crest, the migratory population of cells that arise at the dorsal surface of the closing neural tube [45]. Following initial migration along the ventral (somitic) neural crest cell pathway and an attendant series of cell divisions, a subpopulation of crest cells gives rise to committed Schwann cell progenitors. These progenitor cells proliferate in the peripheral ganglia and peripheral nerves in which they soon take up residence, and are thought to pass through several distinct phases prior to their final differentiation (see below) [67,68]. In response to appropriate axonal cues, they eventually differentiate into one of two distinct Schwann cell phenotypes – 'myelinating' and 'non-myelinating'. As their name implies, non-myelinating Schwann cells do not produce myelin, but instead enwrap numerous smaller diameter axons (such as pain and temperature fibers and those of the sympathetic trunk) within individual troughs of Schwann cell membrane. In most mammals (rodents are the best studied), the various phases of Schwann cell differentiation take place during the last half of embryogenesis and the first few weeks of postnatal life.

Progenitor, non-myelinating and myelinating Schwann cells are each characterized by the expression of a distinct set of gene products. The phenotype of progenitor Schwann cells, also referred to as Schwann cell precursors, has been most carefully analyzed in the developing peripheral nerves of rodents [69]. Like most migratory trunk neural crest cells, these cells express relatively high levels of the low affinity p75 nerve growth factor (NGF) receptor. Within the nerve, their commitment to a Schwann cell fate appears to be marked by the acquired expression of the gene encoding growth-associated protein 43 (GAP-43), which is activated before embryonic day 14 in rats, and which is not expressed by multipotent neural crest cells themselves. The first distinctive marker of Schwann cells to appear in peripheral nerve development is the calcium binding protein S100, whose expression is activated about two days later (around E16 in the rat sciatic nerve) [69]. Schwann cell progenitors also express a variety of other markers that are not significantly expressed at later times by myelinating cells; these include certain voltage-sensitive sodium channels, the transcription factor c-*jun*, and the cell adhesion proteins N-CAM and L1. In addition, these cells also appear to express very low but clearly detectable levels of at least some end-stage myelin genes. The best example of this is seen for P_0 in chick neural crest derivatives, where a sensitive P_0 antibody, together with PCR techniques, has been used to detect P_0 expression in neural crest cells at very early stages in their migration from the neural tube [70]. It is possible that this low level of expression simply reflects a 'preparatory' activation of the chromosomal region around the P_0 gene, which will be expressed at massively higher levels much later in development.

11.4.2 MYELINATING VERSUS NON-MYELINATING SCHWANN CELLS

Late in embryogenesis (in the nerves of mice and rats) developing Schwann cells reach a critical decision point, at which they adopt either a final myelinating or a non-myelinating phenotype. The genes expressed at high levels by the former encode the unique myelin genes described above (e.g. the P_0 and *MBP* genes). In contrast, non-myelinating Schwann cells in mature nerves, with certain exceptions, express the same repertoire of markers as Schwann cell progenitors. That is, they are positive for expression of p75, NCAM etc., but are to a first approximation negative for the major myelin genes. This finding has led to the notion that non-myelinating Schwann cells are to some extent 'stalled out' in the differentiation pathway that normally leads to myelination. Although there is validity to this view, it is also true that mature non-myelinating Schwann cells eventually express certain markers that are *not* characteristic of Schwann cell progenitors, including the intermediate filament protein GFAP and galactocerebrocide (GalC), which is often used as a marker of a myelinating phenotype. It is important to note that the alternative Schwann cell phenotype – the myelin-forming cell – involves *both* the high level activation of myelin genes and the concomitant down-regulation of the genes that mark Schwann cell progenitors and mature non-myelinating cells. Thus, mature myelinating cells are both P_0^- and MBP-positive, and at the same time negative for p75 and NCAM.

Several lines of evidence suggest that the choice of a myelinating versus a non-myelinating cell fate is imposed on Schwann cells by their association with axons. The features of the axon that control Schwann cell phenotype are not well understood in molecular terms, but one important parameter is axon diameter [71]. Contact with a small diameter axon (< 1 μm) almost invariably results in differentiation into a non-myelinating Schwann cell, whereas contact with a large diameter axon (> 1 μm) results in a myelin-forming cell. It is possible that these phenomena reflect the action of a myelination inducer whose concentration on the axonal surface is fixed per unit area, and that a critical threshold of signaling delivered through this inducer must be achieved in order to result in myelination. Thus, developing Schwann cells in contact with small diameter axons would be subjected to sub-threshold levels of the inducer, and would 'stall out' in the myelination differentiation pathway. Both the establishment of the myelinating phenotype and its maintenance depend on continuous contact with axons. If fully differentiated myelinating Schwann cells are deprived of axonal contact (e.g. when axons degenerate following transection of a myelinated peripheral nerve), they are observed to de-differentiate back to a progenitor cell phenotype [72, 73]. Thus, in contrast to terminally differentiated cells such as neurons, Schwann cells exhibit a remarkable degree of phenotypic plasticity, which is thought to be a crucial feature enabling these cells to promote peripheral nerve regeneration.

11.4.3   SIGNAL TRANSDUCTION EVENTS

Although the molecules underlying axonal regulation of Schwann cell phenotype are largely unknown, it is now clear that elevation of intracellular cyclic AMP (cAMP) in Schwann cells cultured *in vitro* mimics many of the effects of axons on Schwann cells *in vivo* [74]. Thus, expression of myelin genes is up-regulated by cAMP elevation in cultured cells at the same time that expression of many early genes (e.g. *GAP-43* and c-*jun*) is markedly *down*-regulated. The down-regulation of early genes is in most cases pronounced, whereas the up-regulation of myelin genes is less so. Similarly, under appropriate conditions, cAMP is a potent Schwann cell mitogen, an effect that also mimics that of axons [75].

These and other observations support the notion that cAMP is an important second messenger in axonal signaling.

In addition to gene expression, axons also regulate Schwann cell proliferation. At least three distinct phases of Schwann cell division can be defined [76, 77]. As mentioned above, the first of these occurs embryonically during the period when committed Schwann cell progenitors expand in number to populate peripheral nerves. This phase ends well prior to the initiation of myelin formation. A second phase ensues during the period that precedes the onset of myelination, occurring as a transient burst of proliferation that lasts for several days during the late embryonic and early neonatal period in rodents. Following this period, Schwann cells (both myelinating and non-myelinating) become quiescent. A third phase of proliferation may occur in response to peripheral nerve injury or transection. This phase is also transient, and as described above, results in Schwann cell de-differentiation. At least three polypeptide mitogens – platelet-derived growth factor (PDGF), basic fibroblast growth factor (bFGF) and glial growth factor (GGF) – are likely to underlie one or more of these proliferative phases [78]. All of these molecules act as soluble, diffusible Schwann cell mitogens *in vitro*. Their action is markedly potentiated by elevation of intracellular cAMP, a mitogen that works exclusively by up-regulating expression of the PDGF, bFGF and GGF receptors [75]. In addition to its effects as a soluble protein, GGF is also expressed *in vivo* as a transmembrane protein [79] and recent experiments suggest that this membrane-bound form of GGF is the long-studied neurite mitogen active on Schwann cells in culture [80, 81]. Together, these results suggest that neurons regulate Schwann cell proliferation both by providing mitogenic ligands and by up-regulating Schwann cell expression of the receptors for these ligands.

11.4.4   OLIGODENDROCYTE DIFFERENTIATION

Oligodendrocytes arise from a progenitor cell that is often referred to as the O-2A cell [82]. This progenitor is bipotential in culture, where it gives rise to either oligodendrocytes or type-2 astrocytes, depending on culture conditions. The existence of type-2 astrocytes *in vivo* remains controversial, however – there is little evidence that cells with this molecular phenotype actually arise *in vivo*, and the progenitor may in fact only give rise to oligodendrocytes in the developing CNS. Oligodendrocyte progenitors appear to originate in precisely delimited locations within the early neural tube, and then to migrate, much as Schwann cell progenitors do in the PNS, to their final sites of differentiation.

The initial site of oligodendrocyte progenitor specification in the developing spinal cord has been inferred from *in situ* hybridization analyses with probes for either the PDGFα receptor (expressed by oligodendrocyte progenitors *in vitro* and *in vivo*) or for certain myelination markers such as O1, O4, CNP and DM-20, the 'early' form of PLP [83, 84]. These studies have localized early progenitors to two symmetric pools of cells in the mid-ventral thoracic and cervical spinal cord at around embryonic day 14 in the rat; these pools rapidly enlarge and give rise to migratory, dividing progeny. These cells are very similar in their morphology, migratory activity and proliferation to their O-2A counterparts *in vitro*. As for Schwann cells, proliferation of oligodendrocyte progenitors during their migration is robust. Similarly, oligodendrocyte progenitors divide in response to some of the same growth factors that regulate Schwann cell division (e.g. PDGF and bFGF) [85]. In marked contrast to Schwann cells, however, differentiation of oligodendrocytes into myelin-forming cells in culture is largely independent of the presence or absence of axons, and the role of cAMP in this process is apparently marginal. In neuron-free cultures, oligodendrocyte progenitor cells follow a time course of differentiation (the so-called 'developmental clock') that is very similar to the time course observed in the animal, and give rise to oligodendrocytes that eventually express the myelin genes at high levels and that elaborate extensive sheets of myelin-like membrane. Although oligodendrocytes cultured under appropriate conditions *in vitro* differentiate, their survival and differentiation *in vivo* (at least in the developing optic nerve) clearly depend on the presence of factors provided by axons [85]. Careful analysis of the time course of expression of various markers, particularly GalC and the myelin proteins, together with well-described changes in cell morphology and proliferation state, have delimited intermediate stages of oligodendrocyte development prior to their full differentiation as myelin-forming cells [86]. Once committed to a myelinating phenotype, oligodendrocytes are not obviously able to de-differentiate, and thus exhibit little of the phenotypic plasticity displayed by Schwann cells.

11.4.5 TRANSCRIPTIONAL CONTROL OF SCHWANN CELL AND OLIGODENDROCYTE DEVELOPMENT

During myelination, a large battery of myelin-specific genes that were previously dormant become coordinately activated. In the case of the major myelin genes, this activation results in exceptionally high levels of expression. In principle, elevation of myelin protein expression could be achieved by two distinct mechanisms: transcriptional (the production of messenger RNA) and post-transcriptional (e.g. regulation of the stability or translation of messenger RNA). Although evidence does exist for some degree of post-transcriptional regulation [87], these mechanisms are not sufficient to account for the dramatic qualitative shifts in myelin gene expression that occur during the onset of myelination.

A commonly used approach for identifying transcription factors is to first identify the regions of DNA that regulate gene expression [88]. These regulatory regions, which typically lie immediately upstream of protein coding regions and contain the transcription factor binding sites needed for expression of a gene, have been analyzed *in vivo* for the *MBP* [89], *PLP* [90], and P_0 [91] genes. The upstream (5' flanking) regulatory regions of these genes have been shown to direct appropriate expression of heterologous reporter genes when tested in transgenic animals. A consistent finding of the MBP transgenic experiments reported thus far has been the relatively poor expression of transgenes in Schwann cells compared to oligodendrocytes, although native MBP is well expressed in both cell types. This suggests that a separate enhancer may be required for Schwann cell expression, and that this enhancer may not be located immediately 5' to the gene [89, 92, 93]. The 5' P_0 regulatory region is clearly capable of directing quantitative Schwann cell-specific expression of reporter genes when transfected into cultured cells or expressed in transgenic mice, although expression levels in mice have been highly variable from line to line. None the less, this DNA fragment has served as an effective tool for the targeting of transgenes specifically to myelinating Schwann cells, with a developmental time course of expression that mirrors that of the endogenous P_0 gene [91, 94].

11.4.6 TRANSCRIPTION FACTORS

The identification and analysis of transcription factors that directly regulate expression of myelin-specific genes is still at an early stage, but several proteins of interest have thus far been studied. The first of these is a POU domain transcription factor designated SCIP (an acronym for suppressed cAMP inducible POU), which was discovered using an approach designed to identify POU domain proteins expressed in myelinating cells [73, 95]. Also known as Oct-6 and testes-1, SCIP is expressed throughout the developing embryonic nervous system, and later becomes restricted in its expression to limited cell types, including Schwann cells and oligodendrocytes; it is strongly induced in cultured Schwann cells by cAMP. Its transient developmental expression within these cells *in vivo* is particularly interesting – SCIP is detectable in late-dividing Schwann cell (and oligodendrocyte) progenitors and in 'pro-myelinating' cells that have left the cell cycle but not yet differentiated, but is not found in mature myelinating cells. Consistent with this pattern of expression, SCIP acts as a transcriptional repressor of myelin-specific genes in transfection assays, and a dominant-negative antagonist of the wild-type SCIP protein, when expressed in Schwann cells in transgenic mice, triggers premature Schwann cell differentiation and hypermyelination [96, 97]. Thus, SCIP may serve to hold developing Schwann cells in an immature, pre-differentiated phenotype.

A second transcription factor of interest is MyTI (for myelin transcription factor I), which was isolated using a binding site from the PLP promoter that was known to be important for promoter activity *in vitro* [98]. MyTI is a member of a class of transcriptional regulators that contain a motif known as the zinc finger. MyTI expression is highly enriched in the developing nervous system, and precedes the onset of myelination in the CNS, consistent with its presumed role in PLP gene expression. Binding experiments demonstrated that MyTI binds specifically to sites in the PLP promoter that are essential for promoter activity in glial cells. Like SCIP, MyTI expression is relatively low in fully differentiated oligodendrocytes, but appears to be expressed at its highest levels in proliferative O-2A progenitors.

A transcription factor with an expression pattern that is more consistent with a role in myelin gene activation is Gtx (for glial- and testis-specific homeobox gene) [99]. As its name suggests, Gtx is expressed in glial cells and in the testes. In primary glial cell cultures and in the animal, Gtx is clearly expressed by CNS glia; in culture, Gtx expression can be detected in both oligodendrocytes and astrocytes. *In vivo*, Gtx expression correlates strongly with CNS myelination, and is detectable throughout CNS white matter, particularly in areas of high nerve fiber content, such as the corpus callosum and internal capsule. The highest levels of Gtx expression occur in the adult – i.e. in fully differentiated myelinating cells.

Finally, another zinc finger with a demonstrated importance to Schwann cell differentiation and peripheral myelination is Krox-20. Although this protein is expressed in a variety of cell types in development, a major site of expression late in embryogenesis and in the early postnatal period (in mice and rats) is Schwann cells of the developing PNS. The mouse *Krox-20* gene has been insertionally inactivated (again through homologous recombination in ES cells), and mice that are homozygous for this Krox-20 mutation develop a severe postnatal peripheral neuropathy due to a nearly complete absence of myelination in what would normally be heavily myelinated nerves (e.g. the sciatic) [100]. Analysis of myelin gene expression in these nerves reveals that early markers of myelination (e.g. GalC and MAG) are present, but that later markers (e.g. P_0 and MBP) are not. It is thus a distinct possibility that Krox-20 might directly participate in the activation of late myelin genes.

11.5 Conclusions

The development of myelin-forming cells provides a particularly dramatic example of neuron–glial interaction leading to specialized gene expression and cellular differentiation. In the case of myelination, the differentiative events set in motion by this interaction lead to the formation of an organelle that is absolutely essential to higher nervous system function. There is perhaps no better proof of the importance of myelin than the debilitation suffered by patients with demyelinating disease. The destruction of myelin that occurs in MS results from circumstances in which an attack against the myelin sheath and the cells that form it overrides the normal inductive interactions that transpire between between neurons and glia.

As detailed above, progress in the areas of the molecular cloning of myelin-specific genes and the analysis of their expression and mutation in a range of demyelinating diseases, both spontaneous and inherited, has been spectacular. A detailed understanding of the signal transduction molecules and events that regulate the differentiation of myelinating Schwann cells and oligodendrocytes still eludes us, however, and is an important goal for the next phase of research into the molecular mechanisms of myelination.

References

1. Mikol, D.D., Gulcher, J.R. and Stefansson, K. (1990) The oligodendrocyte-myelin glycoprotein belongs to a distinct family of proteins and contains the HNK-1 carbohydrate. *J. Cell Biol.*, **110**, 471–9.
2. Bernier, L., Alverez, F., Norgard, E.M. (1987) Molecular cloning of a 2′,3′-cyclic nucleotide 3′-phosphodiesterase: mRNAs with different 5′ ends encode the same set of proteins in nervous and lymphoid tissues. *J. Neurosci.*, **7**, 2704–10.
3. Kurihara, R., Fowler, A.V. and Takahashi, Y. (1987) cDMA cloning and amino acid sequence of bovine brain 2′,3′-cyclic nucleotide 3′-phosphodiesterase. *J. Biol. Chem.*, **262**, 3256–61.
4. Vogel, U.S. and Thompson, R.J. (1987) Nucleotide sequence of bovine retina 2′,3′-cyclic nucleotide 3′-phosphohydrolase. *Nucleic Acids Res.*, **15**, 7204.
5. Gardinier, M.V., Amiguet, P., Linington, C. and Matthieu, J.M. (1992) Myelin/oligodendrocyte glycoprotein is a unique member of the immunoglobulin superfamily. *J. Neurosci. Res.*, **33**, 177–87.
6. Narayanan, V., Barbosa, E., Reed, R. and Tennekoon, G. (1988) Characterization of a cloned cDNA encoding rabbit myelin P2 protein. *J. Biol. Chem.*, **263**, 8332–7.
7. Schaeren-Wiemers, N., Schaefer, C., Valenzuela, D.M., Yancopoulos, G.D. and Schwab, M.E. (1995) Identification of new oligodendrocyte- and myelin-specific genes by a differential screening approach. *J. Neurochem.*, **65**, 10–22.
8. Greenfield, S., Brostoff, S., Eylar, E.H. and Morell, P. (1973) Protein composition of myelin of the peripheral nervous system. *J. Neurochem*, **20**, 1207–16.
9. Waehneldt, T.V., Matthieu, J.-M. and Jeserich, G. (1986) Appearance of myelin proteins during vertebrate evolution. *Neurochem. Int.*, **9**, 463–74.
10. Lemke, G. and Axel, R. (1985) Isolation and sequence of a cDNA encoding the major structural protein of peripheral myelin. *Cell*, **40**, 501–8.
11. Lemke, G., Lamar, E. and Patterson, J. (1988) Isolation and analysis of the gene encoding peripheral myelin protein zero. *Neuron*, **1**, 73–83.
12. Filbin, M.T., Walsh, F.S., Trapp, B.D., Pizzey, J.A. and Tennekoon, G.I. (1990) Role of myelin P_0 protein as a homophilic adhesion molecule. *Nature*, **344**, 871–2.
13. D'Urso, D., Brophy, P.J., Staugaitis, S.M. (1990) Protein zero of peripheral nerve myelin: biosynthesis, membrane insertion, and evidence of homotypic interaction *Neuron*, **4**, 449–60.

14. Giese, K.P., Martini, R., Lemke, G., Soriano, P. and Schachner, M. (1992) Disruption of the P_0 gene in mice leads to hypomyelination, abnormal expression of recognition molecules, and degeneration of myelin and axons. *Cell*, **71**, 565–76.

15. Nave, K.-A. and Milner, R.J. (1989) Proteolipid proteins: structure and genetic expression in normal and myelin-deficient mice. *Crit. Rev. Neurobiol.*, **5**, 65–91.

16. Milner, R.J., Lai, C., Nave, K.A. *et al.* (1985) Nucleotide sequences of two mRNAs for rat brain myelin proteolipid protein. *Cell*, **42**, 931–9.

17. Yan, Y., Lagenaur, C. and Narayanan, V. (1993) Molecular cloning of M6: identification of a PLP/DM20 gene family. *Neuron*, **11**(3), 423–31.

18. Kitagawa, K., Sinoway, M.P., Yang, C., Gould, R.M. and Colman, D.R. (1993) A proteolipid protein gene family: expression in sharks and rays and possible evolution from an ancestral gene encoding a pore-forming polypeptide. *Neuron*, **11**(3), 433–48.

19. Popot, J.L., Pham Dinh, D. and Dautigny, A. (1991) Major myelin proteolipid: the 4-alpha-helix topology. *J. Membrane Biol.*, **120**, 233–46.

20. Hudson, L.D. (1990) Molecular genetics of X-linked mutants. *Ann. NY Acad. Sci.* **605**, 155–65.

21. Nave, K.-A., Bloom, F. and Milner, R. (1987) A single nucleotide difference in the gene for myelin proteolipid protein defines the *jimpy* mutation in mouse. *J. Neurochem.*, **49**, 1873–7.

22. Macklin, W., Gardiner, M., King K. and Kampf, K. (1987) An AG→GG transition at a splice site in the myelin proteolipid protein gene in *jimpy* mice results in the removal of an exon. *FEBS Lett.*, **223**, 417–21.

23. Gencic, S. and Hudson, L. (1989) Conservative amino acid substitution in the myelin proteolipid protein of *jimpy^{msd}* mice. *J. Neurosci.*, **10**, 117–24.

24. Simons, R. and Riordan, J.R. (1990) The myelin-deficient rat has a single base substitution in the third exon of the myelin proteolipid protein gene. *J. Neurochem.* **54**(3), 1079–81.

25. Nadon, N.L., Duncan, I.D. and Hudson, L.D. (1990) A point mutation in the proteolipid protein gene of the 'shaking pup' interrupts oligodendrocyte development. *Development*, **110**, 529–37.

26. Griffiths, I.R., Scott, I., McCulloch, M.C. (1990) *Rumpshaker* mouse: a new X-linked mutation affecting myelination: evidence for a defect in PLP expression. *J. Neurocytol*, **19**, 273–83.

27. Schneider, A., Montague, P., Griffiths, I. *et al.* (1992) Uncoupling of hypomyelination and glial cell death by a mutation in the proteolipid protein gene. *Nature*, **358**, 758–61.

28. Rapin, I. (1989) Pelizaeus–Merzbacher disease, in *Merritt's Textbook of Neurology*, 8th edn (ed. L.P. Rowland), Philadelphia, Lea & Febiger, pp. 557–8.

29. Hudson, L., Puckett, C., Berndt, J., Chan, J. and Gencic, S. (1989) Mutation of the proteolipid protein (PLP) gene in a human X-linked myelin disorder. *Proc. Natl Acad. Sci. USA*, **86**, 8128–131.

30. Gencic, S., Abuelo, D., Ambler, M. and Hudson, L. (1989) Pelizaeus–Merzbacher disease: an X-linked neurologic disorder of myelin metabolism with a novel mutation in the gene encoding proteolipid protein. *J. Hum. Genet.*, **45**, 435–42.

31. Trofatter, J., Dlouhy, S., DeMyer, W. *et al.* (1989) Pelizaeus–Merzbacher disease: tight linkage to proteolipid protein (PLP) gene exon variant. *Proc. Natl Acad. Sci. USA*, **86**, 9427–30.

32. Ikenaka, K., Kagawa, T. and Mikoshiba, K. (1992) Selective expression of DM-20, an alternatively spliced myelin proteolipid protein gene product, in developing nervous system and in nonglial cells. *J. Neurochem.*, **58**, 2248–53.

33. Fanarraga, M.L., Griffiths, I.R., McCulloch, M.C. (1992) *Rumpshaker*: an X-linked mutation causing hypomyelination: developmental differences in myelination and glial cells between the optic nerve and spinal cord. *Glia*, **5**, 161–70.

34. Campagnoni, A.T. (1988) Molecular biology of myelin proteins from the central nervous system. *J. Neurochem*, **51**, 1–14.

35. Pribyl, T.M., Campagnoni, C.W., Kampf, K. *et al.* (1993) The human myelin basic protein gene is included within a 179-kilobase transcription unit: expression in the immune and central nervous systems. *Proc. Natl. Acad. Sci. USA*, **90**, 10695–9.

36. Roach, A., Takahashi, N., Pravtcheva, D. *et al.* (1985) Chromosomal mapping of the mouse myelin basic protein gene and structure and transcription of the partially deleted gene in *shiverer* mutant mice. *Cell*, **42**, 149–55.

37. Molineaux, S., Engh, H., deFerra, F., Hudson, L. and Lazzarini, R. (1986) Recombination within the myelin basic protein gene created the dysmyelinating *shiverer* mouse mutation. *Proc. Natl Acad. Sci. USA*, **83**: 7542–6.

38. Readhead, C., Popko, B., Takahashi, N. *et al.* (1987) Expression of a myelin basic protein gene in transgenic shiverer mice: correction of the dysmyelinating phenotype. *Cell*, **48**, 703–12.

39. Kimura, M., Sato, M., Akatsuka, A. *et al.* (1989) Restoration of myelin formation by a single type of myelin basic protein in transgenic *shiverer* mice. *Proc. Natl Acad. Sci. USA*, **86**, 5661–5.

40. Edwards, A.M., Ross, N.W., Ulmer, J.B. and Braun, P.E. (1989) Interaction of myelin basic protein and proteolipid protein. *J. Neurosci. Res.*, **22**, 97–102.

41. Martini, R., Mohajeri, M.H., Kasper, S., Giese, K.P. and Schachner, M. (1995) Mice doubly deficient in the genes for P_0 and myelin basic protein show that both proteins contribute to the formation of the major dense line in peripheral nerve myelin. *J. Neurosci.*, **15**, 4488–95.

42. Arquint, M., Roder, J., Loo-Sar, C. *et al.* (1987) Molecular cloning and primary structure of myelin-associated glycoprotein. *Proc. Natl Acad. Sci. USA*, **84**, 600–4.

43. Lai, C., Brow, M.A., Nave, K.-A. *et al.* (1987) Two forms of 1B236/myelin-associated glycoprotein, a cell adhesion molecule for postnatal development, are produced by alternative splicing. *Proc. Natl Acad. Sci. USA*, **84**, 4227–341.

44. Salzer, J.L., Holmes, W.P. and Colman, D.R. (1987) The amino acid sequences of the myelin-associated glycoprotein: homology to the immunoglobulin gene superfamily. *J. Cell. Biol.*, **104**, 957–65.

45. Lemke, G. (1992) Myelin and myelination in *An Introduction of Molecular Neurobiology*, Sunderland, Sinauer, pp. 281–312.

46. Li, C., Tropak, M.B., Gerlai, R. *et al.* (1994) Myelination in the absence of myelin-associated glycoprotein. *Nature*, **369**, 747–50.

47. Montag, D., Giese, K.P., Bartsch, U. H. *et al.* (1994) Mice deficient for the myelin-associated glycoprotein show subtle abnormalities in myelin. *Neuron*, **13**, 229–46.

48. Manfioletti, G., Ruaro, M.E., Del Sal, G. *et al.* (1990) A growth arrest-specific gene codes for a membrane protein. *Mol. Cell. Biol.*, **10**, 2924–30.

49. Spreyer, P., Kuhn, G., Hanemann, C.O. *et al.* (1991) Axon-regulated expression of a Schwann cell transcript that is homolgous to a 'growth-arrest-specific' gene. *EMBO J.*, **10**, 3661–8.

50. Welcher, A.A., Suter, U., De Leon, M., Snipes, G.J. and Shooter, E.M. (1991) A myelin protein is encoded by the homologue of a growth arrest-specific gene. *Proc. Natl Acad. Sci. USA*, **88**, 7195–99.

51. Snipes, G.J., Suter, U., Welcher, A.A. and Shooter, E.M. (1992) Characterization of a novel peripheral nervous system myelin protein (PMP22/SR13). *J. Cell Biol.*, **117**, 225–38.

52. Patel, P.I. and Lupski, J.R. (1994) Charcot–Marie–Tooth disease: a new paradigm for the mechanism of inherited disease. *Trends Genet.*, **10**, 128–33.

53. Davisson, M.T. and Roderick, T.H. (1978) *Cytogenet. Cell Genet.*, **22**, 552–64.

54. Falconer, D.S. (1951) Two new mutants, Trembler and Reeler, with neurological actions in the house mouse (*Mus musculus*). *J. Genet.*, **50**, 192–201.

55. Aguayo, A.J., Attiwell, M., Trecarten, J., Perkins, S. and Bray, G.M. (1977) Abnormal myelination in transplanted Trembler mouse Schwann cells. *Nature*, **265**, 73–6.

56. Henry, E.W. and Sidman, R.L. (1988) Long lives for homozygous *Trembler* mutant mice despite virtual absence of peripheral nerve myelin. *Science*, **241**, 344–6.

57. Suter, U., Welcher, A.A., Ozcelik, T. *et al.* (1992) *Trembler* mouse carries a point mutation in a myelin gene. *Nature*, **365**, 241–4.

58. Suter, U., Moskow, J.J., Welcher, A.A. *et al.* (1992) A leucine-to-proline mutation in the putative first transmembrane domain of the 22-kDa peripheral myelin protein in the Trembler-J mouse. *Proc. Natl. Acad. Sci. USA*, **89**, 4382–6.

59. Vance, J.M., Barker, D., Yamaoka, L.H. *et al.* (1991) Localization of Charcot–Marie–Tooth disease Type 1a to chromosome 17p11.2. *Genomics*, **9**, 623–8.

60. Valentijn, L.J., Bolhuis, P.A., Zorn, I. *et al.* (1992) The peripheral myelin gene *PMP-22/GAS-3* is duplicated in Charcot–Marie–Tooth disease type 1a. *Nature Genet.*, **1**, 166–70.

61. Pleasure, D.E. and Schotland, D.L. (1989) Hereditary neuropathies, in *Merritt's Textbook of Neurology*, 8th edn, (ed. L.P. Rowland), Philadelphia, Lea & Febiger, pp. 604–5.

62. Matsunami, N., Smith, B., Ballard, L. *et al.* (1992) Peripheral myelin protein-22 gene maps in the duplication in chromosome 17p11.2 associated with Charcot–Marie–Tooth 1a. *Nature Genet.*, **1**, 176–9.

63. Patel, P.I., Roa, B.B., Welcher, A.A. *et al.* (1992) The gene for peripheral myelin protein PMP-22 is a candidate for Charcot–Marie–Tooth disease type 1a. *Nature Genet.*, **1**, 159–65.

64. Timmerman, V., Nelis, E., Van Hul, W. (1992) The peripheral myelin protein gene PMP-22 is contained within the Charcot–Marie–Tooth disease type 1a duplication. *Nature Genet.*, **1**, 171–5.

65. Chance, P.F., Alderson, M.K., Leppig, K.A. *et al.* (1993) DNA deletion associated with hereditary neuropathy with liability to pressure palsies. *Cell*, **72**, 143–51.

66. Su, Y., Brooks, D.G., Li, L. *et al.* (1993) Myelin protein zero gene mutated in Charcot–Marie–Tooth type 1B patients. *Proc. Natl Acad. Sci. USA*, **90**, 10856–60.

67. Mirsky, R. and Jessen, K.R. (1990) Schwann cell development and the regulation of myelination. *Semin. Neurosci.*, **2**, 423–35.

68. Jessen, K.R. and Mirsky, R. (1994) Neural development. Fate diverted. *Curr. Biol.*, **4**, 824–7.

69. Jessen, K.R., Brennan, A., Morgan, L. *et al.* (1994) The Schwann cell precursor and its fate: a study of cell death and differentiation during gliogenesis in rat embryonic nerves. *Neuron*, **12**, 509–27.

70. Bhattacharyya, A., Frank, E., Ratner, N. and Brackenbury, R. (1991) P_0 is an early marker of the Schwann cell lineage in chickens. *Neuron*, 7, 831–44.

71. Voyvodic. J.T. (1989) Target size regulates calibre and myelination of sympathetic axons. *Nature*, 342, 430–3.

72. Trapp, B.D., Hauer, P. and Lemke, G. (1988) Axonal regulation of myelin protein mRNA levels in actively myelinating Schwann cells. *J. Neurosci.*, 8, 3515–21.

73. Monuki, E.S., Weinmaster, G., Kuhn, R. and Lemke, G. (1989) SCIP: a glial POU domain gene regulated by cyclic AMP. *Neuron*, 3, 783–93.

74. Lemke, G. and Chao, M. (1988) Axons regulate Schwann cell expression of the major myelin and NGF receptor genes. *Development*, 102, 499–504.

75. Weinmaster, G. and Lemke, G. (1990) Cell-specific cyclic AMP-mediated induction of the PDGF receptor. *EMBO J.*, 9, 915–20.

76. Bradley, W.G. and Asbury, A.K. (1970) Duration of synthesis phase in neurilemma cells in mouse sciatic nerve during degeneration. *Exp. Neurol.*, 26, 275–82.

77. Brown, M.J. and Asbury, A.K. (1981) Schwann cell proliferation in the postnatal mouse: timing and topography. *Exp. Neurol.*, 74, 170–86.

78. Lemke, G. (1990) Glial growth factors. *Sem. Neurosci.*, 2, 437–43.

79. Marchionni, M.A., Gooderal, A.D., Chen, M.S. *et al.* (1993) Glial growth factors are alternatively spliced erbB2 ligands expressed in the nervous system. *Nature* 362, 312–18.

80. Salzer, J.L., Williams, A.K., Glaser, L. and Bunge, R.P. (1980). Characterization of the stimulation and specificity of the response to a neurite membrane fraction. *J. Cell Biol.*, 84, 753–66.

81. Salzer, J.L., Bunge, R.P. and Glaser, L. (1980) Evidence for the surface localization of the neurite mitogen. *J. Cell Biol.*, 84, 767–78.

82. Richardson, W.D., Raff, M. and Noble, M. (1990) The oligodendrocyte-type-2-astrocyte lineage. *Semin. Neurosci.*, 2, 445–54.

83. Pringle, N.P. and Richardson, W.D. (1993) A singularity of PDGF alpha-receptor expression in the dorsoventral axis of the neural tube may define the origin of the oligodendrocyte lineage. *Development*, 117, 525–33.

84. Yu, W.P., Collarini, E.J., Pringle, N.P. and Richardson, W.D. (1994) Embryonic expression of myelin genes: evidence for a focal source of oligodendrocyte precursors in the ventricular zone of the neural tube. *Neuron*, 12(6), 1353–62.

85. Barres, B.A. and Raff, M.C. (1994) Control of oligodendrocyte number in the developing rat optic nerve. *Neuron*, 12, 935–42.

86. Kiernan, B.W. and ffrench-Constant, C. (1993) Oligodendrocyte precursor (O-2A progenitor cell) migration; a model system for the study of cell migration in the nervous system. *Development (Suppl.)*, pp. 219–25.

87. Hudson, L.D. (1990) Molecular biology of myelin proteins in the central and peripheral nervous systems. *Semin. Neurosci.*, 2, 483–96.

88. Lemke, G. (1992) Gene regulation in the nervous system, in *An Introduction of Molecular Neurobiology*, Sunderland, Sinauer, pp. 313–54.

89. Foran, D.R. and Peterson, A.C. (1992) Myelin acquisition in the central nervous system of the mouse revealed byan MBP-Lac Z transgene. *J. Neurosci.*, 12, 4890–7.

90. Wight, P.A., Duchala, C.S., Readhead, C. and Macklin, W.B. (1993) A myelin proteolipid protein-LacZ fusion protein is developmentally regulated and targeted to the myelin membrane in transgenic mice. *J. Cell Biol.*, 123, 443–54.

91. Messing, A., Behringer, R.R., Hammang, J.P. *et al.* (1992) P_0 promoter directs expression of reporter and toxin genes to Schwann cells of transgenic mice. *Neuron*, 8, 507–20.

92. Katsuki, M., Sato, M., Kimura, M. *et al.* (1988) Conversion of normal behavior to *shiverer* by myelin basic protein antisense cDNA in transgenic mice. *Science*, 241, 593–5.

93. Gow, A., Friedrich, V.L. Jr and Lazzarini, R.A. (1992) Myelin basic protein gene contains separate enhancers for oligodendrocyte and Schwann cell expression. *J. Cell Biol.*, 119, 605–16.

94. Messing, A., Behringer, R.R. Wrabetz, L. *et al.* (1994) Hypomyelinating peripheral neuropathies and schwannomas in transgenic mice expressing SV40 T-antigen. *J. Neurosci.*, 14, 3533–9.

95. Monuki, E.S., Kuhn, R., Weinmaster, G., Trapp, B.D. and Lemke, G. (1990) Expression and activity of the POU transcription factor SCIP. *Science*, 249, 1300–3.

96. Monuki, E.S., Kuhn, R. and Lemke, G. (1993) Repression of the myelin P_0 gene by the POU transcription factor SCIP. *Mech. Dev.*, 42, 15–32.

97. Weinstein, D., Burrola, P. and Lemke, G. (1995) Premature Schwann cell differentiation and hypermyelination in mice expressing a targeted antagonist of the POU transcription factor SCIP. *Mol. Cell. Neurosci.*, 6, 212–9.

98. Kim, J.G. and Hudson, L.D. (1992) Novel member of the zinc finger superfamily: a C_2-HC finger that recognizes a glia-specific gene. *Mol. Cell. Biol.*, 12, 5632–9.

99. Komuro, I., Schalling, M., Jahn, L. *et al.* (1993) *Gtx*: a novel murine homeobox-containing gene, expressed specifically in glial cells of the brain and germ cells of testis, has a transcriptional repressor activity *in vitro* for a serum-inducible promoter. *EMBO J.*, 12, 1387–401.

100. Topilko, P., Schneider-Maunoury, S., Levi, G. *et al.* (1994) Krox-20 controls myelination in the peripheral nervous system. *Nature*, 371, 796–9.

12 PATHOPHYSIOLOGY OF THE DEMYELINATED NERVE FIBRE

E. Michael Sedgwick

This chapter is about the changes in nerve conduction as a result of demyelination and how they may relate to some of the symptoms and signs of multiple sclerosis (MS). This involves a consideration of the fast voltage-dependent sodium and potassium channels and their disposition on the normal and demyelinated nerve.

It has become clear that considerable modifications occur in the axons to restore conduction through the demyelinated section; some patients seem to do this better than others. There is the possibility of therapeutic intervention at this level and the activity of the ion channels can be modified by a number of agents. Some have been tried therapeutically with modest and temporary success as yet.

12.1 Nerve conduction

The ionic basis of nerve conduction is now well known but was determined by studies of continuous conduction in the squid giant axon. Mammalian myelinated fibres show variations which are important for an understanding of the pathophysiology of demyelination [1]. Unlike squid axon, myelinated nerve conduction is saltatory, where the depolarization leaps from one node of Ranvier to the next [2–4]. This property is conferred by myelination and loss of myelin is the cardinal histopathological feature of multiple sclerosis (MS). Saltatory conduction allows conduction velocities up to 10 times faster than by continuous conduction in a nerve of equivalent size and fast trains of impulses can be carried, the energy requirements of which are also lower.

Myelinated fibres have two to five nodes per millimetre and the excitation process at a node takes about 20 μs. At the excited node, sodium channels in the membrane open and the rapid inflow of sodium ions produces an inward current. Local circuits operate and there is a balancing outward current through the resting membrane which, if large enough, will excite it. The insulating properties of myelin direct the local current to cross the membrane at the next node and it is here that excitation occurs. The outward current normally builds up quickly but is dependent upon the resistive and capacitative properties of the membrane, which are altered by demyelination.

Depolarization at one node produces more current than is necessary for depolarization at the next by a factor of 5–7. Tasaki [5] estimated that there would be enough longitudinal current to allow the impulse to jump two inactive nodes and excite the third. Normally there is an adequate safety factor for transmission; this can be defined as ratio of the current available for excitation of the next node to the current required to excite the node. A safety factor of 1 will just allow conduction whereas if it falls below 1 conduction will fail. Normally it is about 5.

In squid axon the action potential is terminated by opening of the potassium channels which generate a repolarizing potential. In mammalian myelinated nerve fibres repolarization is by inactivation of the Na^+ channels. Potassium channels, however, have a role in repolarization of demyelinated fibres.

12.1.1 ION CHANNELS

The characteristics of ion channels, their molecular biology, electrophysiology and their number and disposition on the axonal membrane have been determined in recent times. Sodium channels can be visualized as intramembranous particles in freeze fracture electron micrographs and by a ferric ion–ferrocyanide histochemical reaction. Saxitoxin binds externally to the alpha subunit but not to intracellular units of the Na^+ channel and can be used in conjunction with agents which can be assayed. Immunolocalization has been used and electrophysiological techniques, including patch clamping.

Whatever method is used, it is clear that sodium ion channels are concentrated at the node with a density of up to 50 times that of the internodal membrane. There are at least 1000 channels μm^{-2} at the node and 20 μm^{-2} in the internode.

Multiple Sclerosis: Clinical and pathogenetic basis. Edited by Cedric S. Raine, Henry F. McFarland and Wallace W. Tourtellotte. Published in 1997 by Chapman & Hall, London. ISBN 0 412 30890 8.

Potassium channels cannot be visualized but electrophysiological observations suggest that fast K^+ channels are concentrated in the paranodal region with a density of six times that at the node. Because their overall density is low, with relative paucity at the node, and because most of them are covered by myelin, they play little or no part in repolarization in normal conduction. These and the slow K^+ channels are exposed by acute demyelination and then are active in repolarization.[6, 7].

The ion channels in human nerve have the same characteristics as those in other mammals and interspecies differences in nerve physiology are thought to be due to differences in density and distribution of these channels along the membrane[8]. Although different forms of ion channels are known to co-exist, e.g. forms of the acetylcholine receptor in muscle, there is no evidence that alterations of ion channel type are involved in the pathophysiology of MS.

Ion channels are produced in the neuron and transported along the axon by fast axonal transport. Local application of colchicine, which blocks fast transport, results in a vast accumulation of channels proximal to the block[9]. The metabolic burden of sustaining channels in a long axon must be considerable, especially if their half-life really is only 1–3 days as has been estimated[10]. Degradation is most likely by internalization and lysis.

Astrocytes extend cytoplasmic processes to make a close physical association with nodes[11] and these cells have Na^+ channels in their membranes[12]. This has led to speculation that astrocytes may contribute Na^+ channels to the axon to maintain a high concentration at the node or, alternatively, they may be involved in channel breakdown[13, 14]. The astrocyte may provide some signal for the axon cytoskeleton to fix channels at this location.

Prior to oligodendroglial cell ensheathment of axons in the developing nervous system, Na^+ channels are randomly distributed at low density in the membrane with node-like foci developing after ensheathment but before compact myelination[15, 16]. There is intense research activity into the axon–glial interaction with respect to ion channels, but we must turn our attention to the demyelinated axon.

12.2   The demyelinated axon

Experimental focal demyelination can be produced by many means, but diphtheria toxin, lysolecithin and ethidium, a trypanosomicide in veterinary use, have been used in conjunction with electrophysiological recordings.

An area of demyelination has been shown to produce conduction block with survival of the distal part

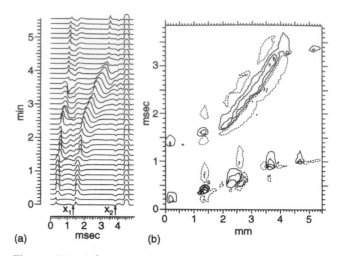

Figure 12.1 Saltatory and continuous conduction. (*a*) A plot of local currents accompanying an action potential in a partially demyelinated rat ventral root. One fibre shows saltatory conduction throughout, the other shows saltatory conduction replaced by slow and continuous conduction over a segment. (*b*) Plots of the membrane currents of the fibres showing the currents located at the nodes except during continuous conduction. (Reproduced from Bostock and Sears, 1978[21], with permission.)

of the axon in which conduction is normal after it has been stimulated. Slowing of conduction has been shown with return to normal velocity downstream of the demyelinated segment. This has the effect of producing temporal dispersion of a volley of impulses in a population of axons. Figure 12.1 shows saltatory conduction and continuous conduction in fibres in rat ventral root which was experimentally demyelinated by local injection of diphtheria toxin a few days earlier.

In addition, there are other, less obvious disturbances of nerve conduction. Some fibres may have a safety factor close to 1 so that they may or may not conduct depending on environmental conditions; these are sometimes referred to as 'knife edge' fibres. Minor changes in extra-axonal environment can determine whether the knife edge fibres conduct or not. A patient with a large number of such fibres will show fluctuation in symptomatology independently of MS pathology.

Demyelinated fibres may show ectopic generation of impulses either spontaneously or because of increased mechanical sensitivity[17]. This activity has been studied extensively in peripheral nerves (see review by Devor[18], but less so in central axons.

Ephaptic transmission has been observed in experimental situations where action potentials in demyelinated fibres excite neighbouring myelinated fibres and cross-talk between dysmyelinated fibres may occur, although this was not seen in one study on peripheral nerve[19].

After demyelination, an area of axon low in Na⁺
channels is exposed and the action current declines to
a level at which propagation can no longer be sustained, i.e. a safety factor less than 1. In experimentally demyelinated fibres (diphtheria toxin acting on
rat ventral root fibres), a period of conduction block
was followed by slow continuous conduction at 5% or
less of normal appearing at 4–6 days and before
remyelination had begun [20, 21]. Morphological studies indicated that the membrane had developed an
increased density of Na⁺ channels.

Experiments in other preparations suggest that the
high density foci of channels can remain for a long
time after demyelination [22] and they do not diffuse
laterally into the internodal region [23]. It has been
demonstrated that increased synthesis of Na⁺ channels
can be triggered, and an increase in saxitoxin binding
sites has been noted in demyelinated tracts of multiple
sclerosis patients [24].

It is not clear how the redistribution of Na⁺ channels occurs. The finding that channels may remain in
high density foci after demyelination suggests that the
internodal region must acquire new channels. Are
these from the neuron and carried by axonal transport
or are they inserted by neighbouring astrocytes? As the
pathological process damages the glial cells, the second
alternative seems unlikely. Channels probably do not
migrate laterally from high density foci as they are
fixed in place by the cytoskeleton. What is the trigger
for the neuron to produce more channels and what,
exactly, decides their location in the membrane? Developmentally, the high density foci of channels appear
after ensheathment by oligodendroglia but before the
formation of myelin. These processes will be studied in
the next few years and the details will have important
therapeutic implications in MS and many other diseases of the central and peripheral nervous system.

Genetically dysmyelinated animals give important
insights into the relationship between myelin producing cells and axonal conduction. In myelin deficient
rats, which form no compact myelin but still have
wrapped axons, optic nerve conducts five times slower
than normal yet has approximately the same overall
density of Na⁺ channels [25]. *Shiverer* mice with a *shi*
gene on chromosome 18 have oligodendrocytes which
wrap axonal membranes but lack myelin basic protein.
These animals have two to four times as many Na⁺
channels as normal [26]. It is suggested that a myelin
basic protein-associated transmembrane signal down-
regulates the Na⁺ channels in normal animals.

12.2.1 COMPUTER MODELS OF AXONS

Studies on partially demyelinated fibres, aided by
computer simulations, have revealed a number of
interesting characteristics. Conduction is slowed and, if

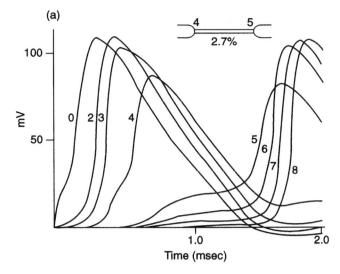

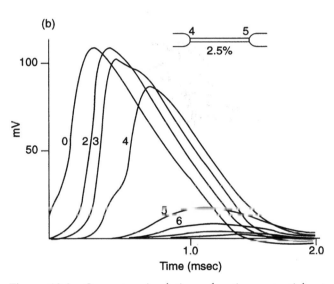

Figure 12.2 Computer simulation of action potentials at
eight nodes of Ranvier. (*a*), A fibre partially demyelinated
between nodes 4 and 5 shows the delay in activation of node
5; (*b*) this fibre is more severely demyelinated and conduction
is blocked between nodes 4 and 5. The inset diagrams indicate
the degree of myelination of the model fibre. Reproduced from
Koles and Rasminsky, 1972 [27], with permission.)

demyelination is sufficient, blocked completely. Figure
12.2 (*a*), from a computer simulation study by Koles
and Rasminsky [27], shows the action potential in
eight successive nodes with demyelination between
nodes 4 and 5. There is a slight delay in conduction
between 3 and 4, a marked delay between 4 and 5, but
the action potential picks up speed thereafter. Figure
12.2 (*b*) represents a more severely demyelinated fibre
in which conduction is blocked after node 4.

The study by Schauf and Davis [28] illustrates the
extreme temperature dependence of partially demyelin-

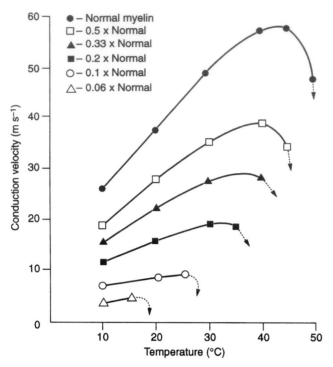

Figure 12.3 Partially demyelinated axons are sensitive to temperature change as shown in these plots of computer modelled fibres. Some fibres show conduction block close to body temperature. (Reproduced from Schauf and Davis, 1974 [28], with permission.)

ated fibres. Figure 12.3 shows the relationship between conduction velocity and temperature in fibres with different degrees of demyelination and also the temperature at which conduction is totally blocked. Fibres with about one-fifth of their normal myelin are blocked at physiological temperatures. Calcium ion concentration is rather critical, in that blocked conduction can be restored by lowering the calcium ion concentration. Increasing pH has a similar effect.

12.2.2 TRANSMISSION OF TRAINS OF IMPULSES

Transmission of trains of impulses is impaired in partially demyelinated fibres. This is not merely a reflection of a prolonged refractory period, but seems to relate to a progressive reduction in current generation at the node before the demyelination and possibly a reduction in excitability of the affected nodes. Transmission can block at low rates of excitation, well within the normal physiological range of frequencies, which can be 300/second and above in the dorsal column fibres.

In central demyelinated fibres potassium channels are exposed [20] and because of their role in repolarizing the membrane, their activation acts against the already weakened depolarizing action of the few Na$^+$ channels. Their action leaves a hyperpolarization after an impulse which tends to limit high frequency trains of pulses.

Ectopic impulses have been observed from demyelinated axons. Fibres in a plaque of demyelination can generate impulses spontaneously and they are very sensitive to slight mechanical deformation, which can produce a shower of impulses travelling in both directions from the plaque [29]. In chronic (3–4 week) lesions produced by ethidium bromide, Felts *et al.* [30] recorded, intra-axonally, bursts of impulses superimposed on slow depolarizing potentials. They speculated that there may be an excessive accumulation of K$^+$ in the paranodal region which leads to an inward current through the K$^+$ channels sufficient to trigger action potentials. Ectopic impulses are also known to be generated in fibres whose K$^+$ channels have been blocked [31] where inward Na$^+$ are the agents of the inward current.

12.3 Clinical implications (Table 12.1)

The laboratory studies on demyelinated fibres go some way towards explaining many of the clinical phenomena observed in MS patients. Weakness, numbness and other symptoms can be attributed to blocked conduction or to fibres which have degenerated. It is thought that the marked variability in neurological deficit often found in MS could be due to conduction in partially demyelinated fibres being unstable due to critical safety factors. Such fibres would conduct if conditions

Table 12.1 Consequences of central demyelination and MS

Nerve conduction	Clinical manifestation
Slow conduction	Stereoscopic vision Delayed EP Flicker fusion frequency reduced
Blocked conduction	Negative symptoms and signs Absent or small EPs
Decreased safety factor	Uhthoff's phenomenon Reduced flicker fusion frequency Intrasubject variability
Ephaptic transmission	Spasms, myokymia ?Pain
Ectopic impulses	Paraesthesiae Spasms Myokymia
Mechanical sensitivity	Lhermitte's sign Phosphenes

were favourable, e.g. low temperature, low calcium and no long trains of impulses. Generation of spurious impulses and extreme mechanical sensitivity of demyelinated fibres may explain symptoms such as paraesthesiae and flashing lights or phosphenes. Lhermitte's sign, a tingling sensation in the body elicited by neck flexion or extension, is thought to be due to mechanical deformation of the cord evoking impulses in demyelinated sensory fibres.

Slowed conduction does not appear to produce much in the way of clinical deficit. The central nervous system seems to have evolved so that precise timing of neuronal events is not normally important. Peripheral nerve conduction varies considerably with temperature in normal subjects and patients with profound peripheral nerve slowing have no great deficit due to slowing as opposed to axonal degeneration. Slowed conduction is of more importance to the clinician as a diagnostic marker.

12.3.1 OPTIC NEURITIS (ON)

Optic neuritis (ON) provides a good clinical model of demyelination as the nerves and demyelinating lesion can be seen on MRI and tested electrophysiologically as well as clinically [32] (Chapter 2). Halliday *et al.* have documented the course of events attending an attack of ON [33, 34]. In the acute phase, visual acuity may fall from normal to no perception of light and recover to normal or near normal over a few days. If visual acuity is severely reduced, no clear visual evoked potential (VEP) can be recorded or it is very delayed even within days of the onset of symptoms, suggesting that both conduction block and demyelination are early and rapid events. As acuity recovers so does the VEP amplitude, but the P100 component remains delayed. It seems that conduction is blocked in many fibres during acute ON when swelling of the disc and optic nerve occur as well as demyelination. The MRI image shows gadolinium enhancement at that time, indicating active inflammation [35] (Chapter 3). Reduction of the swelling is accompanied by return of the VEP or improvement in amplitude and loss of enhancement on MRI. Conduction block is presumed to result from demyelination plus oedema and the accompanying metabolic and pressure disturbances. McDonald [36] has speculated that conduction block may be hastened by the presence of interleukins which could interfere with ion channel function. Restoration of conduction occurs as the swelling subsides but the latency of the VEP may remain permanently delayed as a result of an episode of ON.

A delayed VEP is not an inevitable sequel of an attack of ON. Matthews *et al.* [37] recorded delayed VEPs in only 81% of patients within 3 months of an attack of ON: it is now accepted that the VEP latency

can return to the normal range in 10–20% of patients after ON [38]. However, a delayed VEP usually persists despite complete recovery of visual function as tested by acuity, ophthalmoscopy, field plotting and colour vision. Recovery of a delayed VEP to normal is more common in children. Kriss [39] found 55% of children had normal VEPs when measured a mean of 8 years after the initial episode of optic neuritis.

The delay seen in the VEP P100 after optic neuritis and in MS ranges from 10 to 100 ms. McDonald [40] estimated from autopsy studies that the average length of a plaque of demyelination in the optic nerve was 10 mm and 50 nodes would be expected in that length. Conduction velocity in the fine (3 μm diameter) fibres from the macula was estimated at $10\,\mathrm{m\,s^{-1}}$ and if demyelination can slow conduction by 25 times, then a delay of 24 ms would ensue. It is not certain whether this degree of slowing occurs in optic nerves before conduction block develops. The optic nerve in the myelin-deficient rat conducts five times slower than normal [25].

12.4 Provocative tests

The present model of demyelinated axons predicts that the knife edge fibres with low safety factors can be reversibly blocked. Fluctuations in the symptomatology in MS, including the Uhthoff phenomenon, are thought to reflect the changing state of these fibres. Uhthoff [41] described four patients with MS who developed amblyopia after exercise. Fluctuations in MS symptoms related to exercise or rise in body temperature are now referred to as Uhthoff's phenomenon and heat stress enjoyed a vogue as a diagnostic test for a while [42].

12.4.1 UHTHOFF'S PHENOMENON

The visual evoked potential (VEP) in a subject with Uhthoff's amblyopic phenomenon should show a reduction in amplitude with increasing temperature as more fibres are blocked, with restoration of amplitude as cooling occurs. A few studies have been done and all agree that there is no significant change in amplitude or latency of the VEP of normal subjects with a rise in body temperature due to heating or exercise [43–47]. Patients with MS frequently showed a reduction in amplitude of the VEP with a rise in temperature. Persson and Sachs [45] compared patients with Uhthoff's phenomenon with other MS patients who had delayed VEP but no Uhthoff's symptoms. Amplitude of P100 fell by 68% in the Uhthoff group but not at all in the others, whereas latencies were unchanged. The prediction of the model of demyelinated axons is therefore fulfilled in some patients. The conduction block has been attributed to a rise in temperature but other factors have not been excluded. Many patients with apparently equally disturbed optic nerve function, as judged by the VEP, did not show Uhthoff's phenomenon or a change in VEP amplitude. The model would have to account for the apparent resistance of axons in these patients in terms of them having safety factors well above 1.

The reverse situation, reduction in body temperature, has been less extensively studied, but many patients improve transiently [48, 49]. It is not unusual for patients to report the temporary beneficial effects of a cold shower.

Lepore [50] warns that Uhthoff's symptom can occur in other forms of optic neuropathy, including compressive lesions, so it is not a reliable indicator of demyelination.

12.4.2 Na CHANNEL BLOCK

If demyelinated fibres conduct with low safety factors due to rearrangement of Na^+ channels then a silent lesion may be unmasked by blocking a few of the Na^+ channels. Sakurai et al. [51] tested this hypothesis by administering lidocaine, a short-lived Na^+ channel blocker which crosses the blood–brain barrier, to patients with MS and others with optic atrophy due to axonal neuropathies. Only the MS patients showed changes, with reduction in amplitude of VEPs and reduction in visual function; colour vision tests showed the greatest changes. The authors point out that other drugs in common use have an effect on Na^+ channels and clinicians should be aware that they may affect MS patients adversely.

12.5 Therapeutic strategies

Consideration of the functional properties of demyelinated fibres leads to new therapeutic possibilities. Conduction in demyelinated fibres could be improved by increasing the time for which the sodium channels opened or by inactivating the potassium channels. There are a number of drugs and toxins employed in isolated preparations and in animals but these have not so far been considered safe enough for human use. 4-aminopyridine inactivates the potassium channels and has been shown to restore conduction of isolated demyelinated fibres [19, 52].

Brever et al. [53] administered 3, 4-diaminopyridine, which blocks fast K^+ channels, to MS patients. The rationale is that the exposed K^+ channels on the axon oppose conduction by repolarizing the membrane, and blocking these channels will allow the action current to develop for longer so that the adverse changes in

membrane capacitance may be overcome and the chances of continuous conduction increased. They found a reversible shortening of the latency of the VEP in 2 of 6 patients by 10 ms or so. The patients improved temporarily but paraesthesiae were a troublesome side-effect. Sensory fibres, unlike motor fibres, are prone to generate bursts of impulses when K^+ channels are blocked. Another trial using 4-aminopyridine in 12 MS males showed neurological improvement in vision and motor function in 10 with no serious side-effects [54].

Digoxin, which blocks the hyperpolarizing Na/K pump and would be predicted to increase the chance of conduction in knife edge fibres, also produces small and temporary improvement in MS patients [55].

Temporary functional changes in MS have also been reported after oral phosphate to reduce Ca^{2+}, after bicarbonate and edetate (EDTA) – both these agents produce a microenvironment more favourable to conduction by knife edge fibres [56, 57].

The ideal therapeutic solution is to restore the axons to their normal myelinated state, which happens in peripheral nerve disorders and results in restoration of a normal pattern of ion channels and complete clinical recovery. Remyelination generally does not occur to a great extent in MS but could it occur if healthy glial cells were transplanted into the plaque? Utzschneider et al. [58] recently transplanted myelin-forming glial cells into the myelin-deficient regions in rat spinal cord and demonstrated improved conduction velocity and conduction through the demyelinated area.

While these studies do not represent a therapeutic breakthrough, they do demonstrate that some of the neurological deficits in MS are amenable to modification by manipulation of axons, and offer the expectation of progress in the future.

12.6 Conclusions

The axon in MS undergoes considerable changes which help towards restoration of function but also induce some functional characteristics responsible for the varied symptomatology seen in the disease. Realization of the dynamic changes in axons and the possibilities of modification of axonal function offers an opportunity for therapy but achievements are limited to date. An understanding of the control of production, destruction and distribution of ion channels will enable other therapeutic interventions and will, no doubt, be relevant to a number of other neurological conditions.

One area, entered by neither the author nor other workers, is that of the changes in the terminal branches of an axon following conduction block. Do the branches of the terminal tree die back? Are the synapses capable of liberating transmitter in the usual quantities? Are there still the same number of synapses? Neurobiologists are learning about the plasticity of synaptic populations and just how widely the Hebbian principle applies. Animal experiments show that the number and efficiency of synapses from one source depends on their use, and firm contact on the target neuron is only maintained in competition with synapses from other sources. Disuse results in some degree of takeover by nearby active synapses.

Work on neuromuscular relationships has shown some of the extent to which nerve impulses can modify the post-synaptic structure (muscle) by changing gene expression and metabolism. Research on the neurons 'downstream' from demyelinated axons will, I believe, produce important insights and practical benefits.

References

1. Waxman, S.G., Kocsis, J.D. and Stys, P.K. (1995) *The Axon: Structure, Function and Pathophysiology*. New York, Oxford University Press.
2. Tasaki, I. and Takeuchi, T. (1941) Der am Ranvierischen Knoten ent stehende Aktionsstrom unde seine Bedeutung für die Erregungsteitung. *Pfluger Arch. Eur. J. Physiol.*, **244**, 696–711.
3. Tasaki, I. and Takeuchi, T. (1942) Weitere Studien Uber den Aktionsstrom der markhaltigen Nervenfaser und über die elektrosaltatorische übertragung des nervenimpulses. *Pfluger Arch. Eur. J. Physiol.*, **245**, 764–82.
4. Huxley, A.F. and Stamfli, R. (1949) Evidence for saltatory conduction in peripheral myelinated nerve fibres. *J. Physiol. (Lond.)*, **108**, 316–39.
5. Tasaki, I. (1953) Properties of myelinated fibres in frog sciatic nerve and in spinal cord as examined with microelectrodes. *Jpn J. Physiol.*, **3**, 73.
6. Black, J.A., Kocsis, J.D. and Waxman, S.G. (1990) Ion channel organization of the myelinated fibre. *Trends Neurosci.*, **11**, 48–54.
7. Meiri, H., Baum, Z. and Rosenthal, Y. (1989) Dynamic changes in sodium channels at demyelinated axons. *Progr. Neurobiol.*, **32**, 159–79.
8. Scholz, A., Reid, G., Vogel, W. and Bostock, H. (1993) Ion channels in human axons. *J. Neurophysiol.*, **70**, 1274–9.
9. Liverant, S. and Meiri, H. (1990) Colchicine prevents recovery of nerve conduction at chronic demyelination. *Brain Res.*, **519**, 50–6.
10. Schmidt, J.W. and Catterall, W.A. (1986) Biosynthesis and processing of the alpha subunit of the voltage-sensitive sodium channel in rat brain neurons. *Cell*, **46**, 437–45.
11. Raine, C.S. (1984) On the association between perinodal astrocytic processes and the node of Ranvier in the central nervous system. *J. Neurocytol.*, **13**, 21–7.
12. Black, J.A., Friedman, B., Waxman, S.G., Elmer, L.W. and Angelides, K.J. (1989) Immuno-ultrastructural localization of sodium channels at nodes of Ranvier and perinodal astrocytes in rat optic nerve. *Proc. Roy. Soc. Lond. B*, **238**, 39–51.
13. Gray, P.T. and Ritchie, J.M. (1985) Ion channels in Schwann and glial cells. *Trends Neurosci.*, **8**, 411–15.
14. Bevan, S., Chiu, S.Y., Gray, P.T. and Ritchie, J.M. (1985) The presence of voltage-gated sodium, potassium and chloride channels in rat cultured astrocytes. *Proc. Roy. Soc. Lond. B*, **225**, 229–313.
15. Black, J.A., Friedman, B., Waxman, S.G., Elmer, L.W. and Angelides, K.J. (1982) Rat optic nerve: freeze fracture studies during development of myelinated axons. *Brain Res.*, **250**, 1–10.
16. Waxman, S.G. (1982) Current concepts in neurology: membranes, myelin and the pathophysiology of multiple sclerosis. *N. Engl. J. Med.*, **306**, 1529–33.
17. Smith, K.J. and McDonald, W.I. (1980) Spontaneous and mechanically evoked activity due to central demyelinating lesion. *Nature*, **286**, 154–5.
18. Devor, M. (1995) Abnormal excitability in injured axons, in *The Axon* (eds S.G. Waxman, J.D. Kocsis, and P.K. Stys), New York, Oxford University Press, pp. 530–52.
19. Targ, E.F. and Kocsis, J.D. (1985) 4-aminopyridine leads to restoration of conduction in demyelinated rat sciatic nerve. *Brain Res*, **328**, 358–61.
20. Bostock, H. and Sears, T.A. (1976) Continuous conduction in demyelinated mammalian nerve fibres. *Nature*, **263**, 786–7.
21. Bostock, H. and Sears, T.A. (1978) The internodal axon membrane: electrical excitability and continuous conduction in segmental demyelination. *J. Physiol. (Lond.)*, **280**, 273–301.
22. Shrager, P. (1989) Sodium channels in single demyelinated mammalian axons. *Brain Res.*, **483**, 149–54.
23. Eun-hye, J. and Angelides, K.J. (1993) Clustering and mobility of voltage-dependent sodium channels during myelination. *J. Neurosci.*, **13**, 2993–3005.
24. Moll, C., Mourre, C., Lazdunski, M. and Ulrich, J. (1991) Increase of sodium channels in demyelinated lesions of multiple sclerosis. *Brain Res.*, **556**, 311–16.
25. Utzschneider, D.A., Thio, C., Sontheimer, H. *et al.* (1993) Action potential conduction and sodium channel content in the optic nerve of the myelin-deficient rat. *Proc. Roy. Soc. Lond. B*, **254**, 245–50.
26. Noebels, J.L., Marcom, P.K. and Jalilion-Tehrani, M. H. (1990) Sodium channel density in hypomyelinated brain increased by myelin basic protein gene deletion. *Nature*, **352**, 431–4.
27. Koles, Z.J. and Rasminsky, M. (1972) A computer simulation of conduction in demyelinated nerve fibres. *J. Physiol.*, **227**, 351–64.
28. Schauf, C.L. and Davis, F.A. (1974) Impulse conduction in multiple sclerosis: a theoretical basis for modification by temperature and pharmacological agents. *J. Neurol. Neurosurg. Psychiatry*, **37**, 152–61.
29. Smith, K.J. and McDonald, W.I. (1980) Spontaneous and mechanically evoked activity due to central demyelinating lesion. *Nature*, **286**, 154–5.
30. Felts, P.A. and Smith, K.J. (1991) Conduction properties of central nerve fibres remyelinated by Schwann cells. *Brain Res.*, **574**, 178–92.
31. Targ, E.F. and Kocsis, J.D. (1986) Action potential characteristics of demyelinated rat sciatic nerve following application of 4-aminopyridine. *Brain Res.*, **363**, 1–9.
32. Halliday, A.M., McDonald, W.I. and Mushin, J. (1972) Delayed visual evoked response in optic neuritis. *Lancet*, **i**, 982–5.
33. Halliday, A.M. and McDonald, W.I. (1977) Pathophysiology of demyelinating disease. *Br. Med. Bull.*, **33**, 21–7.
34. Halliday, A.M. (1993) *Evoked Potentials in Clinical Testing*, Edinburgh, Churchill Livingstone.
35. Youl, B.D., Turano, G. and Miller, D.H. (1991) The pathophysiology of acute optic neuritis: an association of gadolinium leakage with clinical and electrophysiological deficits. *Brain*, **114**, 2437–50.
36. McDonald, W.I. (1994) The pathological and clinical dynamics of multiple sclerosis. *J. Neuropathol. Experi. Neurol.*, **53**, 338–43.
37. Matthews, W.B. and Small, D.G. (1979) Serial recording of visual and somatosensory evoked potentials in multiple sclerosis. *J. Neurol. Sci.*, **40**, 11–21.
38. Hely, M.A., McManis, P.G., Walsh, J.C. and McLeod, J.G. (1986) Visual-evoked potentials and ophthalmological examination in optic neuritis: a follow-up study. *J. Neurol. Sci.*, **75**, 275–83.
39. Kriss, A., Francis, D.A., Cuendet, F. *et al.* (1988) Recovery after optic neuritis in childhood. *J. Neurol. Neurosurg. Psychiatry*, **51**, 1253–8.
40. McDonald W.I. (1977) Pathophysiology of conduction time in central nerve fibres, in *Visual Evoked Potentials in Man: New Developments* (ed. J.E. Desmedt), Oxford, Clarendon Press, pp. 427–37.
41. Uhthoff, W. (1890) Unterschungen uber die bei der multiplen Herdsklerose vorkommendem Augenstrorungen. *Archiv. Psychiatr. Nervenkrankh.*, **21**, 303–410.
42. Guthrie, T.C. and Nelson, D.A. (1995) Influence of temperature changes on multiple sclerosis: critical review of mechanisms and research potential. *J. Neurol. Sci.*, **129**, 1–8.
43. Regan, D., Murray, J.T. and Silver, R. (1977) Effect of body temperature on visual evoked potential delay and visual perception in multiple sclerosis. *J. Neurol. Neurosurg. Psychiatry*, **40**, 1083–91.
44. Persson, H.E. and Sachs, C. (1978) Provoked visual impairment in multiple sclerosis studied by visual evoked potentials. *Electroencephalogr. Clin. Neurophysiol.*, **44**, 664–8.
45. Persson, H.E. and Sachs, C. (1981) Visual evoked potentials elicited by pattern reversal during provoked visual impairment in multiple sclerosis. *Brain*, **104**, 369–82.
46. Matthews, W.B., Read, D.J. and Pountney, E. (1979) Effect of raising body temperature on visual and somatosensory evoked potentials in patients with multiple sclerosis. *J. Neurol. Neurosurg. Psychiatry*, **42**, 250–5.
47. Bajada, S., Mastaglia, F.L., Block, J.L. and Collins, D.W.K. (1980) Effects of induced hyperthermia on visual evoked potentials and saccade parameters in normal subjects and multiple sclerosis patients. *J. Neurol. Neurosurg. Psychiatry*, **43**, 849–52.
48. Watson, C.W. (1959) Effect of lowering of body temperature on the symptoms and signs of multiple sclerosis. *N. Engl. J. Med.*, **261**, 1253–9.
49. Honan, W.P., Heron, J.R., Foster, D.H. and Snelgar, R.S. (1987) Paradoxical effects of temperature in multiple sclerosis. *J. Neurol. Neurosurg. Psychiatry*, **50**, 1160–4.
50. Lepore, F.E. (1994) Uhthoff's symptom in disorders of the anterior visual pathways. *Neurology*, **44**, 1036–8.
51. Sakurai, M., Mannen, T., Kanazawa, I. and Tanabe, H. (1992) Lidocaine unmasks silent demyelinative lesions in multiple sclerosis. *Neurology*, **42**, 2088–93.

52. Sherratt, R.M., Bostock, H. and Sears, T.A. (1980) Effects of 4-aminopyridine on normal and demyelinating mammalian nerve fibres. *Nature*, **283**, 570–2.

53. Brever, C.T., Leslie, J., Camenga, D.L., Panitch, H. S. and Johnson, K.P. (1990) Preliminary trial of 3,4-diaminopyridine in patients with multiple sclerosis. *Ann. Neurol.*, **27**, 421–7.

54. Stefoski, D., Davis, F.A., Faut, M. and Schauf, C.L. (1987) 4-Aminopyridine improves clinical signs in multiple sclerosis. *Ann. Neurol.*, **21**, 71–7.

55. Kaji, R., Heppel, L. and Sumner, A.J. (1990) Effect of digitalis on clinical symptoms and conduction variables in patients with multiple sclerosis. *Ann. Neurol.*, **28**, 582–4.

56. Becker, F.O., Michael, J.A. and Davis, F.A. (1974) Acute effects of oral phosphate on visual function in multiple sclerosis. *Neurology*, **24**, 601–7.

57. Davis, F.A., Becker, F.O., Michael, J.A. and Sorenson, E. (1970) Effect of intravenous sodium bicarbonate, disodium edetate (Na$_2$EDTA) and hyperventilation on visual and oculomotor signs in multiple sclerosis. *J. Neurol. Neurosurg. Psychiatry*, **33**, 723–32.

58. Utzschneider, D.A., Archer, D.R., Duncan, I.R., Waxman, S.G. and Kocsis, J.D. (1994) Transplantation of myelin-forming cells enhances impulse conduction in amyelinated spinal cord axons in the myelin deficient rat. *Proc. Natl Acad. Sci.*, **91**, 53–7.

13 GENETIC INFLUENCES IN MULTIPLE SCLEROSIS

Henry F. McFarland, Roland Martin and Dale E. McFarlin

13.1 Introduction

Multiple sclerosis (MS) is generally thought to be caused by an autoimmune process. However, the target of the abnormal immune response, the factors influencing susceptibility and the events that initiate the disease are largely unknown. Extrapolation from results obtained using experimental models and from epidemiological studies of MS have variably supported a strong environmental event or implicated an important role for genetic make-up as the principal factor influencing susceptibility. As our understanding of genetic influences on disease susceptibility, especially complex diseases such as MS, improves, the likelihood that susceptibility for MS is closely, if not entirely, linked to genetic factors increases. The evidence for a genetic influence is based on several different sets of data. In this chapter, the existing evidence for a genetic influence based on genetic epidemiology will be examined. Next, an examination of the types of approaches appropriate for analysis of complex traits or diseases, along with a discussion of the strengths and weaknesses of these approaches, will be discussed. Finally, the results of various studies examining the relationship between MS and particular genes will be evaluated along with a discussion of the implications of association between MS and genes which encode for MHC molecules in an autoimmune disease. The methodology being used in current studies employing molecular techniques to screen the entire human genome will also be reviewed. Although few data are available, several important studies of genetic linkage in MS are under way in the United States, Canada and the UK. This chapter will attempt to provide a critical assessment of the approaches used in studies of this type in order to provide the reader with sufficient background to evaluate new findings as they emerge.

13.2 Genetic epidemiology

It has long been recognized that the geographic distribution of MS is not similar between regions: some geographic areas, such as the Orkney and Shetland Islands off the northern coast of Scotland, have an extremely high prevalence (up to 200/100 000), while other areas such as the southern United States have a very low prevalence (10/100 000). A detailed examination of the incidence and prevalence in various geographic regions can be found in the literature [1, 2] (see also Chapter 7). In general, in the northern hemisphere, a north–south gradient has been described, with the prevalence higher in the north. An unresolved issue is whether the epidemiology points to an environmental or genetic influence or both. Some investigators [3, 4] have suggested that the north–south gradient seen in the United States represents the proclivity for individuals from regions of Europe with a high incidence of MS to migrate to northern regions of the US. In contrast, individuals from regions of Europe with a low incidence of MS have tended to migrate to southern regions of the US.

In addition to the north–south gradient, evidence for an environmental influence has been based on migration studies. Two such studies have been particularly important in providing support for a role for environmental factors on susceptibility to MS. In 1962, a study of the prevalence of MS among native inhabitants of Israel in comparison to immigrants to the country indicated that when individuals migrate from a high-risk area (Europe) to a low-risk area (Israel), the age of migration influences the risk of the migrants [5]. Individuals migrating before the age of 15 took on the risk of their new home, while individuals migrating after the age of 15 took their high risk with them. A study of immigrants to South Africa from Europe has also indicated that the immigrants seem to

Multiple Sclerosis: Clinical and pathogenetic basis. Edited by Cedric S. Raine, Henry F. McFarland and Wallace W. Tourtellotte. Published in 1997 by Chapman & Hall, London. ISBN 0 412 30890 8.

adopt the low risk associated with South Africa [6]. A more recent study of the effect of migration involves an examination of individuals from the West Indies born in the United Kingdom. The results have suggested that the risk to these individuals is much greater than the risk of MS in the West Indies [7]. Although these studies are provocative and are widely accepted, the strength of the data is influenced by a number of important methodological issues. The results of the epidemiological studies of MS have been examined in detail by Sadovnick and Ebers [4] and they have suggested that the conclusions drawn for the migration studies must be viewed with caution. The conclusions are based on relatively small numbers of affected individuals. Also, a question remains regarding the degree to which the immigrating population reflects the population in the country of origin. Often, migrating populations will represent a subset of the native population and the prevalence figures for that native population might not be fully applicable to the migrating population.

Support for an environmental influence is also derived from reports of epidemics of MS, and the most influential of these studies has been the description of an epidemic of MS in the Faroe Islands beginning after occupation by British troops during the Second World War [8]. Epidemiological studies of MS are reviewed in detail in Chapter 7.

Other epidemiological studies have tended to provide support for the importance of the genetic background in influencing susceptibility to MS. For example, the prevalence of MS is low (2/100 000) among Japanese living in Japan, and although Japanese people living on the Pacific coast of the United States show a slightly higher prevalence (6.7/100 000), it is still considerably lower than that for Caucasians living in California (30/100 100) [9]. A similar example is the difference in prevalence between Hungarians of caucasian descent (37/100 000) and Hungarian gypsies (2/100 000) [10]. It must be noted that in addition to genetic factors, life-style differences could contribute to the findings in both of these studies. The most recent study to examine the relative influence of genetic and environmental factors in susceptibility to MS has evaluated families that have adopted children [11]. Two questions were examined. First, if the adopted individual has MS, is there increased risk for other family members developing disease, and secondly, if there are affected members in a family with an adopted individual is the risk to the adopted sibling the same as the non-adopted siblings? The answer to both questions is that the risk appears more closely related to the genetic background than to just living in a family that has one or more individuals affected with MS. It is important to note, however, that these findings do not eliminate an important role of environ-

ment: they do indicate that genetic background seems to contribute to the effect of the environmental influence if it exists. In summary, current assessment of epidemiological evidence seems to provide as much support for a genetic influence as for an environmental influence. It is not unlikely that both contribute to susceptibility.

13.2.1 FAMILY STUDIES

Shortly after Charcot's initial description of multiple sclerosis, Eichhorst [12] reported the disease in a mother and her son. Since that early report numerous studies of the familial occurrence of MS have been undertaken. Sadovnick *et al.*, in an extensive examination of the frequency of MS among family members of MS patients in Canada, reported that approximately 19% of the patients, based on clinical criteria, had an affected relative [13, 14]. These investigators have evaluated the life-time risk for relatives of an MS patient: for a first-degree relative of an affected individual the life-time risk may be as high as 5% while that for individuals without a family history is approximately 0.2%. Life-time risk is a figure derived from calculating the accumulated risk, based on the incidence of the disease, over the period of high risk for developing the disease. The risk is greatest for sibs of affected individuals, especially sisters, and decreases in second- and third-degree relatives. For example, if the affected member is female the life-time risk for a sister is 5.65, for a brother, 2.27, for a daughter, 4.96, and for a first cousin, 2.37. Although the increased familial incidence could be due to either an environmental or a genetic influence, the increased incidence found in second-and third-degree relatives generally favors a genetic factor. The examination of linkage in multiplex families will be discussed later in this chapter.

13.2.2 TWINS

The use of twins to distinguish environmental from genetic influences in disease has a long history. Diseases with a strong genetic influence should result in a higher concordance rate in monozygotic twins than in dyzygotic twins since the MZ twins are genetically identical while DZ twins are only as genetically similar as other siblings. In distinction, since DZ twins would be expected to have a more common environment that non-twin sibs, diseases with an important environmental influence would be expected to result in a concordance rate which would be generally similar in MZ and DZ twins. Despite this seemingly simple model, twin studies have been the subject of considerable debate as to the potential for methodical errors and interpretation

Table 13.1 Comparison of concordance rates for MS in monozygotic and dizygotic twins

| Investigator | Concordance | | Reference |
	Monozygotic	Dizygotic	
MacKay and Myrianthopoulos[a]	6/39 (15%)	3/29 (10%)	[15]
Bobwick et al.[a]	1/5 (20%)	0/4 (0%)	[16]
Currier and Eldridge[a,b]	8/22 (36%)	3/26 (11%)	[17]
		2 sets unlike sex	
Williams et al.[a,b]	6/12 (50%)	2/12 (17%)	[18]
McFarland et al.[a,b]	10/14 (71%)	2/12 (17%)	[19]
Heltberg and Holm	8/23 (35%)	2/29 (7%)	[20]
Kinnunen et al.	2/8 (25%)	0/6 (0%)	[21]
Ebers et al.	7/25 (28%)	1/40 (2.5%)	[22, 23]
Mumford et al.			[24]
French Twin Study Group[a]	1/17 (6%)	1/41 (2.4%)	[25]

[a] Study subject to ascertainment bias.
[b] Three studies of overlapping patient cohort.

of results. The most problematic issue involves how twins are identified for studies. If a study is not a true population-based study, meaning that all MS patients in a given geographic population with a twin are identified, the study may be subject to what is termed ascertainment bias, which means that the results of a study may be biased by the methods used to identify the study population. In studies of twins it is more likely to identify concordant sets since the critical criterion is a twin having MS, and if both twins have MS the likelihood of identifying the set is increased. It has been argued that it is also more likely to identify MZ twins and female twins. With these cautions, what are the results of twin studies in MS? An overview is presented in Table 13.1.

The first study of significant size, by Mackay and Myrianthopoulos, examined 60 sets of twins and found a slight but non-significant increase in concordance in MZ twins[15]. A subsequent study of twins with military service records reported a 20% concordance in MZ twins and none in DZ twins[16]. A study of 51 twin sets in the US identified by advertisement found a concordance rate of 36% in MZ twins and 12% in DZ twins[17]. A portion of this cohort, 12 MZ and 12 DZ sets, was studied with detailed clinical evaluation and a concordance rate of 50% was found in the MZ twins while a rate of 17% was found in the DZ twins[18]. Each of these studies was flawed in study design which no doubt resulted in a disproportionate number of MZ twins and concordant sets. However, 5-year follow-up of the cohort reported by Williams et al. indicated that two of the six MZ discordant sets became concordant while the six DZ sets did not change[19], strengthening the argument that concordance was indeed greater in the MZ twins. Only a handful of twin studies escape

serious design flaws. Two such studies include those of Heltberg and Holm[20] and Kinnunen et al.[21], which reported a concordance rate of 35% and 25% respectively in MZ twins and a concordance rate of 7% and 0% in DZ twins. Although the larger Canadian[22, 23] and British studies[24] were not totally population-based, both were extremely well designed and went to extensive lengths to achieve full ascertainment. Importantly, the concordance rates in these two studies ranged from 21 to 30.8% in MZ twins while the rate in DZ twins ranged from 3.3 to 4.7%, a rate similar to that in non-twin siblings. The results from these latter two studies probably represent the most accurate assessment of concordance for MS in twins, at least in North America and the UK.

The four twin studies outlined above have each examined concordance in geographic regions known to have a high incidence of MS and reflect an important genetic influence in these populations. In distinction to the twin studies just described, a study of twins in France has reported a similar concordance rate in MZ and DZ twins; both rates were approximately those found in DZ twins and non-twin siblings in the other large family studies[25]. The explanation for the differences between the results of the French study and others discussed above may be methodological, since in the French study ascertainment was by advertisement. However, ascertainment bias is generally expected to result in an over-representation of concordant sets. It has also been suggested that the differences between the results of these various studies are within the expected variation and therefore not meaningful[26]. An alternative explanation is that genetic influence is more pronounced in regions with higher prevalence. Since the prevalence for MS is lower in

France than in Scandinavia, Canada or the UK, the magnitude of the genetic influence may be less. If it is postulated that MS is a multigenic disease with susceptibility influenced by multiple genes, the prevalence of MS may increase with the strength of the genetic influence in the population.

Experimental evidence for this hypothesis comes from studies of an animal model for lupus nephritis [27]. The F_1 progeny of New Zealand Black (NZB) mice and New Zealand White (NZW) mice, but not the parental strains, develop anti-nuclear antibodies and severe renal disease. Genes known to contribute to disease include the NZW MHC and probably a gene on chromosome 4 of the NZB mouse. To identify other genes contributing to disease a backcross analysis was performed and 6 NZB loci which influence disease were identified. In another set of backcross experiments various F_1 cohorts were generated. The surprising finding was that the incidence of disease differed substantially between cohorts: in some nearly 100% developed severe disease, some had very low incidence of disease and others were intermediate in susceptibility. Next, the results of this and other studies using similar methods to examine the lupus model indicate that the likelihood of disease increases as the number of susceptibility genes in the cohort increases. Importantly, it seems that susceptibility is influenced more by the number of susceptibility genes than by the actual function of the individual genes. Thus, animals with any combination of two susceptibility genes will have a similar incidence of disease [28]. It appears that phenotypic expression of disease under multigenic influence depends on the epistatic interactions between these genes, which, depending on the number of genes and their effects can result in various degrees of clinical expression. Similar experimental results have been obtained using the animal model of insulin-dependent diabetes mellitus (IDDM) [29], in which 10 disease-susceptibility-influencing loci have been identified. It is, therefore, important to re-evaluate twin studies in light of these elegant animal experiments demonstrating a polygenic effect of disease susceptibility and a threshold effect due to gene interactions. Results from the studies of lupus and IDDM models raise two important points. They establish that a disease incidence of less than 100% can occur in genetically identical individuals and that the variation in phenotypic expression of disease is not necessarily due to environmental factors or to modifications of the genetic influence occurring after inheritance of the germline, such as somatic mutations. If environmental factors are removed from consideration, the concordance rate in MZ twins provides an estimate of genotypic penetrance – the proportion of genetically identical individuals that will express the phenotype. However, the highly outbred genetics in humans may preclude an accurate assessment of genotypic penetrance.

13.3 Methodology in the analysis of complex diseases

The rapid technological advances in molecular genetics have resulted in remarkable progress in exploring diseases following Mendelian recessive or dominant inheritance. Examples of neurological diseases which have been successfully mapped include Huntington's chorea, spinal muscle atrophy and muscular dystrophy. However, it is known that most diseases do not follow Mendelian genetics and lack a clear correlation between genotype and phenotype. Phenotypic variation can occur in diseases linked to a single gene because of incomplete penetrance. An additional cause of phenotypic variation, and the one most relevant to a discussion of MS, is polygenic inheritance. As reflected by results of family and twin studies discussed above, the genetic influence in MS is most consistent with a polygenic influence, with multiple genes possibly exerting a threshold effect on susceptibility, similar to that seen in the experimental lupus model. Only recently have geneticists begun serious efforts to unravel complex diseases, and with the rapidly evolving techniques in molecular biology it is expected that, for many diseases, progress may be swift. However, an epistatic interaction between multiple susceptibility genes could prove extremely difficult to unravel in the outbred human population.

The initial step in dissecting complex diseases is to carefully examine the genetic epidemiology in order to estimate the sample sizes needed to have a reasonable chance of defining the genetic components of the disease. For example, the success of genetic mapping will increase as the relative risk for the disease increases. The empirical risk can be examined for kin of an affected individual and compared to the risk or incidence in the general population. This empirical risk has been called relative risk. In a disease such as MS with a non-constant age of onset, the most accurate assessment of risk will use age-adjusted recurrence risk or risk adjusted for age of onset of the disease, as is done in assessing life-time risk. As indicated above, twin studies are also extremely important in the assessment of risk. Finally, efforts need to be directed at fitting the inheritance pattern of the disease to known models of inheritance. This approach, known as segregation analysis, is helpful in defining the approaches which will be useful in analyzing the DNA based studies. Considerable effort has been made over the years to fit MS inheritance to various models of inheritance. An early report by Mackay and Myrianthopoulos [15] suggested an autosomal recessive inheritance. It is now clear that this is incorrect. A number of other inheritance patterns have been assessed [30] but have not shown much promise. One report [31] has suggested inheritance based on homozygosity for a recessive gene and a dominant gene on the X chromosome and with low penetrance. This suggestion awaits confirmation.

All of these genetic epidemiological studies, and especially those involving segregation analysis, can be influenced by characteristics of the disease leading to errors in ascertainment of affected and unaffected individuals. In this regard, MS poses some particular problems. Often diagnostic uncertainty can exist in patients. More difficult is establishing unaffected individuals. Since the age of high risk extends from late teens to the mid 50s, an individual cannot be considered unaffected with much certainty until past the age of high risk. In addition, it is known that many patients will have very mild or clinically silent forms of the disease and studies of unaffected members of MS multiplex families using MRI have reported that the incidence of unaffected individuals having MRI abnormalities may be as high as 10% [32, 33]. While MRI abnormalities do not establish that these individuals have MS, it may raise important questions as to whether they should be considered unaffected. The analysis of some complex diseases has used very restrictive criteria regarding the clinical characteristics of the disease in order to define as homogeneous a population as possible. Even this is difficult in MS, since variability in the clinical course is a hallmark of the disease. One important issue that has probably not received sufficient attention in MS is that the results of genetic studies in a disease can vary depending on the ethnic populations. This issue will be discussed in conjunction with the association studies but it is clear that the disease can be associated with different HLA genes in different geographic and ethnic populations. Thus, the results of genetic studies may well vary depending on whether they are done in ethnically heterogeneous or homogeneous populations; in regard to the latter, results of linkage or association studies may differ from population to population.

13.4 Relationship between genetic markers and MS

13.4.1 METHODS

Before examining evidence linking MS to particular genes it is important to have an understanding of the strengths and weaknesses of various methods used to assess the relationship between genotype and phenotype. Three major approaches have been used: those that test inheritance of a particular gene with a model of inheritance, those that examine allele sharing without a predetermined model, and association studies that look for association of genotype with affected individuals in a case-control population.

Linkage analysis

Linkage analysis has, traditionally, been the most commonly used approach to examine a relationship between a gene or genetic marker and disease. First, an inheritance model which incorporates the gene frequency, penetrance and other parameters is chosen for testing. Next, the experimental linkage data are tested against the proposed model and compared to a model representing the null hypothesis that no linkage exists. This process results in a likelihood ratio expressed as a **lod score**. Generally lod scores of 3 or greater are considered significant but in complex diseases lower lod scores may warrant consideration. The principal weakness of linkage analysis is that, in complex diseases, the choice of models is problematic and success of the method depends on selection of an appropriate model. Despite this problem, linkage analysis has been used to analyze diseases due to multiple genes. For example, this method was used in a recent report of a Finnish study [34] indicating that MS is linked to two genes, one for HLA and a second for myelin basic protein, but this observation has not been confirmed by other investigators.

Allele-sharing methods

Allele-sharing methods are based on determining whether a genetic marker is shared by affected members of a pedigree. The important difference between linkage analysis and allele-sharing methods is that the latter do not require that a model be specified since allele-sharing methods are model-free [35]. Two allele-sharing methods are **sib pair analysis** and the **affected pedigree member** (APM) method [36]. Sib pair analysis in its purest form depends on determining whether siblings in a pedigree inherit an identical allele or genetic marker. To establish that it is the same locus, it is necessary to establish that the locus is **identical by descent** (IDB), meaning that the locus comes from the same parent. This requires the parents of the affected individual to be available for genetic typing and limits the number of families that can be considered useful. If sufficient polymorphic markers exist on the chromosome, IDB can often be inferred. In distinction to sib pair analysis, APM analyzes sharing of a locus or marker independent of IDB.

Association studies

Association studies, which are designed to examine whether an association exists between a disease and a particular genetic marker, have been, until recently, the most common type of genetic study done in MS. Starting in the late 1970s, many investigators began to study the relationship between HLA antigens and MS. The data derived from these studies will be reviewed below, but it is important first to evaluate the strength and weaknesses of association studies in the analysis of a genetic influence.

The major attraction to association studies is their simplicity: one compares the frequency of a genetic marker in the affected population to that in a control population. The greatest weakness of association studies probably involves the choice of control groups. Not uncommonly the incidence of a genetic marker in MS is compared to controls derived from populations which may differ in ethnicity. Problems with control groups are particularly common when association studies are done in a highly heterogeneous population, such as that of the United States, and less common when done in more homogeneous populations, such as in Scandinavia. In any association study care must be taken to ensure that a marker seemingly associated with disease is not simply a market that is found in high frequency in a particular ethnic or geographic population which has high risk for the disease. If a particular HLA gene is over-represented in an ethnic population with high risk for a particular disease, an association study could conclude that the HLA gene was associated with disease unless the control group had identical ethnic characteristics. For example, a study of MS, a disease most

common in individuals of northern European descent, could easily reach erroneous conclusions if the control group used a random US population, which could be considerably more ethnically diverse. Even when studies are done in countries that may seem homogeneous with respect to ethnicity, the methodology must be reviewed carefully. For example, if control groups consist of blood donors, it is possible that ethnically diverse groups, even though they represent a small portion of the total population, may be over-represented in blood donor populations.

If an association between a genetic marker and a disease is found, the significance of that association is usually not known. In most cases (and certainly this is true in MS) there may be only a weak association with disease, and this may be alternatively interpreted as reflecting a marker that is in genetic dysequilibrium with a marker more tightly linked to disease, or reflecting a marker that represents one of many genes that contribute to increased susceptibility. Association studies alone cannot distinguish these two possibilities.

Since each of the approaches to analyzing genetic influence has strengths and weaknesses, a combination of several techniques is needed in the analysis of complex diseases such as MS in order to have a reasonable chance to identify relevant genes affecting susceptibility.

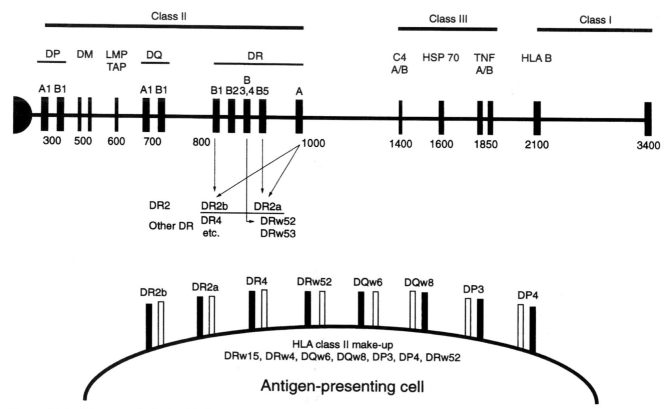

Figure 13.1   Diagram of relationship between genes encoding for HLA class I and class II molecules and the expression of the molecules on cell membranes.

Methods used in molecular genetics

The molecular biological techniques used to study genetics have evolved rapidly over the past few years. The first generation of molecular studies employed a technique known as **restriction fragment length polymorphisms** (RFLPs). This technique is based on the observation that certain enzymes known as restriction enzymes target different DNA segments and will cut the DNA when that sequence is present. Through trial and error (if the sequence of the gene is not known) an enzyme may be found that will distinguish two or more allelic forms of a gene since each will have a different sequence and will give different size fragments after being cut by the enzyme. Thus, one allele may produce a large fragment while a second allele might result in two fragments of smaller size. The use of RFLP analysis has been largely replaced by **polymerase chain reaction** (PCR). This technique allows the amplification of small amounts of DNA. Since the unique sequence of individual alleles is becoming known, PCR can be used to identify those sequences specific for a particular allele. In addition, some studies have sequenced the entire region of interest.

Currently considerable effort is directed at identification of unknown genes that may contribute to susceptibility. This approach requires the screening of the entire human genome. One of the most commonly used techniques is based on the observation that certain sequences that are characterized by certain bases being repeated for short stretches occur throughout the genome. These markers can be used to examine the relationship between different portions of each chromosome with occurrence of disease. Once a general area of interest is identified, the region can be studied in more detail, including sequencing of the region.

13.4.2 STUDIES OF SPECIFIC GENETIC MARKERS AND MS

HLA region – chromosome 6

The human HLA genes are located on chromosome 6 and represent the equivalent of the major histocompatibility region (MHC) in animals. The organization of the HLA region is shown in Figure 13.1. It should be noted that a large number of different HLA molecules are expressed on the surface of cells, particularly antigen-presenting cells that express class II molecules. Also, a number of genes other than those commonly thought of as HLA molecules are found in the HLA region.

HLA

The two groups of proteins encoded in the HLA region that have been of particular interest in MS are HLA class I and class II molecules. HLA class I molecules (HLA A, B and C) consist of a polymorphic alpha chain combined with the conserved beta-2 microglobulin. HLA class II molecules (HLA DR, DQ, DP) consist of a relatively conserved alpha chain and the more polymorphic beta chain. HLA class I molecules are expressed on the surface of almost all cells and are responsible for presenting antigen to HLA class I-restricted T cells which express CD8. HLA class II molecules are expressed on a more limited range of cells and are found primarily on cells known as antigen-presenting cells that are able to present antigen to class II-restricted $CD4^+$ T cells. Recognition of antigen by $CD4^+$ T cells is the initial event in the induction of either a cellular or humoral immune response. Thus the expression of HLA class II molecules and their ability to bind and present antigens, especially self antigens, is central to concepts of autoimmune disease. The role of HLA molecules in the immune response will be discussed in more detail in Chapter 14.

In order to understand the extensive and often conflicting data on the relationship between HLA class II molecules and MS it is necessary to understand the structure and nomenclature of class II molecules. The DR, DQ and DP regions consist of one expressed gene encoding for the alpha chain and one or more expressed genes encoding for a beta chain. For each haplotype (there is one on each chromosome 6) one DQ and one DP alpha/beta chain complex is expressed. In distinction, for HLA DR the alpha chain combines with two different beta chains, meaning that for each haplotype two DR molecules are expressed (DR1 and DR8 express only one). For most of the DR genotypes one of the expressed beta chains is polymorphic while the second (which may be beta 3, 4 or 5 depending on the haplotype) is conserved and results in a limited number of Drw 54/53 phenotypes for each of the DR types (except DR1 and DR2). In the DR2 haplotype, which is important since it is associated with MS, both beta chains are polymorphic and result in two molecules, DR2a (DRalpha + DRbeta *0101) and DR2b (DRalpha + DRbeta *1501), both of which are probably important in presenting antigen and differ in regard to the characteristics of the peptides they can bind. Thus, in an individual who inherits two different HLA haplotypes, four DR molecules, two DQ molecules and two DP molecules will be expressed. An important issue regarding the evaluation of the literature dealing with the relationship between HLA molecules or genes and MS is that there has been considerable change in the nomenclature for HLA molecules and especially HLA class II molecules over the past 10 years. The changes in nomenclature have paralleled the use of more sensitive methods for HLA typing. Until recently, most typing was done using serological techniques that were dependent on antibodies specific for the various HLA molecules. Over time more specific antibodies were

Table 13.2 Representative associations between various HLA markers and multiple sclerosis

Population	Association	Reference
Mixed	A3, B7	[37, 38]
Mixed	DR2	[39]
Mexican	DRw6	[42]
Japanese	DRw6	[43]
Arabian	DR4	[41]
Sardinian	DR4	[40]
Norwegian	Association with particular DQB1 sequences	[45]
Norwegian	DQA1 with Glu at position 34	[46]
Swedish	Both RR and first-degree progressive -Drw15, Dqw6	[47, 49]
	RR associated with DRw17, DQw2	
	First-degree progressive with DR4, DQw8	
Norwegian	Both RR and first-degree progressive -Drw15, Dqw6	[50]
	RR associated with DRw17, DQw2	
	First-degree progressive with DR4, Dqw8 not confirmed	
	Association with DQB1 sequences or DQA1 Glu34 *not* confirmed	
French Canadians and mixed ethnic caucasians	Association with DR2 haplotype (DRB1*1501, DQA1*0102, DQB1*0602	[51]
	DQB1 sequences and DQA1 Glu34 linked to haplotype not disease	
	Association with DQB1 Leu26 in French Canadians but *not* mixed caucasians	

identified leading to splits of HLA types. For example, DR2 is now split into DRw 15 and DRw16. Additional specificities have been identified using cellular typing techniques so that DRw 15 could be split into Dw2 and Dw12. Because of the strong linkage disequilibrium between DR15 and DQw6 it has often been unclear if cellular reactivities were due to the DR or DQ molecule. Over the past few years HLA molecules have been characterized at the molecular level and most HLA typing is now done using the sensitive molecular techniques which allow precise identification of alpha and beta chains. Thus, the DR15, Dw2, DQw6 haplotype is represented by the DRB1*1501, DRB5*0101, DQA1*0102, DQB1*0602 genotype.

Since the 1970s the association between HLA class I and class II antigens has been examined extensively. A summary of some of the important observations is outlined in Table 13.2. This table does not include every study dealing with this issue; instead, it points out some of the trends that have evolved from studies of the relationship between HLA and MS. Initial association studies indicated a very weak association between HLA class I antigens, HLA A3 and B7 with MS [37, 38]. Subsequently, a stronger association with HLA class II molecules and, in particular, DR2 (reviewed in [39], and with DQw6 (previously DQw1), has been reported. These associations have been found in individuals of northern European descent. In other geographic and ethnic populations other associations have been identified; HLA DR4 has been reported to be associated with MS in Italians and Arabs [40, 41] and DR6 has been associated with MS in Mexican and

Japanese patients [37, 42, 43]. The association between DR4 and MS in Japan remains controversial. An association with DPw4 has been reported in Scandinavia [44], but has generally not been confirmed in more recent studies.

As indicated above, the genes for HLA3, B7, DR15, DQw6 are in linkage dysequilibrium, meaning that they segregate together more frequently than expected by chance. Recent studies have examined the association between MS and HLA genes at the molecular level. A study of Norwegian MS patients reported that patients expressing DR15, DR4 or DR6 expressed HLA-DQβ chains that had similar polymorphic regions in the portion of the molecule that would be involved in antigen presentation [45]. The importance of DQ was also strengthened by evidence from the same investigators demonstrating that the DQA1 chain in MS commonly has a glutamine at position 34 [46]. In addition, a study of Swedish MS patients has reported an association with DQB1 chains that contain a glycine at position 86 [47]. This observation has recently been confirmed in a population of Italian MS patients [Massacesi, L., personal communication].

Some studies have reported associations strengthened by the inheritence of a combined HLA haplotype. An association with DRB1*1501 and DRB1*0401 has been reported in Belgian MS patients and an increased susceptibility associated with amino acids at positions 11, 13 and 71 of DRB1 was suggested with some genotypes producing a protective effect [48]. Since these amino acid residues are in the binding groove, a relationship with antigen presentation is likely. Analyses of HLA associations in the MS populations in Sweden or Norway have reported a strong association between the DRw15, DQw6 haplotype and MS, but in addition reported additional associations which differed in patients with RR MS as compared to first-degree progressive MS [49, 50]. These findings have been extended and the RR MS has been reported to be associated with a second haplotype (in addition to DRw15, DQw6), consisting of DRw17 (previously DR3), DQw2 while the first-degree progressive disease was associated with DR4, DQw8. Importantly, this later study of MS in Norway failed to confirm an association with particular DQB1 chain sequences or with a glutamine at position 34. However, a study of Canadian MS patients has demonstrated a difference between French Canadians and patients of mixed ethic background [51]. Both populations showed an association with the DRw15, DQw6 haplotype, which supports an influence of DQB1 on susceptibility, but the French Canadians also tended to have a DQB1 chain that has a leucine at position 26. The Canadian MS patients also were found to have an association with particular DQB1 chain sequences, as reported previously in Norwegian patients [45], and a glutamine at position 34 of the DQA1 chain, as reported in another study of Norwegian patients [46], but this association was found to be secondary to the association with the DRw15, DQw6 haplotype. Thus, when the associations were examined using a two-allele linkage method, it was found that the unique characteristics of the DQB1 and DQA1 chains were associated with the MS haplotype and did not have a primary association with disease. A similar finding was reported by other investigators [52]. These findings bring up several important points. First, as mentioned previously, the control group used for association studies is extremely important and a failure to use a control group that is ethnically identical to the study population can yield misleading interpretations of findings. Secondly, the association of the leucine at position 26 of the DQB1 chain in the French Canadians but not other Canadian MS patients indicates that multiple class II characteristics may influence susceptibility.

Although there is some disagreement on the specific associations between HLA class II molecules and MS, the evidence for an association is extremely strong. The differences between studies may represent separate susceptibility genes operating in distinct populations, as has been suggested by the study of French Canadians. Despite the evidence for an association, the influence of genes in the class II region is modest. It is estimated from various studies that the relative risk for individuals bearing the class II molecules discussed above is between 2 and 3. Thus, the genes most likely represent only one of many genes influencing susceptibility.

The implications of weak disease associations have been examined in the context of complex psychiatric disease, and two general interpretations can be considered [53]. The first is that the genetic marker is in linkage dysequilibrium with a gene required for disease and the second is that the gene showing association represents a susceptibility gene. If association reflects linkage dysequilibrium with a necessary gene, evidence for linkage of the gene will generally be found in formal linkage analysis. If linkage is not identified, the gene is more likely a susceptibility gene not necessary for disease but increasing the risk for disease. Thus, linkage analysis of HLA genes in MS is important in establishing the importance of HLA in MS. Initially, several investigators presented evidence supporting linkage (reviewed in [54]). These studies have been faulted, however, for methodological flaws. Subsequent attempts to demonstrate linkage of HLA with affected members of multiplex families have produced conflicting results. Several studies employing sib pair analysis [54–56] have failed to demonstrate an increase in HLA DR2 (DR15) sharing in affected sibs that reaches a high degree of significance. In contrast, linkage analysis of DQA and DQB in a group of Finnish families [57, 58] did report linkage using IBD analysis. These same families were found to show linkage with a MBP locus and this point will be discussed below in more detail. The results of the various linkage studies raise two important points. First, differences between different geographic and ethnic populations may exist and this aspect must be considered in analyzing results of genetic studies in MS. Secondly, the general lack of evidence supporting linkage, in the presence of evidence supporting weak but positive association between HLA DR and/or DQ and MS, may not only be due to ethnic differences but may also suggest that these genes may influence susceptibility but are not necessary for disease. With respect to HLA class II genes, it is attractive to postulate that the ability of certain class II molecules to present certain antigens could increase the risk or susceptibility for disease. Consistent with this hypothesis, a recent study examining segregation of the DR2, Dw2, DQw15 haplotype in MS families has suggested that the haplotype is a risk factor for MS and, importantly, is not merely a marker for the northern European populations generally at high risk for MS [59].

Although most attention has focused on the HLA genes in the HLA region of chromosome 6, there are other genes in the HLA complex that could contribute to susceptibility. As can be noted from Figure 13.1, genes encoding for TNF, some components of complement and genes important for antigen processing and presentation, TAP and LMP are also found in the HLA complex. Thus, it is possible that the association with the HLA complex could reflect an association with one of these other genes rather than HLA class II genes.

Tumor necrosis factor (TNF)

As discussed in detail in Chapter 15, proinflammatory cytokines, particularly gamma interferon and tumor necrosis factor alpha (TNFα), are thought to contribute to the evolution of the MS lesion. Not only could TNFα produce up-regulation of HLA class II molecules within the CNS and increase expression of cell adhesion molecules on endothelial cells and glial cells, but it may also directly result in damage to myelin. In addition, the genes of TNF are located within the HLA region on chromosome 6. Thus, if the HLA association findings are interpreted as reflecting a gene in linkage dysequilibrium with disease (which is unlikely as discussed above), TNF would represent a reasonable possibility. One study using an RFLP to examine the association between MS and TNF failed to find an association, but the ability of this RFLP to demonstrate polymorphisms in the TNF region of chromosome 6 was limited [60]. A subsequent study examining more pleomorphic markers also failed to find an association [61]. Because of the potential importance of TNF in the MS lesion, additional studies are needed to further define this region of the HLA region.

Tap 1 and Tap 2

HLA class I-restricted CD8 + T cells recognize cytosolic antigens which are transported from the cytoplasm into the endoplasmic reticulum where they become associated with class I alpha chain molecules. Peptides after transport into the endoplasmic reticulum (ER) are loaded on to the alpha chain of the HLA class I molecule which, in turn, associates with beta 2 microglobulin and is transported through the Golgi apparatus to the cell membrane. Transport of the peptides from the cytoplasm to the ER is mediated by the tap 1 and tap 2 transport proteins. The genes for the tap proteins are located in the HLA class II region between the genes for DP and DQ. The tap genes have been shown to be polymorphic and these polymorphisms have been used by several investigators to examine an association between MS and tap genes. A number of studies have now been conducted in various MS populations, and although the methodology has differed among these studies all have failed to identify an association [62–66]. These negative results have important implications other than indicating that tap genes fail to influence susceptibility for MS. The lack of association indicates that the portion of the class II haplotype that is in linkage disequilibrium and that does generally show an association with disease does not extend to the tap region of the chromosome.

Localization of important HLA class II genes

It has been postulated that the weak association between HLA DR and DQ in MS may indicate that these associations merely reflect associations with genes in close proximity to genes that may show a stronger correlation with disease. If the positive and negative associations between various genes in the HLA region are examined they indicate that the relevant region of the HLA region is probably found in a region telomeric to the TAP region and centromeric to the class III region, since no association has been found for the C4 region [67]. Consequently, it is likely that the HLA class II genes are responsible for influencing susceptibility.

T cell receptor genes

Since multiple genes most likely influence susceptibility for MS and since the strongest association identified to date has been for genes encoding for HLA class II molecules that are responsible for presenting antigen to T cells, other genes encoding for elements of the trimolecular complex, especially those for the alpha and beta chains of the TCR, would be strong candidates for influencing susceptibility and for possibly interacting with the penetrance of genes for class II molecules. Additional support for the role of TCR genes influencing susceptibility for MS comes from studies of the experimental autoimmune demyelinating disease experimental allergic encephalomyelitis (EAE). As discussed Chapter 14, dealing with immunological mechanisms in MS, the trimolecular complex which consists of the MHC molecule, antigen bound to the MHC binding groove and the T cell receptor, is central to induction of EAE. In some strains of mice and in Lewis rats, encephalitogenic T cells induced with the encephalitogen myelin basic protein (MBP), have a restricted TCR expression; almost all encephalitogenic T cells use Vβ8. Although these findings do not reflect a germline difference in these animals, they do emphasize the importance of the TCR in disease.

The TCR is a highly polymorphic heterodimer consisting of an alpha and a beta chain (Figure 13.2). The alpha chain includes a constant region, a junctional region and a variable region. The beta chain consists of a constant region, a junctional region, a diversity region and a variable region. The diversity of the TCR is derived from the recombination of different C, J, (D) and V region genes. The highly polymorphic region involved in recognition of antigen, known as the CDR3 region, is formed by the junction of the V, (D), J and C region genes. While the number of C and D genes is small, more than 100 Vα and Vβ genes have been identified.

The examination of the relationship between the TCR and MS has occurred at two different levels. First, an association or linkage of TCR genes to disease has been examined and will be discussed below. These studies focus on the relationship between germline genes and disease. A second approach has been to examine the TCRs used by T cells that are

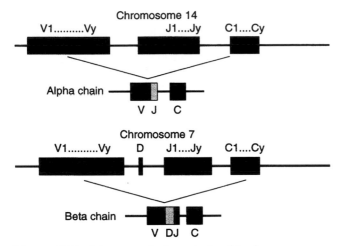

Figure 13.2 Diagram of the relationship between genes encoding for the components of the alpha and beta chains of the T cell receptor and expression of the T cell receptor on T cells.

specific for antigens such as MBP which might contribute to disease. As a variant of this second approach, TCR sequences have been examined in MS lesions in an effort to identify unique TCR usage in MS. The results of these studies are discussed in Chapter 15. TCR usage is important in assessing the significance of a particular TCR in disease but are not directly related to genetic susceptibility unless a TCR chain found to be overused in a particular T cell response is also found to be associated with disease when analyzed at the germline level.

Initially, an association between alleles encoding for Vα and MS was reported in patients who were DRw15[68]. An association with Vα polymorphisms was supported by a subsequent study of MS and myasthenia gravis[69]. However, a number of studies have re-examined the relationship between Vα and MS and have failed to find an association[70–72]. The importance of a susceptibility locus within the TCR Vβ region was initially indicated by results of a sib pair analysis which indicated that one Vβ haplotype was shared to an extent greater than expected[73]. This was followed by an analysis of allelic forms of Vβ8, Vβ11 and Cβ using RFLPs that identified a haplotype involving the genes for these regions in patients with chronic progressive MS[74–76] This association was greater when DR15 patients were compared to DR15 control individuals, again raising the possibility of an interaction between TCR loci and those for HLA class II. However, the association was weak, resulting in a relative risk of only 3.2 in the DR2 positive individuals. Subsequent studies examining the association between TCR Vβ and MS have yielded conflicting results. A study of Spanish MS patients reported an association between Vβ 8 and 11 and MS[77]. In contrast, a study of Swedish MS patients using methods identical to those used in previous studies failed to demonstrate an association even in patients who were DR15[78]. A failure to identify an association has also been reported from a study of French and Belgian MS patients[79, 80]. Further, no evidence of linkage between TCR Vβ and MS could be identified in a study of families in the United States[81].

The explanation for these conflicting results relating to an association between genes for the TCR and MS are uncertain and have been the subject of a recent review[82]. Several possibilities, mentioned previously as potential problems in genetic studies, should be considered. Most important, association studies in mixed ethnic populations can can yield misleading results if differences in ethnic make-up between the control and patient populations exist. An interaction between TCRβ and the DR15 haplotype has been examined recently[26] and has demonstrated a small but significant relationship supporting the possibility of an epistatic interaction between these loci. Consequently, it is likely that an association between TCR genes and MS may exist but that it is extremely weak. This would suggest that TCR genes may represent one of several set of genes that contribute to susceptibility but are neither necessary nor sufficient for disease. If it is postulated that recognition of an antigen or group of antigens is a critical aspect of MS, it is understandable that the ability of the HLA class II molecule to bind and present antigen will contribute to susceptibility. Since the ability of the TCR to recognize the antigen/HLA complex is influenced by the hypervariable region which is generated by the interaction of genes encoding for the variable, junctional and diversity regions of the molecule, it is not unexpected that if any association with variable region genes is found it would be weaker than the association with class II molecules.

Immunoglobulin genes

Several years ago an association was reported between MS and genes encoding for a highly polymorphic region of the constant region of the heavy chain of IgG known as the GM locus[83]. A subsequent report identified a protective effect associated with a different GM phenotype[84]. Subsequently a study of French MS patients reported an increased risk for developing disease in individuals sharing both HLA DR2 and a certain GM haplotype[85]. Since this initial report, most subsequent studies have failed to confirm these initial observations[86–88]. It is now known that there are substantial variations in GM frequencies in different ethnic populations. Thus, as has been mentioned previously, considerable risk exists in conducting association studies unless the ethnic make-up of the two study samples is identical. A recent examination of associations between MS and Ig polymorphisms has also failed to identify a relationship with GM but did find a relationship with a gene coding for a locus on the variable region of IgG VH-2[87]. The association has been confirmed by the same investigators but a linkage to disease in families could not be identified[88]. In distinction, a study of MS patients in the United Kingdom has reported a trend towards linkage[26]. Together these results indicate a positive but weak association between Ig V region polymorphisms and MS. If antibody contributes to the demyelination in the MS lesion, genes influencing biological characteristics of Ig could represent one aspect of susceptibility. Additional studies are needed to resolve the relationship between Ig loci and MS.

Myelin basic protein

Of all of the myelin proteins which have been shown to be encephalitogenic, myelin basic protein (MBP) has been the most extensively studied owing partly to the ease with which it can be purified. Consequently, it is not surprising that MBP has been extensively studied as a potential autoantigen in MS. The results of these studies are complicated and are reviewed in detail in Chapter 15. In brief, MBP-reactive T cells can be demonstrated in both healthy controls as well as patients. Although MBP-specific T cells are not specific for MS they may still represent one component of the disease. Thus regulation of MBP expression could represent one factor influencing susceptibility for MS. Polymorphisms have been identified in the up-stream regulatory region of MBP. Initially studies comparing a patient population with controls reported an association between a polymorphism in the 5′ region and MS[89]. Subsequent family studies demonstrated linkage of this region with disease [34, 90]. However, numerous other studies have failed to confirm this observation [91–94]. If an association exists, it is no doubt very weak.

A number of other myelin antigens, including myelin oligodendrocyte glycoprotein (MOG), 2-3-cyclic nucleotide-3-phosphodiesterase (CNPase) and proteolipid protein (PLP) have been found to be encephalitogenic in various experimental animals. Mutations in PLP which is encoded on the X chromosome result in a defect in myelination which in humans produces Pelizaeus–Merzbacher disease. A relationship between the genes encoding these proteins and susceptibility for MS has not been investigated extensively.

Mitochondrial genes

Mitochondria are subcellular organelles that are responsible for oxidative phosphorylation and contain a 16.6 kilobase segment of DNA. This DNA encodes for a small number of proteins involved in the respiratory chain. Although both sperm and oocytes contain mitochondria, mitochondrial DNA is only maternally transmitted. Since maternal transmission of MS is more frequently observed a role for mitochondrial DNA has been attractive. More specific interest in mitochondrial DNA has come from the recent demonstration of a mutation in mitochondrial DNA in Leber's hereditary optic neuropathy (LHON), which can resemble optic neuritis and is transmitted by females. A small number of patients with an illness that has features of both LHON and MS have been reported and a mutation in mitochondrial DNA similar to that seen in Leper's disease was identified[95]. These patients had bilateral optic neuritis but in addition other symptoms suggesting MS. They also had MRI abnormalities (seven of the eight patients), but had relatives diagnosed as LHON. A subsequent study of a large population of MS patients looking at mutations in mitochondrial DNA has failed to identify the mutation associated with LHON or other mutations that would not be expected to occur normally[96]. In contrast, some patients with marked visual involvement consistent with LHON but with other neurological involvement suggesting MS have been identified and found to have various mitochondrial DNA mutations. Overall, these findings do not provide a compelling argument for a role for mitochondrial DNA in MS. They do raise the possibility of a subset of patients which may have a disease resembling MS and characterized by visual loss which is associated with mutations in mitochondrial DNA; this would provide additional evidence for heterogeneity with respect to both genetic influence and clinical features in MS. Disease heterogeneity has long been suspected because of the differing clinical patterns of disease, such as the primary-progressive form of MS. Consideration of disease heterogeneity must be given consideration in designing studies of either the cause or treatment of MS.

Other genes

Associations between MS and genes other than those discussed above have also been reported but generally lack confirmation. An early report described an association between MS and a gene for a component of complement, C3, encoded on chromosome 19[97]. A subsequent study failed to confirm this observation [98]. A second marker, alpha-1-antitrypsin, also found on chromosome 19, has been reported to be associated with MS[99]. Again, a subsequent study has failed to confirm this association[97]. If an association exists with either of these genes it is very weak. It is possible that weak associations such as these may point to another gene on chromosome 19 that will have a stronger association.

Gene mapping

As mentioned previously, several groups of investigators have initiated large detailed analyses of the entire genome in families with MS in order to identify regions of the genome contributing to susceptibility. The results from three of these studies, which evaluated a total of 324 sib pairs, one from the US and France, one from Canada and one from the United Kingdom, have recently been published [100, 101, 103]. Each of these studies used highly pleomorphic markers distributed throughout the genome to identify genes influencing susceptibility. The results of these studies have confirmed many of the points made earlier in this chapter. No single gene or region with a strong linkage to MS susceptibility was identified, suggesting that MS is a disease in which multiple genes have a relative effect on susceptibility and that no single gene is either necessary or sufficient for disease. Instead, as in the animal models discussed previously, multiple genes probably can have partial effects resulting in small increases in susceptibility. Two of the studies [100, 101] identified a gene in the MHC or HLA region of chromosome 6 as having the strongest association, and the third study [102] found a similar but weaker linkage after analysis of a second and third data set. These findings both support the relative importance of HLA molecules in influencing susceptibility and also demonstrated the care that must be taken in the analysis of genetic studies; to rule out a region as contributing to susceptibility, large numbers of sib pairs must be studied. Thus, if a linkage or association is not found the results must be interpreted with caution.

Three other possible regions of interest, located on chromosomes 5, 7 and 17, were identified in one or more of the studies as having a possible association. A fourth study examined Finnish families for linkage to three regions of the genome that have been linked to susceptibility to EAE [104]. The study of genetic susceptibility in EAE used a similar approach to that used in the human studies described above. Microsatellite markers were used to study the entire genome in mice back-crossed to generate animals with variable susceptibility. Three regions other than MHC were identified which seemed linked to susceptibility. The corresponding human region would be on chromosome 5, and linkage to a marker on chromosome 5 was identified in the Finnish study.

As mentioned earlier in the chapter, the relative genetic influence may differ in various geographic regions, making identification of relevant genes even more difficult in studies with relatively limited numbers of families and from diverse genetic backgrounds. Although these results may seem disappointing, as cooperation between investigators increases and standardization of genetic markers improves, the ability to pinpoint genes with influence on susceptibility will also improve.

13.5 Summary

As discussed, considerable evidence points to a strong genetic influence on susceptibility in MS. In fact, recent studies of multigenic influences in animal models indicate that the effect of multiple susceptibility genes acting epistatically are capable of producing less than 100% penetrance of disease even in animals that are genetically identical. Thus, it is possible that genetic influence alone, without implicating an environmental factor, could account for susceptibility for MS. If a strong genetic influence exits for susceptibility for MS, why has the genetic factor been so difficult to identify? First, the tools that have led to rapid progress in identifying relevant genes in diseases with inheritance following mendelian genetics are not sufficiently powerful to unravel the genetic influence in complex diseases such as MS. Secondly, compared to some other complex diseases such as IDDM, MS has characteristics that make the problem more difficult. These include a broad age of onset, lack of a specific diagnostic test, and great variation in clinical course, raising the possibility of disease heterogeneity. In addition, genetic factors may influence the clinical course as well as susceptibility. Despite these difficulties, rapid progress is being made in establishing analytical approaches for examining complex diseases. Combined with the exponential progress in molecular genetics it is likely that increased understanding of genetic factors in MS will evolve rapidly.

References

1. Kurtzke, J.F. (1985) Epidemiology of multiple sclerosis, in *Handbook of Clinical Neurology, 3* (revised series) (ed. J.C. Koetsier), *Demyelinating Diseases*, Amsterdam, Elsevier, pp. 259–87.
2. Compston, A. (1994) The epidemiology of multiple sclerosis: principles, achievements and recommendations. *Ann. Neurol.*, pp. S211–S217.
3. Ebers, G.C. and Sadovnick, A.D. (1994) The role of genetic factors in multiple sclerosis susceptibility. *J. Neuroimmunol.*, pp. 1–17.
4. Sadovnick, A.D. and Ebers, G.C. (1993) Epidemiology of multiple sclerosis: a critical overview. *Can. J. Neurol. Sci.*, pp. 17–29.
5. Alter, M., Leibowitz, U. and Spear, J. (1966) Risk of multiple sclerosis related to age of migration to Israel. *Arch. Neurol.*, pp. 110–13.
6. Dean, G. (1967) Annual incidence, prevalence and mortality of MS in white South African-born and white immigrants to South Africa. *Br. Med. J.*, pp. 724–6.
7. Elian, M., Nightingale, S. and Dean, G. (1990) Multiple sclerosis among the United Kingdom born children of immigrants from the Indian Subcontinent. *J. Neurol. Neurosurg. Psychiatry*, pp. 906–11.
8. Kurtzke, J.F. and Hyllested, K. (1986) Multiple sclerosis in the Faroe Islands I. Clinical update, transmission, and the nature of MS. *Neurology*, pp. 307–28.
9. Detels R., Visscher, B., Malmgren, M. et al. (1977) Evidence for susceptibility to multiple sclerosis in Japanese Americans. *Am. J. Epidemiol.*, pp. 303–10.
10. Kalman, B., Takacs, K., Gyodi, E. et al. (1991) Sclerosis multiplex in gypsies. *Acta Neurol. Scand.*, pp. 181–5.
11. Ebers, G.C., Sadovnick, A.D. and Risch, N.J. (1995) A genetic basis for familial aggregation in multiple sclerosis. *Nature*, pp. 150–1.
12. Eichhorst, H. (1913) Multiple sklerose und spastische spinalparalyse. *Med. Klin.*, pp. 1617–19.
13. Sadovnick, A.D., Baird, P.A. and Ward, R.II. (1988) Multiple sclerosis: updated risk for relatives. *Am. J. Med. Genet.*, pp. 533–41.
14. Sadovnick, A.D. (1993) Familial recurrence risks and inheritance of multiple sclerosis. *Curr. Opin. Neurol. Neurosurg.*, pp. 189–94.

15. MacKay, R.P. and Myrianthopoulos, N.C. (1966) Multiple sclerosis in twins and their relatives: final report. *Arch. Neurol. Psych.*, pp. 449–52.

16. Bobowick, A.R., Kurtzke, J.F. and Brody, J.A. (1978) Twin study of multiple sclerosis: an epidemiological inquiry. *Neurology*, pp. 978–87.

17. Currier, R.D. and Eldridge, R. (1982) Possible risk factors in multiple sclerosis as found in a national twin study. *Arch. Neurol.*, pp. 140–4.

18. Williams, A., Eldridge, R., McFarland, H. and McFarlin, D.E. (1980) Multiple sclerosis in twins. *Neurology*, pp. 1139–47.

19. McFarland, H.F., Eldridge, R. and McFarlin, D.E. (1984) Family and twin studies in multiple sclerosis. *Ann. NY Acad. Sci.*, pp. 118–20.

20. Heltberg, A. and Holm, N.V. (1982) Concordance in twins and recurrence in sibships in multiple sclerosis. *Lancet*, pp. 1068.

21. Kinnunen, E., Juntunen, J. and Ketonen, L. (1988) Genetic susceptibility to multiple sclerosis: a co-twin study of a nationwide study. *Arch. Neurol.*, pp. 1108–11.

22. Ebers, G.C., Bulman, D.E. and Sadovnick, A.D. (1986) A population based study of multiple sclerosis in twins. *N. Engl. J. Med.*, pp. 1638–42.

23. Sadovnick, A.D., Armstrong, H., Rice, G. and Ebers, G.C. (1992) A population based study of multiple sclerosis in twins: update. *Ann. Neurol.*, pp. 281–5.

24. Mumford, C.J., Wood, N.W., Kellar-Wood, H. *et al.* (1994) The British Isles survey of multiple sclerosis in twins. *Neurology*, pp. 11–15.

25. French Research Group on Multiple Sclerosis (1992) Multiple sclerosis in 54 twinships: concordance rate is independent of zygosity. *Ann Neurol.*, pp. 724–7.

26. Compston, D.A.S., Kellar Wood, H., Roberston, N., Sawcer, S. and Wood, W. (1995) Genes and susceptibility to multiple sclerosis. *Acta Neurol. Scand.*, pp. 43–51.

27. Drake, C.G., Rozzo, S.J., Hirschfeld, H.F. *et al.* (1994) Analysis of the New Zealand black contribution to lupus-like renal disease. *J. Immunol.*, pp. 2441–7.

28. Morel, L., Rudofsky, O.H., Longmate, J.A., Schiffenbauer, J. and Wakeland, E.K. (1994) Polygenic control of susceptibility to murine systemic lupus erythematosus. *Immunity*, pp. 219–23.

29. Risch, N., Ghosh, S. and Todd, J.A. (1993) Statistical evaluation of multiple-locus linkage data in experimental species and its relevance to human studies: application to nonobese diabetic (NOD) mouse and human insulin-dependent diabetes mellitus (IDDM). *Am. J. Hum. Genet.*, pp. 702–14.

30. Sadovnick, A.D., Bulman, D. and Ebers, G.C. (1991) Parent–child concordance in multiple sclerosis. *Ann. Neurol.*, pp. 252–5.

31. Lord, D. and O'Farrell, A.G.O. (1990) The inheritance of MS susceptibility. *Irish J. Med.*, pp. 1–20.

32. Tienari, P.J., Salonen, O., Wikstrom, J., Valanne, L. and Palo, J. (1992) Familial multiple sclerosis: MRI findings in clinically affected and unaffected siblings. *J. Neurol. Neurosurg. Psychiatry*, pp. 883–6.

33. Lynch, S.G., Rose, J.W. and Smoker, W. (1990) MRI in familial multiple sclerosis. *Neurology*, pp. 900–3.

34. Tienari, P.J., Terwilliger, J.D., Ott, J., Palo, J. and Peltonen, L. (1994) Two-locus linkage analysis in multiple sclerosis (MS). *Genomics*, pp. 320–5.

35. Lander, E.S. and Schork, N.J. (1994) Genetic dissection of complex traits. *Science*, pp. 2037–47.

36. Weeks, D.E. and Hardy, L.D. (1995) The affected-pedigree-member method: power to detect linkage. *Hum. Hered.*, pp. 13–24.

37. Batchelor, J.R., Compston, D.A.S. and McDonald, W.I. (1978) The significance of the association between HLA and multiple sclerosis. *Br. Med. Bull.*, pp. 279–84.

38. Jersild, C., Sveigaard, A. and Fog, T. (1972) HLA antigens and multiple sclerosis. *Lancet*, pp. 1240–1.

39. Olerup, O. and Hillert, J. (1991) HLA class II associated genetic susceptibility in multiple sclerosis: a critical evaluation. *Tissue Antigen*, pp. 1–15.

40. Kurdi, A., Ayesh, I., Addallat, A. *et al.* (1977) Different B-lymphocyte alloantigens associated with multiple sclerosis in Arabs and northern Europeans. *Lancet*, pp. 1123–5.

41. Marrosu, H.G., Muntoni, F., Murru, M.R. *et al.* (1988) Sardinian multiple sclerosis is associated with HLA-DR4: a serological and molecular analysis. *Neurology*, pp. 1749–53.

42. Gorodezky, C., Najera, R., Rangel, B.E. *et al.* (1986) Immunogenetic profile of multiple sclerosis in Mexicans. *Hum. Immunol.*, pp. 364–74.

43. Naito, S., Kuroiwa, Y., Itoyama, T. *et al.* (1978) HLA and Japanese MS. *Tissue Antigens*, pp. 19–24.

44. Odum, N., Hyldig-Nielsen, J.J. and Morling, N. (1988) HLA-DP antigens are involved in the susceptibility to multiple sclerosis. *Tissue Antigens*, pp. 235–7.

45. Vartdal, F., Sollid, L.M., Vandvik, B., Markussen, G. and Thorsby, E. (1989) Patients with multiple sclerosis carry DQB1 genes which encode shared polymorphic aminoacid sequences. *Hum. Immunol.*, pp. 103–10.

46. Spurkland, A., Ronningen, K.S., Vandvik, B., Thorsby, E. and Vardal, F. (1991) HLA-DQA1 and HLA-DQB1 genes may jointly determine susceptibility to develop multiple sclerosis. *Hum. Immunol.*, pp. 69–75.

47. Allen, M., Sandberg-Wollheim, M., Sjogren, K. *et al.* (1994) Association of susceptibility to multiple sclerosis in Sweden with HLA class II DRB1 and DQB1 alleles. *Hum. Immunol.*, pp. 41–8.

48. Ghabanbasani, M.Z., Gu, X.X., Spaepen, M. *et al.* (1995) Importance of HLA-DRB1 and DQA1 genes and of the amino acid polymorphisms in the functional domain of DR beta 1 chain in multiple sclerosis. *J. Neuroimmunol.*, pp. 77–82.

49. Olerup, O., Hillert, J., Frederikson, S. *et al.* (1989) Primary chronic progressive and relapsing remitting multiple sclerosis: two immunogenetically distinct disease entities. *Proc. Natl Acad. Sci.*, pp. 7113–17.

50. Hillert, J., Gronning, M., Nyland, H., Link, H. and Olerup, O. (1992) An immunogenetic heterogeneity in multiple sclerosis. *J. Neurol. Neurosurg. Psychiatry*, pp. 887–90.

51. Haegert, D.G. and Francis, G.S. (1993) HLA-DQ polymorphisms do not explain HLA class II associations with multiple sclerosis in two Canadian patient groups. *Neurology*, pp. 1207–10.

52. Olerup, O. and Hillert, J. (1991) HLA class II-associated genetic susceptibility in multiple sclerosis: a critical evaluation. *Tissue Antigens*, pp. 1–15.

53. Hodge, S.E. (1994) What association analysis can and cannot tell us about genetics of complex disease. *Am. J. Med. Genet.*, pp. 318–23.

54. Kellar-Wood, H.F., Wood, N.W., Holmans, P. *et al.* (1995) Multiple sclerosis and the HLA-D region: linkage and association studies. *J. Neuroimmunol.*, pp. 183–90.

55. Ebers, G.C., Paty, D.W., Stiller, C.R. *et al.* (1982) HLA typing in sibling pairs with multiple sclerosis. *Lancet*, pp. 88–90.

56. Govaerts, A., Gony, J., Martin-Mondiere, C. *et al.* (1985) HLA and multiple sclerosis: population and family studies. *Tissue Antigens*, pp. 187–99.

57. Tienari, P.J., Wikstrom, J., Koskimies, S. *et al.* (1993) Reappraisal of HLA in multiple sclerosis: close linkage in multiplex families. *Eur. J. Hum. Genet.*, pp. 257–68.

58. Tienari, P.J. (1994) Multiple sclerosis: multiple etiologies, multiple genes? *Ann. Med.*, pp. 259–69.

59. Hauser, S.L., Fleischnick, E. and Weiner, H.L. (1989) Extended major histocompatibility complex haplotypes in patients with multiple sclerosis. *Neurology*, pp. 275–7.

60. Fugger, L.M., Morling, N. and Sandberg-Wolheim, M. (1990) Tumor necrosis factor alpha gene polymorphism in multiple sclerosis and optic neuritis. *J. Neuroimmunol.*, pp. 85–8.

61. Lepage, V., Lamm, L.U. and Charron, D. (1993) Molecular aspects of HLA class II and some autoimmune diseases. *Eur. J. Immunogenet.*, pp. 153–64.

62. Liblau, R., van Endert, P.M., Sandberg-Wollheim, M. *et al.* (1993) Antigen processing gene polymorphisms in HLA-DR2 multiple sclerosis. *Neurology*, pp. 1192–7.

63. Kellar-Wood, H.F., Powis, S.H., Gray, J. and Compston D.A. (1994) MHC-encoded TAP1 and TAP2 dimorphisms in multiple sclerosis. *Tissue Antigens*, pp. 129–32.

64. Vandevyver, C., Stinissen, P., Cassiman, J.J. and Raus J. (1994) TAP 1 and TAP 2 transporter gene polymorphisms in multiple sclerosis: no evidence for disease association with TAP. *J. Neuroimmunol.*, pp. 35–40.

65. Middleton, D., Megaw, G., Cullen, C. *et al.* (1994) TAP1 and TAP2 polymorphism in multiple sclerosis patients. *Hum. Immunol.*, pp. 131–4.

66. Bell, R.B. and Ramachandran, S. (1995) The relationship of TAP1 and TAP2 dimorphisms to multiple sclerosis susceptibility. *J. Neuroimmunol.*, pp. 201–4.

67. Hillert, J. and Olerup, O. (1993) Multiple sclerosis is associated with genes within or close to the HLA-DR-DQ subregion on a normal DR15, DQ6, Dw2 haplotype. *Neurology*, pp. 163–8.

68. Martell, M., Marcadet, A. and Strominger, J. (1987) T cell receptor alpha genes might be involved in multiple sclerosis genetic susceptibility. *CR Acad. Sci.*, pp. 105–10.

69. Oksenberg, J.R., Sherritt, M., Begovich, A.B. and Steinman, L. (1989) T cell receptor V alpha and C alpha alleles associated with multiple sclerosis and myasthenia gravis. *Proc. Natl Acad. Sci.*, pp. 988–92.

70. Eoli, M., Wood, N.W., Kellar-Wood, H.F. *et al.* (1994) No linkage between multiple sclerosis and the T cell receptor alpha chain locus. *J. Neurol. Sci.*, pp. 32–7.

71. Hashimoto, L.L., Mak, T.W. and Ebers, G.C. (1992) T cell receptor alpha chain polymorphisms in multiple sclerosis. *J. Neuroimmunol.*, pp. 41–8.

72. Lynch, S.G., Rose, J.W., Petajan, J.H. and Leppert, M. (1992) Discordance of the T-cell receptor alpha-chain gene in familial multiple sclerosis. *Neurology*, pp. 839–44.

73. Seboun, E., Robinson, M.A., Doolittle, T.H. and Kindt, T. (1989) A susceptibility locus for multiple sclerosis is linked to the T cell receptor beta chain complex. *Cell*, pp. 1095–100.

74. Beall, S.S., Concannon, P., Charmely, P. *et al.* (1989) The germline repertoire of T cell receptor beta chain genes in patients with chronic progressive multiple sclerosis. *J. Neuroimmunol.*, pp. 59–66.

75. Charmely, P., Beall, S.S., Concannon, P., Hood, L. and Gatti, R.A. (1991) Further localization of a multiple sclerosis susceptibility gene on chromosome 7q using a new T cell receptor beta-chain DNA polymorphism. *J. Neuroimmunol.*, pp. 231–41.

76. Beall, S.S., Biddison, W.E., McFarlin, D.E., McFarland, H.F. and Hood, L.E. (1993) Susceptibility for multiple sclerosis is determined, in part, by inheritance of a 175-kb region of the TcR V beta chain locus and HLA class II genes. *J. Neuroimmunol.*, pp. 53–60.

77. Martinez-Naves, E., Victoria-Gutierrez, M., Uria, D.F. and Lopez-Larrea, C. (1993) The germline repertoire of T cell receptor beta-chain genes in multiple sclerosis patients from Spain. *J. Neuroimmunol.*, pp. 9–13.

78. Hillert, J., Leng, C. and Olerup, O. (1991) No association with germline T cell receptor beta chain alleles or haplotypes in Swedish patients with multiple sclerosis. *J. Neuroimmunol.*, pp. 141–7.

79. Vandevyver, C., Buyse, I., Philippaerts, L. *et al.* (1994) HLA and T-cell receptor polymorphisms in Belgian multiple sclerosis patients: no evidence for disease association with the T-cell receptor. *J. Neuroimmunol.*, pp. 25–32.

80. Fugger, L., Sandberg-Wollheim, M., Morling, N., Ryder, L.P. and Svejgaard, A. (1990) The germline repertoire of T-cell receptor beta chain genes in patients with relapsing remitting multiple sclerosis or optic neuritis. *Immunogenetics*, pp. 278–80.

81. Lynch, S.G., Rose, J.W., Petajan, J.H. *et al.* (1991) Discordance of T-cell receptor beta-chain genes in familial multiple sclerosis. *Ann. Neurol.*, pp. 402–10.

82. Hillert, J. and Olerup, O. (1992) Germ-line polymorphism of TCR genes and disease susceptibility – fact or hypothesis? *Immunol. Today*, pp. 47–9.

83. Pandy, J.P., Goust, J.M. and Salier, J.P. (1981) Immunoglobulin G heavy chain (GM) allotypes in multiple sclerosis. *J. Clin. Invest.*, pp. 1797–800.

84. Steinman, L. (1992) Autoimmune disease and the nervous system (Editorial). *West. J. Med.*, pp. 664–6.

85. Propert, D.N., Bernard, C.C.A. and Simons, M.J. (1982) Gm allotypes in multiple sclerosis. *J. Immunogenet.*, pp. 359–61.

86. Gaiser, C.N., Johnson, M.J., deLange, G., Rasenti, L. and Steinman, L. (1987) Susceptibility to multiple sclerosis associated with immunoglobulin gamma 3 restriction length polymorphism. *J. Clin. Invest.*, pp. 309–13.

87. Walter, M.A., Gibson, W.T., Ebers, G.C. and Cox, D.W. (1991) Susceptibility to multiple sclerosis is associated with the proximal immunoglobulin heavy chain region. *J. Clin. Invest.*, pp. 1266–73.

88. Hashimoto, L.L., Walter, M.A., Cox, D.W. and Ebers, G.C. (1993) Immunoglobulin heavy chain variable region polymorphisms and multiple sclerosis susceptibility. *J. Neuroimmunol.*, pp. 77–83.

89. Boylan, K., Takahashi, N. and Paty, D. (1990) DNA length polymorphism 5' to the myelin basic protein gene is associated with multiple sclerosis. *Ann. Neurol.*, pp. 291–7.

90. Tienari, P.J., Wikstrom, J., Sajantila, A., Palo, J. and Peltonen, L. (1992) Genetic susceptibility to multiple sclerosis linked to myelin basic protein gene. *Lancet*, pp. 987–91.

91. Rose, J., Gerken, S., Lynch, S. *et al.* (1993) Genetic susceptibility in familial multiple sclerosis not linked to the myelin basic protein gene. *Lancet*, pp. 1179–81.

92. Graham, C.A., Kirk, C.W., Nevin, N.C. *et al.* (1993) Lack of association between myelin basic protein gene microsatellite and multiple sclerosis (Letter). *Lancet*, pp. 1596

93. Wood, N.W., Holmans, P., Clayton, D., Robertson, N. and Compston, D.A. (1994) No linkage or association between multiple sclerosis and the myelin basic protein gene in affected sibling pairs. *J. Neurol. Neurosurg. Psychiatry*, pp. 1191–4.

94. Eoli, M., Pandolfo, M., Milanese, C. *et al.* (1994) The myelin basic protein gene is not a major susceptibility locus for multiple sclerosis in Italian patients. *J. Neurol.*, pp. 615–19.

95. Harding, A.E., Sweeney, M.G., Miller, D.H. *et al.* (1992) Occurrence of a multiple sclerosis-like illness in women who have a Leber's hereditary optic neuropathy mitochondrial DNA mutation. *Brain*, pp. 979–89.

96. Kellar-Wood, H., Robertson, N., Govan, G.G., Compston, D.A. and Harding, A.E. (1994) Leber's hereditary optic neuropathy mitochondrial DNA mutations in multiple sclerosis. *Ann. Neurol.*, pp. 109–12.

97. Francis, D.A., Klouda, P.T. and Brazier, D.M. (1988) Alpha-antitrypsin types in multiple sclerosis and lack of interaction with the Gm marker *J. Immunogenet.*, pp. 251–5.

98. Bulman, D.E., Armstrong, H. and Ebers, G.C. (1991) Allele frequency of the third component of complement (C3) in MS patients. *J. Neurol. Neurosurg. Psychiatry*, pp. 554–5.

99. McCombe, P.A., Clark, P., Frith, J.A. *et al.* (1985) Alpha-1-antitrypsin phenotypes in demyelinating disease. *Ann. Neurol.*, pp. 514–16.

100. Sawcer, S., Jones, H.B., Feakes, R. *et al.* (1996) A genome screen in multiple sclerosis reveals susceptibility loci on chromosome 6p21 and 17q22. *Nature Genet.*, **13**, 461–3.

101. The Multiple Sclerosis Genetics Group (1996) A complete genomic screen for multiple sclerosis underscores a role for the major histocompatibility complex. *Nature Genet.*, **13**, 467–71.

102. Ebers, G.C., Kukay, K., Bulman, D.E., *et al.* (1996) A full genome search in multiple sclerosis. *Nature Genet.*, **13**, 472–6.

103. Kuokkanen, S., Sundvall, M., Terwilliger, J.D. *et al.* (1996) A putative vulnerability locus to multiple sclerosis maps to 5p14-p12 in a region syntenic to the murine locus Eae2. *Nature Genet.*, **13**, 477–80.

104. Sundvall, M., Jirholt, J., Yang, H. *et al.* (1996) Identification of a murine locus associated with susceptibility to chronic experimental autoimmune encephalomyelitis. *Nature Genet.*, **10**, 313–17.

14 IMMUNOLOGY OF MULTIPLE SCLEROSIS AND EXPERIMENTAL ALLERGIC ENCEPHALOMYELITIS

Roland Martin and Henry F. McFarland

14.1 Introduction

The etiology of multiple sclerosis (MS) is still unknown, but it is currently widely accepted that a T cell-mediated autoimmune response is involved in the demyelinating process. Evidence for this hypothesis stems from findings gathered in epidemiologic, genetic, histopathologic and immunologic studies. The composition of central nervous system (CNS) white matter infiltrates consisting primarily of lymphocytes and monocytes, the association with genes relevant to immune responses, the similarities with experimental, immune-mediated demyelinating diseases as well as the response to immunosuppressive and immunomodulatory treatments all support an autoimmune pathogenesis. During recent years, the understanding of the immunological mechanisms involved in demyelination has advanced greatly through the investigation of experimental allergic encephalomyelitis (EAE), an animal model of multiple sclerosis induced by injection of myelin components into susceptible animal strains. The characterization of the human T cell-mediated immune response against myelin components as well as the possible effector stages of demyelination has followed these paths. Furthermore, the introduction of magnetic resonance imaging (MRI) as a direct measure of inflammatory activity *in vivo* has allowed a better understanding of the sequential events involved in lesion formation. Finally, studies of new immunomodulatory treatments, in particular interferon beta (IFN-β), have resulted in more effective interventions with fewer side-effects than conventional immunosuppression. This chapter will summarize the most important immunologic findings which have been made during recent years in both EAE and MS research. We will try to relate them to the clinical disease courses and phenotypes and discuss their implications for immunomodulatory treatments of MS.

14.2 Evidence that multiple sclerosis is an autoimmune disease

Although the possibility that MS is caused by a single infectious agent, preferably a virus, cannot be excluded, intensive research in this direction has not disclosed such an agent. Numerous viruses, including measles virus, parainfluenza virus, herpes simplex virus and, laterly, human T lymphotropic retrovirus type 1 (HTLV-1) and human herpes virus type 6 have been implicated in the etiology of MS [1, 2], but these reports could later not be confirmed or are still under investigation. At present, epidemiological as well as immunological data suggest that a number of viruses are able to induce disease or relapses of established disease, but that this only occurs in genetically susceptible individuals. Once the induction by this as yet undefined event/s has happened, an autoimmune pathogenesis directed against myelin antigens is most likely to be involved in disease progression. This view is supported by a number of findings which will be outlined briefly below. Detailed descriptions of these aspects of MS will be presented elsewhere in this book.

14.2.1 GENETIC FACTORS – EPIDEMIOLOGY

The prevalence of MS is not evenly distributed throughout the world. In general, prevalence rates increase with latitudes in both hemispheres. MS is virtually absent in populations living around the Equator whereas up to 200/100 000 individuals are affected in northern European countries [3]. This increase of disease in populations living in zones with moderate or colder climates has been attributed to both environmental and genetic factors. With respect to environment, differences in infectious agents found in these areas, socioeconomic and hygiene standards as well as

Multiple Sclerosis: Clinical and pathogenetic basis. Edited by Cedric S. Raine, Henry F. McFarland and Wallace W. Tourtellotte. Published in 1997 by Chapman & Hall, London. ISBN 0 412 30890 8.

nutrition and vaccination policies are candidates that could contribute to susceptibility. There are, however, exceptions to these rules, such as Hungarian gypsies, Yakuts or Inuit, to name only a few, who have much lower prevalence rates than other populations living in the same areas. It is very difficult to assess, however, whether these disparities are due to genetic differences or to different exogenous factors [4, 5].

In addition to showing variations in prevalence rates, epidemiological studies have pointed out that relapses may be induced by viral infections [6], whereas other factors such as trauma or stress could not reliably be related to exacerbations. Further support for a causal relation of infectious agents with induction of disease stems from the study of local epidemics, for example the one on the Faroe Islands that has been documented by Kurtzke, which supposedly started with the arrival on the Islands of British troops during the Second World War [3]. As mentioned before, however, a specific virus or other infectious agent could not consistently be linked to MS.

Besides environmental influences, it has become increasingly clear that disease susceptibility to develop MS is influenced by genetic factors. Similar to other autoimmune diseases, population, family and twin studies have supported this notion. Depending on the ethnic background, prevalence rates for MS are, for example, much higher in caucasian than Asian, Indian or African populations, even if the respective groups live in similar geographic locations. Furthermore, the risk to develop MS is about 20 times higher for first-degree family members of MS patients, with the highest risk carried by daughters of affected mothers [7]. Identical twin sets are concordant for MS in about 25–35% [8], clearly underscoring that genetic factors are involved in conferring disease susceptibility. The fact that substantially less than 100% of the identical twin sets are concordant, however, also shows that genetic background alone is not sufficient to develop disease, but that exogenous factors are also required. Among the candidate susceptibility genes that have been examined over the years, the best evidence exists for an association between genes of the major histocompatibility complex (MHC; or HLA gene complex in humans) and MS. In caucasian MS patients, HLA-DR15 Dw2 and -DQw6 are closest associated with disease [9]. In populations with lower prevalences, such as Japanese, Mediterranean and Arabic MS patients, other HLA-class II genes, in particular HLA-DR4 and -DR6 have also been found to be related to disease susceptibility (summarized in [2]). Whether other genes, such as those of the immunoglobulin heavy chain locus, of the myelin basic protein (MBP) gene or of the T cell receptor (TCR) alpha or beta chain are related is currently a matter of intensive research, but not yet clear (for details see Chapter 13 on genetics of MS). In summary, we currently believe that a number of genes contribute to disease susceptibility, but even if all these genes are carried by an individual, exogenous factors are required to induce disease.

14.2.2 CHARACTERISTICS OF THE MS LESION

Predilection sites of the lesions or plaques characteristic of MS are the areas of postcapillary venules in the periventricular white matter, the optic nerve and tract, the corpus callosum and the brain stem. Depending on the length of the disease course and the current stage – active versus non-active–various stages of the lesions may be seen adjacent to each other. Early plaques are characterized by blood–brain barrier (BBB) leakage, immunoglobulin secretion and fresh inflammatory infiltrates consisting of CD4$^+$ and CD8$^+$ T lymphocytes, monocytes/macrophages, plasma cells and various degrees of minor populations such as γ/δ T cells [10–12]. These early lesions tend to be well demarcated and show loss of myelin, with axons being less affected. Expression of adhesion molecules such as intercellular adhesion molecule-1 (ICAM-1; CD54) and vascular cell adhesion molecule-1 (VCAM-1; CD106), which have both been implicated in migration of activated T cells into the parenchyma, is not significantly different from constitutive levels, but VCAM-1-positive endothelial cells and T cells expressing their ligand very late antigen-4 (VLA-4; CD49d/CD29) are elevated in chronic active stages [13], suggesting a role during the propagation of disease. Besides the cellular infiltrates, the secretion of various proinflammatory (interferon gamma, IFN-γ, tumor necrosis factor/lymphotoxin, TNFα/β; interleukin 1, IL-1) and anti-inflammatory (interleukin 4, IL-4; interleukin 10, IL-10; transforming growth factor beta, TGFβ) cytokines and the presence of reactive oxygen and nitrogen intermediates, effector molecules released by activated monocytes, strongly supports the idea that MS is an immunologically mediated disease. The acute inflammatory stage of the lesion usually resolves within a few weeks. It is currently not understood why some lesions disappear almost completely with good remyelination whereas in others glial scar tissue and axonal loss dominate, resulting in the classical sclerotic white matter lesion that is described by the term multiple sclerosis. For further details on the histopathology of the EAE lesion see Chapter 15 or a number of excellent reviews [10–12].

14.2.3 LESSONS FROM EXPERIMENTAL AUTOIMMUNE ENCEPHALOMYELITIS (EAE)

Definition of EAE

EAE is an acute or chronic-relapsing inflammatory demyelinating disease of the CNS which is characterized by inflammatory and demyelinating white matter foci of various intensity [2, 14]. Following Rivers's demonstration that post-vaccinal encephalomyelitis after rabies vaccination can be induced by the injection of spinal cord homogenates alone [15], extensive research showed that EAE can be induced in a number of susceptible inbred animal strains by injection of whole white matter or single myelin proteins such as MBP or proteolipid protein (PLP) in complete Freund's adjuvant [16]. Transfer experiments with either humoral or cellular components from affected animals into naive recipients clearly established that EAE is a T cell-mediated autoimmune disease [17]. Following the initial observations that demyelinating diseases can be induced in experimental animals by injection of myelin components, different animal species and strains, various myelin components and modes of induction have been employed to create a number of EAE models which differ substantially in terms of disease course, clinical phenotype and pathology [16, 18, 19]. Although these findings will not be addressed in this chapter, we would like to outline the characteristics of different EAE models as well as the important hallmarks of EAE research in order to allow a better understanding of immunological studies in MS.

Different EAE models in various susceptible animal species and strains

Initial studies of various outbred rodent strains showed that their susceptibility to develop EAE differed considerably [16]. During subsequent years, it became clear through extensive backcrossing experiments that resistance or susceptibility for EAE in inbred rodent strains, including mice, rats and guinea pigs, was primarily associated with their MHC-class II background [16], but, similar to the multigenic influences suspected in MS, other gene loci as well as gender differences are involved in EAE susceptibility [20, 21]. With respect to the different EAE models and their relevance to MS, it is often criticized that none reflects the entire clinical and pathological picture of MS. Indeed, the course and pathology of EAE vary considerably among different rodent strains or other species. In Lewis rats, for example, a monophasic disease without relapses is observed, and pathology is characterized by acute inflammation with predilection sites in the brain stem and lumbar cord, but notably with very limited or no demyelination [22]. Recently, a severe, chronic-relapsing and demyelinating type of EAE was shown in DA rats after injection of whole myelin [22,23]. In mice, monophasic or chronic-relapsing models with perivascular inflammation, demyelination and remyelination have been described [14, 17, 24]. When animals were examined during later stages of disease, lesions of various stages of inflammation, demyelination and glial scarring like the typical MS plaques were observed [14].

Chronic-relapsing EAE induced in strain 13 guinea pigs is another useful model, but due to the paucity of immunological tools available for guinea pigs, mouse and rat models have gained more and more importance during the last decade. EAE has also been examined in primates. In macaques and rhesus monkeys, the disease is more reminiscent of acute disseminated or post infectious encephalomyelitis than MS and histologically characterized by a hemorrhagic leucoencephalitis (L. Massacesi and S. Hauser, personal communication), whereas a chronic-relapsing EAE can be induced in marmosets with whole myelin [25]. The latter model seems particularly useful, since inflammatory and demyelinating foci show the same distribution pattern as in MS, i.e. the spinal cord and periventricular white matter, the inflammatory activity can be followed by MRI and adoptive transfer studies are feasible since heterozygous twins show placental chimerism [25]. The factors responsible for the differences in clinical course and phenotype and in pathology are still poorly understood and will be discussed further below. However, it is clear from clinical experience that MS also presents in at least two major types, relapsing-remitting (RR-MS) and primary chronic progressive MS (PP-MS). Moreover, special forms of MS such as Devic's disease, which presents with demyelination primarily in the spinal cord and the optic nerve, exist. Furthermore, with increasing MRI data it becomes obvious that lesion distribution, i.e. brain, cerebellum or spinal cord, number of acute inflammatory foci with blood-brain barrier leakage or lesions which are dominated by axonal loss and glial scarring and little inflammation may differ in individual patients. With this in mind, one should not expect one EAE model to reflect every aspect of MS. Acute Lewis rat EAE, which is characterized by inflammation, may therefore be useful to study one pathogenetic part of MS – the early phase which leaves little residual damage – whereas other models may be more suitable to examine later stages.

Factors contributing to disease susceptibility and type

As mentioned previously, the MHC class II background is an important factor contributing to disease susceptibility. During recent years, the study of MHC–peptide interactions at the molecular level has allowed for a better understanding of how MHC alleles confer susceptibility. It is now clear that the binding affinity of an antigenic peptide to a given MHC allele is a critical factor which determines T cell immunogenicity and is also important for encephalitogenicity [26]. However, genetic studies [20, 21], experiments examining T cell reactivity and encephalitogenicity with mouse strains expressing the same class II allele on different backgrounds [26], as well as backcrossing experiments, for example of various class II alleles on to the Lewis rat background [27], have shown that genes other than those coding for MHC alleles are also relevant for the susceptibility to develop EAE. The genetic studies mentioned before have employed microsatellite markers to determine disease-associated loci, but the products of these loci are not known [20, 21]. In Lewis rats, which are highly susceptible to EAE when compared to Brown Norway rats, neuroendocrine factors are thought to be involved, and it has been demonstrated that endogenous corticosteroids modulate lymphoproliferation and susceptibility to EAE in the latter rat strain [28].

Another important variable is the antigen which is used for inducing EAE. Proteolipid protein (PLP) and MBP are the major protein components of myelin (see below) and have been studied most extensively as encephalitogens [16, 29, 30]. Together with myelin lipids they assure the highly organized structure of compact myelin. The propensity of an animal strain to mount a cellular or humoral response against one of the myelin proteins and the cellular localization of this protein may both be important for the type of disease. MBP, for example, is a cytosolic protein and therefore not easily accessible to antibodies. A T cell-mediated response to MBP is therefore critical for initiating the disease process. Consequently, immunization with MBP in an animal which tends to develop a strong delayed type hypersensitivity response like the Lewis rat is more likely to show T cell infiltration, but few or no antibodies. When antibodies against myelin oligodendroglial glycoprotein (MOG), a minor myelin glycoprotein exposed on the outer surface of oligodendrocytes, are added after induction of EAE by MBP, marked demyelination is observed [31]. In another rat strain, the DA strain, induction of EAE by whole myelin results in a T cell response against MBP, but also antibody secretion to MOG [23]. Clinically and pathologically, EAE in these animals is severe, runs a chronic-relapsing course and is characterized by inflammation and demyelination [23].

If one asks the question why one animal strain responds to a certain encephalitogen whereas another does not, it has to be taken into account that EAE experiments are performed with inbred animal strains. The T cell response against one particular myelin peptide (see below) may be mediated initially by a small population of T cells with restricted fine specificity and TCR usage [17]. If T cells with the T cell receptor (TCR) variable chain which would be employed in recognition of the complex of MHC and encephalitogenic peptide are deleted in this strain due to expression of an endogenous retrovirus with superantigen activity, this strain may not respond to one particular peptide, but readily develop EAE if another myelin protein is used. Clearly, such a mechanism is less likely in outbred populations, but this possibility only documents that factors other than MHC may influence reactivity to

myelin antigens. Genes coding for proinflammatory cytokines, myelin proteins, costimulatory and adhesion molecules, to name only a few, are all good candidates for factors contributing to disease susceptibility. Genetic as well as functional immunological studies will hopefully soon allow us to understand better their importance for the disease.

Characteristics of encephalitogenic T cells in EAE

To describe in detail the findings made in recent years on encephalitogenic T cells in EAE goes beyond the scope of this chapter. The reader is therefore referred to excellent reviews about this subject [17, 32], but we will briefly describe the most important aspects of encephalitogenic T cells since this research has potentially great importance for understanding the autoimmune pathogenesis of MS.

Transfer experiments with either humoral or cellular components from affected animals into naive recipients clearly established that EAE is a T cell-mediated autoimmune disease [17]. Furthermore, encephalitogenic T cells capable of inducing EAE could be generated from peripheral blood lymphocytes in vitro [33], an important observation that indicated that autoreactive T cells are part of the normal T cell repertoire and not deleted during thymic selection. During the last ten years, EAE became the most extensively studied model for any human autoimmune disease. It is now clear that encephalitogenic T cells belong to the CD4 subset and usually also express the T helper-1 phenotype (secrete IFN-γ and TNFα/β) [17, 34]. Their fine specificity, MHC restriction and TCR expression have been characterized in detail. In the various susceptible animal strains, such as SJL and PL mice or Lewis rats to name only a few, susceptibility to develop EAE is related to the expression of certain MHC-class genes (IA^s, IA^u, RT1B^1) [18], and encephalitogenic CD4$^+$ T cells recognize myelin antigens in the context of these class II molecules. Furthermore, if EAE is induced, for example in SJL mice by injection of MBP, a certain MBP peptide dominates the encephalitogenic response (MBP (89–100) [35]), whereas different MBP peptides are encephalitogenic in mouse strains expressing different MHC class II molecules (MBP (Ac1–9) in PL or B10.PL mice, [17]). Thus, the molecular interaction of autoantigenic peptide with a disease-associated MHC molecule apparently influences the effector T cell response. When the third player of this so-called trimolecular complex consisting of MHC molecule, antigenic peptide and TCR, was examined, a striking observation was made. In certain susceptible animal strains (for example the PL mouse or the Lewis rat) the majority of the encephalitogenic T cells, at least during the initial response, expressed only a very limited numer of TCR variable chains, in particular Vβ8.2 [36–39]. Interestingly, the

TCR chains expressed by encephalitogenic T cells from PL and B10.PL mice as well as from Lewis rats expressed not only the same variable chains, but also similar junctional regions of the TCR, areas that are supposed to contact the antigenic peptide embedded in the MHC binding groove [39]. Further reports have shown that the initial response to the inducing myelin antigen which is directed against one epitope and carried by T cells expressing a limited number of TCR molecules may broaden later in terms of fine specificity and TCR usage [40, 41]. This process, which is referred to as epitope spreading, results in broadening of the immune response in later stages of the disease [40, 41]. Intra- and intermolecular spreading leads to a more diverse autoimmune response with recognition of different dominant and subdominant epitopes of one or several myelin proteins [40, 41]. It is conceivable that therapeutic interventions which specifically target T cells directed at one myelin peptide are less likely to be effective at this stage. This may be a major problem in designing specific immunotherapies for MS (see below), since the neurologist will usually see the patient long after the disease process has been initiated.

Pathogenesis of demyelination in EAE

Based on studies of EAE, the current concept of how demyelinating lesions develop can be summarized as follows. Autoreactive T cells are constantly part of the mature T cell repertoire and even if they are present in extremely high numbers, which has been shown in elegant transgenic mouse models [42], an exogenous inducing event (either the injection of myelin antigen in adjuvant or an infectious agent) is necessary to set the stage for disease development. This phase involves not only the appropriate activation of autoantigen-specific T cells in the periphery by the inducing myelin antigen in the presence of costimulatory signals [43], but also the up-regulation of adhesion molecules on both T cells (LFA-1 and VLA-4 [44, 45]) and cerebrovascular endothelial cells (ICAM-1 and VCAM-1, see above). Only activated T cells are able to transmigrate through the BBB into the CNS parenchyma [46], where they activate resident glial cells and also attract further influx of monocytes and non-specific T cells through the secretion of proinflammatory cytokines, in particular IL-12, IFN-γ and TNF α/β [47, 48]. Damage to myelin sheaths and oligodendrocytes is probably mediated by direct toxic effects of TNF α/β, but also by toxic oxygen and nitrogen intermediates such as O_2^- and NO, which are released by activated monocytes [49]. In addition to these T cell- and macrophage-mediated toxicities, antibodies against myelin antigens that are accessible on the surface of the myelin sheath and the oligodendrocyte, in particular MOG, may further enhance demyelination [31]. Passively recruited inflammatory cells rapidly

disappear, whereas myelin-specific T cells can be detected in the lesions for longer periods of time [50]. Down-regulation of inflammatory activity in the lesion probably involves both programmed cell death [51] and secretion of anti-inflammatory cytokine such as IL-4, IL-10 and TGFβ [52–56]. IL-4, IL-10 and TGFβ expression have been shown to increase when the inflammatory activity of the lesion decreases, and all four cytokines were able to ameliorate the course of EAE when administered therapeutically (see below). Considerably fewer data exist about which mechanisms determine the outcome of myelin repair. It was shown both in EAE and MS that the extent of oligodendrocyte damage varies with the stage of disease, that remyelination is usually incomplete and that the quantitative and qualitative composition of remyelinated areas is different from normal myelin [57]. Whether differences in the expression of the various myelin components, such as different isoforms and post-translationally modified forms of MBP which are physicochemically different from 18.5 kD MBP, contribute to future vulnerability of remyelinated areas is currently less clear but a topic of intensive research.

Therapeutic strategies in EAE

Finally, it should be mentioned that EAE has not only allowed for a better understanding of the pathogenetic events leading to demyelination, but also been crucial to the design of a wide spectrum of therapeutic modalities that range from highly specific interventions targeting the trimolecular complex to less specific approaches which interfere with migration of encephalitogenic T cells into the CNS or with effector stages of the demyelination. In summary, the therapeutic strategies can be grouped into those that affect the initial events of antigen presentation to encephalitogenic T cells, the activation of these T cells or their migration into the target tissue. Furthermore, therapies have been developed which alter the function of encephalitogenic T cells, those which employ the inhibition of proinflammatory cytokines or the enhancement of regulatory cytokines. In addition, different routes of administering myelin proteins or peptides have been shown to be therapeutically effective.

Therapies targeting the trimolecular complex and the initial events of activation include the administration of antibodies against the TCR expressed by encephalitogenic T cells [58], vaccination with either whole inactivated encephalitogenic T cells [59] or peptide fragments derived from the CDR3- [60] or CDR2 [61] regions of these TCR. Other approaches target the MHC molecule either by modified antigenic peptides or unrelated high-affinity binding peptides that compete with the binding of encephalitogenic peptide to the MHC molecule [62]. Recently, this approach has been abandoned and replaced by altered peptide ligands (APL), encephalitogenic peptides modified at their TCR contact residues, in a way that results in partial activation, antagonism or anergy of encephalitogenic T cells and results in down-regulation of EAE[63,64]. The mechanisms operative after administration of APL peptides *in vivo* are not entirely clear yet. However, this approach has gained widespread interest following the demonstration that APL peptides may induce T cell populations which secrete regulatory cytokines upon stimulation by the native peptide[65] or may decrease the ratio of IFN-γ/IL-4 secreted by encephalitogenic TH0 cells[66]. Furthermore, antibodies and soluble receptors against adhesion molecules[44], costimulatory molecules[67,68] and against proinflammatory cytokines such as TNFβ and IL-12 [47,48], the administration of soluble TNF receptors[69], the inhibition of TNF and IFN-γ secretion by phosphodiesterase type IV inhibitors[70,71] as well as the administration or induction of anti-inflammatory cytokines such as IL-4, IL-10, IL-13 and TGFβ [53,54,72–74] were used to treat EAE. Finally, different routes to administer encephalitogenic peptide or protein such as oral, intranasal or intravenous application were shown to be therapeutically effective in EAE[75–77]. Depending on the dose of orally or intranasally administered myelin protein or other autoantigens, a state of anergy or the induction of T cells which secrete immunoregulatory cytokines such as IL-4 or TGFβ resulted[75–77]. Oral tolerization with peptide was also able to cause unresponsiveness to other determinants or whole encephalitogenic protein[76], and this resistance could adoptively be transferred to naive animals[78]. Different from the oral route, intravenous administration of high doses of MBP led to programmed cell death or apoptosis of encephalitogenic T cells and subsequently, improvement of EAE[79].

Although this list is far from being complete, it underscores that the pathogenetic concepts that evolved from the studies of EAE can be used to design effective immunotherapies. Consequently, there is considerable interest to confirm these findings in MS and translate them into specific immunotherapies.

Despite the elegant studies in EAE, it has often been criticized that it is an artificial system and that the various EAE models only reflect parts of the disease process. As mentioned before, the best example for this criticism is the EAE observed in Lewis rats. Following injection of MBP or transfer of MBP-specific, encephalitogenic T cells, Lewis rats develop a monophasic disease characterized by dense lymphomonocytic infiltrates in the brain stem and lumbar spinal cord; however, the hallmark of MS, demyelination, is absent[80]. In addition, no further relapses can be induced in Lewis rats once they have recovered from disease. Therefore, Lewis rat EAE serves as an equivalent to the initial stages of lesion development (BBB breakdown and cellular infiltration) during MS. The factors that are necessary for perpetuating disease and for developing demyelination are apparently absent in Lewis rats, and, in addition, this strain seems to have an efficient immunoregulation that prevents further relapses. Other EAE models, such as the chronic relapsing disease seen in guinea pigs or active or adoptive transfer EAE in the SJL mouse that can either be induced by MBP or by PLP, resemble MS more closely and show not only the chronic relapsing-remitting course, but also all the histopathological characteristics of MS [14,81].

Despite the enormous progress that we made during the past decade, it becomes clear from the above summary of the most important findings in EAE research that we are far from understanding all the factors involved. However, the authors are convinced that EAE will continue to be the best model in which to study pathogenetic as well as therapeutic aspects of demyelinating diseases of the CNS experimentally, and the observations made in this model will be relevant for MS.

14.2.4 IMMUNOMODULATORY AND IMMUNOSUPPRESSIVE TREATMENTS OF MS

The various established and experimental treatments of MS will be addressed in more detail later. At this point, they will only be mentioned to further support the hypothesis that MS is an immunologically mediated disease. For the past decades, corticosteroids have become the treatment of choice for exacerbations of MS. Their potent unspecific anti-inflammatory and immunosuppressive effects rapidly block the inflammatory stage of the lesion and lead to closing of the BBB[82]. As a result, the exacerbations are shortened and less severe. However, corticosteroids have no effect on the long-term course of the disease and cannot be given continuously due to their severe side-effects during long-term treatment. Other immunosuppressive treatments such as cyclophosphamide effectively inhibit inflammatory activity as visualized by the decrease in gadolinium contrast-enhancing lesions, but their long-term effects, especially during later stages of the disease, are not yet clear. Recently, more specific immunomodulatory treatments have been introduced. IFN-β, a drug with both antiviral and immunomodulatory activities, has been shown to decrease exacerbation rates and inflammatory activity in the CNS significantly, and was therefore approved as a treatment of MS[83–85]. Its action is primarily due to antagonistic effects on IFN-γ, which up-regulates MHC molecules, is involved in recruitment and differentiation of inflammatory cells and activates macrophages.

In summary, the association with immunologically relevant genes, the composition of CNS infiltrates of T cells, B cells and macrophages, the parallels to EAE and the response to immunosuppressive and immunomodulatory therapies support our hypothesis that MS is an immunologically mediated disease.

14.3 Are infectious agents causing MS?

As mentioned before, epidemiological studies have linked viral infections to exacerbations of MS [6], and the demonstration of local 'epidemics' or flare-ups of MS [3] as well as the concordance rates of considerably less than 100% in identical twin sets all suggest an as yet unknown exogenous trigger of the disease. Over the past decades, a number of viruses, including herpes viruses, paramyxoviruses and retroviruses such as human T lymphotropic retrovirus type 1 (HTLV-1), have been linked with MS [2, 86], but careful follow-up could not confirm a universal role of one of these viruses as the etiologic agent of MS. As the latest candidate, human herpes virus type 6 (HHV-6) has been implicated as a potential candidate following the demonstration of viral genome in oligodendrocytes only in MS brains [87].

Viruses are clearly the most likely candidates as triggers of MS for a number of reasons. They could cause demyelinating diseases by the following mechanisms (for summary see [2]):

- Viral infection and direct lysis of oligodendrocytes – experimental infection with mouse hepatitis virus or the infection with JC virus during progressive multifocal leucoencephalopathy are examples.
- Immune-mediated damage of virus-infected oligodendrocytes – subacute sclerosing panencephalitis, Theiler's virus-induced encephalomyelitis (TMEV), infection of Lewis rats with both the mouse hepatitis virus (JHM) or a rat-adapted strain of measles virus, and visna, a lentivirus-induced leucoencephalomyelitis of sheep, are examples.
- 'Bystander demyelination' – the immune activation by a neurotropic or other virus leads to cytokine release, up-regulation of adhesion and MHC molecules and activation of myelin-specific T cells.
- Virus-induced autoimmune demyelination – post-infectious encephalomyelitis is an example and usually develops days to weeks after a viral infection. It is thought to be mediated by myelin-specific T cells which are activated by viral antigens similar to myelin antigens either at the amino acid sequence [88] or at the structural level, which is recognized by autoreactive T cells [89].

It becomes clear from this list that the interaction of virus and host is dependent on a number of factors and that both players can influence the outcome of such an infection. Factors important on the side of the virus are tissue and cell tropism, cytopathogenicity, mode of viral spread, influence of the viral infection on cellular metabolism such as antigen processing and presentation as well as interference with protein expression, for example of MHC antigens, to name only a few. On the host's side, its propensity to mount a strong and rapid immune response against an invading virus will determine whether a virus is able to spread to the CNS. As soon as CNS cells such as glial cells or neurons are infected, it will again depend on the cytopathogenicity and the host's response whether infected cells are damaged by the infecting virus or by cytotoxic T cells which lyze infected cells in order to limit further viral spread. It is known from infections with viruses of relatively low cytopathogenicity such as mumps virus that infections in immunosuppressed hosts will not lead to overt clinical manifestation. Individuals who mount a strong cell-mediated immune response against mumps virus, however, will suffer from organ manifestation such as parotitis, pancreatitis or meningitis. In this instance, the inflammation in certain organs is mediated by the immune response rather than the virus itself. In contrast, individuals with a low or absent cell-mediated immune response against the virus will not show acute organ manifestations, but on the other hand have a higher likelihood of not completely eliminating the respective virus. One of the most important factors that determines the strength of such virus-specific immune responses is the MHC/HLA background of the host, but other at present less well understood factors certainly also influence the outcome of an infection, i.e. whether the immune response is primarily mediated by $CD8^+$ and $CD4^+$ TH1 cells or by $CD4^+$ TH2 cells and antibody secretion. In addition to these immunological factors of the host, the vulnerability of the target tissue will also determine whether a virus-specific immune response is protective and advantageous to the host at the same time. Especially in the CNS, where neurons are arrested in G0 and cannot enter the cell cycle again after differentiation, a cell-mediated immune response that eliminates virus-infected cells would clearly be to the disadvantage of the host, whereas the situation is completely different in rapidly dividing tissues such as lymphoid cells or epithelia. Although we cannot cover each aspect of virus and host that might influence the outcome of a viral infection, it is obvious from both human virus-induced demyelinating disease as well as from experimental models that viruses are excellent candidates as causes of MS. It is very possible that different forms of MS are caused by different agents and that type of course, i.e. relapsing-remitting (RR-MS) versus primary chronic progressive (PP-MS), and acuity of disease are influenced by the type of the infecting agent as well as by the host's immune response against the respective infectious agent. This also implies that searching for candidate viruses further on is certainly important, but that studies that try to understand the interaction of virus and host might be even more relevant.

14.4 Characterization of the autoimmune response against candidate myelin antigens

Initial experiments in post-vaccinational encephalomyelitis (PVE) and EAE employed whole spinal cord homogenate to induce disease [15, 90]. Since pathology of MS, PVE and EAE indicates that components of the white matter, either the myelin sheath or/and the oligodendrocyte itself, are the target of the demyelinating immunological process, we will briefly summarize the composition of normal myelin and mention some of the differences that may be found in diseased myelin. The structure and function of myelin are described in excellent reviews elsewhere [91, 92]. CNS myelin, which is at question in this review, consists of about 75–80% lipids and 20–25% proteins [92]. The highly hydrophobic PLP (50%) and the basic MBP (25–30%) are most important with respect to the relative abundance in CNS myelin. 2′,3′-cyclic nucleotide 3′-phospodiesterase (CNPase), myelin-associated glycoprotein (MAG) and MOG each contribute to less than 3% of whole myelin protein content. Besides these proteins, a number of other, less abundant proteins have recently been implicated in disease. These include αB-crystallin, a small heat shock protein that is found at high concentrations in the eye lens, and transaldolase-H (TAL-H), an enzyme expressed in oligodendrocytes [93]. PLP and MBP, due to their physicochemical characteristics, primarily serve structural functions. PLP is integrated in the myelin membrane which it spans by several transmembrane loops. MBP, in contrast, is a cytosolic protein that interacts with acidic lipids at the inner surface of the myelin membrane and stabilizes the tight lamellar structure of the myelin sheath. MAG and MOG are located in the periaxonal space of the myelin sheath and the myelin membrane at the surface of oligodendrocytes, respectively. Whether CNPase, a protein which, like MBP, is found in the cytoplasm of oligodendrocytes, primarily serves structural purposes or is important due to its enzymatic function is not clear at present, since its natural substrate, 2′,3′-cyclic nucleotides, is not found in oligodendrocytes. Besides this complexity, a number of myelin proteins occur in different size isoforms and charge isomers [94–96] Depending on differential splicing of the seven exons, four size isoforms of MBP can, for example, be demonstrated [95]. Although the 18.5 kD isoform is clearly the most important, their relative amounts and time of occurrence vary not only during myelination, but also later during remyelination. Further, posttranslational modifications, i.e. phosphorylation, methylation or arginine to citrulline modifications, are described for MBP [96]. It has recently been demonstrated that amino acids (aa) encoded by exon 2 of MBP, which is only expressed in the 21.5 kD isoform, may not only serve as a target for human MBP-specific T cells,

but exon 2 is also able to induce EAE in SJL mice [97, 98]. Further, C8, a post-translationally modified isoform of the 18.5 kD MBP, contains six arginine to citrulline modifications and has a neutral pH [96]. C8 is not only expressed at relatively higher amounts during early myelination and contributes up to 30% of MBP in mature myelin, but also increases in abundance during the course of MS [99]. T cells that specifically recognize C8 have been isolated from MS patients as well as from healthy controls (see below). Thus not only the major myelin proteins, MBP and PLP, and their size isomers, but also minor myelin components and posttranslational modifications may be the target of the autoimmune response. Further, the location of the myelin components – at the surface of oligodendrocytes and the myelin sheath versus in the cytoplasm – and their accessibility to humoral components may determine their relative importance in humoral, i.e. antibody-mediated, and cellular immune responses.

14.5 T cell-mediated immune responses against myelin antigens

Over the past two decades, it has been firmly established that autoimmune demyelinating disease in the various experimental animal systems is induced and can be transferred by T lymphocytes of the CD4 subset [17]. The latest evidence for this concept stems from mice which carried a transgenic MBP-specific T cell receptor and, at the same time, lacked the RAG genes, recombinases required for the generation of both B and T cell responses [100]. These animals are unable to generate any antibodies or mount a T cell-mediated immune response against antigens other than the MBP peptide which is recognized by the transgenic TCR. Since a high percentage of these animals developed spontaneous EAE, it was clear that one encephalitogenic T cell population carrying one TCR is able to mediate disease in the complete absence of other T cells or antibodies [100].

Following the early studies in EAE, the examination of immune responses in MS also focused on T lymphocytes. Some of the initial experiments indicated that autoreactivity in MS might be due to more general defects in immunoregulation [101, 102]. The increased immunoglobulin synthesis, for example, was ascribed to a lack in soluble suppressor activity either because of defective $CD8^+$ T cell function or a lack of a subset of $CD4^+$ T cells that was termed suppressor-inducer cells. Although a defective reactivity of MS patients against a specific antigen, i.e. measles virus, was also documented [103], most of this research was done in antigen-unspecific, mitogen-driven systems and conclusions as to the importance of specific cells or antigens were therefore difficult. In addition, the heterogeneity of CD4$^+$ T cells and their differentiation into various subtypes, i.e. TH1, TH2 and TH0 cells, depending on their cytokine profiles, was not known during times when the initial studies were performed. With our increasing knowledge of the immune system in general and the detailed characterization of the encephalitogenic T cells in EAE, a number of neuroimmunologists started to examine the human T cell response against those myelin antigens which had been demonstrated to be encephalitogenic in EAE. Unlike EAE though, in human studies as to whether myelin-specific T cells are related to MS we have to rely on indirect evidence, since the test that established encephalitogenicity in EAE, i.e. the direct transfer of T cells, is obviously not possible.

Researchers have therefore addressed the following questions in order to establish the importance of myelin-specific T cells in humans:

1. Does the frequency of T cells with specificity for one or several myelin antigens differ between patients and controls?
2. What is the fine specificity of myelin-reactive T cells and does this differ between patients and controls?
3. Which restriction elements are used by myelin-specific T cells?
4. Is there a unique or restricted TCR usage in peripheral blood lymphocytes (PBL) or T cells infiltrating the CNS of MS patients?
5. Are there differences in phenotype and function in myelin-specific T cells derived from patients and controls?

We shall not be able to cover every aspect of the studies of human myelin-specific T cells in great detail, but will try to outline the path MS research has taken by examining MBP-specific T cells first. Later, human T cell reactivity to other myelin antigens will also be covered, and important reviews and original literature will be cited.

14.5.1 T CELL REACTIVITY AGAINST MYELIN BASIC PROTEIN (MBP)

Although MBP is less abundant in CNS myelin than PLP and also appears in peripheral myelin, early studies in both EAE and MS largely focused on this myelin component. We believe that this is primarily due to the fact that MBP is considerably easier to isolate from myelin, and therefore availability of the protein and knowledge about its physicochemical characteristics, gene organization and amino acid sequence preceded that of other myelin components. Most of the immunological research on MBP has focused on the major 18.5 kD isoform, but it has been shown in recent years that other isoforms and post-translational modifications of MBP may also be a target of the autoimmune T cell response. Reactivity against the latter forms of MBP will be mentioned at the end of the section on MBP-specific T cells.

Frequency of MBP-specific T cells

With the above questions it was expected that differences in frequencies might be found in patients. A number of interesting observations were made during these studies. The first striking observation that was already made more than ten years ago was the demonstration of MBP-specific T cells not only in peripheral blood of MS patients, but also in normal individuals [104]. This result was later confirmed by a large number of groups and highlighted that autoantigen-specific T cells are far from being completely deleted during thymic selection processes, but can easily be demonstrated in the peripheral blood in healthy individuals [105–108]. When the frequencies of MBP-specific T cells were later determined in both PBL and CSF, different frequencies were observed depending on the techniques used, i.e. enumeration of IFN-γ secreting cells by ELISPOT [109, 110] or using tritiated thymidine uptake as a measure for proliferation [105–108]. The numbers ranged between 2.7×10^{-5} (PBL) and 185×10^{-5} (CSF) (IFN-γ secreting cells by ELISPOT following stimulation with MBP [110]) and 0.68×10^{-5} to 0.5×10^{-7} (antigen-specific proliferation [107–111]). The question why considerably higher numbers of MBP-specific T cells are detected by using IFN-γ secretion as a readout is currently not resolved, but the comparison of frequencies in MS patients and controls showed higher frequencies in the MS patients [107, 109, 110], although some studies failed to confirm these results [108, 111]. The negative results could be due to the fact that patients and controls were not matched well enough for HLA type, age and sex and that the patients' blood had been isolated more often during remissions or phases of little disease activity; but stratification for disease status and type of disease was performed neither in the studies showing differences nor in those which failed to show them. To eliminate at least the differences in genetic background, frequencies were also compared between affected and unaffected family members [112] and even between identical twins discordant and concordant for disease [111]. Similar frequencies were observed in the family members regardless of disease [112]. In identical twins, the frequencies differed between different sets but not between individuals of the same set [111]. The latter observation indicated that the frequency of MBP-specific T cells may be linked to the immunogenetic background of an individual and thus be a prerequisite rather than a consequence of disease development. Such a hypothesis will, however, require broader confirmation. Further evidence for an involvement of MBP-specific T cells in

MS stems from analyzing *in vivo* activated cells from the peripheral blood. When PBL lymphocytes were pre-cultivated with IL-2 in order to selectively expand those cells that had been activated *in vivo* rather than *in vitro* and tested for antigen specificity and frequency, higher numbers of activated MBP- and PLP-specific T cells were found in MS patients [113]. Furthermore, the demonstration of *in vivo* activated hprt- mutant T cells with specificity for MBP in MS patients [114], suggests that such cells are not merely an epiphenomenon, but were rather stimulated *in vivo* by exposure to either MBP released into the circulation, by nonspecific stimuli such as bacterial superantigens or by foreign antigens with sequence or structural similarities with MBP peptides.

Fine specificity of MBP-specific T cells

Following the observation that different MBP peptides are encephalitogenic in different animal strains for EAE, the fine specificity of human MBP-specific T cell lines (TCL) was studied. Since encephalitogenic TCL could be generated *in vitro* by repeated antigenic stimulation, and since these TCL recognized the portion of MBP that was found to be encephalitogenic in this particular strain, for example MBP (68–84) in Lewis rats [33], human TCL have also been established from bulk populations [106]. Mapping the fine specificity of these bulk-derived long-term TCL [106] or of TCL that had been generated by seeding limiting cell numbers (i.e. 2×10^5 cells; split well technique) with overlapping peptides spanning the entire sequence of MBP demonstrated that TCL from both MS patients and controls preferentially recognized three areas of MBP [106–112, 115, 116]. These immunodominant areas are located in the N-terminus, but even more in the middle (aa 83–102) and C-terminus (approximately aa 140–170) of the MBP molecule [106–112, 115–118]. In DR2-positive MS patients, peptide 84–102 was immunodominant, whereas the C-terminal peptide 143–168 appeared to be equally important in DRw11-positive MS patients and healthy controls [107]. The importance of the middle region was further supported by the finding that it is recognized by MBP-specific TCL in the context of a number of different HLA-DR molecules, particularly those that are associated with MS (HLA-DR15, -DR4 and -DR6 [116]. Further examination of TCL specific for MBP peptide (87–106) with truncated and Ala-substituted peptides revealed a number of nested epitopes in this area and a considerable degree of heterogeneity [119].

The above findings about the fine specificity of MBP-specific TCL are again disappointing at first, since similar specificities are observed in both MS patients and controls and since TCL are heterogeneous even when TCL with specificity for one peptide are examined.

However, it is important to note that the areas of MBP which are immunodominant in humans are the same as those which are encephalitogenic in a number of different animal strains susceptible to EAE [2, 17]. The middle region (aa 89–101), for example, is encephalitogenic not only in SJL mice, but also in Lewis rats. AA (Ac1–9) and 153–170 are encephalitogenic in PL and B10.PL mice and rhesus monkeys respectively. These similarities suggest either similarities in the processing and presentation of MBP in different species which result in presentation of the same areas of MBP in the peptide binding groove of the respective MHC-class II molecule and/or common binding requirements of the disease-associated MHC-class II molecules in the animals susceptible to EAE and in MS patients (see below). It also argues for the usefulness of EAE and probably means that at least some of the analogies that have been made between encephalitogenic, MBP-specific T cells and MBP-specific T cells derived from MS patients are valid.

Besides heterogeneity in the response against the 18.5 kD isoform of MBP, it has recently been shown that aa derived from exon 2 of the MBP gene and expressed only in the 21.5 kD MBP isoform, as well as post-translationally modified forms of MBP, can also specifically be recognized by TCL established from MS patients as well as controls [98, 120].

In summary, no striking differences in terms of fine specificity of MBP-specific T cells have been described in MS patients and controls. However, immunodominant regions of MBP exist in the N-terminus, middle and C-terminus of the molecule, and these might be important since they overlap with areas of MBP which are encephalitogenic in animals. The diversity in fine specificity that was demonstrated in patients with longstanding disease is again reminiscent of epitope spreading in EAE. However, a more limited number of T cell specificities has been found in earlier stages and may persist over longer periods of time in patients with milder disease [121].

HLA restriction of MBP-specific T cells

It has been mentioned before that susceptibility to develop EAE is under the control of MHC-class II molecules and that the genes with the strongest association with MS belong to the HLA class II complex, i.e. HLA-DR15 and -DQw6 in caucasians. The analysis of the molecular interaction between HLA molecules and antigenic peptides has recently been elucidated by X-ray crystallography, sequencing of self peptides released from HLA molecules and by peptide binding studies [122–124]. For HLA class II molecules, these studies demonstrated that interactions of the floor and α-helical walls of the peptide binding groove with the carbon backbone of the antigenic peptide contribute most of the binding energy [123]. In addition, the side chains of aa in defined anchor positions of the peptide contact the various pockets of the groove and are important for positioning the peptide. It was concluded from these structural interactions and from disease associations with certain HLA-DR or -DQ alleles that the hypervariable regions of HLA class II molecules are responsible for binding particular pathogenetically relevant autoantigens.

The HLA restriction of human MBP-specific TCL was tested by using antibodies against HLA class I molecules, HLA-DR, -DP or -DQ to block antigen-specific proliferation or cytotoxicity, but also by matching antigen-presenting cells (APC) for certain alleles. Due to the high polymorphism of the HLA system and the coexpression of up to four HLA-DR alleles on the surface of cells of an individual heterozygous for HLA-DR, it was sometimes only possible to determine the restriction with murine or human fibroblasts transfected with cDNAs for certain HLA DR alleles. The overall consensus from these studies was that the vast majority of MBP-specific T cells are restricted by HLA-DR molecules [105–108, 115, 125]. Only a minority of cell lines recognized MBP peptides in the context of either HLA-DQ or even less -DP [105, 107]. Those HLA-DR molecules that had been shown by genetic studies to be associated with MS, i.e. DR15, DR4 and DR6, were most often found to serve as the restriction element, and, in addition, each of them was able to present up to nine different MBP peptides [105–108, 115, 125]. It has already been mentioned that the immunodominant regions of MBP, peptides (87–106) or (84–102) and (152–170) can, in turn, be presented by a variety of different HLA-DR molecules [116, 126]   and   HLA-DQw6   (MBP (84–102) [107]. Thus, there is not only the ability of the HLA-DR molecule to present several MBP peptides, but the complexity is expanded by 'promiscuous binding' of some peptides to a number of different alleles. Recent experiments that addressed the interaction of the immunodominant peptide (87–99) or (84–102) and overlapping MBP peptides to different HLA-DR alleles at the molecular level [127, 128] demonstrated that certain amino acids of the peptide serve as anchors to the HLA molecule. Furthermore, it was shown that immunodominant peptides, i.e. those peptides which are recognized by large numbers of T cells, bind with higher affinities to the relevant HLA-DR molecule than others [126–128]. When large numbers of TCL from MS patients and controls were compared for HLA restriction, again no major differences between patients and controls were observed, but in both groups and also in identical twins discordant and concordant for MS a clear ranking was seen [111]. The HLA-DR molecules which are associated closest with MS served most often as restriction element, i.e. DR2 (DR15) > DR4 > DR6 > other alleles.

As mentioned before, in most DR haplotypes two heterodimers encoded by DRα paired with a DRB1 gene product and DRα paired with a DRB3–5 gene product are coexpressed. It was therefore of interest to find out which of the two DR heterodimers coexpressed in the MS-associated HLA-DR15 haplotype – DRα paired with DRB1*1501 (DR2b) or DRα paired with DRB5*0101 (DR2a) – is more important in restricting MBP-specific T cell responses. Initial reports showed that both DR2a and DR2b are able to present MBP peptides [115, 129]. One report claimed that DR2b may be more important because only TCL specific for MBP (80–99) from MS patients were restricted by DR2b, whereas DR2a was able to present different peptides to TCL from both MS patients and controls [115]. When cytotoxic MBP-specific TCL were examined, most of them were restricted by DR2a [129]. These studies were both compromised by the small numbers of lines studied, and although another report also claimed that DR2b might be more relevant in restricting MBP-specific T cell responses, our own data with over 50 different MBP-specific TCL which are either restricted by DR2a or DR2b (Vergelli et al., manuscript in preparation) show that both molecules restrict about equal numbers of TCL. In agreement with binding studies, however, DR2b primarily binds MBP peptide (83–99) and serves as restriction element for lines specific for this peptide, whereas DR2a binds a number of different peptides and accordingly restricts cell lines with a number of specificities, in particular for the middle (87–99) and the C-terminal region (135–155) of the molecule [126] (M. Kalbus et al., unpublished results). The immunodominant MBP peptide (87–106) or (84–102) contains the peptide binding motifs of DR2a and DR2b overlapping each other [127, 128]. This finding not only explains the high binding affinity to both alleles, but probably also why this peptide is immunodominant in the human MBP-specific T cell response.

Taken together, HLA-DR molecules serve as the primary restriction elements in the human MBP-specific response. MS-associated HLA-DR molecules are most often found as restriction elements and their binding requirements apparently determine immunodominance. The observation that MS-associated HLA-DR molecules preferentially bind those MBP peptides which have been found to be encephalitogenic in animals susceptible for EAE again underlines similarities in the interaction between MHC-class II molecule, autoantigenic peptide and T cell response in MS and EAE.

T cell receptor usage of MBP-specific T cells

The description of a restricted TCR variable chain usage in encephalitogenic T cells and the therapeutic implications of this finding, which led to a number of highly specific therapies directed against the TCR, has also raised great hopes to study TCR expression in human MBP-specific T cells. Early reports seemed to confirm the observations made in Lewis rat and PL- and B10.PL mouse EAE and demonstrated restricted usage of a few TCR Vβ chains in MBP (84–102)-specific T cells (Vβ17 and Vβ12 [130]) or in MBP-specific T cells in general from MS patients (Vβ5.2 and Vβ6.1 [131]. Another report documented limited TCR usage in MBP-specific TCL derived from one, but not between different individuals [132]. Differences in the patient populations as well as in the specificity and restriction of the TCL make it hard to compare the data. Furthermore, each of these studies differed from the others in the chains that were found over-represented. Additional reports addressed the question as to whether the response of TCL specific for one MBP peptide is restricted in fine specificity and TCR variable chain usage. Both documented a considerable degree of heterogeneity in fine specificity and V-chain usage [119, 133]. Heterogeneity of TCR V chain expression was also reported from families and twins [112] and also when the TCR beta chain rearrangements of 17 (152–170)-specific and DR13-restricted T cell clones derived from one MS patient were examined [134].

The analysis of the structural interactions of the TCR molecule with the MHC–peptide complex has shown that the complementarity determining region (CDR) 3 which is represented by the boundary between variable, N-additions, joining (or diversity and joining for the beta chain) and constant regions is primarily contacting the antigenic peptide [135]. CDR1, CDR2, both hyper-variable regions located in the variable chain, however, interact either with the HLA molecule (CDR1) alone or together with the peptide (CDR2) [136]. At first, it was concluded from these findings that, if a specific autoantigen in the context of one or a few HLA molecules is involved in the pathogenesis of MS, similarities should be found in the CDR3 regions of MBP-specific TCL. When this aspect of MBP-specific TCL was analyzed in detail, it again became clear that there is no general overutilization of one specific TCR CDR3 region [137]. However, the observation that similar CDR3 regions are expressed by DR2a-restricted and MBP (87–106)-specific TCL [116] (Vergelli et al., submitted for publication), by in vivo activated MBP-specific hprt-TCL [138] as well as by TCR from encephalitogenic mouse and rat TCL [138] and also in the brains of MS patients [139] (see below), led to the hypothesis that the immunodominant MBP peptide and certain TCR CDR3 regions are involved in the pathogenesis of MS, at least in a subgroup of MS patients.

The involvement of the TCR repertoire in the disease process found further support in studies performed with short-term TCL in identical twins. When peripheral blood lymphocytes were stimulated several times either by tetanus toxoid or MBP before the Vα chain profile of

the cell lines was compared, considerable differences were observed in the profiles of the affected twin compared to the unaffected twin [140]. In identical twins concordant for disease as well as in healthy twins the profiles were very similar, consistent with the idea that the selection of the TCR repertoire is driven by the HLA background. The results from the discordant twins showed that the TCR repertoire of the affected individual, despite the identical genetic background, was either skewed before or during the chronic disease process. It was therefore concluded from these results that T cells and their TCR are related to the disease process.

One of the TCR Vα chains which was frequently detected in the above study was Vα8 [140]. As a follow-up, Utz and colleagues therefore asked the question whether the CDR3 sequences of these Vα8-expressing TCL were similar or different at the various stages of disease [137]. The most important observation from this report was a trend towards increasing heterogeneity in patients with severe and long-standing disease as opposed to early and mild disease [137]. This suggests that the heterogeneity of T cells and their specificity broaden during the disease process, and although other reports could show that single MBP peptide-specific TCL and their receptors can be isolated over long periods of time from the blood of individual patients [141], it is unlikely that both peptide specificity and TCR usage are restricted in later stages of the disease.

A number of remarks should be made with respect to the current knowledge about TCR usage of MBP-specific T cells. Although the degree of restriction in either V chain usage or expression of CDR3 sequences has certainly been overestimated by initial studies, a number of the above findings support the idea that MBP-specific T cells may be related to disease in a subgroup of patients. However, most of the reports are compromised by the small number of individuals and TCL studied as well as the lack of stratification for clinical type and stage of disease. Participants of the TCR workshop held in Leiden during the International Congress of Neuroimmunology (Amsterdam, 1994) have therefore launched an initiative to collect TCR sequence information on well-defined TCL. It is hoped that we will understand the role of MBP-specific TCR with MHC–peptide better as soon as more data from larger samples of MS patients and TCL becomes available, and as soon as researchers have succeeded in clarifying the three-dimensional interaction between TCR molecule and MHC–peptide complex at the molecular level.

T cell receptor usage in MS lesions

As opposed to EAE, where the antigenic peptide that induces disease is well known, we do not at present understand which antigen/s induce MS. Furthermore, it was often argued that the analysis of MBP-specific TCL generated from activated peripheral blood T cells or even just from PBL does not necessarily reflect which cells are present in the MS lesion. This notion is supported by data derived from EAE where it was shown that, in contrast to the peripheral blood, encephalitogenic T cells and their TCR are easily detectable at early stages in the inflammatory CNS lesion and, during that time, contribute the majority of infiltrating cells. Subsequently, passive recruitment of other cells with unknown specificity predominated whereas encephalitogenic T cells appeared to stay in the lesion for longer periods of time and were therefore easier to detect again at this point[50]. Although activation of myelin-specific T cells is thought to happen in the periphery, it was hoped that the analysis of TCR expression in CNS lesions during MS might show restricted usage and thus allow the association of certain TCR chains or CDR3 regions with the disease process. It is clear that such a question could not be approached systematically in humans and that one would probably not be able to analyze MS plaques at defined stages of disease. Despite these concerns, several investigators have studied TCR expression in MS brains obtained from autopsy tissue[139, 142, 143]. One of these reports described a limited Vα chain usage with only two to four rearranged Vα chains in three MS brains[142]. Vα10 was present in plaques in all three brains, Vα8 and 12 in two brains each[142]. Further studies documented a limited expression of Vα and Vβ chains in chronic but not in acute inflammatory plaques[143], and also a limited degree of heterogeneity in Vα and Vβ chain expression (Vβ5.2 and −6.1) and, in particular, the presence of defined CDR3 sequences in patients with the MS-associated HLA haplotype DRB1*1501, DRB5*0101, DQA1*0102 and DQB1*0602[139]. Since these brain-derived transcripts were shared in part with the CDR3 region of a Vβ5.2-expressing DR2a-restricted MBP (87–106)-specific cytotoxic TCL[116], it was concluded that T cells specific for the immunodominant MBP peptide, expressing a specific junctional region and restricted by DR15, are involved in the pathogenesis of MS[139].

Although TCR expression in the brain clearly needs further study, the initial results provide a lead for future directions of research. It will be particularly important to determine whether TCR expression in the peripheral blood correlates with that in the CNS and whether TCR sequences are indeed linked to antigen-specific T cell clones.

Phenotype and function of MBP-specific T cells

We have mentioned before that encephalitogenic T cells in EAE primarily belong to the TH1 subtype and that the expression of certain adhesion molecules is required for encephalitogenicity[44, 144]. Since targeting the cytokines released by encephalitogenic TH1 T cells (IFN-γ and TNFα/β) or their adhesion molecules (VLA-4 and LFA-1) resulted in ameliorating disease, considerable interest focused on these aspects of human myelin-reactive T cells, too. One of the reasons was the hope that even if the antigen specificity of human disease-related T cells could not be defined, one might still be able to design therapeutic interventions that interfere with their migration into the CNS or their effector functions. Two pieces of evidence support this reasoning. First, although given only to a small number of patients the therapeutic application of IFN-γ resulted in an increase in exacerbation rate and therefore had to be terminated[145]. Secondly, a number of reports documented that TNFα levels in blood and CSF are elevated in MS patients and related to disease activity[146, 147]. Thirdly, increased levels of IL-2 have also been observed in MS patients[148]. Although these results are not unquestioned, they seem to support a role of TH1 cytokines in MS.

When MBP-specific T cells were analyzed for their phenotype and function, the vast majority of cell lines which had been established by stimulation with whole MBP was found to express CD4[106, 125, 149]. Since exogenous proteins are processed primarily via the exogenous or endocytic processing pathway and presented in the context of HLA class II molecules to CD4+, class II-restricted T cells, this was not surprising. Further analysis demonstrated that MBP-specific CD4+ T cells, similar to encephalitogenic TCL in EAE, often belong to the TH1 subtype[149], although TH0 and TH2 cell lines, i.e. TCL that secrete IL-4 and/or IL-10 in addition to IFN-γ and TNFα, are also observed (Hemmer et al., in press). Another function of cells that has been linked to encephalitogenicity in EAE, cytotoxicity, is also frequently found in CD4+, MBP-specific T cells[106, 125, 149]. Although such MBP-specific CD4+ TH1 cells are found in both patients and controls, their similarities with T cells capable of mediating EAE suggests that they are involved in the pathogenesis of MS. Furthermore, elevated levels of IFN-γ-and IL-2-secreting cells in both peripheral blood and CSF as well as elevated levels of several adhesion molecules, including VLA3–6, LFA-1, LFA-3, CD2 and of CD26 and CD44 on CSF T cells support the concept that T cell activation is critical for autoimmune pathogenesis[150].

The detection of immunoregulatory cytokines such as IL-4- and TGFβ-secreting T cells by ELISPOT in the CSF of patients with optic neuritis[151] or by analyzing supernatants and message from PLP-specific T cell clones that had been isolated from times with low disease activity, i.e. remissions, documents that it is critical at what stage of the disease they are isolated[152]. Interestingly, the lymphokine secretion patterns of the cells clones in the latter study did not change during the *in vitro* propagation, suggesting that the tissue culture of cell lines may not bias the phenotype of cells, as was often anticipated previously.

The improved understanding of interactions between HLA class I molecules and processing and presentation of proteins in the class I-associated endogenous processing pathway allowed the definition of binding motifs that are required for peptides in order to bind to a specific HLA class I molecule [153]. With this knowledge it became possible to screen different myelin antigens for the presence of such binding motifs, and consequently it was possible to establish CD8$^+$, HLA class I-restricted TCL against a number of myelin antigens, including MBP [154]. CD8$^+$ T cells have been detected in MS plaques and although there is much less evidence for a direct role of CD8$^+$ T cells in the pathogenesis of EAE or MS, such cells could either be important in immunoregulation or damage oligodendrocytes directly. The latter hypothesis should be addressed by future studies since oligodendrocytes do not express HLA class II molecules. It is therefore currently believed that damage to oligodendrocytes or myelin sheaths is primarily mediated either by antibody-mediated cellular cytotoxicity, by complement-mediated lysis, by reactive oxygen or nitrogen intermediates derived from macrophages or by TNFα/β derived from CD4$^+$ TH1 cells and macrophages. Direct T cell-mediated damage to oligodendrocytes can be mediated by CD8$^+$ class I-restricted T cells, but usually not by CD4$^+$ T cells. A CD4$^+$ T cell population that mediates a novel type of MHC-unrestricted lysis of oligodendrocytes was, however, recently demonstrated [155].

Clearly, these questions whether and to what extent the processing and presentation of MBP or other myelin antigens is responsible for the predominance of certain cell types, whether certain lymphokine secretion patterns can consistently be linked to certain disease types and stages, and the role of CD8$^+$ T cells and other phenotypes in contributing to disease need to be pursued in more detail in the future.

14.5.2   T CELL REACTIVITY AGAINST OTHER MYELIN ANTIGENS OR ANTIGENS EXPRESSED IN MS LESIONS

MBP represents the myelin antigen that is by far the best investigated in both EAE and MS. This is probably related to the ease with which MBP can be isolated in sufficient amounts from white matter material. Furthermore, its good solubility facilitates its use in studies of humoral and cellular immunity. With increasing understanding of the physicochemical and biological characteristics of other myelin proteins, as well as with knowledge about the encoding genes, myelin proteins such as PLP, MAG, MOG and a few other minor proteins have gained more and more attention. For some of these

antigens, in particular PLP, encephalitogenicity has already been demonstrated [156]. Furthermore, size isoforms [98] and charge isomers [120] have been investigated. Although we will not address these studies in similar detail as MBP, the most important observations will be summarized and discussed.

Proteolipid protein (PLP)

Due to its extreme hydrophobicity, PLP is not only more difficult to isolate but also causes problems in tissue culture, since it will quickly precipitate when put in aqueous solutions. An early study failed to demonstrate PLP-specific T cells in peripheral blood, CSF or brain lesions [157]. During recent years, a number of investigators succeeded in establishing PLP-specific TCL from PBL or documented PLP-specific T cells in peripheral blood and CSF [158–161]. Usually these cell lines are responding only weakly to whole PLP [158–160]. Whether this is due to difficulties of APC in processing PLP or to other reasons is currently not clear. When synthetic peptides from either extracellular or cytosolic loops of the protein were used to establish PLP-specific TCL, a marked increase in stimulatory capacity was shown and two peptides, PLP (40–60) and -(89–106), were recognized by larger numbers of TCL from both MS patients and controls and can thus be considered immunodominant [159, 160]. Initially, the choice of peptides seemed arbitrary and was therefore often criticized. However, it turned out that the hydrophilic stretches of the protein from which the peptides had been derived, and in particular the immunodominant regions, contained peptide binding motifs for MS-associated HLA-DR alleles and could be shown to bind with high affinity to HLA-DR2a and -DR2b (C. Pelfrey, A.B. Vogt *et al.*, manuscript submitted). With respect to phenotype and function, PLP-specific TCL are very similar to MBP-specific TCL. A high percentage of these CD4$^+$ TCL show cytotoxic activity and the majority are restricted by HLA-DR molecules [159, 160]. PLP-specific clones with different TH subtypes have been isolated during times of different clinical activity [152]. TH1-like cells dominated during clinical exacerbations, whereas cells isolated during remissions secreted primarily IL-4 and IL-10 [152]. It is currently not completely clear whether the response to PLP is stronger in MS patients as compared to controls, but elevated frequencies of PLP-specific T cells have been found in CSF and blood [161] and also in the fraction of *in vivo*-activated T cells [113].

Myelin oligodendroglia glycoprotein (MOG)

The description of the administration of antibodies against MOG resulting in demyelination in the otherwise purely inflammatory Lewis rat EAE led to the examination of T cell reactivity against MOG. In two recent studies, strong responses against MOG were observed [162, 163]. When the reactivity of PBL derived from MS patients and controls against the myelin antigens MAG, MOG, PLP and MBP was compared in primary proliferative assays, 50% of the patients, but only one out of 16 controls reacted against MOG [163]. Reactivity to other myelin antigens tested was marginal.

Myelin-associated glycoprotein (MAG)

MAG-specific antibodies are related to a subgroup of polyneuropathies associated with monoclonal gammopathies, but their involvement in MS has been addressed only in a few smaller studies [164–166]. One demonstrated low-level reactivity in a subgroup of patients with active disease [164], another reactivity in 7 of 11 patients [166]. Finally, elevated precursor frequencies have been observed in CSF and blood of MS patients [165].

αB-crystallin

Unlike the above-mentioned reports, which used purified myelin proteins for cellular immune studies, an interesting and novel approach was applied by van Noort and co-workers [167, 168]. They separated myelin obtained from MS brains or normal white matter by HPLC and established short-term TCL against the various fractions. Interestingly, the strongest and most consistent T cell reactivity in MS patients and controls was directed against a minor protein component which was later identified as αB-crystallin, a 23 kD heat shock protein, which is expressed in highest concentration in the eye lens but also in other tissues [168]. The demonstration of αB-crystallin expression in glial cells in MS plaques led to the hypothesis that αB-crystallin expression is induced during the CNS inflammatory process by as yet unknown mechanisms and that T cells directed against this protein are pathogenetically relevant in MS [168]. Further studies to assess the encephalitogenic potential of this protein and to characterize αB-crystallin-specific T cells in more detail are currently under way (J.M. van Noort, personal communication).

Transaldolase-H (TAL-H)

Perl and co-workers described reactivity to an enzyme expressed in oligodendrocytes, transaldolase-H (TAL-H), [93, 169]. Searching for endogenous retroviral sequences in MS they found a highly repetitive retrotransposable element with limited sequence homology to human T-cell leukemia virus and a related endogenous retroviral sequence, HRES-1 [93]. This repetitive element is part of the coding sequence of the human transaldolase gene. Humoral and cellular reactivity against this protein was subsequently examined both in CSF and peripheral blood from MS patients [169]. Reactivity of T cells was tested in primary proliferative assays. As expected, reactivity was low, but attempts to confirm these responses with larger numbers of patients and at the clonal level are under way (A. Perl, personal communication).

2′-3′-cyclic nucleotide-3′-phosphodiesterase (CNPase)

Our own studies with recombinant CNPase, with CNPase isolated from porcine and bovine brain as well as with CNPase peptides that have been chosen based on the presence of MHC-binding motifs for DR2a, DR2b and DR4 Dw4 indicate that CNPase-specific CD4+ T cells can be isolated from both MS patients and controls (A. Riethmüller et al., M. Kalbus et al., M. Rösener et al., manuscripts in preparation). We currently do not know whether the response to CNPase differs between patients and controls, but studies to address this point as well as the encephalitogenicity of this myelin component are currently being performed.

The research on T cell reactivity against myelin antigens can be summarized as follows. Besides the well-defined T cell response against MBP, T cell reactivity directed against each myelin component that has been examined so far could be demonstrated. These cells primarily belong to the CD4 population, are often cytotoxic, HLA-DR-restricted and may be grouped into various T helper subtypes depending on the disease activity at the time of isolation. However, CD8+, HLA class I-restricted T cells specific for MAG, MOG, PLP and MBP have also been established, although, based on observations in EAE, their pathogenic role is less clear. If we consider that disease susceptibility in EAE is under the control of MHC background and that not every myelin antigen is encephalitogenic in each strain, we anticipate that different myelin components may be relevant during the initial stages in individual patients based on their immunogenetic differences. The data available so far are often not comparable with respect to antigen preparations, patient demographics and tissue culture conditions applied. It is therefore difficult to determine at present which myelin antigen is most important in individuals or in groups of patients, and also in early as opposed to late stages of the disease. Although the information on this subject may seem exhaustive already to the reader, more data on well-defined groups of patients and disease stages, in particular the very early monosymptomatic form of MS, are clearly required.

14.5.3 INVOLVEMENT OF γ/δ T CELLS

T cells bearing the γ/δ T cell receptor have been found in demyelinated CNS plaques in MS patients [170–172]. The biological role of these cells is currently not clear, but it has been speculated that at least a fraction of them are directed against heat shock proteins (HSP), a group of proteins which serve important functions during stress arising from various causes. HSP are, for example, expressed by macrophages in inflammatory lesions, and it has been shown that HSP-specific T cells are able to lyze HSP-expressing macrophages[173]. This observation has gained wide attention since several HSP species are highly conserved in phylogeny and, for example, HSP derived from mycobacteria share common sequences with human HSP. It was therefore hypothesized that T cells directed against bacterial HSP might cross-react with human HSP expressed in inflammatory tissues, and that this might eventually lead to autoimmunity. The colocalization of γ/δ T cells and HSP 65 + oligodendrocytes in MS lesions has further supported this idea[170]. A number of studies have addressed the question whether there is restricted TCR usage in γ/δ T cells in MS plaques of various stages[170–172, 174]. While two reports demonstrated a predominance of Vδ2-Jδ1 rearrangements in active and chronic lesions[171, 172], another found a limited diversity of Vδ2-Jδ3 TCR in chronic active lesions from several patients[174]. Interestingly, identical junctional sequences were found in Vδ2-Jδ3 transcripts from all 9 patients examined. These data argue for clonal expansion of a subpopulation of γ/δ T cells in MS lesions which could be driven by an as yet unknown antigen. These interesting observations should be followed up. It will be interesting to see whether a specific antigen such as an HSP serves as the target for γ/δ T cells in MS.

14.6   Involvement of antibody-mediated immune responses in MS

It has been known for decades that intrathecal secretion of oligoclonal antibodies is one of the hallmarks of MS[175, 176]. These oligoclonal bands (OCB) are found in CSF and CNS tissue[176], are present in more than 90% of MS patients and are currently used as a diagnostic laboratory marker supporting the diagnosis of MS. Similar to other diagnostic tests, these OCB are, however, not specific for MS, but are also found in any chronic inflammatory CNS process of infectious (chronic viral or bacterial meningitis such as CNS Lyme disease) or autoimmune origin (for example CNS lupus erythematosus). Numerous attempts to find a single antigen against which these antibody bands are directed have failed, although it was shown that single bands are specific for viral, bacterial or self antigens. It is therefore not clear whether the intrathecal immunoglobulin synthesis is driven by disease-related T cells or rather by cells that are passively recruited into the CNS after the pathogenetically relevant, probably myelin-specific, T cells entered first. As mentioned before, the administration of MOG-specific antibodies in EAE leads to

widespread demyelination[31], and therefore it was of particular interest whether CSF antibodies react with myelin antigens. Although not confirmed by other groups yet, the secretion of MBP-specific immunoglobulins (Ig) reacting with MBP peptides in the middle of the molecule (61–105) was demonstrated by using a sensitive radioimmunoassay in about 95% of MS patients[177, 178]. A small percentage of patients showed secretion of antibodies against PLP in the same study[178]. When the specificity of the CSF B cell response was examined directly, reactivity against MBP, PLP and MOG was found[161, 162]. Interestingly, MBP-specific B cells were again specific for the area of MBP (70–89) which was found immunodominant in the study mentioned above[179]. CSF Ig may cross-react with both pentapeptides derived from MBP and Epstein–Barr virus nuclear antigen (EBNA), suggesting that molecular mimicry could be relevant in the humoral immune response[180].

The importance and specificity of antibody secretion in the CSF of MS patients has been studied extensively and is certainly not covered in detail in this review. Considering the information from EAE and MS research so far, T cells are apparently the principal mediator of disease, but myelin-specific antibodies, particularly against those myelin proteins that are easily accessible such as MOG and MAG, could play a role in determining the extent of demyelination and remyelination in plaques of various stages. After almost two decades of intensive research of cellular immunity in MS, it is obvious that we need more information about the B cell response and the specificity and role of antibodies in disease pathogenesis.

14.7   Lessons from magnetic resonance imaging (MRI) during the course of MS

Our understanding about the clinical course of MS and the underlying inflammatory changes in the CNS has changed completely during recent years. While it was believed that relapsing-remitting disease, particularly in the early stages, is characterized by intermittent bouts of inflammatory activity leading to clinical exacerbations, studies of the natural history of MS by serial magnetic resonance imaging (MRI) has shown that inflammatory activity in the CNS can be demonstrated at almost any point, even at times of clinical remission[181]. In addition, the improved imaging techniques are now able to visualize directly structural changes within lesions which lead to persistent damage as shown by T2-weighted images. Furthermore, distribution of free fluid and water bound to macromolecules in lesioned but normal-appearing white matter can be distinguished by different magnetization transfer ratios[182]. Furthermore, axonal loss will result in decreases in N-acetyl aspartate (NAA) shown by magnetic resonance spectroscopy. However, most important, the initial stages of lesion development can now be visualized following administration of the paramagnetic contrast material gadopentate-dimeglumine (gadolinium-DTPA, GD-DTPA) [181, 183]. Active inflammatory lesions are characterized by BBB damage within the lesion. In these areas, GD-DTPA leaks into the CNS tissue and then appears as a hyperintense lesion on T1-weighted post-contrast MRI films [183]. The extent of affected CNS tissue, as measured by area and number of T2-enhancing lesions and GD-contrasting lesions, has proved extremely useful in predicting the prognosis of disease [184] and is related to clinical activity [185]. When MRI lesions are found in optic neuritis patients, the probability of developing MS is about 75–80% whereas it is very low in patients without MRI signs of CNS involvement. The extent of involvement is also a clear predictor of the disease course. Patients with small and few lesions as well as rare GD-contrast enhancement have a much better prognosis than those with numerous large lesions and the demonstration of frequent contrast enhancement. Furthermore, serial MRI scanning at monthly or biweekly intervals over the course of disease has shown that most inflammatory lesions are only active for 2–4 weeks, and that they do not appear continuously but rather in waves which almost resemble sinusoidal functions of different lengths in different patients [183]. Owing to the highly unpredictable clinical course of MS, particularly in the early stages, GD-enhanced, but also T2-weighted MRI is now an accepted measure for disease activity and an effective tool to document the efficacy of novel therapies for MS. Besides the reduction of relapse rate it was primarily the decrease of MRI lesion numbers that led to the rapid approval of recombinant interferon beta (IFN-β 1b) as a treatment for RR-MS by the Food and Drug Administration [83, 84]. Besides these clinical implications, MRI has also proved useful in immunological studies, because disease activity in the CNS can now directly be correlated with immunological markers, for example TNF secretion (see below). Future studies employing these tools are therefore expected to greatly enhance our understanding of the immunological factors involved in disease pathogenesis in general and lesion development in particular.

14.8 Association of immunological markers with disease activity

Following the demonstration that TH1-like, myelin-specific CD4$^+$ T cells mediate EAE via secretion of TNFα and lymphotoxin (LT) [47], considerable research has focused on the question as to whether certain immunological markers can be correlated with disease activity in MS. TNFα/β and IFN-γ are the most likely candidates since they are able to up-regulate MHC and adhesion molecule expression on endothelial and glial cells, activate macrophages, and are involved in recruiting and differentiating TH1 T cells. In addition, TNFα/β is able to damage oligodendroglial cells and myelin sheaths directly [186]. The expression of these cytokines has been demonstrated in both MS and EAE lesions [13]. Furthermore, TNFα levels were found elevated in both serum and CSF of MS patients and positively correlated with disease activity [146]. In a recent study, mRNA expression in PBL for various cytokines was followed in MS patients and compared to MRI documented disease activity [147]. Increased TNFα and LT mRNA levels preceded relapses and inflammatory activity as measured by MRI, whereas the mRNA levels of the inhibitory cytokines IL-10 and TGFβ declined at the same time [147]. As a consequence of TNFα and LT secretion, it is anticipated that the expression of the above-mentioned adhesion and activation markers will also increase, and this has indeed been found when the soluble forms have been measured. Soluble ICAM-1 and E-selectin are elevated in MS sera, soluble VCAM-1 and E-selectin levels increased in the CSF of MS patients [187]. As an indicator of T cell activation, soluble IL-2 receptors could also be detected in the blood of MS patients [148].

Some of these findings have not been confirmed by others. Whether this is due to differences in patient populations, disease stages or assay systems remains to be determined. In summary, there is, however, evidence to suggest that proinflammatory cytokines are correlated to disease activity in MS. In the future it will be necessary to confirm some of these observations in well-stratified patient populations and using MRI as an indicator for inflammatory activity in the CNS.

14.9 Lessons from immunomodulatory and immunosuppressive treatments of MS

As mentioned before, the concept that MS is a disease with an autoimmune pathogenesis is supported by successful treatment with anti-inflammatory and immunosuppressive drugs. Corticosteroids, although not effective in modulating the long-term course of the disease, are the cornerstone in the treatment of relapses. It was recently shown that BBB leakage as visualized by GD-enhanced MRI stops immediately following administration of high-dose intravenous steroids [82]. Although the effects are only moderate and sometimes controversial, a number of immunosuppressive drugs, including cyclophosphamide and methotrexate, have been used to treat more severe courses of disease. Depending on the poor predictability of the natural course of disease, it is extremely difficult to assess the efficacy of these drugs. As mentioned above, this will improve with the inclusion of MRI as a readout in future clinical trials. However, in later stages of the disease, factors other than new inflammatory bouts may become more important in determining the disease course and in these stages it may therefore happen that an immunosuppressant is found ineffective. These factors include axonal loss, destruction of local cytoarchitecture within a plaque due to astroglial scarring and exhaustion of the oligodendrocytes to remyelinate. It is clear that immunosuppression will not improve these latter mechanisms, but it will probably nevertheless be necessary in order to avoid new inflammation with all its consequences.

During the last few years new treatment modalities have been tried besides steroids and immunosuppression by chemotherapy. The administration of IFN-γ led to a marked increase in exacerbations in a small trial and was therefore immediately stopped [145]. This observation supports the concept that MS is mediated by TH1-like T cells. IFN-β, however, which counteracts a number of the effects of IFN-γ, in particular the up-regulation of MHC and adhesion molecules and the recruitment and activation of other inflammatory cells, was shown to lower the exacerbation rate, the relapse-free intervals and also the inflammatory activity shown by MRI [83–85]. The drug was therefore quickly approved as a treatment of RR-MS and is already in wide use. Other more subtle immunomodulatory treatments are currently being tested. Copolymer-1 (COP-1), a synthetic polypeptide consisting of a random sequence of four amino acids, blocks antigen presentation by competing with antigenic peptides for the MHC-binding groove [188]. A multicenter trial demonstrated that COP-1 is almost as efficient as IFN-β in early RR-MS, and it is expected that it will also be licensed in the near future [189].

Numerous other trials are under way or currently being planned. Most of the experimental therapies evolved from EAE research and include the administration of inhibitory cytokines such as TGFβ or IL-4, soluble receptors of proinflammatory cytokines such as TNF, antibodies against adhesion molecules and drugs that block the secretion of proinflammatory cytokines such as inhibitors of specific types of phosphodiesterases. Besides relatively unspecific immunomodulation, therapies that target the trimolecular complex of potentially disease-related T cells directly include T cell vaccination or TCR peptide vaccination and the use of altered peptide ligands, i.e. antigenic peptides that are modified in such a way that they antagonize effector functions of autoreactive T cells *in vitro* and *in vivo*.

14.10 Future perspectives

Despite the enormous progress that has been made in the research into EAE and virus-induced demyelinating diseases, it is amazing how little we know about the immunology of MS. The current hypothesis that MS is an immune-mediated disease is supported by many observations which have been outlined above, but whatever piece of the puzzle we look at, it is clear that we are far from seeing the whole picture. Most of the problems stem from the difficulties in proving hypotheses which have been generated in EAE. In MS we deal with patients with different immunogenetic backgrounds, we do not know when their disease started and what course it will take. To assess the importance of immunological factors such as myelin-reactive T cells or their TCR, to name only one example, we have to rely on indirect evidence such as frequencies of cells or over-representation of certain TCR sequences. Furthermore, a few genetic studies as well as clinical and MRI data suggest that the two major disease types – relapsing-remitting and primary chronic progressive MS – might be different entities. The data that try to link certain myelin antigens to disease pathogenesis are often either controversial or based on small patient populations and techniques which make it hard to compare them with other reports.

Besides all this criticism, there is no doubt that we have made progress in understanding some of the factors involved. It has, for example, been confirmed by all the genetic studies that certain HLA genes are associated with disease. Also, immunological as well as clinical and MRI data support the idea that MS, like EAE, is mediated by TH1-like T cells and that we can use this information to develop new treatments. Numerous questions are still open: for example, what induces disease? Is it one specific as yet unknown infectious agent or a number of common ones that we have known for a long time? Are immunoregulatory mechanisms more important than the mere reactivity with one or several myelin antigens, because we all bear T cells reactive to any myelin antigen as part of our natural T cell repertoire? Are there common reactivity patterns against certain myelin antigens comparable to what is known from EAE, and can we then specifically modify this autoimmune response? Which factors determine the extent of remyelination and astroglial scarring and how can we influence them?

This list addresses only a few obvious questions. With our rapidly increasing knowledge in immunology, neuroimaging and neurobiology at the molecular level and in more complex systems, there is hope, however, that we will answer some of them in the near future.

ACKNOWLEDGMENT

R. Martin is a Heisenberg Fellow of the Deutsche Forschungsgemeinschaft (Ma 965/4–1).

References

1. McFarlin, D.E. and McFarland, H.F. (1982) Multiple sclerosis (Part 1). *N. Engl. J. Med.*, **307**, 1183–8.
2. Martin, R., McFarland, H.F. and McFarlin, D.E. (1992) Immunological aspects of demyelinating diseases. *Annu. Rev. Immunol.*, **10**, 153–87.
3. Kurtzke, J.F. (1985) Epidemiology of multiple sclerosis, in *Handbook of Clinical Neurology 3 (revised series), Demyelinating Diseases* (eds P.J. Vinken, G.W. Bruyn, H.L. Klawans and J.C. Koetsier), Amsterdam/New York, Elsevier, pp. 259–87.
4. Waksman, B.H. and Reynolds, W.E. (1984) Minireview: multiple sclerosis as a disease of immune regulation. *Proc. Soc. Exp. Biol. Med.*, **175**, 282–94.
5. Palffy, G. (1982) MS in Hungary, including Gypsy population, in *Multiple Sclerosis East and West* (eds. Y. Kuroiwa and L.T. Kurland) Basle, Karger, pp. 149–57.
6. Sibley, W.A., Bamford, C.R. and Clark, K. (1985) Clinical viral infections and multiple sclerosis. *Lancet*, **i**, 1 1313–15.
7. Sadovnick, A.D., Baird, P.A. and Ward, R.A. (1988) Multiple sclerosis: updated risks for relatives. *Am. J. Med. Genet.*, **29**, 533–41.
8. Sadovnick, A.D., Armstrong, H., Rice, G.P. *et al.* (1993) A population-based study of multiple sclerosis in twins: update. *Ann. Neurol.*, **33**, 281–5.
9. Vartdal, F., Sollid, L.M., Vandvik, B., Markussen, G. and Thorsby, E. (1989) Patients with multiple sclerosis carry DQB1 genes which encode shared polymorphic aminoacid sequences. *Hum. Immunol.*, **25**, 103–10.
10. Prineas, J.W. (1985) The neuropathology of multiple sclerosis, in *Handbook of Clinical Neurology 3 (revised series), Demyelinating Diseases* (eds P.J. Vinken, G.W. Bruyn, H.L. Klawans and J.C. Koetsier.) Amsterdam/New York, Elsevier, pp. 213–57.
11. Raine, C.S. and Scheinberg, L.C. (1988) On the immunopathology of plaque development and repair in multiple sclerosis. *J. Neuroimmunol.*, **20**, 189–201.
12. Raine, C.S. (1994) Multiple sclerosis: immune system molecule expression in the central nervous system. *J. Neuropathol. Exp. Neurol.*, **53**, 328–37.
13. Cannella, B. and Raine, C.S. (1995) The adhesion molecule and cytokine profile of multiple sclerosis lesions. *Ann. Neurol.*, **37**, 424–35.
14. Raine, C.S. (1983) Multiple sclerosis and chronic relapsing EAE: comparative ultrastructural neuropathology, in *Multiple Sclerosis* (eds J F Hallpike, C.W. Adams and W.W. Tourtellotte), Baltimore, MD, Williams and Wilkins, pp. 413–78.
15. Rivers, T.M., Sprunt, D.H. and Berry, G.P. (1933) Observations on attempts to produce acute disseminated encephalomyelitis in monkeys. *J. Exp. Med.*, **58**, 39–53.
16. Fritz, R.B. and McFarlin, D.E. (1989) Encephalitogenic epitopes of myelin basic protein, in *Antigenic Determinants and Immune Response* (ed. E.E. Sercarz) (*Chem. Immunol.*, **46**), Basle, Karger, pp. 101–25.
17. Zamvil, S.S. and Steinman, L. (1990) The T lymphocyte in experimental allergic encephalomyelitis. *Annu. Rev. Immunol.*, **8**, 579–621.
18. Fritz, R.B., Skeen, M.J., Jen-Chou, C.H., Garcia, M. and Egorov, I.K. (1985) Major histocompatibility complex-linked control of the murine immune response to myelin basic protein. *J. Immunol.*, **134**, 2328 32.
19. Martin, R. and McFarland, H.F. (1995) Immunological aspects of experimental allergic encephalomyelitis and multiple sclerosis. *CRC. Lab. Sci.*, **32**, 121–82.
20. Baker, D., Rosenwasser, O.A., O'Neill, J.K. and Turk, J.L. (1995) Genetic analysis of experimental allergic encephalomyelitis in mice. *J. Immunol.*, **155**, 4046–51.
21. Sundvall, M., Jirholt, J., Yang, H.T. *et al.* (1995) Identification of murine loci associated with susceptibility to chronic experimental autoimmune encephalomyelitis. *Nat. Genet.*, **10**, 313–17.
22. Stepaniak, J.A., Gould, K.E., Sun, D. and Swanborg, R.H. (1995) A comparative study of experimental autoimmune encephalomyelitis in Lewis and DA rats. *J. Immunol.*, **155**, 2762–9.
23. Lorentzen, J.C., Issazadeh, S., Storch, M. *et al.* (1995) Protracted, relapsing and demyelinating experimental autoimmune encephalomyelitis in DA rats immunized with syngeneic spinal cord and incomplete Freund's adjuvant. *J. Neuroimmunol.*, **63**, 193–205.
24. Steinman, L. (1995) Escape from 'horror autotoxicus': pathogenesis and treatment of autoimmune disease. *Cell*, **80**, 7–10.
25. Massacesi, L., Joshi, N., Lee, P.D. *et al.* (1992) Experimental allergic encephalomyelitis in cynomolgus monkeys. Quantitation of T cell responses in peripheral blood. *J. Clin. Invest.*, **90**, 399–404.
26. Greer, J.M., Sobel, R.A., Sette, A. *et al.* (1996) Immunogenic and encephalitogenic epitope clusters of myelin proteolipid protein. *J. Immunol.*, **156**, 371–9.
27. Mustafa, M., Vingsbo, C., Olsson, T. *et al.* (1993). The major histocompatibility complex influences myelin basic protein 63–88-induced T cell cytokine profile and experimental autoimmune encephalomyelitis. *Eur. J. Immunol.*, **23**, 3089–95.
28. Peers, S.H., Duncan, G.S., Flower, R.J. and Bolton, C. (1995) Endogenous corticosteroids modulate lymphoproliferation and susceptibility to experimental allergic encephalomyelitis in the Brown Norway rat. *Int. Arch. Allergy. Immunol.*, **106**, 20–4.
29. Tuohy, V.K., Lu, Z., Sobel, R.A., Laursen, R.A. and Lees, M.B. (1988) A synthetic peptide from myelin proteolipid protein induces experimental allergic encephalomyelitis. *J. Immunol.*, **141**, 1126–30.
30. Yamamura, T., Namikawa, T., Endoh, M., Kunishita, T. and Tabira, T. (1986) Experimental allergic encephalomyelitis induced by proteolipid apoprotein in Lewis rats. *J. Neuroimmunol.*, **12**, 143–53.
31. Linington, C., Bradl, M., Lassmann, H., Brunner, C. and Vass, K. (1988) Augmentation of demyelination in rat acute allergic encephalomyelitis by circulating mouse monoclonal antibodies directed against a myelin/oligodendrocyte glycoprotein. *Am. J. Pathol.*, **130**, 443–54.
32. Urban, J.L., Horvath, S.J. and Hood, L. (1989) Autoimmune T cells: immune recognition of normal and variant peptide epitopes and peptide-based therapy. *Cell*, **59**, 257 71.
33. Schlüsener, H. and Wekerle, H. (1985) Autoaggressive T lymphocyte lines recognize the encephalitogenic region of myelin basic protein; *in vitro* selection from unprimed rat T lymphocyte populations. *J. Immunol.*, **135**, 3128–33.
34. Acha-Orbea, H., Steinman, L., McDevitt, H.O. (1989) T cell receptors in murine autoimmune diseases. *Annu. Rev. Immunol.*, **7**, 371–406.
35. Sakai, K., Zamvil, S.S., Mitchell, D.J. *et al.* (1989) Prevention of experimental encephalomyelitis with peptides that block interaction of T cells with major histocompatibility complex proteins. *Proc. Natl Acad. Sci. USA*, **86**, 9470–4.
36. Acha Orbea, H., Mitchell, L., Timmermann, L. *et al.* (1988) Limited heterogeneity of T cell receptors from lymphocytes mediating autoimmune encephalomyelitis allows specific immune intervention. *Cell*, **54**, 263–73.
37. Urban, J.L., Kumar, V., Kono, D.H. *et al.* (1988) Restricted use of the T cell receptor V genes in murine autoimmune encephalomyelitis raises possibilities for antibody therapy. *Cell*, **54**, 577–92.
38. Chluba, J., Steeg, C., Becker, A., Wekerle, H. and Epplen, J.T. (1989) T cell receptor β chain usage in myelin basic protein-specific rat T lymphocytes. *Eur. J. Immunol.*, **19**, 279–84.
39. Burns, F.R., Li, X., Shen, N. *et al.* (1989) Both rat and mouse T cell receptors specific for the encephalitogenic determinant of myelin basic protein use similar Vα and Vβ chain genes even though the major histocompatibility complex and encephalitogenic determinants being recognized are different. *J. Exp. Med.*, **169**, 27–39.
40. Lehmann, P.V., Forsthuber, T., Miller, A. and Sercarz E.E. (1992) Spreading of T-cell autoimmunity to cryptic determinants of an autoantigen. *Nature*, **358**, 155–7.
41. McRae, B.L., Vanderlugt, C.L., Dal Canto, M. and Miller, S.D. (1995) Functional evidence for epitope spreading in the relapsing pathology of experimental autoimmune encephalomyelitis. *J. Exp. Med.*, **182**, 75–85.
42. Goverman, J., Woods, A., Larson, L. *et al.* (1993) Transgenic mice that express a myelin basic protein-specific T cell receptor develop spontaneous autoimmunity. *Cell*, **72**, 551–60.
43. Schwartz, R.H. (1992) Costimulation of T lymphocytes: the role of CD28, CTLA-4, and B7/BB1 in interleukin production and immunotherapy. *Cell*, **71**, 1065.
44. Baron, J.L., Madri, J.A., Ruddle, N.H., Hashim, G. and Janeway, C.A. (1993) Surface expression of α4 integrin by CD4 T cells is required for their entry into brain parenchyma. *J. Exp. Med.*, **177**, 57–68.
45. Cannella, B., Cross, A.H. and Raine, C.S. (1990) Upregulation and coexpression of adhesion molecules correlate with relapsing autoimmune demyelination in the central nervous system. *J. Exp. Med.*, **172**, 1521–4.
46. Wekerle, H., Linington, C., Lassmann, H. and Meyermann, R. (1986) Cellular immune reactivity within the CNS. *Trends Neurosci.*, **9**, 271–7.
47. Ruddle, N.H., Bergman, C.M., McGrath, K.M. *et al.* (1990) An antibody to lymphotoxin and tumor necrosis factor prevents transfer of experimental allergic encephalomyelitis. *J. Exp. Med.*, **172**(4), 1193–200.
48. Leonard, J.P., Waldburger, K.E. and Goldman, S.J. (1995) Prevention of experimental autoimmune encephalomyelitis by antibodies against interleukin 12. *J. Exp. Med.*, **181**, 381–6.
49. Cross, A.H., Misko, T.P., Lin, R.F. *et al.* (1994) Aminoguanidine, an inhibitor of inducible nitric oxide synthase, ameliorates experimental autoimmune encephalomyelitis in SJL mice. *J. Clin. Invest.*, **93**, 2684–90.
50. Offner, H., Buenafe, A.C., Vainiene, M. *et al.* (1993) Where, when, and how to detect biased expression of disease-relevant Vβ genes in rats with experimental autoimmune encephalomyelitis. *J. Immunol.*, **151**, 506–17.

51. Schmied, M., Breitschopf, H., Gold, R. *et al.* Apoptosis of T lymphocytes in experimental autoimmune encephalomyelitis: evidence for programmed cell death as a mechanism to control inflammation in the brain. *Am. J. Pathol.*, **143**, 446–52.

52. Racke, M.K., Cannella, B., Albert, P. *et al.* (1992). Evidence of endogenous regulatory function of transforming growth factor-β1 in experimental allergic encephalomyelitis. *Int. Immunol.*, **4**, 615–20.

53. Racke, M.K., Bonomo, A., Scott, D.E. *et al.* (1994) Cytokine-induced immune deviation as a therapy for inflammatory autoimmune disease. *J. Exp. Med.*, **180**, 1961–6.

54. Rott, O., Fleischer, B. and Cash, E. (1994) Interleukin-10 prevents experimental allergic encephalomyelitis in rats. *Eur. J. Immunol.*, **24**, 1434–40.

55. Issazadeh, S., Mustafa, M., Ljungdahl, Å. *et al.* (1995) Interferon-γ, interleukin-4 and transforming growth factor β in experimental autoimmune encephalomyelitis in Lewis rats: dynamics of cellular mRNA expression in the central nervous system and lymphoid cells. *J. Neurosci. Res.*, **40**, 579–90.

56. Issazadeh, S., Ljungdahl, Å., Höjeberg, B., Mustafa, M. and Olsson, T. (1995) Cytokine production in the central nervous system of Lewis rats with experimental autoimmune encephalomyelitis: dynamics of mRNA expression for interleukin-10, interleukin-12, cytolysin, tumor necrosis factor α and tumor necrosis factor β. *J. Neuroimmunol.*, **61**, 205–12.

57. Brück, W., Schmied, M., Suchanek, G. *et al.* (1994) Oligodendrocytes in the early course of multiple sclerosis. *Ann. Neurol.*, **35**, 65–73.

58. Zaller, D.M., Osman, G, Kanagawa, O. and Hood, L. (1990) Prevention and treatment of murine experimental allergic encephalomyelitis with T cell receptor V beta-specific antibodies. *J. Exp. Med.*, **171**, 1943–55.

59. Ben Nun, A., Wekerle, H. and Cohen, I.R. (1981) Vaccination against autoimmune encephalomyelitis with T-lymphocyte line cells reactive against myelin basic protein. *Nature*, **293**, 60–1.

60. Howell, M.D., Winters, S.T., Olee, T. *et al.* (1989) Vaccination against experimental allergic autoimmune encephalomyelitis with T cell receptor peptides. *Science*, **246**, 668–70.

61. Vandenbark, A.A., Hashim, G. and Offner, H. (1989) Immunization with a synthetic T-cell receptor V-region peptide against experimental autoimmune encephalomyelitis. *Nature*, **341**, 541–4.

62. Lamont, A.G., Sette, A., Fujinami, R. *et al.* (1990). Inhibition of experimental autoimmune encephalomyelitis induction in SJL/J mice by using a peptide with high affinity for IA^S molecules. *J. Immunol.*, **145**, 1687–93.

63. Karin, N., Mitchell, D.J., Brocke, S., Ling, N. and Steinman, L. (1994) Reversal of experimental autoimmune encephalomyelitis by a soluble peptide variant of a myelin basic protein epitope: T cell receptor antagonism and reduction of interferon γ and tumor necrosis factor α production. *J. Exp. Med.*, **180**, 2227–37.

64. Kuchroo, V.K., Greer, J.M., Kaul, D. *et al.* (1994) A single TCR antagonist peptide inhibits experimental allergic encephalomyelitis mediated by a diverse T cell repertoire. *J. Immunol.*, **153**, 3326–36.

65. Nicholson, L.B., Greer, J.M., Sobel, R.A., Lees, M.B. and Kuchroo, V.K. (1995) An altered peptide ligand mediates immune deviation and prevents autoimmune encephalomyelitis. *Immunity*, **3**, 397–405.

66. Brocke, S., Gijbels, K., Allegretta, M. *et al.* (1996) Dynamics of autoimmune T cell infiltration: reversal of paralysis and disappearance of inflammation following treatment of experimental encephalomyelitis with a myelin basic protein peptide analog. *Nature*, **379**, 343–6.

67. Kuchroo, V.K., Prabhu Das, M., Brown, J.A. *et al.* (1995) B7-1 and B7-2 costimulatory molecules activate differentially the Th1/Th2 developmental pathways: application to autoimmune disease therapy. *Cell*, **80**, 707–18.

68. Racke, M.K., Scott, D.E., Quigley, L. *et al.* (1995) Distinct roles for B7–1 (CD80) and B7.2 (CD86) in the initiation of experimental allergic encephalomyelitis. *J. Clin. Invest.*, **96**, 2195–203.

69. Selmaj, K., Papierz, W., Glabinski, A. and Kohno, T. (1995) Prevention of chronic relapsing experimental autoimmune encephalomyelitis by soluble tumor necrosis factor receptor I. *J. Neuroimmunol.*, **56**, 135–41.

70. Sommer, N., Löschmann, P.A., Northoff, G.H. *et al.* (1995) The antidepressant rolipram suppresses cytokine production and prevents autoimmune encephalomyelitis. *Nature Med.*, **1**, 244–8.

71. Genain, C.P., Roberts, T., Davis, R.L. *et al.* (1995) Prevention of autoimmune demyelination in non-human primates by a cAMP-specific phosphodiesterase inhibitor. *Proc. Natl Acad. Sci. USA*, **92**, 3601–5.

72. Racke, M.K., Dhib-Jalbut, S., Cannella, B. *et al.* (1991) Prevention and treatment of chronic relapsing experimental allergic encephalomyelitis by transforming growth factor-β1. *J. Immunol.*, **146**, 3012–17.

73. Cash, E., Minty, A., Ferrara, P. *et al.* (1994) Macrophage-inactivation by IL-13 suppresses experimental autoimmune encephalomyelitis in rats. *J. Immunol.*, **153**, 4258–67.

74. Racke, M.K., Burnett, D., Pak, S.-H. *et al.* (1995) Retinoid treatment of experimental allergic encephalomyelitis. IL-4 production correlates with improved disease course. *J. Immunol.*, **154**, 450–8.

75. Whitacre, C.C., Gienapp, I.E., Orosz, C.G. and Bitar, D.M. (1991) Oral tolerance in experimental autoimmune encephalomyelitis. III. Evidence for clonal anergy. *J. Immunol.*, **147**, 2155–63.

76. Metzler, B. and Wraith, D.C. (1993) Inhibition of experimental autoim-

mune encephalomyelitis by inhalation but not oral administration of the encephalitogenic peptide: influence of MHC binding affinity. *Int. Immunol.*, **5**, 1159–65.

77. Chen, Y., Inobe, J.-I., Marks, R. *et al.* (1995) Peripheral deletion of antigen-reactive T cells in oral tolerance. *Nature*, **376**, 177–80.

78. Gregerson, D.S., Obritsch, W.F. and Donoso, L.A. (1993) Oral tolerance in experimental autoimmune uveoretinitis. Distinct mechanisms of resistance are induced by low dose vs. high dose feeding protocols. *J. Immunol.*, **151**, 5751–61.

79. Critchfield, J.M., Racke, M.K., Zúñiga-Pflücker, J.C. *et al.* (1994) T cell deletion in high antigen dose therapy of autoimmune encephalomyelitis. *Science*, **263**, 1139–43.

80. Wekerle, H., Kojima, K., Lannes-Vieira, J., Lassmann, H. and Linington, C. (1994) Animal models. *Ann. Neurol.*, **36**, S47–53.

81. Pettinelli, C.B. and McFarlin, D.E. (1981) Adoptive transfer of experimental allergic encephalomyelitis in SJL/J mice after *in vivo* activation of lymph node cells by myelin basic protein: requirement for Lyt- 1 + 2- T lymphocytes. *J. Immunol.*, **127**, 1420–3.

82. Burnham, J.A., Wright, R.R., Dreisbach, J. and Murray, R.S. (1991) The effect of high-dose steroids on MRI gadolinium enhancement in acute demyelinating lesions. *Neurology*, **41**, 1349–54.

83. Paty, D.W., Li, D.K.B., The UBC MS/MRI Study Group and the IFNβ Multiple Sclerosis Study Group (1993) Interferon beta-1b is effective in relapsing-remitting multiple sclerosis. II. MRI analysis results of a multicenter, randomized, double-blind, placebo-controlled trial. *Neurology*, **43**, 662–7.

84. The IFNβ Multiple Sclerosis Study Group (1993) Interferon beta-1b is effective in relapsing-remitting multiple sclerosis. I Clinical results of a multicenter, randomized, double-blind, placebo-controlled trial. *Neurology*, **43**, 655–61.

85. Stone, L.A., Frank, J.A., Albert, P.S. *et al.* (1995) The effect of interferon-β on blood–brain-barrier disruptions demonstrated by contrast-enhanced magnetic resonance imaging in relapsing-remitting multiple sclerosis. *Ann. Neurol.*, **37**, 611–19.

86. Johnson, R.T. (1985) Viral aspects of multiple sclerosis, in *Handbook of Clinical Neurology 3* (revised series), *Demyelinating Disorders* (eds P.J. Vinken, G.W. Bruyn, H.L. Klawans and J.C. Koetsier) Amsterdam/New York, Elsevier, pp. 319–36.

87. Challoner, P.B., Smith, K.T., Parker, J.D. *et al.* (1995) Plaque-associated expression of human herpesvirus 6 in multiple sclerosis. *Proc. Natl Acad. Sci. USA*, **92**, 7440–4.

88. Fujinami, R.S. and Oldstone, M.B.A. (1985) Amino acid homology between the encephalitogenic site of myelin basic protein and virus: mechanism for autoimmunity. *Science*, **230**, 1043–5.

89. Wucherpfennig, K.W. and Strominger, J.L. (1995) Molecular mimicry in T cell-mediated autoimmunity: viral peptides activate human T cell clones specific for myelin basic protein. *Cell*, **80**, 695–705.

90. Remlinger, J. (1905) Accidents paralytiques au cours du traitement antirabique. *Ann. Inst. Pasteur*, **19**, 625–46.

91. Waxman, S.G. (1985) Structure and function of the myelinated fiber, in *Handbook of Clinical Neurology 3* (revised series), *Demyelinating Diseases* (eds P.J. Vinken, G.W. Bruyn, H.L. Klawans and J.C. Koetsier), Amsterdam, New York, Elsevier, pp. 1–28.

92. Williams, K.A. and Deber, C.M. (1993) The structure and function of central nervous system myelin. *CRC Lab. Sci.*, **30**, 29–64.

93. Banki, K., Halladay, D. and Perl, A. (1994) Cloning and expression of the human gene for transaldolase. A novel highly repetitive element constitutes an integral part of the coding sequence. *J. Biol. Chem.*, **269**, 2847–51.

94. Moscarello, M.A. (1990) Myelin basic protein: a dynamically changing structure, in *Dynamic Interactions of Myelin Proteins* (eds G.A. Hashim and M. Moscarello), New York, John Wiley, pp. 25–48.

95. Kamholz, J., Toffenetti, J. and Lazzarini, R.A. (1988) Organization and expression of the human myelin basic protein gene. *J. Neurosci. Res.*, **21**, 62–70.

96. Wood, D.D. and Moscarello, M.A. (1989) The isolation, characterization, and lipid-aggregating properties of a citrulline containing myelin basic protein. *J. Biol. Chem.*, **264**, 5121–7.

97. Segal, B.M., Raine, C.S., McFarlin, D.E., Voskuhl, R.R. and McFarland, H.F. (1994) Experimental allergic encephalomyelitis induced by the peptide encoded by exon 2 of the MBP gene – a peptide implicated in remyelination. *J. Neuroimmunol.*, **51**, 7–19.

98. Voskuhl, R.R., Robinson, E.D., Segal, B.M. *et al.* (1994) HLA restriction and TCR usage of T lymphocytes specific for a novel candidate autoantigen, X2 MBP, in multiple sclerosis. *J. Immunol.*, **153**, 4834–44.

99. Moscarello, M.A., Wood, D.D., Ackerley, C. and Boulias, C. (1994) Myelin in multiple sclerosis is developmentally immature. *J. Clin. Invest.*, **94**, 146–54.

100. Lafaille, J.J., Nagashima, K., Katsuki, M. and Tonegawa, S. (1994) High incidence of spontaneous autoimmune encephalomyelitis in immunodeficient anti-myelin basic protein T cell receptor transgenic mice. *Cell*, **78**, 399–408.

101. Antel, J.P. and Arnason, B.G.W. (1979) Suppressor cell function in multiple sclerosis – correlation with clinical disease activity. *Ann. Neurol.*, **5**, 338–42.

102. Reder, A.T. and Arnason, B.G.W. (1985) Immunology of multiple sclerosis, in *Handbook of Clinical Neurology 3* (revised series), *Demyelinating Diseases* (eds P.J. Vinken, G.W. Bruyn, H.L. Klawans and J.C. Koetsier), Amsterdam/New York Elsevier, pp. 337–95.

103. Jacobson, S.J., Flerlage, M.L. and McFarland, H.F. (1985) Impaired measles virus-specific cytotoxic T-cell response in multiple sclerosis. *J. Exp. Med.*, **162**, 839–50.

104. Burns, J. Rosenzweig, A., Zweiman, B. and Lisak, R.P. (1983) Isolation of myelin basic protein-reactive T-cell lines from normal human blood. *Cell. Immunol.*, **81**, 435–40.

105. Chou, Y.K., Vainiene, M., Whitham, R. *et al.* (1989) Response of human T lymphocyte lines to myelin basic protein: association of dominant epitopes with HLA-class II restriction molecules. *J. Neurol. Sci.*, **23**, 207–16.

106. Martin, R., Jaraquemada, D., Flerlage, M. *et al.* (1990) Fine specificity and HLA restriction of myelin basic protein-specific cytotoxic T cell lines from multiple sclerosis patients and healthy individuals. *J. Immunol.*, **145**, 540–8.

107. Ota, K., Matsui, M., Milford, E.L. *et al.* (1990) T-cell recognition of an immunodominant myelin basic protein epitope in multiple sclerosis. *Nature*, **346**, 183–7.

108. Pette, M., Fujita, K., Kitze, B. *et al.* (1990) Myelin basic protein-specific T lymphocyte lines from MS patients and healthy individuals. *Neurology*, **40**, 1770–6.

109. Olsson, T., Wei Zhi, W., Höjeberg, B. *et al.* (1990) Autoreactive T lymphocytes in multiple sclerosis determined by antigen-induced secretion of interferon-γ. *J. Clin. Invest.*, **86**, 981–5.

110. Olsson, T., Sun, J., Hillert, J. *et al.* (1992) Increased numbers of T cells recognizing multiple myelin basic protein epitopes in multiple sclerosis. *Eur. J. Immunol.*, **22**, 1083–7.

111. Martin, R., Voskuhl, R., Flerlage, M., McFarlin, D.E. and McFarland, H.F. (1993) Myelin basic protein-specific T-cell responses in identical twins discordant or concordant for multiple sclerosis. *Ann. Neurol.*, **34**, 524–35.

112. Joshi, N., Usuku, K. and Hauser, S.L. (1993) The T-cell response to myelin basic protein in familial multiple sclerosis: diversity of fine specificity, restricting elements, and T-cell receptor usage. *Ann. Neurol.*, **34**, 385–93.

113. Zhang, J., Markovic-Plese, S., Lacet, B. *et al.* (1994) Increased frequency of interleukin 2-responsive T cells specific for myelin basic protein in peripheral blood and cerebrospinal fluid of patients with multiple sclerosis. *J. Exp. Med.*, **179**, 973–84.

114. Allegretta, M. Nicklas, J.A., Sriram, S. and Albertini, R.J. (1990) T cells responsive to myelin basic protein in patients with multiple sclerosis. *Science*, **247**, 718–21.

115. Pette, M., Fujita, K., Wilkinson, D. *et al.* (1990) Myelin autoreactivity in multiple sclerosis: recognition of myelin basic protein in the context of HLA-DR2 products by T lymphocytes of multiple sclerosis patients and healthy donors. *Proc. Natl Acad. Sci. USA*, **87**, 7968–72.

116. Martin, R., Howell, M.D., Jaraquemada, D. *et al.* (1991) A myelin basic protein peptide is recognized by cytotoxic T cells in the context of four HLA-DR types associated with multiple sclerosis. *J. Exp. Med.*, **173**(1), 19–24.

117. Richert, J.R., Reuben-Burnside, C.A., Deibler, G.E. and Kies, M.W. (1988) Peptide specificities of myelin basic protein-reactive human T-cell clones. *Neurology*, **38**, 739–42.

118. Richert, J., Robinson, E.D., Deibler, G.E. *et al.* (1989) Evidence for multiple human T cell recognition sites on myelin basic protein. *J. Neuroimmunol.*, **23**, 55–66.

119. Martin, R., Utz, U., Coligan, J.E. *et al.* (1992) Diversity in fine specificity and T cell receptor usage of the human CD4 + cytotoxic T cell response specific for the immunodominant myelin basic protein peptide 87–106. *J. Immunol.*, **148**, 1359–66.

120. Martin, R., Whitaker, J.N., Rhame, L., Goodin, R.R. and McFarland, H.F. (1994) Citrulline-containing myelin basic protein is recognized by T-cell lines derived from multiple sclerosis patients and healthy individuals. *Neurology*, **44**, 123–9.

121. Salvetti, M., Ristori, G., D'Amato, M. *et al.* (1993) Predominant and stable T cell responses to regions of myelin basic protein can be detected in individual patients with multiple sclerosis. *Eur. J. Immunol.*, **23**, 1232–9.

122. Bjorkman, P.J., Saper, M.A., Samraoui, B. *et al.* (1987) Structure of the human class I histocompatibility antigen HLA-A2. *Nature*, **329**, 506–12.

123. Brown, J.H., Jardetzky, T.S., Gorga, J.C. *et al.* (1993) Three-dimensional structure of the human class II histocompatibility antigen HLA-DR1. *Nature*, **364**, 33–9.

124. Falk, K., Rötzschke, O., Deres, K. *et al.* (1990) Isolation and analysis of naturally processed viral peptides as recognized by cytotoxic T cells. *Nature*, **348**, 252–4.

125. Richert, J.R., Robinson, E.D., Deibler, G.E. *et al.* (1989) Human cytotoxic T-cell recognition of a synthetic peptide of myelin basic protein. *Ann. Neurol.*, **26**, 342–6.

126. Valli, A., Sette, A., Kappos, L. *et al.* (1993) Binding of myelin basic protein peptides to human histocompatibility leukocyte antigen class II molecules and their recognition by T cells from multiple sclerosis patients. *J. Clin. Invest.*, **91**, 616–28.

127. Wucherpfennig, K.W., Sette, A., Southwood, S. *et al.* (1994) Structural requirements for binding of an immunodominant myelin basic protein peptide to DR2 isotypes and for its recognition by human T cell clones. *J. Exp. Med.*, **179**, 279–90.

128. Vogt, A.B., Kropshofer, H. Kalbacher, H. *et al.* (1994) Ligand motifs of HLA-DRB5*0101 and DRB1*1501 molecules delineated from self-peptides. *J. Immunol.*, **153**, 1665–73.

129. Jaraquemada, D., Martin, R., Rosen-Bronson, S. *et al.* (1990) HLA-DR2a is the dominant restriction molecule for the cytotoxic T cell response to myelin basic protein in DR2Dw2 individuals. *J. Immunol.*, **145**, 2880–5.

130. Wucherpfennig, K.W., Ota, K., Endo, N. *et al.* (1990) Shared human T cell receptor V beta usage to immunodominant regions of myelin basic protein. *Science*, **248**, 1016–19.

131. Kotzin, B.L., Karuturi, S., Chou, Y.K. *et al.* (1991) Preferential T-cell receptor Vβ-chain variable gene use in myelin basic protein-reactive T-cell clones from patients with multiple sclerosis. *Proc. Natl Acad. Sci. USA*, **88**, 9161–5.

132. Ben Nun, A., Liblau, R.S., Cohen, L. *et al.* (1991) Restricted T-cell receptor Vβ gene usage by myelin basic protein-specific T-cell clones in multiple sclerosis: predominant genes vary in individuals. *Proc. Natl Acad. Sci. USA*, **88**, 2466–70.

133. Giegerich, G., Pette, M., Meinl, E. *et al.* (1992) Diversity of T cell receptor alpha and beta chain genes expressed by human T cells specific for similar myelin basic protein peptide/major histocompatibility complexes. *Eur. J. Immunol.*, **22**(3), 753–8.

134. Richert, J.R., Robinson, E.D., Johnson, A.H. *et al.* (1991) Heterogeneity of the T-cell receptor beta gene rearrangements generated in myelin basic protein-specific T-cell clones isolated from a patient with multiple sclerosis. *Ann. Neurol.*, **29**, 299–306.

135. Jorgensen, J.L., Esser, U., Fazekas de St Groth, B., Reay, P.A. and Davis, M.M. (1992) Mapping T-cell receptor-peptide contacts by variant peptide immunization of single-chain transgenics. *Nature*, **355**, 224–30.

136. Jorgensen, J.L., Reay, P.A., Ehrich, E.W. and Davis, M.M. (1992) Molecular components of T-cell recognition. *Annu. Rev. Immunol.*, **10**, 835–73.

137. Utz, U., Brooks, J.A., McFarland, H.F., Martin, R. and Biddison, W.E. (1994) Heterogeneity of T-cell receptor α-chain complementarity-determining region 3 in myelin basic protein-specific T cells increases with severity of multiple sclerosis. *Proc. Natl Acad. Sci. USA*, **91**, 5567–71.

138. Allegretta, M., Albertini, R.J., Howell, M.D. *et al.* (1994) Homologies between T cell receptor junctional sequences unique to multiple sclerosis and T cells mediating experimental allergic encephalomyelitis. *J. Clin. Invest.*, **94**, 105–9.

139. Oksenberg, J.R., Panzara, M.A., Begovich, A.B. *et al.* (1993) Selection for T-cell receptor Vβ-Dβ-Jβ gene rearrangements with specificity for a myelin basic protein peptide in brain lesions of multiple sclerosis. *Nature*, **362**, 68–70.

140. Utz, U., Biddison, W.E., McFarland, H.F. *et al.* (1993) Skewed T cell receptor repertoire in genetically identical twins with multiple sclerosis correlates with disease. *Nature*, **364**, 243–7.

141. Wucherpfennig, K.W., Zhang, J., Witek, C. *et al.* (1994) Clonal expansion and persistence of human T cells specific for an immunodominant myelin basic protein peptide. *J. Immunol.*, **152**, 5581–92.

142. Oksenberg, J.R., Stuart, S., Begovich, A.B. *et al.* (1990) Limited heterogeneity of rearranged T-cell receptor V alpha transcripts in brains of multiple sclerosis patients. *Nature*, **345**, 344–6.

143. Wucherpfennig, K.W., Newcombe, J., Li, H. *et al.* (1992) T cell receptor Vα-Vβ repertoire and cytokine gene expression in active multiple sclerosis lesions. *J. Exp. Med.*, **175**, 993–1002.

144. Ando, D.G., Clayton, J., Kono, D., Urban, J.L. and Sercarz, E.E. (1989) Encephalitogenic T cells in the B10.PL model of experimental allergic encephalomyelitis (EAE) are of the Th-1 lymphokine subtype. *Cell. Immunol.*, **124**, 132–43.

145. Panitch, H.S., Hirsch, R.L., Schindler, J. and Johnson, K.P. (1987) Treatment of multiple sclerosis with gamma interferon: exacerbations associated with activation of the immune system. *Neurology*, **37**, 1097–102.

146. Sharief, M.K. and Hentges, R. (1991) Association between tumor necrosis factor-α and disease progression in chronic progressive multiple sclerosis. *N. Engl. J. Med.*, **325**, 467–72.

147. Rieckmann, P., Albrecht, M., Kitze, B. *et al.* (1995) Tumor necrosis factor-α messenger RNA expression in patients with relapsing-remitting multiple sclerosis is associated with disease activity. *Ann. Neurol.*, **37**, 82–8.

148. Hartung, H.-P., Hughes, R.A.C., Taylor, W.A. *et al.* (1990) T cell activation in Guillian-Barré syndrome in MS: elevated serum levels of soluble IL-2 receptors. *Neurology*, **40**, 215–18.

149. Voskuhl, R.R., Martin, R., Bergman, C. *et al.* (1993) T helper 1 (TH1) functional phenotype of human myelin basic protein-specific T lymphocytes. *Autoimmunity*, **15**, 137–43.

150. Svenningsson, A., Hansson, G.K., Andersen, O. *et al.* (1993) Adhesion molecule expression on cerebrospinal fluid T lymphocytes: evidence for common recruitment mechanisms in multiple sclerosis, aseptic meningitis, and normal controls. *Ann. Neurol.*, **34**, 155–61.

151. Link, J., Söderström, M., Kostulas, V. *et al.* (1994) Optic neuritis is associated with myelin basic protein and proteolipid protein reactive cells producing interferon-β, interleukin-4 and transforming growth factor-β. *J. Neuroimmunol.*, **49**, 9–18.

152. Correale, J., Gilmore, W., McMillan, M. *et al.* (1995) Patterns of cytokine secretion by autoreactive proteolipid protein-specific T cell clones during the course of multiple sclerosis. *J. Immunol.*, **154**, 2959–68.

153. Rammensee, H.-G., Friede, T. and Stevanovic, S. (1995) MHC ligands and peptide motifs: first listing. *Immunogenetics*, **41**, 178–228.

154. Tsuchida, T., Parker, K.C., Turner, R.V. *et al.* (1994) Autoreactive CD8 + T-cell responses to human myelin protein-derived peptides. *Proc. Natl Acad. Sci. USA*, **91**, 10859–63.

155. Antel, J.P., Williams, K., Blain, M., McRea, E. and McLaurin, J. (1994) Oligodendrocyte lysis by CD4 + T cells independent of tumor necrosis factor. *Ann. Neurol.*, **35**, 341–8.

156. Tuohy, V.K., Lu, Z., Sobel, R.A., Laursen, R.A. and Lees, M.B. (1989) Identification of an encephalitogenic determinant of myelin proteolipid protein for SJL mice. *J. Immunol.*, **142**, 1523–7.

157. Hafler, D.A., Benjamin, D.S., Burks, J. and Weiner, H.L. (1987) Myelin basic protein and proteolipid protein reactivity of brain- and cerebrospinal fluid-derived T cell clones in multiple sclerosis and postinfectious encephalomyelitis. *J. Immunol.*, **139**, 68–72.

158. Trotter, J.L., Hickey, W.F., van der Veen, R.C. and Sulze, L. (1991) Peripheral blood mononuclear cells from multiple sclerosis patients recognize myelin proteolipid protein and selected peptides. *J. Neuroimmunol.*, **33**, 55–62.

159. Pelfrey, C.M., Trotter, J.L., Tranquill, L.R. and McFarland, H.F. (1993) Identification of a novel T cell epitope of human proteolipid protein (residues 40–60) recognized by proliferative and cytolytic CD4 + T cells from multiple sclerosis. *J. Neuroimmunol.*, **46**, 33–42.

160. Pelfrey, C.M., Trotter, J.L., Tranquill, L.R. and McFarland, H.F. (1994) Identification of a second T cell epitope of human proteolipid protein (residues 89–106) recognized by proliferative and cytolytic CD4 + T cells from multiple patients. *J. Neuroimmunol.*, **53**, 153–61.

161. Sun, J.B., Olsson, T., Wang, W.-Z. *et al.* (1991) Autoreactive T and B cells responding to myelin proteolipid protein in multiple sclerosis and controls. *Eur. J. Immunol.*, **21**, 1461–8.

162. Sun, J., Link, H., Olsson, T. *et al.* (1991) T and B cell responses to myelin-oligodendrocyte glycoprotein in multiple sclerosis. *J. Immunol.*, **146**, 1490–5.

163. Kerlero de Rosbo, N., Milo, R., Lees, M.B. *et al.* (1993) Reactivity to myelin antigens in multiple sclerosis. Peripheral blood lymphocytes respond predominantly to myelin oligodendrocyte glycoprotein. *J. Clin. Invest.*, **92**, 2602–8.

164. Johnson, D., Hafler, D.A., Fallis, R.J. *et al.* (1986) Cell-mediated immunity to myelin-associated glycoprotein, proteolipid protein, and myelin basic protein in multiple sclerosis. *J. Neuroimmunol.*, **13**, 99–108.

165. Link, H., Sun, J.-B., Wang, Z. *et al.* (1992) Virus-specific and autoreactive T cells are accumulated in cerebrospinal fluid in multiple sclerosis. *J. Neuroimmunol.*, **38**, 63–74.

166. Zhang, Y.D., Burger, D., Saruhan, M., Jeannet, M. and Steck, A.J. (1993) The T-lymphocyte response against myelin-associated glycoprotein and myelin basic protein in patients. *Neurology*, **43**, 403–7.

167. van Noort, J.M., van Sechel, A., Boon, J. *et al.* (1993) Minor myelin proteins can be major targets for peripheral blood T cells from both multiple sclerosis patients and healthy subjects. *J. Neuroimmunol.*, **46**, 67–72.

168. van Noort, J.M., van Sechel, A.C., Bajramovic, J.J. *et al.* (1995) The small heat-shock protein αB-crystallin as candidate autoantigen in multiple sclerosis. *Nature*, **375**, 798–801.

169. Banki, K., Colombo, E., Sia, F. *et al.* (1994) Oligodendrocyte-specific expression and autoantigenicity of transaldolase in multiple sclerosis. *J. Exp. Med.*, **180**, 1649–63.

170. Selmaj, K., Brosnan, C.F. and Raine, C.S. (1991) Colocalization of lymphocytes bearing gamma delta T-cell receptor and heat shock protein hsp65 + oligodendrocytes in multiple sclerosis. *Proc. Natl Acad. Sci. USA*, **88**, 6452–6.

171. Hvas, J., Oksenberg, J.R., Fernando, R., Steinman, L. and Bernard, C.C. (1993) Gamma delta T cell receptor repertoire in brain lesions of patients with multiple sclerosis. *J. Neuroimmunol.*, **46**, 225–34.

172. Wucherpfennig, K.W., Newcombe, J., Li, H. and Keddy, C. (1992) Gamma delta T cell receptor repertoire in acute multiple sclerosis lesions. *Proc. Natl Acad. Sci. USA*, **89**, 4588–92.

173. Koga, T., Wand-Württenberger, A., DeBruyn, J. *et al.* (1989) T cells against a bacterial heat shock protein recognize stressed macrophages. *Science*, **245**, 1112–15.

174. Battistini, L., Selmaj, K., Kowal, C. *et al.* (1995) Multiple sclerosis: limited diversity of the Vδ2-Jδ3 T-cell receptor in chronic active lesions. *Ann. Neurol.*, **37**, 198–203.

175. Kabat, E.A., Freedman, D.A., Murray, J.P. and Knaub, V. (1950) A study of the cristalline albumin, gamma globulin and total protein in the cerebrospinal fluid of one hundred cases of multiple sclerosis and in other diseases. *Am. J. Med. Sci.*, **219**, 55–64.

176. Tourtellotte, W.W. (1985) The cerebrospinal fluid in multiple sclerosis, in *Handbook of Clinical Neurology 3* (revised series), *Demyelinating Diseases* (eds P.J. Vinken, G.W. Bruyn, H.L. Klawans and J.C. Koetsier), Amsterdam/New York, Elsevier, pp. 79–130.

177. Warren, K.G. and Catz, I. (1992) Synthetic peptide specificity of anti-myelin basic protein from multiple sclerosis cerebrospinal fluid. *J. Neuroimmunol.*, **39** (1–2), 81–9.

178. Warren, K.G., Catz, I., Johnson, E. and Mielke, B. (1994) Anti-myelin basic protein and anti-proteolipid protein specific forms of multiple sclerosis. *Ann. Neurol.*, **35**, 280–9.

179. Martino, G., Olsson, T., Fredrikson, S. *et al.* (1991) Cells producing antibodies specific for myelin basic protein region 70–89 are predominant in cerebrospinal fluid from patients with multiple sclerosis. *Eur. J. Immunol.*, **21**(12), 2971–6.

180. Bray, P.F., Luka, J., Bray, P.F. Culp, K.W. and Schlight, J.P. (1992) Antibodies against Epstein–Barr nuclear antigen (EBNA) in multiple sclerosis CSF, and two pentapeptide sequence identities between EBNA and myelin basic protein. *Neurology*, **42**(9), 1798–804.

181. Harris, J.O., Frank, J.O., Patronas, N., McFarlin, D.E. and McFarland, H.F. (1991) Serial gadolinium-enhanced magnetic resonance imaging scans in patients with early, relapsing-remitting multiple sclerosis: implication for clinical trials and natural history. *Ann. Neurol.*, **29**, 548–55.

182. Gass, A., Barker, G.J., Kidd, D. *et al.* (1994) Correlation of magnetization transfer ratio with clinical disability in multiple sclerosis. *Ann. Neurol.*, **36**, 62–7.

183. McFarland, H.F., Frank, J.A., Albert, P.S. *et al.* (1992) Using gadolinium-enhanced magnetic resonance imaging lesions to monitor disease activity in multiple sclerosis. *Ann. Neurol.*, **32**, 758–66.

184. Filippi, M., Horsfield, M.A., Morrissey, S.P. *et al.* (1994) Quantitative brain MRI lesion load predicts the course of clinically isolated syndromes suggestive of multiple sclerosis. *Neurology*, **44**, 635–41.

185. Smith, M.E., Stone, L.A., Albert, P.S. *et al.* (1993) Clinical worsening in multiple sclerosis is associated with increased frequency and area of gadopentate dimeglumine-enhancing magnetic resonance imaging lesions. *Ann. Neurol.*, **33**, 480–9.

186. Selmaj, K. and Raine, C.S. (1988) Tumor necrosis factor mediates myelin and oligodendrocyte damage *in vitro*. *Ann. Neurol.*, **23**, 339–46.

187. Dore-Duffy, P., Newman, W., Balabanov, R. *et al.* (1995) Circulating, soluble adhesion proteins in cerebrospinal fluid and serum of patients with multiple sclerosis: correlation with clinical activity. *Ann. Neurol.*, **37**, 55–62.

188. Racke, M.K., Martin, R., McFarland, H.F. and Fritz, R.B. (1992) Copolymer-1-induced inhibition of antigen-specific T cell activation: interference with antigen presentation. *J. Neuroimmunol.*, **37**, 75–84.

189. Johnson, K.P., Brooks, B.R., Cohen, J.A. *et al.* (1995) Copolymer 1 reduces relapse rate and improves disability in relapsing-remitting multiple sclerosis: results of a phase III multicenter, double-blind, placebo-controlled trial. *Neurology*, **45**, 1268–76.

15 THE LESION IN MULTIPLE SCLEROSIS AND CHRONIC RELAPSING EXPERIMENTAL ALLERGIC ENCEPHALOMYELITIS: A STRUCTURAL COMPARISON

Cedric S. Raine

15.1 Introduction

15.1.1 PROLOGUE

It is well over a decade since the lesion of multiple sclerosis (MS) and that of chronic relapsing experimental allergic (autoimmune) encephalomyelitis (EAE) in the guinea pig were compared in detail[1,2]. Since that time, quantum leaps have been made in the field of neuropathology, projecting it from a mainly morphologic discipline to one with more of a molecular bent, dependent upon analytical and immunological probes. Concomitant with this trend has been a massive overhaul of our everyday vocabulary and a new heightened awareness of the broad scope of the field, once a territory clearly delimited by disease entities and cellular boundaries. Nevertheless, although our repertoire of applied skills in the nervous system now freely associates between terms barely in existence in the early 1980s – molecules of the major histocompatibility complex (MHC), products of T cell receptor (TCR) genes, cytokine modulation of gene expression, and polymerase chain reaction (PCR), to name but a few – a morphologic framework on which to attach these terms and technologies remains a prerequisite for a comprehensive understanding of disease processes.

With regard to chronic relapsing EAE, the major laboratory tool for MS, the first model[3] was applied in the early 1970s as an innovative approach to MS research and utilized active sensitization of juvenile strain 13 guinea pigs with syngeneic spinal cord tissue[4]. While providing investigators with a reproducible tool with clinical and pathological similarities to MS, the guinea pig model was found to have limitations when it came to immunological analysis and fell short of the standards to which the cellular immunologist was accustomed. In the early 1980s there occurred a redirecting of energies towards the selection of species and development of protocols in which the immunologic terrain was less hazardous. Consequently, for studies on immune-mediated demyelination, the mouse and the rat became the species of choice. After a short period of experimentation with active sensitization[5–9], murine models of chronic demyelination moved more and more towards adoptive-transfer technologies whereby central nervous system (CNS) antigen-specific bulk-isolated lymphocytes[10], T cell lines or T cell clones (e.g.[11]) were administered intravenously into naive recipients. Facilitated by a growing battery of species- and strain-specific molecular and immunologic probes, chronic relapsing EAE in the mouse, while sacrificing some of the structural similarities to the MS lesion seen with the strain 13 guinea pig model, became a widely applied tool for studies on MS. More recently, actively induced and adoptively transferred models of chronic relapsing EAE have been reported in the marmoset[12], forms which hold promise for the further evaluation of the pathology of demyelination in primates and the testing of therapeutic protocols perhaps more relevant to human MS. In light of the now extensively expanded family of EAE models, the overall goal of the following narrative is to present, within the

This chapter is dedicated to the memory of my friend and colleague Dale E. McFarlin MD, who was a key player in the development of chronic relapsing EAE in the mouse and an inspiration to neurologists and neuroimmunologists, young and old, around the world. Dale died on 16 October 1992 at the age of 56.

Multiple Sclerosis: Clinical and pathogenetic basis. Edited by Cedric S. Raine, Henry F. McFarland and Wallace W. Tourtellotte. Published in 1997 by Chapman & Hall, London. ISBN 0 412 30890 8.

same canvas, the comparative neuropathology of the lesions of multiple sclerosis and the currently applied models of chronic relapsing EAE, particularly in the mouse.

15.1.2 AN IMMUNOLOGICAL RATIONALE FOR THE MS PLAQUE

Despite a number of promising leads in support of a viral aetiology, a role for an infectious agent in MS must still remain speculative (see the studies of Johnson[13], Waksman[14], Cook et al.[15], Challoner et al.[16] and Chapter 16). The cumulative image emerging from the many published studies portrays MS as a neurological disorder in which the normal immunological privilege of the CNS has been compromised, where an intra-CNS immune response has been generated and run awry, and where CNS myelin has become the target of immune-mediated damage leaving axons of affected fibres structurally intact but physiologically silent. In the face of an ever-increasing literature on immunological anomalies in MS[17], it is more than likely that both systemic and intra-CNS immunologic (? autoimmune) events play seminal roles both in the initial expression and the perpetuation of the clinical and pathological features of this condition, one of the most enigmatic diseases of the nervous system. Whether the reported immunologic vagaries and their fluctuations might bespeak events of pathogenetic significance to the MS lesion and not merely epiphenomena forms much of the background rationale for what follows.

Although the varied clinical picture innate to MS (see Chapter 1) renders correlation of some of the immunologic findings difficult, the genesis of the demyelinating lesion in MS is best appreciated when presented against the backdrop of growing evidence for an immunogenic process. In this context, and in support of the possibility of both a generalized and an intra-CNS immunological anomaly, large numbers of reports have appeared since the original work of Kabat et al. in 1950[18] which detected an elevated IgG level in the cerebrospinal fluid (CSF) of a significant number of MS subjects. This finding became accepted as indicative of local antibody synthesis within the CNS compartment and is still used as one of the diagnostic criteria for MS (Chapter 5). Also, within the CSF, immunological techniques revealed the presence of free myelin basic protein (MBP) or its fragments and antibodies to MBP[19], phenomena not entirely specific for MS but perhaps indicators of general white matter damage. Within the circulation, numerous investigators, beginning with Oger et al. in 1975[20], documented abnormalities in lymphocyte subpopulations, some of which fluctuated with disease course. The consensus of opinion of the many subsequent studies on circulating lymphocytes in MS is that there is up-regulation of CD4 (helper/inducer) T cells

and down-regulation of CD8 (suppressor/cytotoxic) T cells during relapses, although the specificity and significance of these repeatedly confirmed fluctuations are still debated[21, 22]. Furthermore, there is increasing evidence that certain MHC patterns may be more prevalent among groups of MS subjects (Chapter 14), observations in support of predisposing immunogenetic factors (Chapter 13). Similar factors are implicated in susceptibility to EAE.

While a key role for T lymphocytes in the pathogenesis of the MS lesion is now generally accepted[23], sensitization to myelin antigens (e.g. MBP) in MS has been a hotly debated issue for many years (Chapter 13). With T cell rosetting techniques, early work documented enhanced recognition of MBP by T cells in MS but this response was later found not to be MS specific. With peripheral T cell clones to MBP, a study using a gene mutation technology appeared to indicate increased responsiveness in MS patients[24]. Antibodies against oligodendrocytes in MS were implicated by Abramsky et al. in 1977[25], but these were subsequently found not to be MS specific, the result perhaps of non-specific binding of antibody to Fc receptors. The presence of circulating anti-myelin factors in MS, first demonstrated by Bornstein in 1963[26], has been repeatedly confirmed and shown in vitro to be specific for CNS myelin[27], but unrelated to immunoglobulin[28].

Although the presence of immunoglobulin has long been documented in the MS lesion, its origin being attributed to a defective blood–brain barrier[29–32], specific roles for such immune system components have been difficult to find. With the identification and classification of other immune recognition molecules and their ligands (e.g. TCR, MHC, cytokines and adhesion molecules), and the application of immunopathological technologies to CNS tissue, it has been possible to construct a molecular montage of the MS lesion[33] (Chapter 10). Since the first electron microscope (EM) reports on the subject[34, 35], the superimposition of more sophisticated immunocytological approaches upon fine structural analysis has done much in recent years to broaden our perspective on the genesis of the MS lesion[32, 36–45].

15.1.3 AN IMMUNOLOGICAL MODEL FOR MS

In the absence of a natural non-human counterpart for MS, investigators turned towards the development of different forms of EAE, an autoimmune demyelinating disease of laboratory animals induced by T cell sensitization to myelin antigens. At the time of its introduction in the 1930s by Rivers and co-workers and its later modification by Freund and colleagues[46], EAE was perceived as an acute, fatal, monophasic condition. Historically, EAE has contributed enormously to the understanding of delayed hypersensitivity in general and immune-mediated demyelination in particular [47–53]. In acute EAE, T cell mediation is well proven and roles for antibodies to myelin components have been demonstrated [46]. More recent data suggest some of the encephalitogenicity in EAE to be related to the sharing of common T cell receptor variable regions in some species [54, 55]. Moreover, transgenic mice expressing genes encoding a rearranged TCR specific for MBP [56, 57] have been claimed to develop spontaneous, late-onset EAE in the absence of active or adoptive sensitization, further supporting a key role for the T cell in this condition. Despite the multitude of contributions of acute EAE to immune-mediated myelin pathology, its direct application to MS was limited by its clinical and pathologic dissimilarities to the human disease. Indeed, it was originally developed as a model for post-rabies immunization encephalomyelitis (an iatrogenic condition caused by CNS tissue in the rabies inoculum), and it was only after the observation that this condition resembled the acute form of MS that EAE was elevated to a laboratory counterpart for MS [46, 58]. In spite of its many dissimilarities to MS, acute EAE continues to provide seminal data on fundamental questions in CNS autoimmunity and on a number of therapeutic approaches to MS, such as those involving myelin-related TCR sequences, anti-inflammatory compounds, immunosuppressive modalities and antibodies to immune system molecules (Chapter 18).

Although it had long been realized that a chronic form of EAE might have greater applicability to clinical and pathogenetic mechanisms in MS, prior to 1980 chronic EAE had been reported only sporadically [53]. With one exception, no chronic model had been seriously applied to MS. The exception was the model of chronic EAE of Stone and Lerner [3], a model which, like MS, demonstrated a relapsing course and lesions separated in time and space [4]. A modified version of the same model was subsequently investigated by Lassmann [59] with considerable success. The strain 13 guinea pig model firmly established the clinical and pathologic similarities between chronic relapsing EAE and human MS. The similarities were not only morphologic but also encompassed immunologic, genetic and therapeutic parameters [53]. For example, spontaneous depletion of certain lymphocyte populations from the circulation was shown to occur with clinical onset, changes which fluctuated longitudinally during the course of the disease. From the therapeutic angle, it was found that chronic relapsing EAE in the guinea pig could be suppressed with MBP [60] and successfully treated after onset with MBP combined with a major myelin glycolipid, galactocerebroside – GalC [53, 61]. The latter treatment protocol in the guinea pig model led to enhanced CNS remyelination in affected areas,

the repair correlating with diminished inflammatory activity and clinical improvement. However, the development of a number of rat and mouse forms of chronic relapsing EAE has today somewhat eroded the pre-eminence of the strain 13 guinea pig model (although pathologically the guinea pig lesions remain more like MS lesions), since, as stated above for these species, well-defined immunological and immunogenetic probes are readily available.

15.2 Multiple sclerosis

15.2.1 THE ESTABLISHED LESION

A territory explored repeatedly since its first delineation in the latter half of the nineteenth century, the chronic MS plaque remains a unique enigma of intense interest among neuropathologists [58]. The general neuropathology of the MS plaque, covered elsewhere in this volume (Chapter 9), shows the typical MS plaque to be a chronic silent lesion (both clinically and pathologically), the deserted battlefield of past pathologic events which may have raged for months to decades and during which myelin and oligodendrocytes have been selectively depleted from the affected white matter parenchyma. The plaque area becomes largely taken over by scarring fibrous astrocytes and reactive microglia. Residual inflammatory activity is inconspicuous and in most cases the lesion is a burnt-out silent scar. Myelin loss and fibrous astrogliosis are sometimes centred upon blood vessels, around which it is postulated that the demyelinating process arises as rims of naked axons around perivascular infiltrates (see Figure 15.6a). The coalescence of myriads of such small perivascular zones of demyelination is believed to lead to the chronic MS plaque [62]. However, in most silent MS lesions, the lesion is so large that correlation with blood vessels is impossible. Light microscopic (LM) examination of thin sections from silent (burnt-out) MS lesions reveals areas of gliosis and demyelination ranging from millimetres to several centimetres in diameter, sharply demarcated from adjacent myelinated areas (Figure 15.1a, b) (Chapter 9). The entire neuraxis, from optic nerve to filum terminale, is vulnerable. Myelinated fibres entering a chronic lesion abruptly lose their sheaths, leaving axons to course naked across the affected area. Typically at the perimeters of chronic silent MS lesions, a narrow rim of regenerated myelin (remyelination) is apparent, sometimes associated with a mild degree of oligodendroglial cell hyperplasia (Figures 15.1b, 15.2a, b, 15.3a, b). Axonal sparing is typical but variable in degree, axon survival probably being related to a combination of factors, including lesion age and dimension, the degree of fibrous astrogliosis and the intensity of the inflammation during the formative stages. In general, however, there is invariably

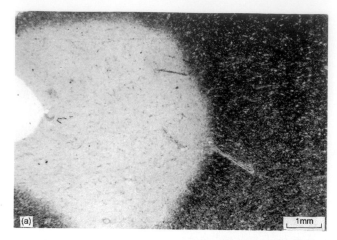

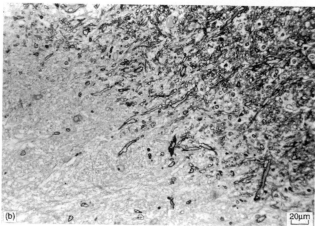

Figure 15.1 (*a*) A small, chronically demyelinated silent MS plaque is shown by LM. Note the sharp demarcation between the circular demyelinated area and the surrounding darkly staining myelinated white matter and the sleeve of demyelination along the vessel leaving the plaque on the right. (One micron section; toluidine blue stain. (*b*) Detail of the same silent lesion to show the abrupt transition from myelinated white matter (*right*, note individual nerve fibres with myelin sheaths, some of the thinner myelinated fibres probably indicative of remyelination) to the demyelinated, fibrous astrogliotic parenchyma of the plaque (*left*). No infiltrating cells are apparent.

significant axonal loss in MS. In areas of severe gliosis, the density of fibres suggests a significant reduction from the original population (Figures 15.2*c*, 15.3*c*, *d*). The commonest cellular component of the chronic MS plaque is the hypertrophic astrocyte, which may be multinucleated (Figure 15.2*d*, 15.3*d*), giving the cell a syncytial appearance. Corpora amylacea, non-specific products of fibrous astrocytes, are present in variable numbers (Figure 15.3*c*). Oligodendrocytes, the myelinating cells of the CNS, are absent from older gliotic areas (Figures 15.1*b*, 15.2*c*, 15.3*d*). Other plaque constituents include the occasional foamy macrophage, scattered microglial cells and blood vessels which may be increased in number. Within the spinal cord, axonal

sparing is usually more apparent than in hemispheric lesions. Naked axons reside as a mosaic in a dense, fibrous astrocytic matrix lacking oligodendrocytes (Figure 15.4*a*). By EM, one is impressed by the geometry and intimate relationships between naked axons and scarring astrocytes (Figure 15.4*b*). Between demyelinated axons, axoglial membrane specializations have been described [63] (Figure 15.4*b*, *inset*). Some processes of fibrous astrocytes are particularly dense due to a more intense accumulation of glial filaments. Desmosomes and gap junctions are common between astroglial cell profiles (Figure 15.4*b*, *inset*). These intercellular membrane specializations probably have physiological significance [64]. Occasionally, silent chronic lesions contain perivascular collections of foamy macrophages and their margins in the absence of any obvious lymphocytic infiltrate (Figures 15.5*a*, *b*), suggestive of ongoing, insidious activity fuelled by locally synthesized factors, namely cytokines. Like hemispheric lesions, spinal cord lesions display a narrow rim of CNS remyelination about their margins and, on rare occasions, some demyelinated CNS axons become invested and myelinated by Schwann cells (Figure 15.5*c*).

With regard to inflammatory cell types, a detailed morphologic study by Prineas and Wright [65] analysed quantitatively macrophages and inflammatory cells in chronic MS lesions. This work showed the parenchymal microglial cell, the ubiquitous macrophage of the CNS, to be prominent and sometimes to contain cytoplasmic membranous stacks, presumably the end-stage of myelin degeneration (see Figure 15.10). In addition, large numbers of plasma cells were apparent. Small lymphocytes were not common but adjacent 'normal' white matter was estimated to contain about 250 small lymphocytes per mm^3, with plasma cells slightly fewer than 200 per mm^3. Immunocytochemistry with phenotypic markers to T cell subsets have since confirmed the paucity of T cells within chronic silent MS lesions [33]. Perivascular infiltrates of T cells, rare to absent in chronic silent lesions, serve as a reliable index of disease activity, sometimes correlating with recent clinical activity (see below).

In MS lesions of all ages, much effort has been devoted to the analysis of lymphocytic populations. By immunocytochemistry, recent inflammation equates with the influx of T cells, predominantly of the CD4+ (helper) phenotype. These decrease in number as the lesion resolves, giving way to more and more CD8+ (suppressor/cytotoxic) T cells. However, the relative distributions of CD4+ and CD8+ T cells in MS lesions is a controversial issue (see [33, 66, 67] and Chapter 10), particularly since the CD4 phenotype, now known to embrace both effector (TH1) and regulatory (TH2) populations distinguishable by cytokine profile only, now renders previous speculations on CD4/CD8 switching a less topical issue. In less active lesions (judged by

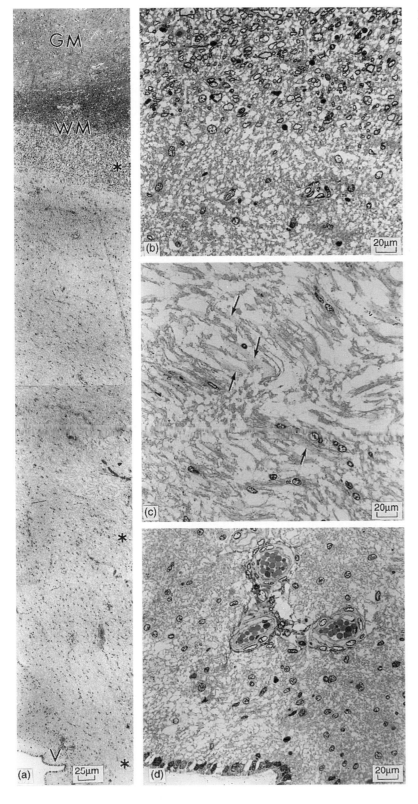

Figure 15.2   (*a*) A strip montage of a chronic silent lesion extends from the ventricular wall (V), traverses a wide expanse of demyelinated white matter to a narrow zone of myelinated subcortical white matter (WM) and overlying cerebral grey matter (GM). The areas at the asterisks are shown in (*b*), (*c*) and (*d*). (One micron epoxy section; toluidine blue stain. (*b*) Detail from the edge of the same lesion, at the level of the uppermost asterisk in (*a*), to show the sharp demarcation between the myelinated subcortical white matter (note myelin sheaths around fibres, *above*) and the fibrous astrogliotic demyelinated lesion, below. Some oligodendroglial hyperplasia may be present in this region, evidenced by the numerous small, round densely staining nuclei. (*c*) Detail of the area indicated by the middle asterisk in (*a*). Note the fibrous astrogliotic parenchyma, the markedly reduced number of naked axons (*arrows*), and the increased extracellular space. The cell nuclei are mainly astroglial. (*d*) Detail of the area at the level of the lowermost asterisk in (*a*), adjacent to the ventricular wall (note ependymal lining, *below*). Axons are not readily apparent within the fibrous astrogliotic matrix, many astroglial nuclei are present and perivascular microglia are seen around the small blood vessels.

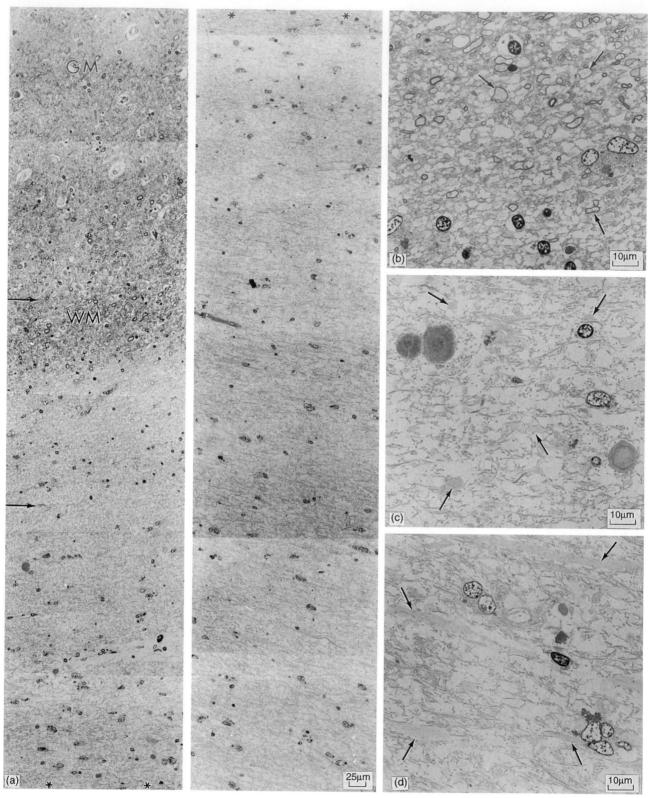

Figure 15.3 (*a*) A strip montage of a chronic silent MS lesion is shown in two adjacent segments (connected at the asterisks), to extend from the cerebral grey matter (GM), across a narrow myelinated area of subcortical white matter (WM) into a broad zone of chronically demyelinated, sclerotic plaque (*lower half, left segment, and entire right hand segment*). Note the absence of an inflammatory component in the lesion and the oligodendroglial hyperplasia marked by the numerous small dark nuclei at the lesion edge (*between arrows*). (One micron epoxy section; toluidine blue stain.) (*b*) Higher magnification from the edge of the same lesion to show myelinated white matter (*above*) meeting demyelinated plaque (*below*). Numerous thinly myelinated (remyelinated) fibres (*arrows*), an hypertrophic astrocyte (*centre, right*) and hyperplastic oligodendrocytes (dense nuclei, *below*) can be discerned. (*c*) Detail of a deeper area of the same lesion to show corpora amylacea (dense, round profiles), scattered naked axons (*arrows*) and increased extracellular space. (*d*) Detail of an even deeper area to show multinucleated astrocytes, demyelinated axons (*arrows*) and overall twig-like appearance of the plaque parenchyma due to the fibrous astrogliosis.

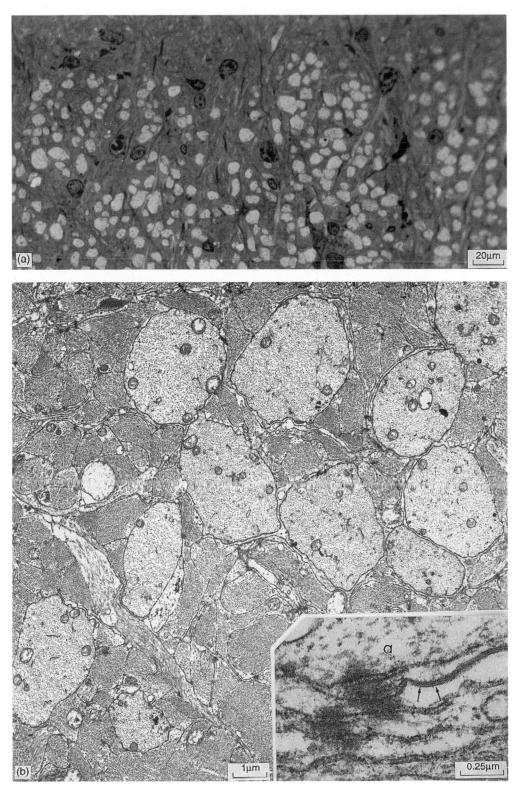

Figure 15.4   (*a*) A light micrograph from a large lesion in the anterior column of the spinal cord at L3 shows impressive sparing of demyelinated axons sectioned transversely (white profiles) embedded in a dense matrix of fibrous astrocytes. (One micron epoxy section; toluidine blue stain.) (*b*) An electron micrograph of the same chronic silent MS lesion shows more clearly the demyelinated axons and the background astroglial scar tissue. *Inset*: an axoglial junction exists between a demyelinated axon (**a**) and an astroglial process. Desmosomes and a gap junction (*arrows*) exist between other astroglial cell processes.

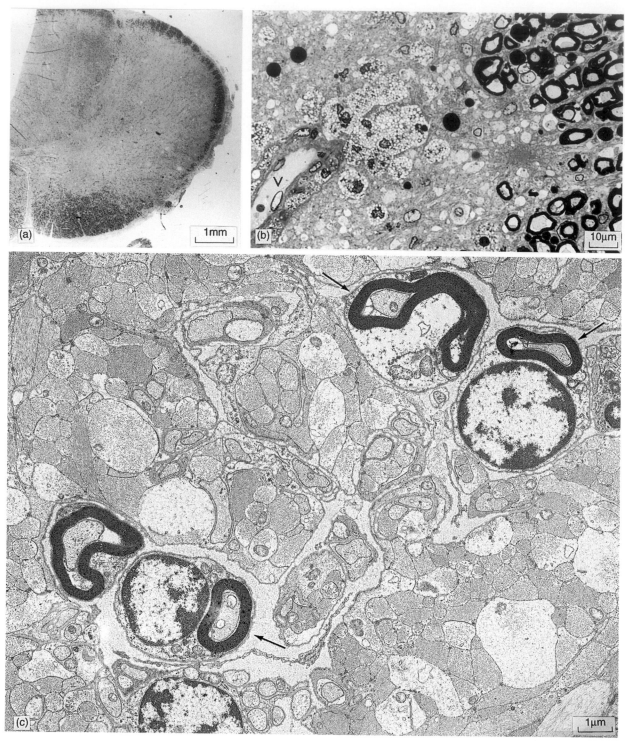

Figure 15.5 (*a*) A hemisection of mid-thoracic spinal cord from a case of chronic MS depicts a massive demyelinated plaque about the subpial margins of which a narrow rim of myelinated white matter is preserved. The dorsal columns lie above, the anterior fissure, below left. (One micron epoxy section; toluidine blue stain. (*b*) Detail of a subpial margin of the same lesion reveals the presence of many lipid-laden macrophages throughout the demyelinated area and around a blood vessel (**v**). These macrophages stained positively for class II MHC. Note the absence of lymphocytes, the demyelinated axons in cross-section, the relatively normal myelin to the right and the densely staining corpora amylacea. (*c*) An area of chronically demyelinated MS plaque in a spinal cord contains Schwann cells which have elaborated PNS-type myelin around CNS axons (*arrows*). Elsewhere, fibrous astroglial cell processes and a few demyelinated CNS axons are apparent.

the decreasing intensity of inflammatory response and increased gliosis), there is a gradual shift in components of perivascular cuffs from high to low numbers of small lymphocytes (T cells, mainly), and to more plasma cells and foamy macrophages. The latter percolate towards blood vessels as lesion activity wanes, to accumulate within the Virchow–Robin space until they exit the CNS (Figure 15.5b). Perivascular (foamy) macrophages are morphologically identical to macrophages in the CNS parenchyma and persist in lesions for long periods, probably of the order of months to years. These cells are considered by some to be the progeny of reactive microglia and their apparent migration to and from the perivascular space suggests that these microglia have a haematogenous origin. This conclusion is also supported from work on other CNS systems [68, 69]. However, a definitive marker to distinguish amoeboid microglia from monocytic macrophages remains to be identified.

Plasma cells and occasional small lymphocytes can be documented in perivascular areas in chronic lesions but polymorphonuclear leukocytes are notably absent, being more associated with acute, haemorrhagic (usually post-infectious) states. Mast cells have been described on a number of occasions in MS but their presence has not been correlated with any disease stage. Since the majority of chronic MS patients eventually succumb to an intercurrent infection (e.g. pneumonia, septicaemia), some of the infiltrating elements seen within the autopsied CNS may be due to the systemic infection, rather than intra-CNS events.

15.2.2   RECENT, ACUTE MS LESIONS

Precisely what distinguishes an 'acute' from a 'chronic' MS plaque, particularly the 'chronic active' type, has been a long-standing bone of contention among neuropathologists. Lesion nosology varies between authors and it is possible that some of the discord, particularly that associated with T cell phenotypes in lesions of different ages [33, 58], might have at its roots differences in lesion classification. Retrospective analysis of several of the reported ultrastructural studies claiming to document 'acute' MS lesions has proved them to have described chronic changes, some of them non-specific for MS. Moreover, it is not altogether impossible that the acute fatal clinical entity known as 'acute MS' may, in the final analysis, prove to be a condition distinct from chronic MS, linked only by a common pathogenetic mechanism.

Reports on acute MS (Marburg-type) are limited in number, no doubt due to the rarity of the condition which is typified by a fatal outcome weeks to months after the onset of a rapidly progressive neurological syndrome. Acute MS lesions are distinct from chronic MS lesions (Chapter 9) (Figures 15.6a, 15.7). They are not confined to the clinical syndrome acute MS but can also be intermingled with chronic lesions in the CNS of patients succumbing to chronic progressive MS with a particularly malignant course. In acute lesions, the parenchyma is loose and highly oedematous (Figures 15.6b, c, 15.7). Astrocytes are intensely hypertrophic, globoid, lack processes and stain faintly for GFAP [45] (Figure 15.6e). They invariably stain strongly for IgG [29–31]. Diffuse parenchymal infiltration and perivascular cuffing are common, mainly by lymphocytes of the T cell lineage (Figures 15.6b, c, d 15.8). There is widespread expression of MHC class II (Figure 15.8b), a macrophage molecule associated with antigen presentation and interactions with T cells of the CD4 phenotype (Figure 15.8). The previously well myelinated parenchyma is reduced to a loosely packed, oedematous zone containing an abundance of myelin debris- and fat-laden macrophages, probably reactive microglial cells (Figures 15.6f, 15.7). Some of the latter that contain recognizable myelin debris (Figures 15.6f, 15.7) stain positively for myelin markers like MBP and are MHC class II+. Axons are much reduced in number. Hypertrophic astrocytes, many of them multinucleated, extend from deep within the lesion into the adjacent normal-appearing white matter but display their globoid form only within the oedematous centre (Figures 15.6e, 15.7). Such globoid astrocytes are not seen in EAE lesions. As the lesion ages, these cells remain hypertrophic but develop processes and become more intensely GFAP+. The major ultrastructural features of the acute MS lesion have been outlined by Lee et al. [43] and Wu and Raine [45].

Myelin destruction involves the rapid lysis of intact myelin into extracellular vesicular arrays [43] – a phenomenon also described in acute EAE [70]. Phagocytosis of myelin is effected by investing macrophages which internalize the myelin debris as it is lysed from the outer layers of the sheath, giving it an attenuated appearance in places. Macrophages (? reactive microglia) involved in myelin breakdown invariably contain the lamellar inclusions described elsewhere (see Figure 15.10). Myelin debris-laden macrophages are often arranged around perivascular cuffs made up mostly of small lymphocytes (Figures 15.6 and 15.8). Hypertrophic astrocytes may also be involved in myelin phagocytosis on rare occasions [43] and may interact with and internalize surviving oligodendrocytes [44, 45, 71] (Chapter 9). Surviving, demyelinated axons are present but difficult to discern due to their reduced number and smaller diameter. Paradoxically, areas of CNS remyelination have been described in acute MS lesions [72, 73] (see below).

Although definition of the precise sequence of immunopathological events during active demyelination in MS plaques awaits clarification, the current

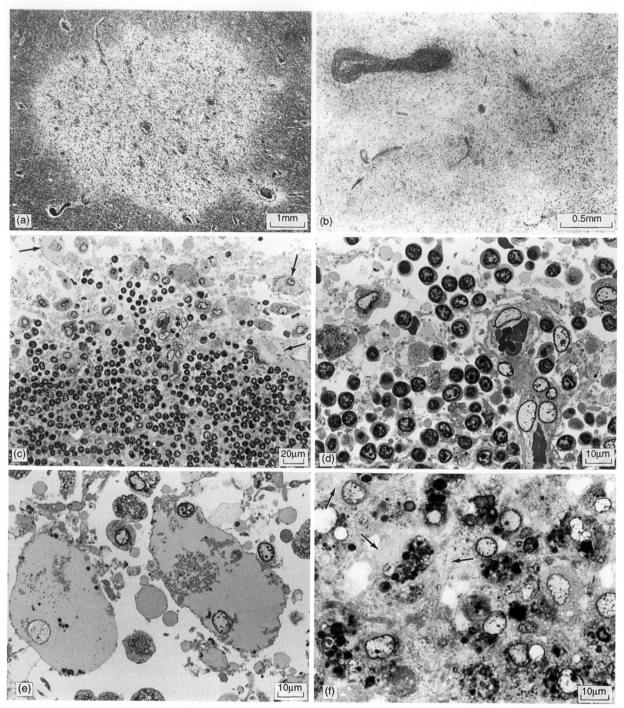

Figure 15.6 (*a*) A small, heavily infiltrated acute lesion from a case of chronic progressive MS is depicted in the centrum semiovale. Note the irregular, ill-defined margin of the plaque and foci of demyelination around perivascular infiltrates (Paraffin section; Luxol fast blue. (*b*) The centre of an acute lesion displays intense inflammation around one vessel and widespread infiltration elsewhere, in addition to demyelination. (One micron epoxy section; toluidine blue. (*c*) Detail of the heavily inflamed vessel in (*b*) reveals small lymphocytes percolating from the Virchow–Robin space into the adjacent demyelinated, oedematous parenchyma. Note the hypertrophic astrocytes (*arrows*) and the lipid-laden macrophages. (*d*) Higher power of (*c*) to show homogeneity among the infiltrating cells. (*e*) Same case, different lesion. Two hypertrophic astrocytes lie in an oedematous, demyelinated CNS parenchyma surrounded by macrophages and astroglial cell processes. The two cells indenting the surface of the hypertrophic astrocyte to the right are oligodendrocytes (Chapter 9). Astroglial hypertrophy and these oligodendroglial associations are not features of the lesion in EAE. (*f*) At the edge of another acute MS lesion, myelin debris-laden macrophages and a few demyelinated axons (*arrows*) can be seen.

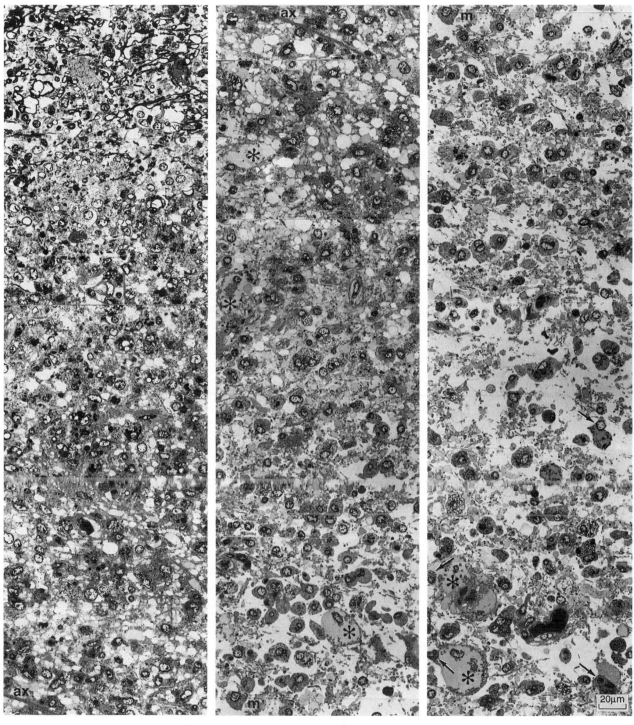

Figure 15.7   A strip montage from the myelinated edge (*top, left segment*) to the oedematous demyelinated centre (*bottom, right segment*) is connected at the naked axon (**ax**) (*bottom left segment and top centre*), and the macrophage (**m**) (*bottom centre segment and top right*). Note the pale hypertrophic astrocytes (*), some of which show surface associations with oligodendrocytes (*arrows*) (Chapter 9). The loosely packed central zone merges into a more compact area of macrophages, hypertrophic astrocytes and poorly differentiated cells before contacting a broad zone of active demyelination characterized by macrophages containing osmiophilic myelin debris and lipid droplets (*centre, left segment*). The myelinated edge of the lesion (*top, left segment*) displays hypertrophic astrocytes and supernumerary oligodendrocytes. (One micron epoxy section; toluidine blue stain.)

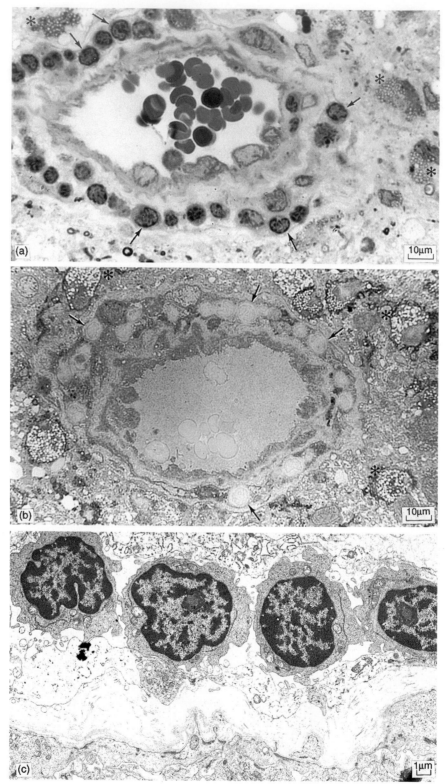

Figure 15.8 (*a*) A perivascular cuff of infiltrating cells from the centre of an acute MS lesion, sampled by biopsy from an 18-year-old female with a 3-month history of neurological signs, depicts a uniform population of small lymphocytes (*arrows*). Lipid-laden macrophages (*) reside in the adjacent demyelinated parenchyma which contains scattered droplets of myelin debris. (One micron epoxy section; toluidine blue stain.) (*b*) A similar section from the same vessel is reacted for class II MHC. Note the class II MHC⁺ macrophages (*) and the class II MHC⁻ small lymphocytes which are probably non-activated T cells (activated T cells and B cells should express class II MHC). (*c*) The same cells are shown by EM.

consensus leans towards a process involving both T and B cells [23] (see also Chapter 10). One implicated process, antibody-dependent cell-mediated demyelination, is believed to involve the binding of specific anti-CNS antibodies to white matter, a phenomenon associated with the local recruitment of lymphocytes. These may also produce soluble mediators (cytokines) which contribute to myelin lysis [74, 75]. Antibody-dependent cell-mediated demyelination may be related not so much to sensitization to a single myelin antigen but rather to a combination of myelin components [53]. This possibility, based upon experimental data [76, 77], involves the T cell arm of the immune response being primed by a protein, e.g. MBP, while the B cell (antibody) response occurs later and is directed against a different component of myelin, e.g. a lipid hapten like GalC. Yet another pathogenetic possibility, emanating from work on EAE by Brosnan et al. [78], relates the myelin loss to a bystander effect exerted by proteinases produced by macrophages stimulated by T cells. While some of the myelin loss may indeed be due to non-specific soluble mediators, a significant role for bystander demyelination during immune-mediated demyelination has been challenged by a number of investigators (see [79]). Using a non-CNS antigen to sensitize animals and lymphocytes responsive to the same antigen, these workers claimed that primary damage to myelin did not accompany the invasion of non-specific lymphocytes into nervous tissue. Similar conclusions have also been reached by other laboratories and it is well known from the literature on human conditions that inflammation in the CNS is not necessarily accompanied by demyelination, inasmuch as there are many viral encephalitides where the CNS is heavily infiltrated with little or no apparent effect on neighboring myelin. In any event, in MS the net result of inflammation is the lysis and phagocytosis of myelin by local macrophages [36, 37, 39, 43, 80]. Related to myelin degradation in acute MS is a phenomenon known as 'receptor-mediated phagocytosis of myelin', whereby myelin sheaths are reduced to extracellular vesicular or lamellar droplets (Figure 15.9a) that associate with clathrin-coated pits on the surface of macrophages and become internalized (Figure 15.9b) [39, 43, 80]. The same phenomenon has been described in chronic active MS and identical appearances occur during acute and relapsing phases of EAE in which the binding of myelin droplets to clathrin-coated pits appears to involve IgG as the ligand (see below).

Other features peculiar to the acute MS lesion include the binding of immunoglobulin by reactive astrocytes and the capping of oligodendrocytes by cytoplasmic processes from astrocytes, the latter perhaps indicative of phagocytosis [30]. In general, oligodendroglial cells appear to survive the active phases of demyelination [37, 72], although an occasional oligodendrocyte undergoing apoptosis can be seen [39] (see Figure 15.12d).

One intriguing aspect of acute and chronic active MS plaques that has emerged from studies of lesions displaying ongoing myelin degradation is the occurrence of CNS remyelination (see below). This regenerative phenomenon proceeds in the face of ongoing myelin destruction [37, 72, 81]. Remyelination in active lesions was also reported on routine LM by Lassmann [2]. What underlies this paradoxical, perhaps abortive reparatory event is not known but it may be related to oligodendrocyte proliferation ('oligodendroglial hyperplasia' in the older literature), occurring particularly at the margins of MS lesions (Chapter 9). More recent analyses suggest oligodendroglial hyperplasia to be the result of the local release of cytokines by infiltrating and/or glial cells. In this regard, interleukin 2 (IL-2), a cytokine claimed to be stimulatory for oligodendrocytes in vitro [82], has been localized at the periphery of the MS lesion [83]. However, the stimulatory effect of IL-2 upon oligodendrocytes remains controversial and awaits confirmation. Also implicated in oligodendroglial hyperplasia is a proliferative effect exerted by locally released immunoglobulin or enzymes in response to myelin degradation. On the other hand, yet to be reconciled is the concomitant presence in active lesions of cytokines like tumour necrosis factor alpha (TNFα) and lymphotoxin (LT) [84–86], mediators with known cytolytic effects upon oligodendrocytes [75, 87]. These paradoxes notwithstanding, CNS remyelination in active lesions appears to bespeak a robust regenerative response at the height of the inflammatory attack, an event perhaps related to the release of soluble mediators with stimulatory activity.

From the inflammatory standpoint, it is well known that CD4+ T cells and class II MHC-expressing cells (microglial cells, macrophages) coexist within the CNS in MS [33]. The expression of MHC molecules within the CNS, a tissue usually negative for MHC II, bestows upon the CNS the ability to interact with T cells, thus compromising its normally immunologically privileged state. The earlier demonstration of class II MHC on endothelial cells in early acute MS lesions and on astrocytes and endothelial cells in vitro led to much speculation that the blood–brain barrier may represent the site of initial lesion activity with endothelial cells serving as antigen-presenting cells. However, later studies on lymphocyte adhesion molecules in situ in acute MS failed to confirm the expression of Ia (MHC II) on endothelial cells although perivascular pericytes were invariably Ia+ [33]. In view of the occurrence of class II MHC in a number of non-MS conditions [88], an immunomodulatory role for endothelial cells in the MS lesion must remain a debatable issue, at least at the level of antigen presentation.

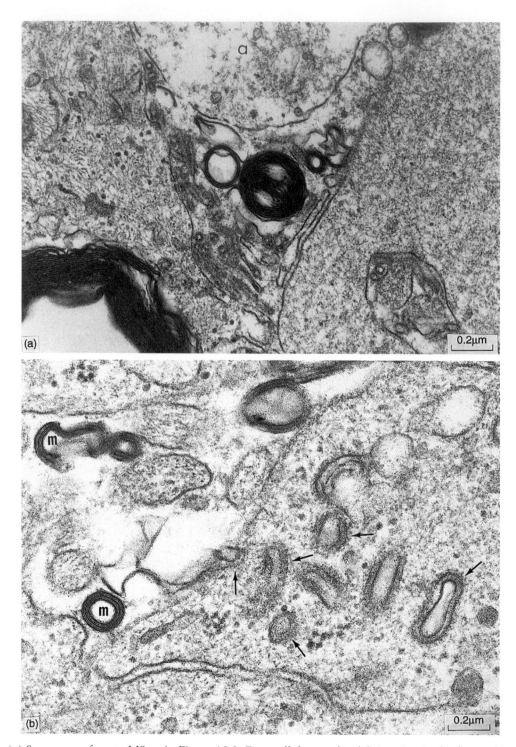

Figure 15.9   (*a*) Same case of acute MS as in Figure 15.8. Extracellular myelin debris exists in the form of lamellar droplets (*centre*) and tubular vesicles with a granular coating. A demyelinated axon (**a**) lies above. (*b*) This EM image from the same case shows extracellular myelin debris (**m**) adjacent to a portion of a microglial cell which is apparently in the process of internalizing a droplet of myelin attached to an elongated, serpiginous, clathrin-coated pit (*arrows*).

15.2.3 THE CHRONIC ACTIVE MS LESION

Ultrastructural studies on chronic active MS lesions have revealed a number of phenomena pertinent to lesion expansion. The edges of such lesions are hypercellular and less well defined than those of the more common chronic silent lesion. There is a diffuse transition from normal white matter to plaque area, a zone which contains macrophages engorged with myelin debris (Figure 15.10a). This myelin debris stains positively with several anti-myelin-related antibodies and oil-red-O and resides mainly within globular macrophages (amoeboid microglia) (Figure 15.10b). An occasional astrocyte may be involved in myelin phagocytosis and surviving oligodendrocytes are common [37].

Typically, ongoing demyelination is encountered. Like acute MS lesions (see above), this involves investment of the affected fibre by the pleated processes of macrophages and lysis of myelin from the outer layers of the sheath. The myelin sheath is gradually thinned as vesicular droplets of apparently normal myelin sheath are separated from the sheath and become internalized by macrophages into membrane-bound phagosomes (Figure 15.11a). The uptake of droplets of myelin into phagosomes involves the above-mentioned phenomenon of receptor-mediated phagocytosis of myelin whereby extracellular myelin fragments become attached to clathrin-coated pits on the surface of macrophages (Figure 15.11a). The normal 11 nm CNS myelin periodicity is reduced to about 6 nm after the myelin leaves the nerve fibres. Immunocytochemical studies by Prineas and Graham [89] suggest that the capping of macrophages by IgG in active MS lesions might be related to myelin phagocytosis. Work by Epstein et al. [90] on rabbits confirmed the occurrence of the same phenomenon in EAE and suggested the existence of a structural ligand between the myelin droplet and the coated pit on the surface of the macrophage. This was later confirmed in the guinea pig model by immunogold staining in a study that showed the structural ligand to be IgG [91]. Whether this denoted opsonization and a role for specific antibody or whether the myelin uptake was effected by non-specific binding of IgG to Fc receptors on macrophages, remains to be elucidated. Attachment of myelin fragments to coated pits on the surface of macrophages appears to be a mechanism peculiar to autoimmune demyelination and a feature that underscores an immune-mediated process in MS. This same pattern of demyelination has also been described in actively induced acute EAE in the SJL/J mouse [5], actively induced chronic relapsing EAE in the SJL/J mouse [9], and adoptively transferred chronic relapsing EAE in SJL/J and PL/J mice [92, 93], conditions in which T cell autoimmunity is well documented.

Although fibrous astrocytes can be seen on rare occasions to be engaged in myelin degradation [43], phagocytic cells are, in most cases, difficult to identify with certainty. The reactive microglial cell, the cell believed to give rise to amoeboid microglia (the foamy cell, compound granular corpuscle, or gitter cell of the older literature), is the major scavenger in the MS lesion. Ultrastructurally, reactive and amoeboid microglia, best seen in chronic active lesions, contain, in addition to free lipid, recognizable myelin debris at various stages of degradation (Figures 15.11b, 15.13). Examination of reactive microglial cells in such lesions reveals within the cytoplasm membranous stacks that are apparently derived from osmiophilic, lipid lamellar arrays (Figure 15.11c), the end-product of myelin degradation. The same profiles have been described during myelin phagocytosis in other conditions [94, 95]. These membranous stacks, claimed to be unusual in MS lesions [36], have been documented in CNS conditions of varied aetiology [96]. The suggestion has also been made that these structures might have a viral origin and be specific for MS [97]. Yet another structural peculiarity associated with microglial cells is the occurrence of short regions of plasmalemma covered with basal lamina-like material underlaid by zones of intense osmiophilia (Figure 15.11b).

Reminders that the recent changes in chronic active MS lesions are superimposed upon areas of long-term damage are present in the form of twig-like scarring astroglial cell processes packed with intermediate filaments (Figures 15.11b, 15.12a, 15.13). The cell bodies of some scarring astrocytes are large and sometimes contain more than one nucleus (a typical feature of silent MS plaques, Figure 15.3d). These cells reside in a neuropil containing naked axons, some of which are dystrophic (Figure 15.13 and see Figure 15.17b). In most chronic active MS lesions, the ever-present perivascular cuffs of infiltrating cells contain cells with a morphology typical of activated lymphocytes. Immunocytochemistry has shown these collections to be rich in T cells of the CD4 (helper) phenotype [23, 33]. The latter features contrast the chronic active lesion with the more typical silent lesion described above.

Encountered frequently along the margins of actively demyelinating chronic lesions are oligodendroglial somata (Figures 15.12a, 15.13). This confirms observations on oligodendroglial persistence and proliferation in acute MS plaques previously recorded by Ibrahim and Adams [98, 99]. The oligodendrocytes are round and reactive (Figure 15.12a). Nevertheless, they retain the immunocytochemical and morphological characteristics of oligodendrocytes, in particular microtubules but no intermediate filaments (Figure 15.13), a rich cytoplasm, a nucleus containing abundant heterochromatin and gap junctions between themselves and adjacent astrocytes (Figure 15.12b, c).

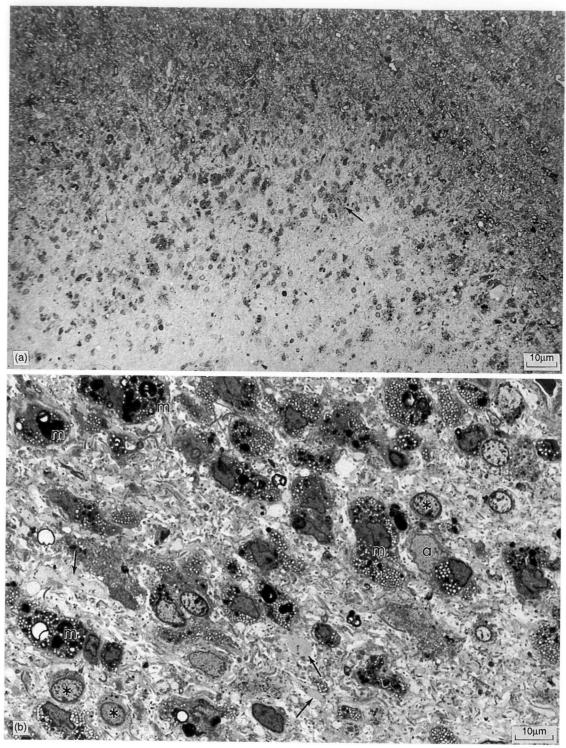

Figure 15.10   (*a*) A one micron epoxy section across the edge of a chronic active MS lesion shows it to possess a less distinct edge than that of a chronic silent lesion (see Figure 15.1*a*), that contains the occasional perivascular cuff of infiltrating cells (*arrow*) and macrophages filled with osmiophilic myelin debris. (*b*) Detail from the demyelinated edge of the same chronic active lesion shows an abundance of myelin- and lipid-laden macrophages (**m**), the occasional hypertrophic astrocyte (**a**) and demyelinated axon (*arrows*), in addition to a fibrous astrogliotic background and several surviving oligodendrocytes (*).

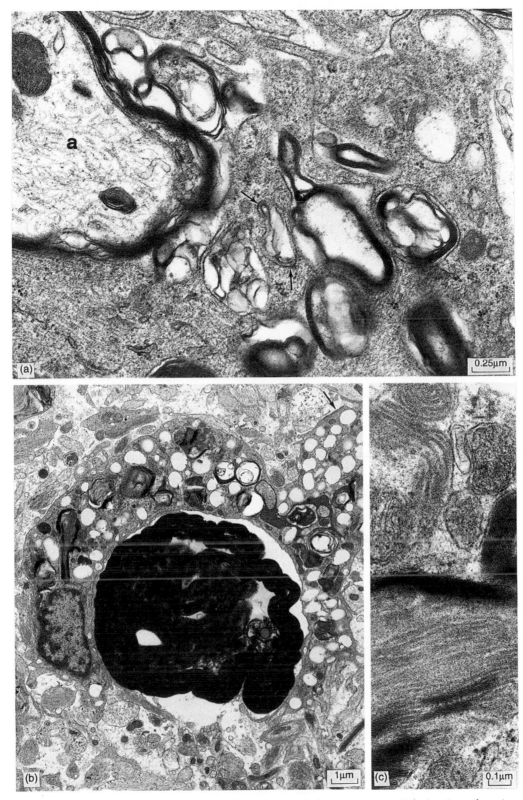

Figure 15.11 (*a*) A myelinated nerve fibre, axon (**a**) (*upper left*) in a chronic active MS lesion is undergoing demyelination following its encompassment by processes from a microglial cell. Myelin is being lysed from the outer layers and the droplets, some attached to coated pits on the invaginated cell surface (*arrows*), are being internalized into phagosomes. (*b*) A foamy macrophage (? reactive microglial cell) is seen in a chronic, active lesion. The cell nucleus lies to the left. A large droplet of myelin debris is almost engorged by the cell and throughout the cytoplasm myelin exists at various stages of degradation. The clear rounded profiles are lipid droplets. A region of thickened plasmalemma is seen to the upper right (*small arrow*). The twig-like denser profiles to the lower right are processes from fibrous astrocytes. (*c*) Detail of the inclusion above the nucleus in (*a*). A late stage in myelin degradation is seen. Stacks of electron dense lamellae are apparently undergoing transformation into the less dense lamellar arrays which are seen as stacked or coiled aggregates. These inclusions are characteristic of CNS myelin breakdown but are not specific for MS.

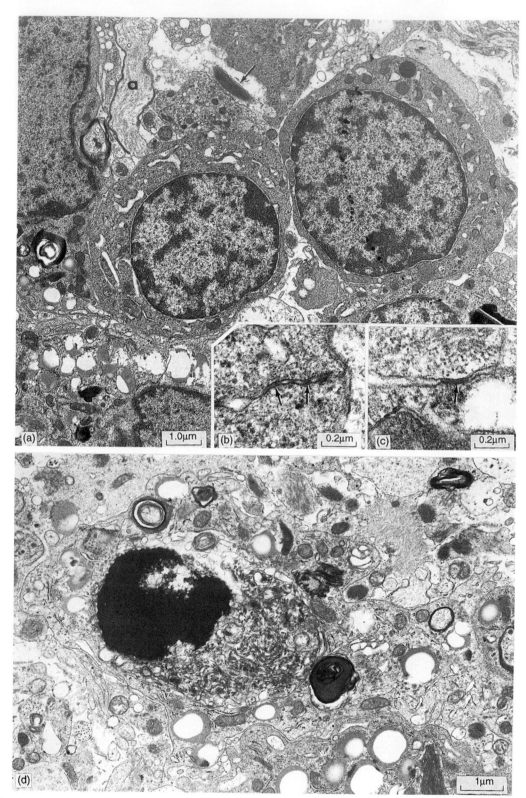

Figure 15.12   (*a*) Two oligodendrocytes reside in an area of myelin breakdown within a chronic active MS lesion. A segment of thin remyelination along an axon (**a**) and a fibrous process from a scarring astrocyte (*arrow*) are shown. A demyelinated axon is closely applied to the oligodendrocyte on the right and an astrocyte lies to the upper left. (*b*) This inset shows the existence of gap junctions (*arrows*) between adjacent oligodendrocytes within the same chronic active MS lesion. (*c*) Another example of a gap junction (*arrow*) between an oligodendrocyte (*below*) and a fibrous astrocyte (*above*), also within a chronic active MS lesion. (*d*) A cell believed to be an oligodendrocyte is undergoing apoptosis within a lesion from a case of acute MS. This is a rare appearance.

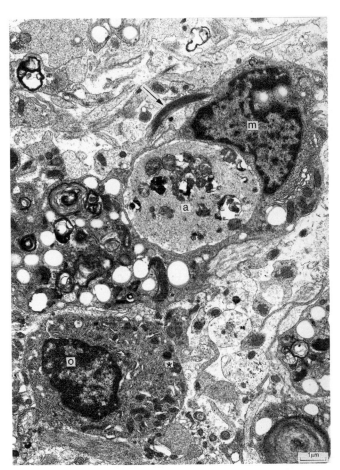

Figure 15.13 (a) Within a zone of ongoing demyelination in a chronic active MS lesion sampled at biopsy, a dystrophic, degenerating demyelinated axon (a) contains accumulations of mitochondria and dense bodies and is surrounded by a reactive microglial cell (m) filled with myelin debris, lipid droplets and lamellar inclusions (Figure 15.11c). Myelin debris is scattered throughout the field and a surviving oligodendrocyte (o) lies to the lower left – note the microtubules at (*). The lesion is fresh and oedematous but evidence of previous activity exists in the form of scarring astroglial processes (arrow).

Moving deeper into the active lesion, scattered oligodendrocytes can be found, sometimes arranged in nests or rows[37]. Taken in concert, these observations support the concept of oligodendroglial proliferation occurring concomitantly with and perhaps in response to myelin destruction[37, 39, 41, 42, 45].

The sequence of pathologic events in the chronic active MS lesion suggests that myelin loss precedes oligodendroglial cell depletion. Although an occasional apoptotic oligodendrocyte is seen[39] (Figure 15.12d), there is no evidence for widespread, primary oligodendrocyte damage, the demise of the cell probably being protracted and insidious. Attempts to document serologic evidence for oligodendroglial involvement have not been met with much support and immunocytochemical studies have shown them not to express

MHC class II[100]. The latter observation rules out oligodendroglia as antigen-presenting cells. The documentation of TCRγ/δ T cells colocalizing with oligodendrocytes expressing heat shock protein 65 (HSP 65) in chronic active MS, lesions[101, 102], raises the intriguing possibility that oligodendrocyte depletion might occur as a later event in MS, the result perhaps of a γ/δ T cell response to HSP 65 (Chapter 9). In addition, the documented association of proliferated oligodendrocytes with hypertrophic astrocytes in demyelinated active lesions[44, 45] may also bespeak oligodendroglial phagocytosis secondary to myelin loss.

Despite a fairly complete pathologic montage of the CNS changes in MS at the ultrastructural level, several nagging, fundamental questions remain. Among these, the roles of cytokines and adhesion molecules on infiltrating cells and CNS endothelium continue to provide the focus of much attention, in addition, of course, to the search for putative aetiologic factor(s). Since several chronic inflammatory conditions have recently been shown to be associated with the expression of lymphoid molecules within the target organ, e.g. the synovium in rheumatoid arthritis[103], a search for high endothelial venule (HEV) markers or other vascular adhesion molecules in the CNS was undertaken in MS[86, 104, 105]. To date, we have been unable to document an adhesion molecule profile specific for MS. The presence of lymphatics and lymphoid tissue within the CNS of MS patients[100] might suggest selective lymphoid trafficking within the CNS. Interestingly, some chronic relapsing EAE models have also revealed collections of organized lymphoid elements (see Figure 15.24) and blood vessels with the features of HEV within the CNS[92, 93, 107], additional features perhaps linking the animal model to MS.

15.2.4   REMYELINATION IN MS

Remyelination as a phenomenon

Loss of myelin from the CNS is no longer considered an inexorable lesion and many studies over the past two decades have convincingly documented CNS remyelination after a variety of insults[58]. Since the first reports on remyelination in MS[35, 108], the phenomenon has been recognized as a feature of both acute and chronic MS lesions. As stated above, remyelination in acute and chronic active MS is associated with oligodendroglial cell proliferation. It occurs typically at the edge of chronic damage and is characterized by the presence of nerve fibres with myelin sheaths disproportionately thin for the diameter of the axon (Figure 15.12a, 15.14–15.16). Remyelination in MS has been documented in detail by Prineas and

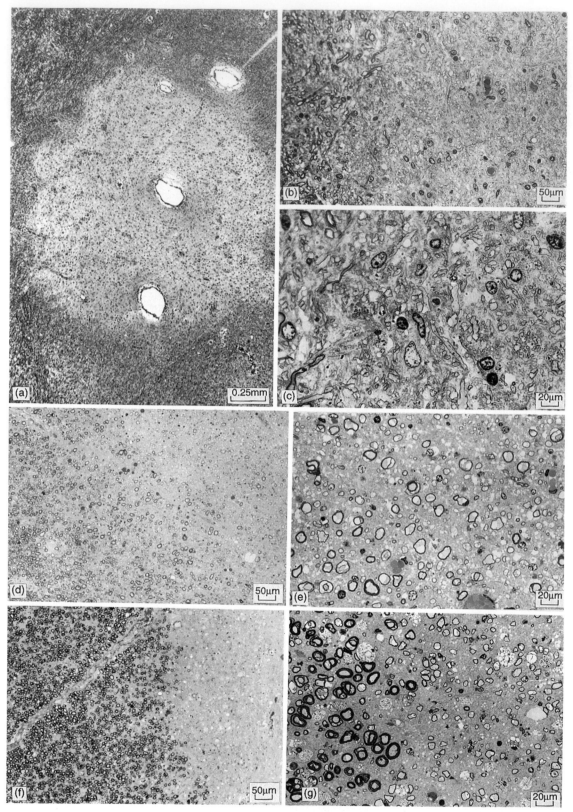

Figure 15.14 (*a*) A remyelinated shadow plaque from a cerebral hemisphere is shown. Note the pale staining for myelin and lack of inflammatory cells. The lesion is hypercellular, probably the result of oligodendroglial hyperplasia. (Paraffin section; Luxol fast blue.) (*b*) The edge of a small shadow plaque (normal white matter to the left) is presented from the centrum semiovale of a case of chronic progressive MS. Thinly remyelinated fibres, a lack of inflammatory activity and glial hyperplasia are apparent in the lesion area. (One micron epoxy section; toluidine blue stain.) (*c*) Detail from the area shown in (*b*), to show the abundance of thinly remyelinated axons. A few unaffected fibres with myelin sheaths of normal thickness are seen to the left. Some oligodendroglial hyperplasia (small, round dense nuclei) is apparent. (*d*) The perimeter of a shadow plaque is shown

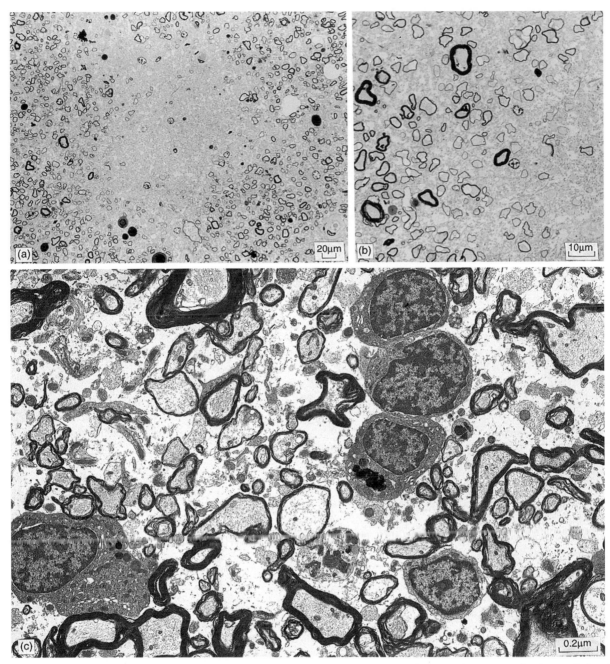

Figure 15.15 (*a*) A small, incompletely remyelinated lesion from the ventro-medial gracile tract at the base of the dorsal columns at T10 presents with an intensely gliotic, demyelinated centre, a rim of remyelination and numerous corpora amylacea (round, dense bodies). (One micron section; toluidine blue stain.) (*b*) At higher magnification, the uniformly thinly remyelinated fibres depicted in (*a*) can be clearly distinguished from fibres with normal myelin thickness. (*c*) EM of a remyelinated lesion in a cerebral hemisphere (biopsy sample) shows thinly remyelinated nerve fibres, fibres with normal myelin sheath thickness, oligodendroglial hyperplasia, extracellular oedema and some fibrous astrogliosis.

Figure 15.14 (*cont.*) within the dorsal column of the spinal cord at L4. More normally myelinated white matter lies to the left; the remyelinated lesion to the right. Similar preparation to (*b*). (*e*) Higher magnification from (*d*). Note the extensive remyelination with myelin sheaths barely half as thick as would have been predicted for axons of these dimensions. Some nerve fibre attrition has probably occurred. (*f*) The perimeter of another lesion in a lumbar dorsal column from a case of chronic progressive MS. Normal white matter is seen to the left and the lesion area to the right is vacuolated. Similar preparation to (*b*). (*g*) Detail from (*f*) to show the normal myelin thickness of unaffected fibres on the left and many remyelinated fibres to the right. Ongoing disease activity is apparent by the presence of many foamy macrophages but lymphocytic infiltration is not a feature.

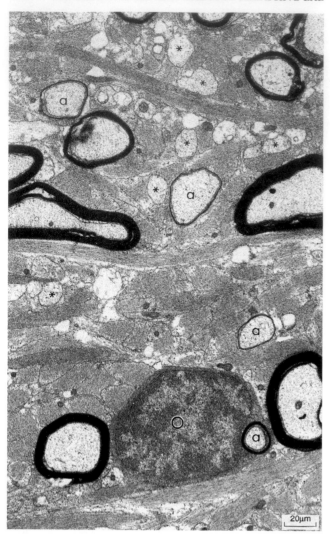

Figure 15.16   Thinly remyelinated nerve fibres (**a**) intermixed with normally myelinated fibres are shown by EM at the periphery of a chronic silent MS plaque. Densely packed processes from fibrotic astroglial cells separate the nerve fibres. One remyelinated fibre is intimately associated with an oligodendroglial cell (**O**). Demyelinated axons (*) can also be seen. (Courtesy of Dr John Prineas. Reproduced from Prineas and Connell, 1978 [80], with permission.)

Connell [109]. In addition to thin myelin, remyelination is associated with attenuation of the myelin sheath, short myelin internodes and aberrant collections of loops of oligodendroglial cell cytoplasm along the length of the axon. That these thin myelin sheaths represent incomplete demyelination is ruled out in most cases by the absence of a prominent macrophage component, a paucity of myelin debris and the occasional attachment of the myelin sheath to oligodendrocytes. Abrupt internodal attenuation of myelin lamellae and uncompacted, isolated loops of oligodendroglial cytoplasm to naked axons further attest to the phenomenon being reparative.

Remyelinated lesions

In addition to their being encountered around the margins of chronic plaques and as islands within active lesions, remyelinated CNS fibres also occur in well-demarcated plaque areas which have been able to remyelinate extensively, possibly after the cessation of a single inflammatory event. These areas correspond to what histologists have traditionally termed 'shadow plaques', a name assigned to discrete areas of myelin pallor situated satellitic to chronic lesions, probably representative of single-hit lesions [46] (Chapter 9) Figure 15.14*a*). This myelin pallor is now believed to be due to the reduced density of myelination (remyelination). Within shadow plaques, myelin sheaths are thin and there is hypercellularity, some of it related to oligodendrocyte hyperplasia (Figures 15.14*b*, *c*, 15.15*c*). Fibrous astrogliosis is usually in evidence. Ultrastructurally, the supernumerary oligodendrocytes display minute gap junctional complexes between one another and between adjacent astroglial elements (Figures 15.12*b* and *c*), perhaps indicative of electrophysiological potential.

In the typical demyelinated plaque, the amount of remyelination encountered is relatively small and probably insignificant at the clinical level. The common failure of deeper areas of such plaques to acquire new myelin is probably related to factors like an inability of oligodendrocytes to penetrate deeper sclerotic demyelinated areas, a gradual decrease in the number of naked axons with time post-demyelination, an unfavourable environment for regeneration in general, and a near absence of oligodendrocytes subsequent to long-term demyelination. Prineas *et al.* [41], in a report confirming oligodendroglial cell proliferation at the edge of active MS lesions [37], raised the interesting possibility that the eventual failure of remyelination might be due to an inappropriate prolonged expression of an early differentiation molecule, HNK-1. A similar study on acute MS by Lee and Raine [100] showed proliferated oligodendrocytes in lesion areas to stain positively for myelin associated glycoprotein (MAG), a myelin component belonging to the immunoglobulin supergene family and another marker of immature oligodendrocytes. In the latter case, it was felt that the expression of MAG was a feature of recent cell derivation rather than persistent expression of the molecule. More recently, oligodendrocytes expressing an MBP isoform present normally only during myelination and involving exon 2 of the MBP gene, have been localized to the perimeter of chronic MS lesions [110]. The presence of MBP exon 2 peptide expression on oligodendrocytes provides the most convincing evidence to date that some oligodendrocytes at the edge of the MS lesion are of recent derivation. Finally, the above-mentioned concept of oligodendrocyte depletion in MS being a later event, related perhaps to their expressing HSP and being colocalized with TCRγ/δ T cells [101, 102], cells which are known to respond in a cytolytic fashion to HSP, affords interesting new avenues still under investigation [111].

Spinal cord lesions in MS are known to display invasion and myelination by Schwann cells [112] (see Figure 15.5c) presumably the result of Schwann cells entering the demyelinated CNS via root entry zones and along the Virchow–Robin spaces of vessels penetrating from the meninges [113]. The PNS is generally spared in MS, although some myelin pathology has been noted [58]. It is unlikely that these PNS changes are related to MS *per se* and probably represent secondary phenomena, perhaps due to nutritional deficits, chronic disability or proximity to large spinal cord lesions.

The permanence of CNS remyelination

Shadow plaques (Figures 15.14a–e) are traditionally presented as areas of quiescence and stability in which, with the cessation of inflammatory activity, the defect in the blood–brain barrier is apparently healed, the demyelinated fibres remyelinated and the regenerated myelin rendered less vulnerable to recurrent disease. However, examination of many shadow plaques reveals that remyelinated areas are equally prone to later demyelination, as are previously unaffected myelinated areas. Evidence for this comes from the observation of shadow plaques that have been subjected to a later wave of inflammatory attack (Figures 15.14f, g, 15.17). The net effect is that the zone of remyelination is once more infiltrated with foamy, class II MHC$^+$ macrophages (Figure 15.17d, e) filled with myelin debris and free lipid (Figures 15.14f, g, 15.17). Shadow plaques both in the cerebral hemispheres and the spinal cord have been seen to come under attack in this manner (Figures 15.14, 15.17). Prineas et al. [73] have described successive episodes of demyelination and remyelination in MS, in much the same manner as has been reported in Balo's concentric sclerosis [114].

Thus, it appears that the restoration of myelin to a demyelinated plaque does not confer upon the tissue an assurance of permanent repair and that later bouts of inflammation are capable of reducing the repaired lesion to a demyelinated state. In retrospect, this is not surprising since evidence exists from the literature that the remyelination and oligodendroglial cell proliferation in acute and chronic active MS lesions are probably transient and that as the lesion expands, these regenerative events are consumed by the relentless inflammatory activity and the scarring process.

15.3 Chronic relapsing experimental allergic encephalomyelitis

15.3.1 THE NEED FOR A CHRONIC MODEL

In the absence of a spontaneous animal analogue, investigators were compelled to develop an ideal laboratory model for MS research. As tools in this regard, immunological, virological, toxic and traumatic parameters were extensively explored. Many of the resultant models simulated in one way or another isolated features of the MS lesion but not one truly encapsulated the entire clinical or pathologic picture of the human disease. The relapsing nature of MS was particularly elusive since most models were monophasic and acute. The model of chronic (relapsing) EAE developed in strain 13 guinea pigs [3, 4, 53] was for many years the best animal model. It had an immunological basis, large CNS lesions, a relapsing clinical course and a low mortality – features highly reminiscent of MS. Today, most work on chronic relapsing EAE involves other more readily available species (mice and rats), that can be applied on a large scale to research into the human disease process. The yet-to-be-explored model of chronic relapsing EAE in the marmoset [115] might provide immunopathologists and clinicians opportunities to examine the disease course with human-related technologies, e.g. MRI. Despite several dissimilarities between the various models and MS (e.g. the need for subcutaneous or intravenous injection of lymphocytes or sensitization against CNS antigens, a more subacute course, lesions never acquiring the dimensions and age of MS lesions), the following paragraphs will show that the various immune-mediated demyelinating models, though not perfect, have much in common with the situation in MS and that they do indeed provide valid tools for the testing of immune-related protocols designed to reduce the CNS inflammation and perhaps enhance repair.

The model of chronic relapsing EAE in strain 13 guinea pigs involves a single subcutaneous sensitization of juveniles in the nuchal region with syngeneic spinal cord tissue in complete Freund's adjuvant (CFA). The ensuing disease usually has a latent period of 1–2 months after this single sensitization, during which subclinical CNS lesions develop before overt signs are manifest [70]. In recent years we have found that this latent period has decreased to 2–3 weeks, a period similar to that associated with the acute form of the disease induced in adults, and that there is some mortality. Clinical signs consist of weight loss, incontinence and paraparesis, sometimes progressing to quadriparesis. These events are rarely fatal and remit to varying degrees, after which relapses occur, as in MS, at irregular intervals over periods of more than three years. Throughout this chronic disease sampling of blood is possible, as is lymph node biopsy and CSF sampling

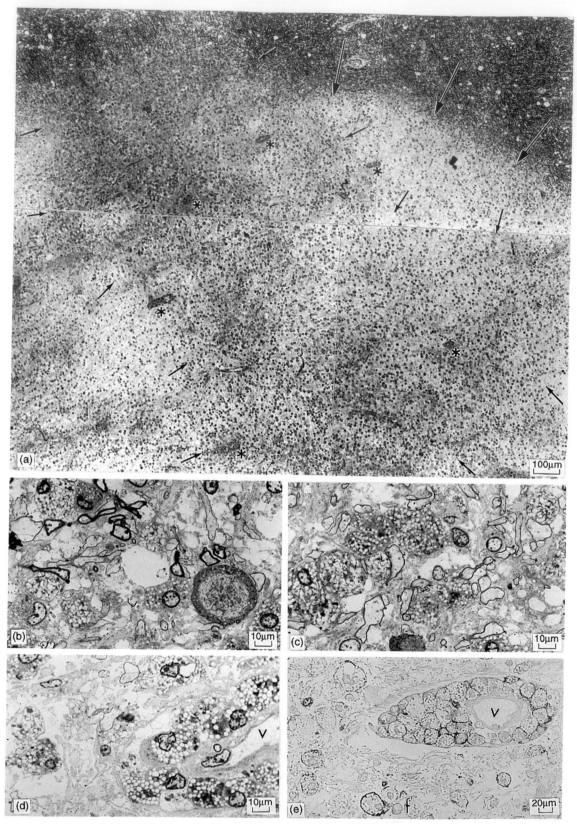

Figure 15.17 (*a*) A montage of the edge of a chronic silent MS lesion (*large arrows*) shows an area of myelin pallor (a shadow plaque, *small arrows*) extending into the main lesion. The shadow plaque contains many perivascular cuffs of infiltrating cells (*) and an overall hypercellularity. (One micron epoxy section; toluidine blue stain. (*b*) At the perimeter of the above shadow plaque, both normal and remyelinated nerve fibres can be seen. More significant is the evidence of recent disease revealed by the presence of foamy macrophages and the large axonal spheroid (*lower right*). (*c*) Deeper into the same shadow plaque, a mixture of remyelinated fibres and foamy macrophages is immediately apparent – evidence of a recurrence of disease activity after remyelination has occurred. An axonal spheroid lies below (*centre*). (*d*) Even deeper, parenchymal and perivascular macrophages with myelin debris and lipid droplets occur in greater numbers and remyelinated fibres are sparse. The vessel lumen is shown at (**v**). (*e*) An epoxy section shows reactivity for class II MHC on the foamy macrophages. Vessel lumen at (**v**). Note the overall absence of infiltrating lymphocytes.

and, ultimately, fresh CNS tissue is available for multidisciplinary study. A similar form of chronic EAE in outbred guinea pigs was later reported by Wisniewski and Keith [116] and Lassmann [59]. Attempts to induce chronic relapsing EAE with MBP (as opposed to whole CNS tissue) have been unsuccessful and have resulted in an acute syndrome which heals and does not relapse. Equally unsuccessful have been attempts to induce chronic disease in strain 13 guinea pigs using adoptive transfer technology. In these experiments, irrespective of whether donor lymphocytes were derived from CNS antigen-sensitized juveniles (for chronic relapsing EAE) or adults (for acute EAE), the outcome was invariably an acute form of EAE [117].

The majority of studies on autoimmune demyelination in recent years have employed rodent species, particularly the mouse. The first ultrastructural studies on mouse EAE, as in most other species, began with an examination of the acute disease induced by active sensitization with an emulsion of whole CNS tissue in adjuvant in combination with booster injections of pertussis vaccine. Ten mouse strains with different H-2 backgrounds were tested. Among these, EAE-susceptible and non-susceptible strains were included [5]. While demyelination was a constant (albeit minor) feature of the acute EAE lesion in the mouse, the inflammatory component was invariably more severe than in the strain 13 guinea pig model and consisted of polymorphonuclear leucocytes (PMNs), fibrin and some haemorrhage. In addition, there was invariably a degenerative component manifested by axonal loss, particularly in subpial zones. Work on EAE in the mouse then turned towards the development of more chronic forms, and in 1981 Brown and McFarlin [7] reported a new model induced in the EAE-susceptible SJL/J mouse (H-2^s) with a protocol involving multiple (usually two or three) subcutaneous sensitizations with whole CNS tissue in adjuvant administered at weekly intervals, after which animals developed a chronic relapsing disease. The neuropathology of this model [9] showed some loss of axons in most lesions, a severe inflammatory response, primary demyelination and remyelination and some sparing of oligodendrocytes. Immunocytochemistry of both the acute and chronic relapsing forms of actively induced EAE in the mouse implicated early expression of class II MHC prior to lesion formation and a predominance of CD4$^+$ (helper) T cells in lesion pathogenesis [33]. A similar actively induced mouse model was reported by Lublin et al. [8] but never subjected to detailed neuropathologic scrutiny.

Regarding similarities to MS, the above murine models left much to be desired in terms of lesion size, topography and degree of axonal sparing. In 1984, Mokhtarian et al. [10] reported on a form of chronic relapsing EAE in the female SJL mouse using adoptive (passive) transfer technology. This model was a modification of the earlier protocol of Pettinelli and McFarlin [118]. Females were selected because they are more susceptible to EAE than males [118a]. The protocol involved the injection into the tail vein of a naive animal of lymph node cells, from syngeneic MBP-injected donors, which had been maintained in vitro for 3–4 days in the presence of MBP. This resulted in recipient mice developing an acute disease 7–10 days post-transfer, a disease from which they recovered. Over the following several months multiple relapses were observed. The ultrastructural neuropathology of this model [92] revealed a picture more fitting a model of primary demyelination (but still with a heavy PMN component in the infiltrates and some vascular damage) and remyelination during remissions. A somewhat similar model was reported later by Lublin [119] but appears not to have been developed or applied. Since donor cells for recipients developing chronic relapsing EAE in our model were derived from mice actively sensitized with MBP in CFA that never got sick, and since MBP does not produce chronic relapsing EAE in the guinea pig, we decided to investigate whether MBP might produce a chronic disease in mice. With many animals tested at different dose levels (100–800 µg MBP), it was found that instead of a demyelinating condition, a chronic relapsing necrotizing encephalomyelitis resulted [120]. Although this condition had a demyelinative component to the lesions, the parenchymal damage was such that it rendered comparison with typical MS lesions difficult. Interestingly, the induction of mouse EAE typically requires a much higher dose of MBP (150 µg) to induce disease than in the guinea pig (50–75 µg), despite the differences in animal size.

As mouse models of EAE became more refined, so did the method of inducing the disease. With long-term cultured T cell lines activated with MBP in vitro, Sakai et al. [121] showed not only that chronic relapsing EAE could be produced in SJL mice, but also that there occurred prolonged up-regulation of class II MHC (Ia) expression on endothelial and infiltrating cells within lesions and this increased during relapses. T cell line-induced chronic relapsing EAE was later extended to work on MBP$^+$ T cell clones and elegantly elaborated upon at the ultrastructural level [11]. The findings complemented in large part those of earlier works [10]. It was found that although there was severe decrease in the numbers of axons in lesions, demyelination was invariably prominent and was especially marked when 'recipient' mice were (a) given whole body X-irradiation, (b) MHC II compatible strains, or (c) congenitally athymic. Although the brunt of the neuropathology of murine chronic EAE has been performed on the SJL/J (H-2^s) strain, other EAE-susceptible haplotypes have provided a number of immunogenetic pointers in the search for the morphologic basis of genetic susceptibility. Among these, the PL/J strain (H-2^u), a strain developing EAE in response to an epitope of the MBP molecule different from that responsible for the disease in the SJL/J strain (H-2^s), has been helpful [93]. While the pathology was very similar except for subtle differences in the degree of demyelination and remyelination, this study had the unusual wrinkle in that lesions related to an unexpected intercurrent viral infection could be distinguished. Thus, it was possible in the same animal to observe lesions due to an immune and an infectious aetiology. In addition, serologic and structural evidence for the virus (mouse hepatitis virus) was detectable. Subsequent studies showed that MBP epitope-specific T cell lines could be used to induce chronic relapsing EAE [122], this work focusing attention upon the need for T cell recognition of haplotype-specific antigenic epitopes for successful disease induction and the phenomenon of epitope spreading during the course of the disease. In all the above mouse models, the pattern of myelin pathology was similar.

The above examples of chronic relapsing EAE were all predicated upon MBP being the major encephalitogen. An observation extending as far back as the early 1950s (e.g. Waksman et al. in 1954 [123]) has been that other protein components of the myelin sheath, most notably proteolipid protein (PLP, the major protein of myelin), might also be encephalitogenic. It has been relatively recently that this has been confirmed. PLP-induced chronic relapsing EAE has now been studied in the guinea pig [124] and in the Lewis rat [125]. This was then confirmed in the BALB/c mouse (a strain with the H-2^k haplotype, normally resistant to EAE induced by MBP) by Endoh et al. [126] and Trotter et al. [127]. Endoh et al. [126] also demonstrated that the 20 kD protein component of PLP, DM20, was also encephalitogenic. The ultrastructural features of the condition in euthymic and athymic mice reconstituted with T cells were similar to models reported above after MBP sensitization. The strategy was then repeated using T cell lines to PLP in SJL mice [128]. Most animals developed acute EAE but a small percentage went on to display relapses. This model was not entirely compatible with the MBP-induced T cell models since priming injections of pertussis vaccine and low dose irradiation were needed to optimize the effects of the T cell lines. Nevertheless, a typical inflammatory demyelinating condition did ensue. In the past 5 years or so we have seen the EAE technology applied to transgenic models in which the effects of different class II MHC gene products on the expression of disease were examined [129], and where mice constructed to express T cell receptors specific for MBP [56, 57] have been claimed to develop EAE either spontaneously or after challenge with pertussis alone.

Among the remaining models of chronic relapsing EAE is a model reported by Lassmann et al. [6] in the Lewis rat. This involved active sensitization with CNS tissue and a disease duration of 4–5 months. A second rat model by Stanley and Pender [130] combined active sensitization with low dose cyclosporin A administration and has been applied in pathophysiological studies. Another model was reported by Tsukada et al. [131] in the guinea pig, using as the encephalitogen purified preparations of cerebral endothelial cell membrane. More recently, two models induced in mice by sensitization with myelin oligodendrocyte glycoprotein (MOG) have been reported [132, 133].

The above increasing collection of models of chronic relapsing EAE serves to document at least five separate trends in the field which have occurred over the past 10 years: first, admittedly perhaps at the expense of a poorer comparison with MS, a move from guinea pig to murine models, a move necessitated by the demand for precise immunologic analysis; secondly, the increased application of adoptive transfer technology and antigen-specific T cells; thirdly, the clear demonstration that MBP is a complex antigen with different epitopes recognized by different TCRs depending upon the genetic make-up of the recipient; fourthly, that other myelin antigens, particularly PLP and MOG, are also encephalitogenic and capable of inducing chronic disease; and fifthly, that with the advent of transgenic and gene depletion (knockout) technologies, we are close to understanding the role

Figure 15.18 (a) Strain 13 guinea pig; chronic relapsing EAE, 20 weeks post-inoculation with whole spinal cord/CFA; one relapse; gross specimen. Note the multiple demyelinated plaques visible along the pial surface of this stretch of lower thoracic/lumbar spinal cord. The plaques are totally disseminated, as is the case in MS (Chapter 9). (b) Paraffin section of thoracic spinal cord from a specimen similar to that in (a) reveals the presence of multiple demyelinated lesions, particularly a large one in the right anterior column. (c) A paraffin section from the brain of another guinea pig sensitized for chronic relapsing EAE 16 weeks earlier, is stained with H&E. Note the large area of inflammation to the right of the ventricle. The hippocampal fibrium hangs into the ventricle and the anterior thalamus is to the left. (d) An adjacent section to (c) is stained with Sudan black for myelin. Note the large demyelinated plaque to the right of the ventricle and the association between areas of demyelination and perivascular infiltrates. (e) A One micron epoxy section from the lumbar spinal cord of a guinea pig sampled during a relapse 5 months post-sensitization, reveals a large demyelinated plaque extending from the anterior to the lateral columns on the right. Perivascular infiltrates are evident along the margins of the lesion, suggestive of recent activity. (f) Higher magnification from (e) shows the extent of demyelination, perivascular cuffs of infiltrating cells and extensive infiltration within the subarachnoid space. (g) A slightly more detailed image from a smaller subpial lesion from an animal with chronic relapsing EAE sampled 18 weeks post-inoculation and 4 weeks after the onset of signs, shows the masses of preserved, demyelinated axons with intervening fibrous astrocytes, the presence of infiltrating cells around some vessels and within the subarachnoid space, and macrophages containing myelin debris.

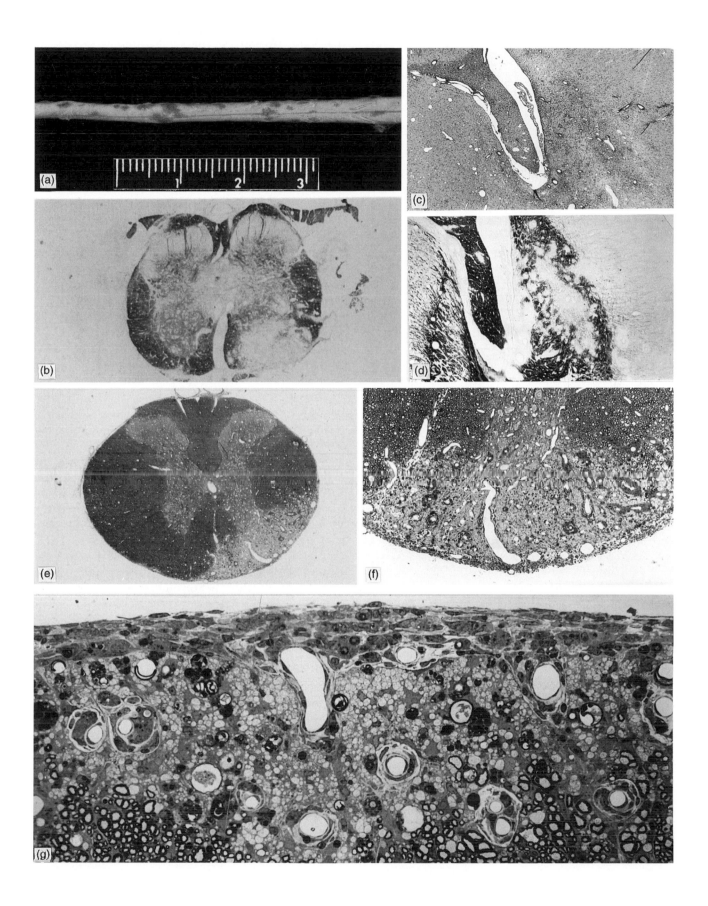

of different immune system molecules in this autoimmune demyelinating condition.

The following paragraphs will delineate where possible the morphologic similarities between these various chronic relapsing models and will compare the picture with that of MS, laid down in the preceding pages. Finally, some applications of these models will be mentioned, particularly as they pertain to the therapy of MS.

15.3.2 LESION TOPOGRAPHY IN COMPARISON TO MS

From the histopathological standpoint, chronic relapsing EAE in the guinea pig resembles MS in many respects (Figure 15.18). In the strain 13 guinea pig model, the CNS disease is most evident in the cerebral and spinal cord white matter in gross specimens (Figure 15.18a). With myelin stains, large foci of demyelination are seen histologically, sometimes extending as a subpial rim (Figures 15.18b, e). Less frequently, large demyelinated plaques are encountered in the deeper white matter, beneath unaffected subpial zones. Lesions in the cerebral hemispheres are equally disseminated and most pronounced in periventricular areas (Figure 15.18b, c). Brain lesions are most common in severely affected animals examined 2–4 months post-inoculation. The brains of less afflicted or more chronic animals display smaller areas of demyelination or shadow (remyelinated) plaques. Invariably, optic nerves are affected in chronic relapsing EAE [134], but unlike the spinal cord (see below), optic nerve lesions rarely reflect relapses and tend to be monophasic. Lesions occur in the PNS in chronic relapsing EAE in guinea pigs, more so than in MS, with involvement heaviest in the proximal (intradural) regions of the spinal nerve roots. There is equal involvement of anterior and posterior roots and dorsal root ganglia are often severely affected. As has been noted previously in chronic EAE in the rabbit [135, 136], PNS fibres remyelinate rapidly and completely, unlike CNS fibres which remyelinate slowly or remain chronically demyelinated.

The topography of lesions in the actively and passively induced mouse models is similar but the lesions are less extensive than in the guinea pig (Figures 15.19a, b). Optic nerves are invariably affected, cerebral white matter lesions are small and involve thin paraventricular zones only, spinal cord lesions are most common in distal segments and are strictly subpial and narrow (Figures 15.19a, b), with some predilection for root entry zones, and there is little or no involvement of the PNS. In the mouse, chronic relapsing EAE is essentially a spinal cord disease, particularly evident at lumbosacral levels. This holds true irrespective of the mode of induction and single sensitization with a crude CNS antigenic emulsion or intravenous injection of an MBP-specific T cell line will both cause a severe disease

mainly of the lower spinal cord. Spinal nerve roots are rarely affected but lesions are seen in dorsal root ganglia. In size and topography, murine EAE lesions compare poorly with typical MS plaques because of their limited extent and subpial distribution but they do retain primary demyelination and remyelination as major features, particularly the adoptively transferred forms (Figures 15.19d, e).

15.3.3 THE ESTABLISHED LESION OF CHRONIC EAE

The typical chronic EAE lesion in the strain 13 guinea pig model (Figures 15.18e, f) is well demarcated from adjacent less affected white matter and not infrequently displays a moderate amount of ongoing inflammation about its margins. The center of the lesion is usually a mosaic of well-preserved naked axons among an increased number of blood vessels with enlarged Virchow–Robin spaces. These perivascular compartments contain fibroblasts, collagen deposits and macrophages (Figure 15.18g). The overlying meninges are usually severely fibrotic, adherent and often attached to the pial surface by glial bridges [113, 137]. Demyelinated fibres are numerous and display a decrease in axonal diameter, a phenomenon also noted in the PNS subsequent to demyelination [135]. There is probably more axonal sparing in the guinea pig model than in MS and much more than that encountered in the mouse models. Ongoing myelin breakdown is manifested by parenchymal and perivascular mononuclear cells containing recognizable myelin debris, most apparent at the margins of lesions (Figures 15.19a, b, 15.20b). These mononuclear cells are the major inflammatory component in old lesions. Plasma cells are common but small lymphocytes are inconspicuous. In the guinea pig, a few PMNs are seen in early acute lesions but are rare in chronic lesions. The presence of abundant gliosis reaffirms the chronicity of the changes and oligodendroglial sparing is apparent [138]. By EM, silent chronic lesions display the anticipated appearances, described in greater detail previously [46, 53], with naked axons embedded in a matrix of fibrillary astrogliosis (Figure 15.20c). In these areas, demyelinated axons possess axoglial membrane specializations (Figure 15.20c, inset) (see [63, 64]), a phenomenon also seen in MS plaques (Figure 15.4c).

A montage of an established chronic EAE lesion (Figure 15.21a) reveals a fibrous astrogliotic centre, fibrotic blood vessels, many of which display a fenestrated endothelium by EM [139], naked axons and axons with thin myelin sheaths (remyelination) towards the edge of the lesion. The presence of myelin debris and the occasional necrotic cell underscores the smouldering nature of the disease process. Such a lesion is typical in chronic animals and is easily distinguished from an expanding lesion (from a relapsing animal) which has a

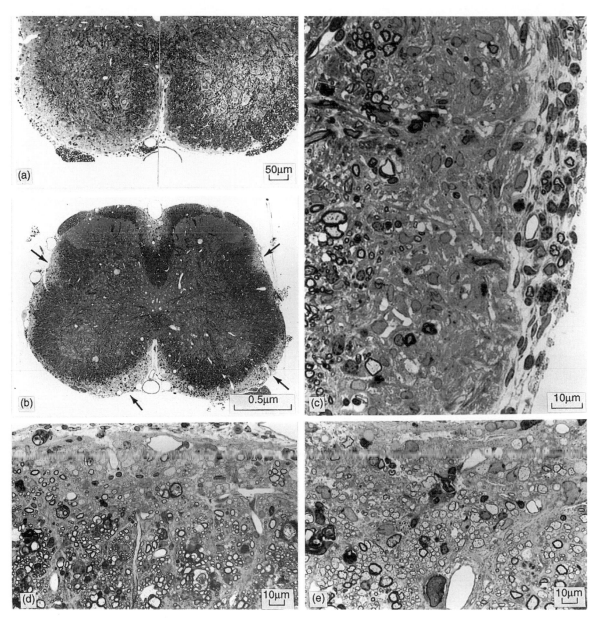

Figure 15.19 (*a*) SJL/J mouse; chronic relapsing EAE, induced by active sensitization with spinal cord tissue; 7 months post-inoculation. A broad zone of subpial demyelination in the lumbar spinal cord involves the anterior and lateral columns, particularly on the left. Inflammatory cells are evident in the subarachnoid space. (One micron epoxy section; toluidine blue.) (*b*) SJL/J mouse; chronic relapsing EAE induced by the adoptive transfer of bulk-isolated, MBP-stimulated lymph node cells; 3 months post-transfer. This section of lumbar spinal cord displays several well demarcated, demyelinated chronic lesions (*arrows*). (*c*) SJL/J mouse; chronic relapsing EAE actively induced by CNS antigen in adjuvant; 7 months post-inoculation. The subpial parenchyma is gliotic and severely depleted of nerve fibres. Some scattered CNS-remyelinated fibres are apparent at the edge of the lesion and heterotopic PNS-myelinated fibres can be seen within the leptomeninges (*right*). (*d*) PL/J mouse; chronic relapsing EAE; 5 months post-transfer of MBP-sensitized lymph node cells. A small subpial lesion from the lumbar spinal cord is shown. Note the many surviving, chronically demyelinated axons in the lesion area and some Wallerian degeneration in the adjacent white matter. (*e*) PL/J mouse; chronic relapsing EAE; adoptive transfer; 9 months post-transfer. Remyelinated axons are seen throughout this subpial lesion. L7 spinal cord.

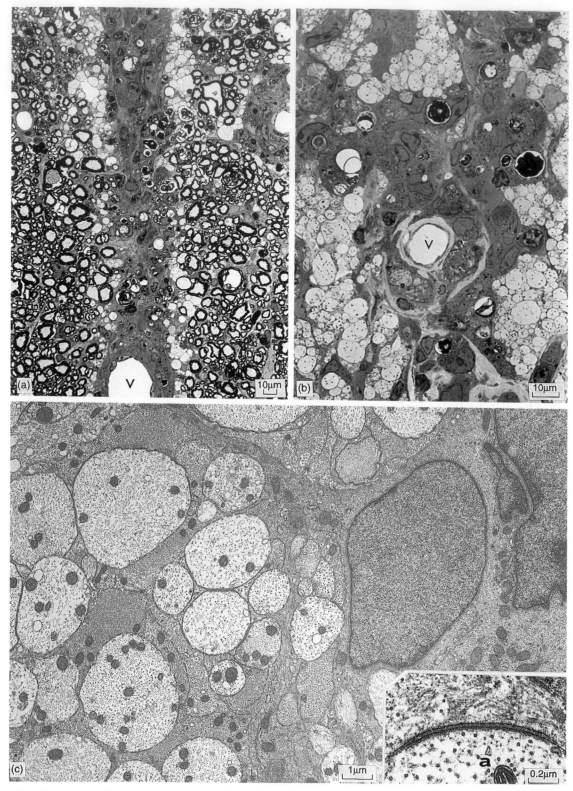

Figure 15.20   (*a*) Strain 13 guinea pig; chronic EAE; 3 months post-sensitization. Within this acute lesion, note the clear association between perivascular inflammation and demyelination. Vessel lumen at (**v**). Macrophages containing undigested myelin debris lie along the rims of demyelination. (*b*) Detail from a spinal cord lesion taken from an animal sampled during a clinical relapse. Perivascular – vessel lumen at (**v**) – and parenchymal inflammation is superimposed upon recently demyelinated areas and macrophages contain myelin debris. (*c*) A typical silent chronic EAE lesion in a strain 13 guinea pig is shown by EM. Note the multinucleated fibrous astrocyte to the right and the gliotic background surrounding the many well-preserved demyelinated axons. *Inset*: an axoglial membrane specialization between an axon (**a**) and an astrocyte (*above*).

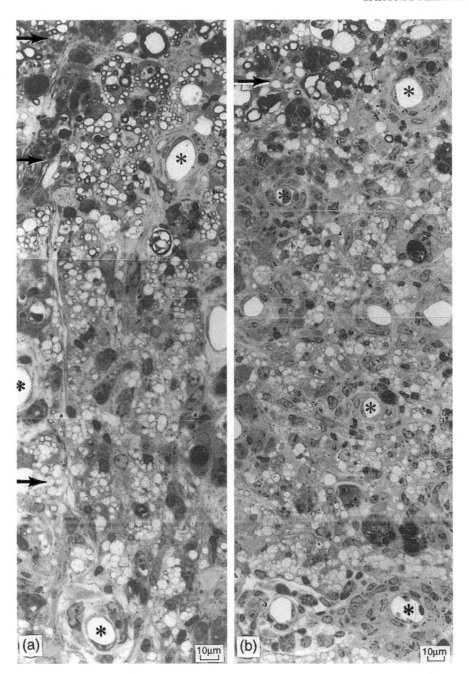

Figure 15.21   (*a*) A montage of a relatively silent EAE plaque in a guinea pig spinal cord extends from the long-term demyelinated centre (*below*) towards more normal white matter (*above*). Note the chronic demyelination and gliosis (*lower arrow*), the rim of remyelination (*middle arrow*) and the more normal white matter (*upper arrow*). Blood vessels (*) display chronic inflammatory changes only, no recent inflammation. (*b*) A montage from an actively demyelinating chronic lesion in the spinal cord of a strain 13 guinea pig, sampled during a relapse. Note how the vessels (*) are surrounded by recent infiltrates, that the parenchyma is more hypercellular, that affected axons are all demyelinated (no remyelination is apparent) and that ongoing myelin breakdown is apparent at the lesion perimeter (*arrow*).

more fleshy texture comprising recent perivascular infiltrates, closely packed, recently demyelinated fibres at the margin (Figure 15.20*b*) and little evidence of remyelination (Figure 15.21*b*).

In the mouse models of chronic relapsing EAE, lesions are intensely gliotic, more depleted of axons and the

extent of demyelination is less spectacular. Lesions from mice in which the disease was induced by active sensitization with CNS emulsions are more destructive, less demyelinative and less widespread (Figure 15.19*b*) than those occurring in the spinal cords of mice in which the disease was adoptively transferred with MBP-

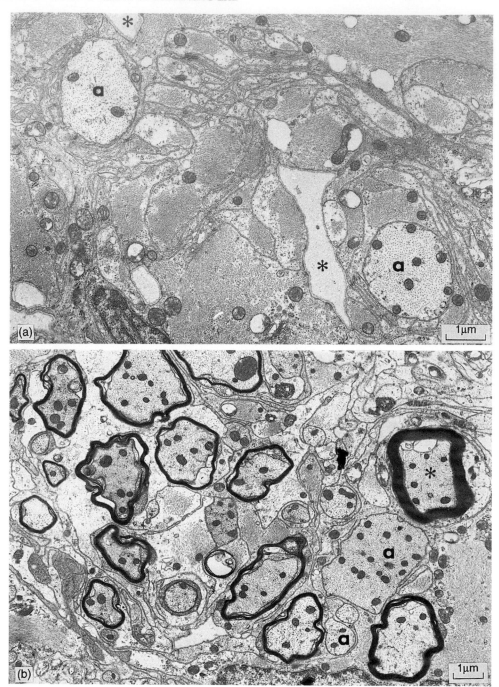

Figure 15.22   (*a*) SJL/J mouse; chronic relapsing EAE; actively induced by CNS antigen; 7 months post-inoculation. By EM, an intensely gliotic subpial CNS parenchyma, two demyelinated axons (**a**), and infoldings or crypts in the glia limitans (*) covered by basal lamina, are apparent. (*b*) SJL/J mouse; adoptive transfer; 3 months post-transfer. A section from the medulla shows a group of CNS-remyelinated nerve fibres lying to the right of a PNS-myelinated CNS axon (*). Note also the demyelinated axons (**a**).

activated lymph node cells (Figure 15.19*c*, *d*). Ultra-structurally, in the actively induced model, chronic lesions display scattered demyelinated axons in a fibrous astrogliotic background (Figure 15.22*a*), the density suggesting axonal loss. Adoptively transferred murine models invariably show more axonal sparing (Figure 15.19*a*) and a proclivity for old lesions to display remyelination (Figure 15.19*e*), of both of the CNS and PNS type (Figure 15.22*b*), as in MS (Figure 15.5*c*). In addition to nerve fibre depletion, vascular damage, haemorrhage, extracellular fibrin, disruption of normal architecture by infoldings of the glia limitans and an abundance of PMNs (neutrophils and eosino-phils) are not uncommon [9, 92, 93, 122], appearances unusual to the MS lesion. However, these features are less prominent (or in the case of vascular damage, virtually absent) in the adoptively transferred model [10].

Commonly present in many murine forms of EAE is the unusual phenomenon of heterotopic regeneration of PNS fibres into the subarachnoid space overlying the spinal cord. Many of these fibres probably emanate from regenerating sprouts from PNS fibres severed at the root entry zones [140]. The same phenomenon also occurs in the guinea pig model, but to a much lesser extent. Although axonal disease is not a prominent feature of the guinea pig model, long-term animals have been described to display some axonal dystrophy and abortive regeneration [141]. Similar dystrophic axons are common in chronic MS plaques, particularly during recurrent activity.

15.3.4   THE ACTIVE PLAQUE IN CHRONIC EAE

In a manner reminiscent of MS, CNS lesions in the guinea pig model reveal a constellation of active, chronic and reparatory events that complement the clinical picture. Examination of CNS lesions sampled during relapsing clinical disease will show large foci of chronic demyelination upon which intense inflammation by large mononuclear cells has been superimposed [142]. Inflammatory changes also occur around marginal areas of chronic lesions where ongoing myelin damage once more becomes a major feature [Figure 15.21b]. Close packing of recently denuded axons predominates in these areas, readily distinguishing this stage of the disease from chronic silent phases [142] and small foci of perivascular cuffs surrounded by recently demyelinated axons [Figure 15.20a].

The intense parenchymal and perivascular infiltration by small lymphocytes in active MS lesions is present but not as pronounced in chronic EAE, being only convincingly observed by immunocytochemistry [46]. Class II MHC expression plays an integral role in these inflammatory events and has been ultrastructurally localized to both endothelial cells and macrophages [143–145]. T cell invasion is more a feature of the early stages of acute EAE. In these areas of recurrent activity in the guinea pig, there is an abundance of plasma cells. PMNs are not prominent. Smaller active lesions in chronic animals are not entirely dissimilar to regions of demyelination occurring in adult strain 13 guinea pigs sensitized for acute EAE [70] where demyelinated lesions consist of narrow rims of naked axons closely associated with inflammatory foci (Figure 15.20a). The latter, as in MS, comprise small lymphocytes and some macrophages early on which eventually give way to macrophages and plasma cells. In acutely demyelinated lesions, affected axons are tightly packed (Figure 15.20b) since the fibrous astrogliosis typical of the chronic lesion (Figures 15.21a, 15.22) has not yet developed.

The mechanism of myelin breakdown in EAE lesions in strain 13 guinea pigs has been described previously and displays many similarities with MS [53, 70]. This process has been analysed in a number of species by several workers and the various patterns of demyelination form the subject of reviews by Raine [146] and Lampert [52]. The previously described phenomenon of myelin stripping by macrophages [147], myelin vesiculation [70, 148] and receptor-mediated phagocytosis of myelin [53, 90, 91] are the most described patterns of myelin breakdown in EAE. Both cell- and antibody-mediated mechanisms are implicated in this process, as is also the case in the acute MS lesion (see above). Longitudinal study of antibody titres in chronic relapsing EAE have shown fluctuations in anti-glial antibodies which correlate with periods of disease worsening [149]. In addition, antibodies against oligodendroglial antigens have been implicated in the induction of relapses in EAE [150]. With the exception of the latter study, the above descriptions apply to the disease occurring in strain 13 guinea pigs. For the sake of completeness, it should be mentioned that similar lesions are also encountered in strain 2 guinea pigs similarly sensitized. Strain 2 is traditionally EAE-resistant. However, prolonged observation of strain 2 animals sensitized for EAE revealed extensive CNS involvement which did not correlate with the clinical picture [151] in that long-term sensitized animals displayed both chronic silent and chronic active lesions with clear evidence of ongoing myelin breakdown. Obviously in this strain the term 'resistance' as it pertains to CNS pathology needs to be re-examined.

Chronic active lesions in the mouse models are less extensive than those seen in the guinea pig. Nevertheless, the same histopathologic scenario is repeated during lesion expansion, albeit on a smaller scale, whereby fresh waves of infiltrating cells enter new and old lesion areas, demyelination of previously unaffected fibres occurs and lesions expand (Figure 15.23b). As in other species like the rabbit (Figure 15.23a), receptor-mediated phagocytosis of myelin is seen with dissociated myelin droplets becoming attached to clathrin-coated pits on the surface of macrophages (Figures 15.23c–f). Therefore, despite marked topographical and histopathological differences between the mouse and the guinea pig, at the level of myelin breakdown the models are identical. That identical patterns are encountered in MS renders these demyelinating models highly relevant to the study of the human disease. It needs to be emphasized that this pattern of myelin degradation is very rapid and lasts only for 1–2 days after the process has commenced, and in acute EAE it is transient and early.

Chronic active or relapsing activity in the guinea pig model has been assumed by some workers to be related to periodic antigen stimulation by antigen depots persisting at the site of injection. While this may be difficult to

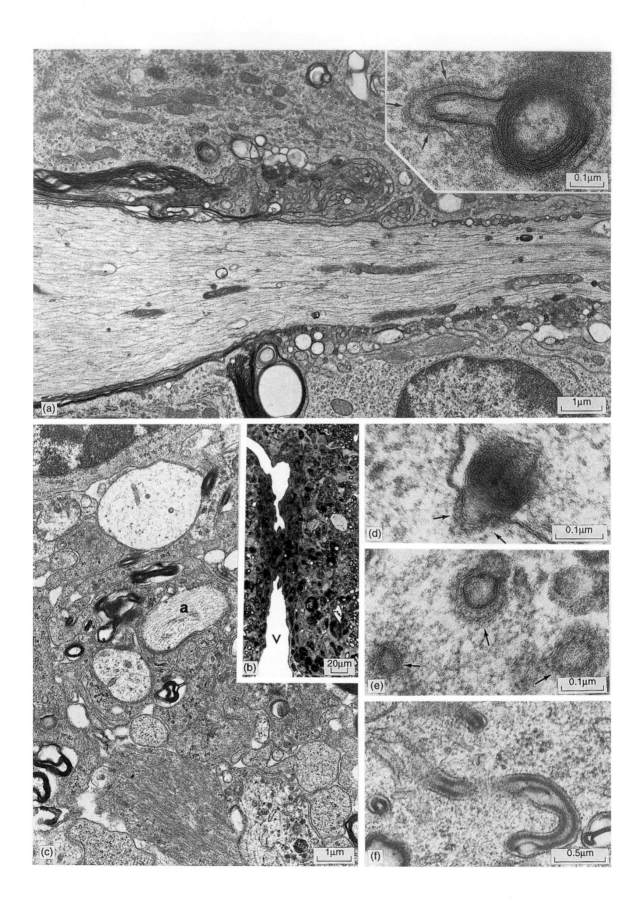

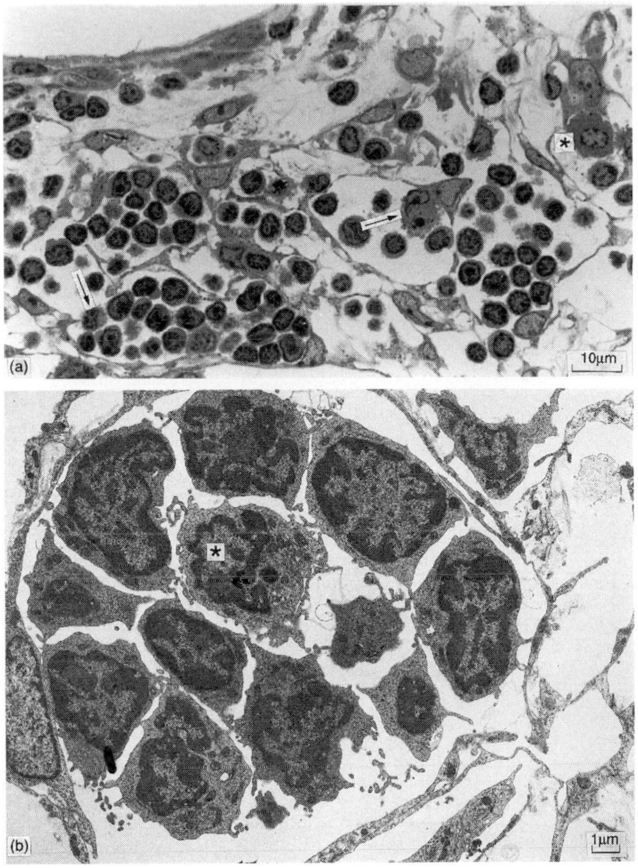

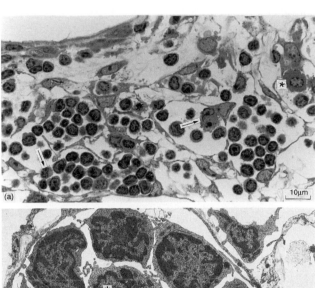

Figure 15.24 (*a*) SJL/J mouse; chronic relapsing EAE; adoptive transfer; 3 months post-transfer. Within the sub-ependymal CNS parenchyma beneath the lateral ventricle of the cerebrum, infiltrates of lymphocytes are seen organized inside sinusoids. Dendritic cells (*arrows*) occur among the lymphocytes, and between the sinusoids, macrophages and plasma cells (*) are found. This type of lymphoid organization within the CNS is reminiscent of lymph node medulla. (*b*) By EM, the same lymphoid deposits present as collections of small lymphocytes aggregated around dendritic cells (*) within sinusoids.

refute in models involving subcutaneous injection of an antigenic emulsion, it does not explain why identical relapses (clinical and structural) occur in the adoptively transferred murine models in which a single intravenous injection of sensitized cells is involved. Therefore, one must seek other explanations. One could be that soon after injection, antigen becomes deposited (or bound) peripherally within draining lymph nodes. Many years ago, the author recalls Byron Waksman relating a series of his own unpublished studies where rabbits were sensitized in a single digit with CNS emulsion and then at various timepoints shortly thereafter the digit was amputated. He found that amputation of the digit before 12 hours after sensitization led to no development of acute EAE, but amputation between 12 and 24 hours (and later) did not affect disease outcome and EAE developed 12–16 days later. These unpublished observations would tend to support the concept of early and persistent antigen deposition in the draining lymphatics.

A second interesting line of evidence has emerged from the above-described murine models [92, 93] where collections of lymphoid elements were encountered within the CNS of relapsing animals. These consisted of sinusoids containing small lymphocytes centred on dendritic cells, with plasma cells and macrophages between the sinusoids (Figures 15.24*a* and *b*) – an appearance highly reminiscent of lymph node medulla, here occurring within the CNS. In some cases, the lymphoid collections comprised aggregates of macrophages containing myelin debris abutting small lymphocytes [93], interactions suggestive of intercellular communication. These appearances support the concept [92] that extra-lymphoid system elements within the target organ might play a role in the perpetuation of the autoimmune disease process. Such was perhaps the implication of a study by Prineas [106] which also described lymphoid elements in the CNS in MS.

Figure 15.23 (*a*) Acute EAE in a rabbit sensitized 14 days earlier with whole CNS tissue in CFA; day of onset of EAE – included to show the image typical of immune-mediated myelin damage. A large diameter myelinated nerve fibre in the lumbar spinal cord is undergoing active demyelination. Processes from an investing macrophage (*arrows*) undermine layers of myelin, reducing them to vesicular droplets that are then internalized by the cell. Note the abrupt decrease in axonal diameter from the point at which myelin is lost from the fibre. *Inset*: detail from a field adjacent to that depicted in (*a*). An extracellular droplet of myelin is being internalized by a macrophage following its attachment to a clathrin-coated pit (*arrows*) on the surface of the cell. (*b*) Mouse chronic relapsing EAE; actively induced; sampled during a relapse. A perivascular infiltrate of haematogenous cells – vessel lumen at (**v**) – is superimposed upon chronic demyelination. (*c*) Same lesion by EM. An axon (**a**) lies among a collection of mononuclear cell processes between which myelin droplets at different stages of internalization are located. Appearances such as these are supportive of recent demyelinative activity, occurring here 30 days post-inoculation. (*d*) PL/J mouse EAE; adoptive transfer; 9 months post-transfer; L7 spinal cord. Three stages of receptor-mediated phagocytosis of myelin are shown in (*d*), (*e*) and (*f*). In (*d*) an extracellular droplet of myelin has become associated with a clathrin-coated pit (*arrows*) on the surface of a macrophage. (*e*) PL/J mouse, chronic relapsing EAE; adoptive transfer, 7 months post-transfer. A glancing section across a macrophage surface shows several ring-like droplets of myelin lying within chambers (*arrows*) surrounded by coated-pit material. Elsewhere, the tangentially sectioned subplasmalemmal web of action filaments can be seen. (*f*) PL/J mouse, chronic relapsing EAE; adoptive transfer, 9 days post-transfer. Vermiform droplets of myelin lie within channels in a macrophage which is engaged in myelin phagocytosis. The channels and adjacent rounded profiles are surrounded by coated pit material.

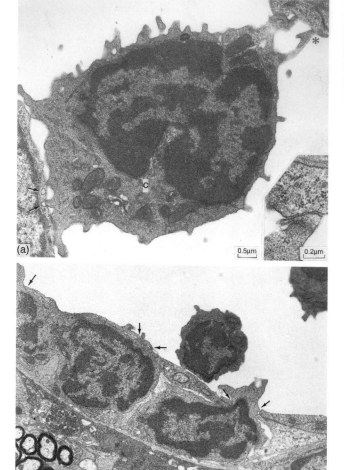

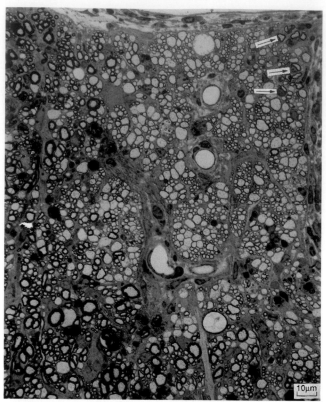

Figure 15.26   A montage of an almost entirely remyelinated chronic EAE lesion in the spinal cord (pial surface above) of a strain 13 guinea pig. The many large diameter axons with disproportionately thin myelin sheaths are typical of remyelination. Note the normal thickness of myelin in the less-affected white matter (*left and below*), the chronic blood vessel changes, and the Schwann cell invasion and PNS myelination (*arrows, upper right*).

Figure 15.25   (*a*) SJL/J mouse; adoptive transfer of a MBP⁺ T cell line; onset of disease; 7 days post-transfer. A small lymphocyte spans a venule with pseudopodia contacting the endothelium on the left at coated pits (*arrows*), and on the right via a gap-junction-like contact (*). The cell contains centrioles (c), suggestive of recent mitosis. *Inset*: detail of the junction at the asterisk. The section has been tilted 40° with a goniometer stage to resolve the membrane specializations. Note the extent of the membrane–membrane association between the lymphocyte (*below*) and the endothelial cell (*above*). (*b*) Same animal as (*a*): lymphocytes are attached to and breach the wall of a venule, seen here at different stages of migration. Note how the cells have interrupted the endothelial lining (*arrows*) and pass directly through the vessel wall and, in the case of the migrating cell on the right, not along the endothelial cell tight junction.

The notion that lymphocytic deposits might become organized within a target organ is not a novel observation and is a feature of many chronic inflammatory conditions [152]. Interpreted in the context of lymphocyte homing, lymphocytic trafficking and adhesion molecule expression, the presence of collections of lymphoid elements in the CNS might denote a role for lymphocyte/endothelial cell interactions whereby HEV or other vascular molecules normally present only in lymphoid tissue become expressed in a non-lymphoid target organ, the CNS. The homing of lymphocytes (both CNS antigen-specific and non-CNS antigen-specific) to the CNS and their unusual affinity to associate with the endothelium of selected vessels in the white matter via unique membrane associations (Figure 15.25*a*), occurring concomitantly with the aberrant expression of lymph node markers and prior to the invasion of the CNS by lymphocytes (Figure 15.25*b*), have been extensively studied [107, 153–156]. The unravelling of these molecular interactions at the CNS endothelial interphase is not only topical and of fundamental importance to CNS inflammation, but may also have important therapeutic ramifications for MS.

15.3.5   REMYELINATION IN CHRONIC EAE

A feature probably reflecting the smaller dimensions of lesions in chronic relapsing EAE (in comparison to MS) is the observation that in the majority of established lesions in the guinea pig remyelination is common, sometimes to the extent that the entire lesion may be repaired (Figure 15.26). Remyelination is readily appar-

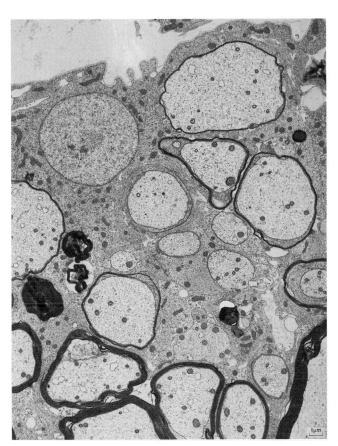

Figure 15.27   By EM, CNS remyelination is typified by thin, sometimes uncompacted myelin sheaths around large axons, here seen in a lesion from the spinal cord of a guinea pig with chronic relapsing EAE for 5 months. Some demyelinated axons are still present. Note the intense fibrous astrogliosis in the background tissue, a few myelin sheaths of normal thickness, the fibrous astroglial cell body and the pial margin of the spinal cord (*upper left*).

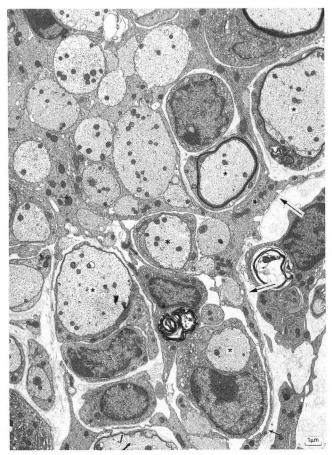

Figure 15.28   The margin of this chronically demyelinated spinal cord lesion from a guinea pig with chronic relapsing EAE demonstrates a phenomenon described in a variety of primary demyelinating conditions, including MS (see **Figure 15.5c**) – Schwann cell invasion and PNS myelination of demyelinated CNS axons. Note the axons (*) undergoing myelination by Schwann cells. Several uncommitted Schwann cells (s) are also present. Chronically demyelinated CNS axons are seen at the upper left and the basal lamina covering the pial surface of the spinal cord lies to the right (*arrows*).

ent structurally when one compares the large axonal diameter and the investing thin myelin sheaths of affected fibres with those of adjacent unaffected fibres. Blood vessels in these lesions may retain evidence of chronic inflammatory activity. By EM, the morphologic criteria of remyelination are readily satisfied (Figure 15.27). Myelin sheaths around large diameter axons are thin, contain varied amounts of oligodendroglial cytoplasm and are sometimes non-compacted. The areas are often associated with increased numbers of oligodendroglial cells and the remyelinated areas possess a fibrous astrogliotic background, as is also the case in MS (Figure 15.16). Such regions of CNS remyelination in EAE animals probably conform to the shadow plaques of MS (Chapter 9). Remyelination is also a constant feature of the chronic murine models although it is less extensive, perhaps due to the smaller lesion diameter and the greater degree of axonal attrition.

Another phenomenon common to both chronic EAE and MS lesions is the incidence of Schwann cell invasion

(Schwannosis) and PNS myelination of CNS axons [142]. Analysis of most established chronic EAE lesions within the spinal cord invariably reveals zones of PNS myelination, most noticeable towards subpial margins of the spinal cord (cf. Figures 15.5c in MS, 15.22b in mouse EAE, and 15.26 in guinea pig EAE). Schwann cell invasion and PNS myelination sometimes precede CNS remyelination and can be seen intermixed with naked CNS axons embedded in a gliotic background (Figure 15.28). Many free (non-committed) Schwann cells reside in these areas and one can only speculate that these cells might eventually seek out and associate with naked segments of CNS axons. The route of entry of these PNS elements has been followed morphologically and attributed to an invasive process from root entry zones and the Virchow–Robin space of penetrating vessels [63]. As has been the experience in MS [112], it

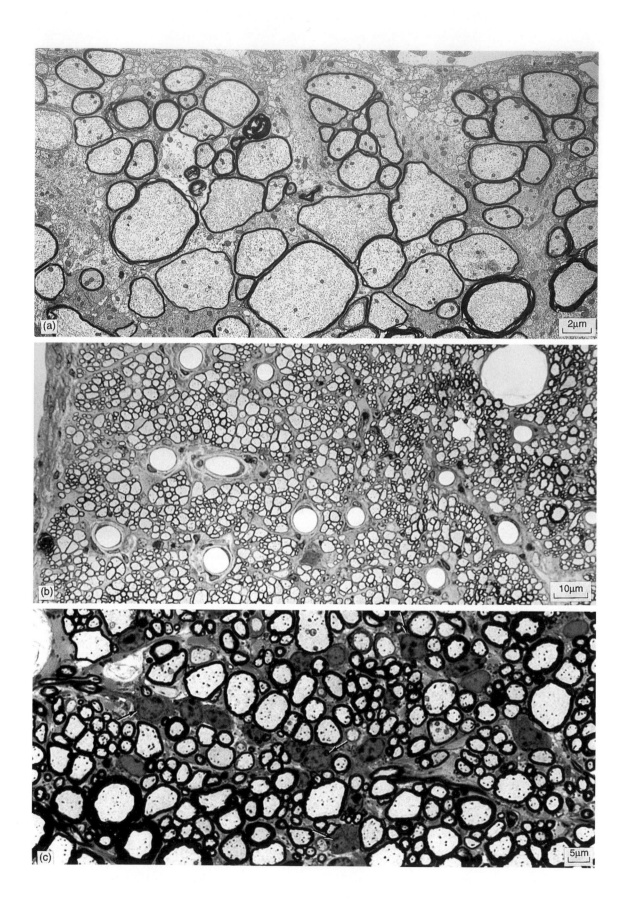

appears that PNS myelination of demyelinated CNS fibres does not correlate with functional improvement.

15.3.6 THERAPEUTIC APPLICATIONS OF THE MODELS TO MS

The availability of chronic demyelinating models in a number of inbred animal species in which the disease process has a latent period and a protracted, relapsing course affords unrivalled opportunities for MS research [53, 157]. With an increasing interest in the administration to MS patients of a vast battery of compounds to thwart the aberrant immune response within the CNS (Chapters 18 and 19), the above models provide valuable adjuncts for clinical trials on humans. With the guinea pig model of EAE, a disease induced by injections of whole spinal cord in CFA, MBP has been shown to be 100% efficacious and suppresses the clinical expression of both acute and chronic EAE when administered in IFA prior to onset of signs [60]. This procedure did not prevent initial lesion formation, but when examined later, the CNS lesions displayed remyelination (Figure 15.29a). It appeared, therefore, that suppression with MBP prevented lesion progression and fostered remyelination. Later studies demonstrated that guinea pigs in which chronic relapsing disease was treated with MBP (i.e. MBP given after the establishment of relapsing disease), showed only transient improvement and disease activity eventually returned [53]. On the other hand, guinea pigs treated with a combination of MBP and GalC in IFA displayed long-lasting clinical stabilization and/or improvement which correlated histologically with oligodendroglial cell proliferation, widespread CNS remyelination and the down-regulation of inflammation in the CNS (Figure 15.29b and c).

The rationale for this MBP/GalC therapy and its outcome in the strain 13 guinea pig model has formed the subject of a number of reviews (see the review by Raine [53]). In short, this therapy involved a vaccination-like series of intramuscular injections of emulsion containing a known amount of MBP and GalC in the appropriate ratio (the same as that occurring in the intact myelin sheath) into large numbers of animals afflicted with chronic relapsing EAE. As stated, the outcome was clinical improvement which correlated with extensive

CNS repair. Later morphometric study confirmed the observations [61] and suggested that the remyelination was effected both by local proliferating oligodendroglial cells and precursor cells which became differentiated during remyelination. Similar results emerged from a modification of the protocol for adoptively transferred murine EAE but the clinical improvement was less striking. The beneficial effect of the MBP/GalC protocol described above in guinea pigs has been confirmed in a murine viral-induced demyelinative disease caused by Theiler's murine encephalomyelitis virus (TMEV) [158]. An extension of this work by Rodriguez and Lennon [159] showed that IgG from animals sensitized with whole myelin has a similar remyelinating effect upon TMEV-induced lesions, particularly in chronic models.

Of potential greater relevance but on which there has been little follow up, is the reported manipulation of acute EAE in the rat using in a therapeutic mode peptides homologous to TCR sequences derived from encephalitogenic T cells [56, 160]. Anti-T cell and anti-Ia (MHC II) monoclonal antibody therapy of chronic EAE in mice (actively induced EAE), has also demonstrated clinical improvement [161–163]. In none of the latter TCR or monoclonal antibody approaches has material been analysed neuropathologically, leaving the findings interesting at the clinical level only. Equally relevant is the application of antibodies to proinflammatory cytokines in the prevention and treatment of murine EAE since cytokines play a major role in the regulation of most immune system molecules. Two studies have reported successful blocking of murine EAE with antibodies to the TH1 pro-inflammatory cytokines TNFα and LT [164, 165]. In addition, treatment of mice, rats and marmosets sensitized for EAE and then given inhibitors of TNFα production also showed that disease development could be abrogated [166, 169]. Modulation of regulatory TH2 cytokine levels has also been shown to have a beneficial outcome on EAE, namely transforming growth factor beta [170], IL-10 [171] and IL-4 [172]. Therapeutic attempts to manipulate EAE with antibodies to adhesion molecules have yielded mixed results. An antibody to the α4β1 integrin (VLA-4) blocked murine EAE effectively [173], while studies on antibodies to ICAM-1 and LFA-1 displayed differing effects [174–177].

Figure 15.29 (a) A spinal cord lesion is shown by EM from a guinea pig with chronic relapsing EAE; 12 weeks post-inoculation. After sensitization with spinal cord tissue in CFA, the disease was suppressed with injections of MBP/IFA prior to onset of signs. Extensive CNS remyelination is apparent to a degree rarely seen in control EAE animals. (b) By LM, a broad zone of CNS remyelination is seen in the spinal cord of a guinea pig with chronic relapsing EAE for 5 months that was then treated for 1 month with injections of MBP/GalC/IFA. Note the remyelination of virtually every affected fibre, the lack of inflammatory activity and, for comparison, the thickness of normal myelin sheaths to the right. The subpial surface of the spinal cord is to the left. (One micron epoxy section; toluidine blue stain). (c) This one micron epoxy section comes from the spinal cord of a guinea pig with chronic relapsing EAE for 24 months which was then treated for one month with injections of MBP/GalC/IFA and sampled two months later (27 mo PI), after the animal had displayed clinical improvement. An area of lesion is shown which displays widespread CNS remyelination and proliferation of oligodendrocytes (arrows). A group of unaffected fibres with myelin sheaths of normal thickness lies below.

15.4 Conclusions and future perspectives

It has been the purview of this author to compare objectively the fine structure of the MS lesion with that of the various forms of chronic relapsing EAE, particularly in the mouse, a species in which the condition had not been fully developed at the time of the last comprehensive reviews on the subject in 1983. It will be clear from the many illustrations that regardless of our skills in the laboratory, a lesion identical to the MS lesion has not yet been produced in animals. The reason for this lies largely in our inability to simulate in a laboratory animal the time frame associated with the development of the typical MS lesion (in many cases measured in decades) or the voracity and scale of the acute MS lesion. Nevertheless, faithful reproductions of selected facets of the various stages of the MS lesion can be reproduced with models of chronic relapsing EAE, feats which are sufficient to convince us that the MS lesion has an immunogenic basis. One myth that commonly permeates the literature is the statement that demyelinated axons are spared in MS and that EAE with lesions displaying fibre depletion is not an appropriate model. In MS, widespread axonal sparing is frequently not the case and most authors couch their evaluation of axonal involvement in the phrase 'relative sparing of axons' (see [58]). It is a fact of life that large numbers of axons are lost from the acute MS lesion and that the number remains depleted as the lesion ages. It is also a fact of life that despite the axonal loss and the intensity of the disease process remyelination frequently occurs. When these observations are set alongside the fact that MS frequently remits clinically, it is clear that compensatory mechanisms must be in place within the CNS that permit functional recovery in the face of significant axonal loss. These are but a few of the many paradoxes that render MS a fascinating challenge.

The oft-times heated debates on the relative attributes of the various animal models of MS, particularly the many forms of EAE, pale in comparison to the questions yet unanswered in MS. The striving, therefore, of researchers to produce models of immune demyelination with total preservation of axons has probably been a somewhat futile goal, a goal with limited relevance to the human condition in which axonal loss is not uncommon. Thus, criticism of some mouse models on the grounds that they display unacceptable degrees of Wallerian degeneration needs to be considered in the context of the present updated image of the typical MS lesion. More important perhaps is the bounty of information emanating from the many seminal studies on immune-mediated demyelination showing the exquisite selectivity of the inflammatory response for the CNS in EAE. It is in this arena that much progress has been made in recent years.

Overall, progress in the analysis of pathogenetic events underlying the establishment of the demyelinated lesion in MS has been slow and sporadic. Subsequent to the pens of Charcot (1868) and Dawson (1916) (see [58]), relatively little new has been added to the pathological picture despite the addition of vast tomes to the literature. Anecdotally, it appears that almost at regular 10-year intervals, theories on the subject of MS go full circle, each cycle introducing a new crop of investigators. In recent years, the pre-eminent position of the previously omnipotent neuropathologist has been usurped somewhat as more multidisciplinary approaches have evolved, to be replaced by the molecular neurobiologist/immunologist. The field today straddles neurology, pathology, neuroscience, biochemistry, immunology, virology and molecular biology. In the light of the enormous degree of informational maturation which has developed amongst these disciplines, it is now becoming possible to arrange in rank order certain significant features of MS lesions which relate to the genesis of the lesion. Some of these are the subject of the preceding paragraphs.

Historically, difficulties in the analysis of clinical, morphological and immunological events in MS with suitably preserved human tissue caused investigators to search for better systems. The novice entering the field today is faced with a healthy choice of models – from immunological and virological to acute and chronic, and *in vivo* and *in vitro*. While the search for new models has sometimes displaced our focus on the human condition, it has been gratifying to witness the emergence of valid therapeutic approaches based upon pilot work on animal models. As an adjunct to studies on the pathogenesis of MS, this laboratory and others have developed over the past three decades a number of immune-mediated chronic relapsing EAE models, models which have proved to share features in common with MS. The expansion in the 1980s of our EAE expertise to the mouse, a species for which there is a wealth of well-defined markers, has compensated for some of the deficiencies inherent in guinea pig models. It has been the major charge of this author to present to the reader the current status of the MS lesion and to compare the findings with the most relevant experimental models. Chronic relapsing EAE has been shown to simulate MS in being age-, sex- and strain-dependent, having a long latent period prior to onset, a progressive, protracted and rarely fatal course which displays relapses, and lesions which are disseminated, demyelinative, large and of different ages. Other parameters of relevance to MS include the requirement for most models of chronic relapsing EAE of a single sensitization only, selected neuropathologic similarities, immunogenetic requirements for susceptibility, the observation of immunologic changes in longitudinal blood and CSF samples, and its promising application as a therapeutic tool.

In a manner probably parallelling CNS lesion activity, circulating lymphocyte values fluctuate with clinical disease in both MS and EAE, as do most other immunologic parameters, and in EAE the first cells to arrive in the CNS appear to be CNS antigen-specific [107, 156]. An area of recent activity in a number of laboratories has been the recognition that lymphocyte trafficking molecules [178] interact in the CNS with adhesion molecules on endothelial cells [105, 153–155]. The expression of these molecules waxes and wanes as the disease develops. It is also recognized that at the blood–brain barrier, lymphocytes and endothelial cells 'are dynamic partners in multiple, complex interactions involving macromolecular and cellular constituents of blood as well as vessel wall components' [179]. It is highly likely that future progress in a number of known or suspected autoimmune conditions will come from understanding the functional status of this interphase as well as the inducibility of the CNS to serve as an adjunct to the immune system. In this regard, many laboratories are turning their attention towards the further characterization of cytokines and their effects upon cells of the nervous system [180]. Families of adhesion molecules like the integrins, immunoglobulins, selectins and addressins, plus a whole bevy yet to be identified (including their respective immune modulators, perhaps a specific lymphocyte homing molecule for CNS endothelium and co-stimulatory molecules), are going to form the major areas of activity in MS and chronic relapsing EAE as we enter the twenty-first century.

Finally, we know that in the case of the MS lesion, more often than not we are looking at the footprints of a disease process long since passed by. We also know that by the appropriate application of the above immunological models, we may come to understand better the mechanisms responsible for or implicated in the changes in the CNS in MS. Bolstered by suggestions from works with molecular probes, experimentation with chronic relapsing EAE continues to target the development of protocols capable of arresting disease progression and fostering repair, the central goals of many laboratories. With this in mind, and since we now know that the demyelinated CNS can be induced to remyelinate extensively, the future is bright for the MS patient and we intend to keep it that way.

ACKNOWLEDGEMENTS

The long-standing close collaboration of Dr Sanford H. Stone (NIAID) led to the many studies on the strain 13 guinea pig model. Drs Robert D. Terry, William T. Norton, Labe C. Scheinberg, Celia F. Brosnan, Wayne Moore, David Snyder, Krzysztof Selmaj, Anne H. Cross, Barbara Cannella, Michael K. Racke, Henry McFarland and the late Murray B. Bornstein and Dale E. McFarlin have each had substantial input into the work described. To all of these colleagues, to my long-established technical team of Everett Swanson, Howard Finch and Miriam Pakingan, and to others too numerous to name, the author extends his sincere thanks.

Supported in part by NIH grants NS 08952, NS 11920 and NS 07098; and by grant RG 1001-I-9 from the National Multiple Sclerosis Society.

The following illustrations have been reproduced with permission. Figure 15.8 from Lee *et al.*, 1990 [43]; Figures 15.9a and b, and Figure 15.12b from Raine and Scheinberg, 1988 [39]; Figures 15.18b and e from Raine *et al.* (1980) in *The Suppression of Multiple Sclerosis and Experimental Allergic Encephalomyelitis* (eds A.N. Davison and M.L. Cuzner), New York, Academic Press, pp. 119–40; Figures 15.19a, 15.22a and 15.23a from Brown *et al.*, 1982 [9]; Figures 15.19b and 15.22b from Raine *et al.*, 1984 [92]; Figures 15.19d and e, 15.23d, e and f from Cross *et al.*, 1987 [93].

References

1. Raine, C.S. (1983) Multiple sclerosis and chronic EAE: comparative ultrastructural neuropathology, in *Multiple Sclerosis* (eds J.F. Hallpike, C.W.M. Adams and W.W. Tourtellotte), London, Chapman & Hall, pp. 413–60.
2. Lassmann, H. (ed.) (1983) *Comparative Neuropathology of Chronic Experimental Allergic Encephalomyelitis and Multiple Sclerosis*, Berlin, Springer.
3. Stone, S.H. and Lerner, E.M. (1965) Chronic disseminated allergic encephalomyelitis in guinea pigs. *Ann. NY Acad. Sci.*, **122**, 227–41.
4. Raine, C.S. and Stone, S.H. (1977) Animal model for multiple sclerosis. Chronic experimental allergic encephalomyelitis in inbred guinea pigs. *NY State J. Med.*, **77**, 1693–6.
5. Raine, C.S., Barnett, L.B., Brown, A., Behar, T. and McFarlin, D.F. (1980) Neuropathology of experimental allergic encephalomyelitis in inbred strains of mice. *Lab. Invest.*, **43**, 150–7.
6. Lassmann, H., Kitz, K. and Wisniewski, H.M. (1980) Chronic relapsing experimental allergic encephalomyelitis in rats and guinea pigs – a comparison, in *Search for the Cause of Multiple Sclerosis and Other Chronic Diseases of the Central Nervous System* (ed. A. Boese), Weinheim, Verlag Chemie, pp. 96–104.
7. Brown, A. and McFarlin, D.E. (1981) Relapsing experimental allergic encephalomyelitis in SJL mouse. *Lab. Invest.*, **45**, 278–85.
8. Lublin, F.D., Maurer, P.H., Berry, R.G. and Tippett, D. (1981) Delayed, relapsing experimental allergic encephalomyelitis in mice. *J. Immunol.*, **26**, 819–22.
9. Brown, A., McFarlin, D.E. and Raine, C.S. (1982) The chronologic neuropathology of relapsing allergic encephalomyelitis in the mouse. *Lab. Invest.*, **46**, 171–85.
10. Mokhtarian, F., McFarlin, D.E. and Raine, C.S. (1984) Adoptive transfer of myelin basic protein sensitized cells produces chronic relapsing demyelinating disease in mice. *Nature (Lond.)*, **309**, 356–8.
11. Tabira, T. and Sakai, K. (1987) Demyelination induced by T cell lines and clones specific for myelin basic protein in mice. *Lab. Invest.*, **55**, 518–25.
12. Massacesi, L., Genain, C.P., Lee-Parritz, D. *et al.* (1995) Actively and passively induced experimental autoimmune encephalomyelitis in common marmosets: a new model for multiple sclerosis. *Ann. Neurol.*, **37**, 519–30.
13. Johnson, R.T. (1985) Viral aspects of multiple sclerosis, in *Handbook of Clinical Neurology*, 3 (revised series), (ed. J.C. Koetsier), Amsterdam, Elsevier, pp. 319–36.
14. Waksman, B.H. (1989) Multiple sclerosis: relationship to a retrovirus? *Nature (Lond.)*, **337**, 599.
15. Cook, S.D., Rohowsky-Kochan, C., Bansil, S. and Dowling, P.C. (1995) Evidence for multiple sclerosis as an infectious disease. *Acta Neurol. Scand. (Suppl.)*, **161**, 34–42.
16. Challoner, P.B., Smith, K.T., Parker, J.D. *et al.* (1995) Plaque-associated expression of human herpesvirus 6 in multiple sclerosis. *Proc. Natl. Acad. Sci. (USA)*, **92**, 7440–4.

17. Reder, A.T. and Arnason, B.G.W. (1985) Immunology of multiple sclerosis, in *Handbook of Clinical Neurology, 3* (revised series) (ed. J.C. Koetsier), Amsterdam, Elsevier, pp. 337–95.

18. Kabat, E.A., Freedman, D.A., Murray, J.P. and Kraub, V. (1950) A study of the crystalline albumin, gammaglobulin and total protein in the cerebrospinal fluid of one hundred cases of multiple sclerosis and in other diseases. *Am. J. Med. Sci.*, **219**, 55–64.

19. Whitaker, J.N. (1984) Indicators of disease activity in multiple sclerosis: studies of myelin basic protein-like materials. *Ann. NY Acad. Sci.*, **436**, 140–50

20. Oger, J.F., Arnason, B.G.W., Wray, S.H. and Kistler, J.P. (1975) A study of B and T cells in multiple sclerosis. *Neurology*, **25**, 444–7.

21. Chofflon, M., Weiner, H.L., Morimoto, C. and Hafler, D.A. (1989) Decrease of suppressor inducer (CD4$^+$2H4$^+$) T cells in multiple sclerosis cerebrospinal fluid. *Ann. Neurol.*, **25**, 494–9.

22. Salonen, R., Ilonen, J., Jageroos, H. *et al.* (1989) Lymphocyte subsets in the cerebrospinal fluid in active multiple sclerosis. *Ann. Neurol.*, **25**, 500–2.

23. Raine, C.S. (1991) Multiple sclerosis: a pivotal role for the T cell in lesion development. *Neuropathol. Appl. Neurobiol.*, **17**, 265–74.

24. Allegretta, M., Nicklas, J.A., Sriram, S. and Albertini, R.J. (1990) T cells responsive to myelin basic protein in patients with multiple sclerosis. *Science*, **247**, 718–21.

25. Abramsky, O., Lisak, R.P., Silberberg, D.H. and Pleasure, D.E. (1977) Antibodies to oligodendroglia in patients with multiple sclerosis. *N. Engl. J. Med.*, **297**, 1207–11.

26. Bornstein, M.B. (1963) A tissue culture approach to demyelinative disorders. *Natl Cancer Inst. Monogr.*, no. 11, 197–214.

27. Bornstein, M.B. and Raine, C.S. (1977) Multiple sclerosis and experimental allergic encephalomyelitis: specific demyelination in vitro. *Neuropathol. Appl. Neurobiol.*, **3**, 359–69.

28. Grundke-Iqbal, I. and Bornstein, M.B. (1979) Multiple sclerosis: immunochemical studies on the demyelinating serum factor. *Brain Res.*, **160**, 489–503.

29. Dubois-Dalcq, M., Shumacher, G. and Sever, J.L. (1973) Acute multiple sclerosis. Electron microscopic evidence for and against a viral agent in the plaques. *Lancet*, **ii**, 1408–11.

30. Prineas, J.W. and Raine, C.S. (1976) Electron microscopy and immunoperoxidase studies of early multiple sclerosis lesions. *Neurology*, **26**, 29–32.

31. Esiri, M.M., Taylor, C.R. and Mason, D.W. (1976) Application of an immunoperoxidase method to a study of the central nervous system: preliminary findings in a study of human formalin-fixed material. *Neuropathol. Appl. Neurobiol.*, **2**, 233–46.

32. Kwon, E.E. and Prineas, J.W. (1995) Blood–brain barrier abnormalities in longstanding multiple sclerosis lesions. An immunohistochemical study. *J. Neuropathol. Exp. Neurol.*, **53**, 617–24.

33. Raine, C.S. (1990) Multiple sclerosis: immunopathologic mechanisms in the progression and resolution of inflammatory demyelination, in *Immunologic Mechanisms in Neurologic and Psychiatric Disease* (ed. B.H. Waksman), Proceedings of the Association for Research in Nervous and Mental Diseases, New York, Raven Press, pp. 37–54.

34. Field, E.J. and Raine, C.S. (1964) Examination of multiple sclerosis biopsy specimens. *Proc. IIIrd Eur. Regional Conf. Electron Microscopy (Prague)*, pp. 189–90.

35. Périer, O. and Grégoire, A. (1965) Electron microscopic features of multiple sclerosis lesions. *Brain*, **88**, 937–52.

36. Prineas, J. (1975) Pathology of the early lesion in multiple sclerosis. *Hum. Pathol.*, **6**, 531–54.

37. Raine, C.S., Scheinberg, L.C. and Waltz, J.M. (1981) Multiple sclerosis: oligodendrocyte survival and proliferation in an active, established lesion. *Lab. Invest.*, **45**, 534–46.

38. Prineas, J. (1985) The neuropathology of multiple sclerosis, in *Handbook of Clinical Neurology, 3* (revised series) (ed. J.C. Koetsier), Amsterdam, Elsevier, pp. 213–57.

39. Raine, C.S. and Scheinberg, L.C. (1988) On the immunopathology of plaque development and repair in multiple sclerosis. *J. Neuroimmunol.*, **120**, 189–201.

40. Sobel, R. (1989) T-lymphocyte subsets in the multiple sclerosis lesion. *Res. Immunol.*, **140**, 209–11.

41. Prineas, J.W., Kwon, E.E., Goldenberg, P.Z. *et al.* (1989) Multiple sclerosis: oligodendrocyte proliferation and differentiation in fresh lesions. *Lab. Invest.*, **61**, 489–503.

42. Lee, S.C. and Raine, C.S. (1989) Multiple sclerosis: oligodendrocytes do not express class II major histocompatibility molecules in active lesions. *J. Neuroimmunol.*, **25**, 261–6.

43. Lee, S.C., Moore, G.R.W., Golenwsky, G. and Raine, C.S. (1990) A role for astroglia in active demyelination suggested by class II MHC expression and ultrastructural study. *J. Neuropathol. Exp. Neurol.*, **49**, 122–36.

44. Prineas, J.W., Kwon, E.E., Goldenberg, P.Z., Cho, E.S. and Sharer, L.R. (1990) Interaction of astrocytes and newly formed oligodendrocytes in resolving multiple sclerosis lesions. *Lab. Invest.*, **63**, 624–36.

45. Wu, E. and Raine, C.S. (1992) Multiple sclerosis: interactions between oligodendrocytes and hypertrophic astrocytes and their occurrence in other, non-demyelinating conditions. *Lab. Invest.*, **67**, 88–99.

46. Raine, C.S. (1985) Experimental allergic encephalomyelitis and experimental allergic neuritis, in *Handbook of Clinical Neurology, 3* (revised series) (ed. J.C. Koetsier), Amsterdam, Elsevier, pp. 429–66.

47. Adams, R.D. (1959) A comparison of the morphology of the human demyelinative diseases and experimental 'allergic' encephalomyelitis, in *Allergic Encephalomyelitis* (eds M.W. Kies and E.C. Alvord), Springfield, IL, C.C. Thomas, pp. 183–209.

48. Waksman, B.H. (1965) Clinical investigations in autosensitization: nervous system. *Ann. NY Acad. Sci.*, **122**, 299–309.

49. Alvord, E.C. (1970) Acute disseminated encephalomyelitis and 'allergic' neuroencephalopathies, in *Handbook of Clinical Neurology, 9* (eds P.J. Vinken and G.W. Bruyn), Amsterdam, North Holland, pp. 500–71.

50. Levine, S. (1974) Hyperacute, neutrophilic, and localized forms of experimental allergic encephalomyelitis: a review. *Acta Neuropathol. (Berlin)*, **28**, 179–89.

51. Paterson, P.Y. (1976) Experimental autoimmune (allergic) encephalomyelitis. Induction, pathogenesis and suppression, in *Textbook of Immunopathology* (eds P.A. Miescher and J.J. Mueller-Eberhard), New York, Grune and Stratton, pp. 179–213.

52. Lampert, P.W. (1983) Fine structure of the demyelinating process, in *Multiple Sclerosis* (eds J.F. Hallpike, C.W.M. Adams and W.W. Tourtellotte), London, Chapman & Hall, pp. 29–46.

53. Raine, C.S. (1984) Biology of disease. The analysis of autoimmune demyelination: its impact upon multiple sclerosis. *Lab. Invest.*, **50**, 608–35.

54. Heber-Katz, E. and Acha-Orbea, H. (1989) The V-region disease hypothesis: evidence from autoimmune encephalomyelitis. *Immunol. Today*, **10**, 164–9.

55. Vandenbark, A.A., Hashim, G. and Offner, H. (1989) Immunization with a synthetic T-cell receptor V-region peptide protects against experimental autoimmune encephalomyelitis. *Nature (Lond.)*, **241**, 541–3.

56. Goverman, J., Woods, A., Larson, L. *et al.* (1993) Transgenic mice that express a myelin basic protein-specific T cell receptor develop spontaneous autoimmunity. *Cell*, **72**, 551–60.

57. Lafaille, J.J., Nagashima, K., Katsuki, M. and Tonegawa, S. (1994) High incidence of spontaneous autoimmune encephalomyelitis in immunodeficient anti-myelin basic protein T cell receptor transgenic mice. *Cell*, **78**, 399–408.

58. Raine, C.S. (1990) Demyelinating diseases, in *Textbook of Neuropathology* (eds R.L. Davis and D.M. Robertson), 2nd edn, Baltimore, Williams and Wilkins, MD, pp. 535–620.

59. Lassmann, H. (1983) Chronic relapsing experimental allergic encephalomyelitis: its value as an experimental model for multiple sclerosis. *J. Neurol.*, **229**, 207–20.

60. Raine, C.S., Traugott, U. and Stone, S.H. (1978) Suppression of chronic allergic encephalomyelitis: relevance to multiple sclerosis. *Science*, **201**, 445–8.

61. Raine, C.S., Moore, G.R.W., Hintzen, R. and Traugott, U. (1988) Induction of oligodendrocyte proliferation and remyelination after chronic demyelination. Relevance to multiple sclerosis. *Lab. Invest.*, **59**, 467–76.

62. Adams, R.D. and Sidman, R.L. (1968) Demyelinative diseases, in *Introduction to Neuropathology* (eds R.D. Adams and R.L. Sidman), New York, McGraw-Hill, pp. 149–70.

63. Raine, C.S. (1978) Membrane specialisations between demyelinated axons and astroglia in chronic EAE lesions and multiple sclerosis plaques. *Nature (Lond.)*, **275**, 326–7.

64. Soffer, D. and Raine, C.S. (1980) Morphologic analysis of axo-glial membrane specialisations in the demyelinated central nervous system. *Brain Res.*, **186**, 301–13.

65. Prineas, J.W. and Wright, R.F. (1978) Macrophages, lymphocytes, and plasma cells in the perivascular compartment in chronic multiple sclerosis. *Lab. Invest.*, **38**, 409–21.

66. Booss, J., Esiri, M., Tourtellotte, W.W. and Mason, D.W. (1983) Immunohistological analysis of T lymphocyte subsets in the central nervous system in chronic progressive multiple sclerosis. *J. Neurol Sci.*, **61**, 219–32.

67. Hauser, S.L., Bhan, A.K., Gilles, F. *et al.* (1986) Immunocytochemical analysis of the cellular infiltrates in multiple sclerosis lesions. *Ann. Neurol.*, **19**, 578–87.

68. Oehmichen, M. (1975) Monocytic origin of microglial cells, in *Mononuclear Phagocytes in Immunity, Infection and Pathology* (ed. F. Van Furth), Oxford, Blackwell, pp. 223–40.

69. Hickey, W.F. and Kimura, H. (1988) Perivascular microglial cells of the CNS are bone marrow-derived and present antigen in vivo. *Science*, **239**, 290–2.

70. Raine, C.S., Snyder, D.H., Valsamis, M.P. and Stone, S.H. (1974) Chronic experimental allergic encephalomyelitis in inbred guinea pigs – an ultrastructural study. *Lab. Invest.*, **31**, 367–80.

71. Ghatak, N.R., Leshner, R.T., Price, A.C. and Felten, W.L. (1989) Remyelination in the human central nervous system. *J. Neuropath. Exp. Neurol.*, **48**, 507–18.

72. Raine, C.S. and Wu, E. (1993) Multiple sclerosis: remyelination in acute lesions. *J. Neuropathol. Exp. Neurol.*, **52**, 199–205.

73. Prineas, J.W., Barnard, R.O., Kwon, E.E., Sharer, L.R. and Cho, E.S. (1993) Multiple sclerosis: remyelination of nascent lesions. *Ann. Neurol.*, **33**, 137–51.

74. Brosnan, C.F., Stoner, G.L., Bloom, B.R. and Wisniewski, H. (1977) Studies on demyelination by activated lymphocytes in the rabbit eye. II. Antibody-dependent cell-mediated demyelination. *J. Immunol.*, **118**, 2103–10.

75. Selmaj, K. and Raine, C.S. (1988) Tumor necrosis factor mediates myelin and oligodendrocyte damage *in vitro*. *Ann. Neurol.*, **23**, 339–46.

76. Raine, C.S., Johnson, A.B., Marcus, D.M., Suzuki, A. and Bornstein, M.B. (1981) Demyelination *in vitro*: absorption studies demonstrate that galactocerebroside is a major target. *J. Neurol. Sci.*, **52**, 117–31.

77. Raine, C.S., Traugott, U., Farooq, M., Bornstein, M.B. and Norton, W.T. (1981) Augmentation of immune mediated demyelination by lipid haptens. *Lab. Invest.*, **45**, 174–82.

78. Brosnan, C.F., Cammer, W., Norton, W.T. and Bloom, B.R. (1980) Proteinase inhibitors suppress experimental allergic encephalomyelitis. *Nature (Lond.)*, **285**, 235–7.

79. Satoh, J. and Tabira, T. (1990) A study of bystander demyelination using T cell lines specific for a non-neural antigen. *Biomed. Res. (India)*, **1**, 25–32.

80. Prineas, J.W. and Connell, F. (1978) The fine structure of chronically active multiple sclerosis plaques. *Neurology*, **28**, 68–75.

81. Prineas, J.W., Barnard, R.O., Ervesz, T. *et al.* (1993) Multiple sclerosis: pathology of recurrent lesions. *Brain*, **116**, 681–93.

82. Benveniste, E.N. and Merrill, J.E. (1986) Stimulation of oligodendroglial proliferation and maturation of interleukin-2. *Nature (Lond.)*, **321**, 610–13.

83. Hofman, F.M., von Hanwehr, R.I., Dinarello, C.A. *et al.* (1986) Immunoregulatory molecules and IL-2 receptors identified in multiple sclerosis brain. *J. Immunol.*, **136**, 3239–45.

84. Hofman, F.M., Hinton, D.R., Johnson, K. and Merrill, J.E. (1989) Tumor necrosis factor identified in multiple sclerosis brain. *J. Exp. Med.*, **170** 607–12.

85. Selmaj, K., Raine, C.S., Cannella, B. and Brosnan, C.F. (1991) Identification of lymphotoxin and tumor necrosis factor in multiple sclerosis lesions. *J. Clin. Invest.*, **87**, 949–54.

86. Cannella, B. and Raine, C.S. (1995) The adhesion molecule/cytokine profile of multiple sclerosis lesions. *Ann. Neurol.*, **37**, 424–35.

87. Selmaj, K., Raine, C.S., Farooq, M., Norton, W.T. and Brosnan, C.F. (1991) Cytokine cytotoxicity against oligodendrocytes: apoptosis induced by lymphotoxin. *J. Immunol.*, **147**, 1522–9.

88. Sobel, R.A. and Ames, M.B. (1988) Major histocompatibility complex molecule expression in the human central nervous system: immunohistochemical analysis of 40 patients. *J. Neuropathol. Exp. Neurol.*, **47**, 19–28.

89. Prineas, J.W. and Graham, J.S. (1981) Multiple sclerosis: capping of surface immunoglobulin G on macrophages engaged in myelin breakdown. *Ann. Neurol.*, **10**, 149–58.

90. Epstein, L.G., Prineas, J.W. and Raine, C.S. (1983) Attachment of myelin to coated pits on macrophages in experimental allergic encephalomyelitis. *J. Neurol. Sci.*, **61**, 341–8.

91. Moore, G.R.W. and Raine, C.S. (1988) Immunogold localization and analysis of IgG in acute experimental allergic encephalomyelitis. *Lab. Invest.*, **59**, 641–8.

92. Raine, C.S., Mokhtarian, F. and McFarlin, D.E. (1984) Adoptively-transferred chronic relapsing experimental allergic encephalomyelitis in the mouse: ultrastructural analysis. *Lab. Invest.*, **51**, 534–50.

93. Cross, A.H., McCarron, R.M., McFarlin, D.E. and Raine, C.S. (1987) Adoptively-transferred acute and chronic relapsing autoimmune encephalomyelitis in the PL/J mouse with observations on altered pathology by intercurrent infection. *Lab. Invest.*, **57**, 499–512.

94. Lampert, P.W. (1968) Fine structural changes of myelin sheaths in the central nervous system, in *Fine Structure and Function of Nervous Tissue* (ed. G.H. Bourne), New York, Academic Press, pp. 187–204.

95. Lassmann, H., Ammerer, H.P. and Kulnig, W. (1978) Ultrastructural sequence of myelin degradation. II. Wallerian degeneration in the rat optic nerve. *Acta Neuropathol. (Berlin)*, **44**, 91–102.

96. Hauw, J.J. and Escourolle, R. (1977) Filamentous and multilamellated cytoplasmic inclusions in progressive multifocal leukoencephalopathy. *Acta Neuropathol. (Berlin)*, **37**, 263–70.

97. Cook, R.D., Flower, R.L.P. and Dutton, N.S. (1986) Light and electron microscopical studies of the immunoperoxidase staining of multiple sclerosis plaques using antisera to a feline-derived agent and to galactocerebroside. *Neuropathol. Appl. Neurobiol.*, **12**, 63–79.

98. Ibrahim, M.Z.M. and Adams, C.W.M. (1963) The relationship between enzyme activity and neuroglia in plaques of multiple sclerosis. *J. Neurol. Neurosurg. Psychiatry*, **26**, 101–10.

99. Ibrahim, M.Z.M. and Adams, C.W.M. (1965) The relation between enzyme activity and neuroglia in early plaques of multiple sclerosis. *J. Pathol. Bacteriol.*, **90**, 239–43.

100. Lee, S.C. and Raine, C.S. (1989) Multiple sclerosis: oligodendrocytes do not express class II major histocompatibility molecules in active lesions. *J. Neuroimmunol.*, **25**, 261–6.

101. Selmaj, K., Brosnan, C.F. and Raine, C.S. (1991) Colocalization of TCR-γδ lymphocytes and hsp-65 ' oligodendrocytes in multiple sclerosis. *Proc. Natl Acad. Sci. (USA)*, **88**, 6452–6.

102. Selmaj, K., Brosnan, C.F. and Raine, C.S. (1992) Expression of heat shock protein-65 by oligodendrocytes *in vivo* and *in vitro*: implications for multiple sclerosis. *Neurology*, **42**, 795–800.

103. Jalkanen, S. (1989) Leukocyte-endothelial cell interaction and the control of leukocyte migration into inflamed synovium. *Springer Semin. Immunopathol.*, **11**, 187–98.

104. Sobel, R.A., Mitchell, M.E. and Fondren, G. (1990) Intercellular adhesion molecule-1 (ICAM-1) in cellular immune reactions in the human central nervous system. *Am. J. Pathol.*, **136**, 1309–16.

105. Raine, C.S. and Cannella, B. (1992) Adhesion molecules and central nervous system inflammation. *Semin. Neurosci.*, **4**, 201–11.

106. Prineas, J.W. (1979) Multiple sclerosis: presence of lymphatic capillaries and lymphoid tissue in the brain and spinal cord. *Science*, **203**, 1123–5.

107. Cross, A.H., Cannella, B., Brosnan, C.F. and Raine, C.S. (1990) Homing to central nervous system vasculature by antigen specific lymphocytes. 1. Localization of ^{14}C-labeled cells during acute, chronic and relapsing experimental allergic acute encephalomyelitis. *Lab. Invest.*, **63**, 162–70.

108. Suzuki, K., Andrews, J.M., Waltz, J.M. and Terry, R.D. (1969) Ultrastructural studies of multiple sclerosis. *Lab. Invest.*, **20**, 444–54.

109. Prineas, J.W. and Connell, F. (1979) Remyelination in multiple sclerosis. *Ann. Neurol.*, **5**, 22–31.

110. Capello, E., Voskuhl, R., McFarland, H.F. and Raine, C.S. (1995) A novel candidate antigen, X2 MBP, in multiple sclerosis (MS) lesions. *J. Neuropathol. Exp. Neurol.*, **54**, 464A.

111. Raine, C.S., Wu. E. and Brosnan, C.F. (1994) The immunologic response of the oligodendrocyte in the active multiple sclerosis lesion, in *A Multidisciplinary Approach to Myelin Diseases* (ed. S. Salvati), New York, Plenum, pp. 143–51.

112. Ghatak, H., Hirano, A., Doron, Y. and Zimmerman, H.M. (1973) Remyelination in MS with peripheral type myelin. *Arch. Neurol. (Chicago)*, **29**, 262–7.

113. Raine, C.S., Traugott, U. and Stone S.H. (1978) Glial bridges and Schwann cell invasion of the CNS during chronic demyelination. *J. Neurocytol.*, **7**, 541–53.

114. Moore, G.R.W., Neumann, P.E., Suzuki, K. *et al.* (1985) Balo's concentric sclerosis: new observations on lesion development. *Ann. Neurol.*, **17**, 604–11.

115. Massacesi, L., Genain, C.P., Lee-Parritz, D. *et al.* (1995) Actively and passively induced experimental autoimmune encephalomyelitis in common marmosets: a new model for multiple sclerosis. *Ann. Neurol.*, **37**, 519–30.

116. Wisniewski, H.N. and Keith, A.B. (1977) Chronic relapsing experimental allergic encephalomyelitis: an experimental model of multiple sclerosis. *Ann. Neurol.*, **1**, 144–7.

117. Stone, S.H., Snyder, D.H. and Raine, C.S. (1983) Adoptive transfer of experimental allergic encephalomyelitis from immature guinea pig donors. *J. Neurol. Sci.*, **60**, 401–9.

118. Pettinelli, C.B. and McFarlin, D.E. (1981) Adoptive transfer of experimental allergic encephalomyelitis in SJL/J mice after *in vitro* activation of lymph node cells by myelin basic protein. Requirement for Lyt 1⁺2⁻ T lymphocytes. *J. Immunol.*, **127**, 1420–3.

118a. Voskuhl, R.R., Pitchekian-Halibi, H., MacKenzie-Graham, A., McFarland, H.F. and Raine, C.S. (1996) Gender differences in autoimmune demyelination in the mouse: implications for multiple sclerosis. *Ann. Neurol.*, **39**, 724–33.

119. Lublin, F.D. (1985) Adoptive transfer of murine relapsing experimental allergic encephalomyelitis. *Ann. Neurol.*, **17**, 188–91.

120. Moore, G.R.W., McCarron, R.M., McFarlin, D.E. and Raine, C.S. (1987) Chronic relapsing necrotizing encephalomyelitis produced by myelin basic protein in mice. *Lab. Invest.*, **57**, 157–67.

121. Sakai, K., Tabira, T., Endoh, M. and Steinman, L. (1986) Ia expression in chronic relapsing experimental allergic encephalomyelitis induced by long-term cultured T cell lines in mice. *Lab. Invest.*, **54**, 345–51.

122. Fallis, R.J., Raine, C.S. and McFarlin, D.E. (1989) Chronic relapsing experimental allergic encephalomyelitis in SJL mice following the adoptive transfer of an epitope-specific T-cell line. *J. Neuroimmunol.*, **22**, 93–106.

123. Waksman, B.H., Porter, H., Lees, M.B., Adams, R.D. and Folch, J. (1954) A study of the chemical nature of components of bovine white matter effective in producing allergic encephalomyelitis in the rabbit. *J. Exp. Med.*, **100**, 451–71.

124. Yoshimura, T., Kunishita, T., Sakai, K. *et al.* (1985) Chronic experimental allergic encephalomyelitis in guinea pigs induced by proteolipid protein. *J. Neurol. Sci.*, **69**, 47–55.

125. Yamamura, T., Namikawa, T., Endoh, M., Kunishita, T. and Tabira, T. (1986) Experimental allergic encephalomyelitis induced by proteolipid apoprotein in Lewis rats. *J. Neuroimmunol.*, **12**, 143–9.

126. Endoh, M., Tabira, T., Kunishita, T. *et al.* (1986) DM-20, a proteolipid apoprotein, is an encephalitogen of acute and relapsing autoimmune encephalomyelitis in mice. *J. Immunol.*, **137**, 3832–5.

127. Trotter, J.L., Clark, H.B., Collins, K.G., Wegeschiede, C.L. and Scarpellini, J.D. (1987) Myelin proteolipid protein induces demyelinating disease in mice. *J. Neurol. Sci.*, **79**, 173–88.

128. Satoh, J., Sakai, K., Endoh, M. *et al.* (1987) Experimental allergic encephalomyelitis mediated by murine encephalitogenic T cell lines specific for myelin proteolipid apoprotein. *J. Immunol.*, **138**, 179–84.

129. Cross, A.H., Ishikawa, S., Raine, C.S. and Diamond, B. (1991) Autoimmune demyelination in transgenic E^d-alpha positive A.CA mice: comparison with E-negative A.CA mice. *Lab. Invest.*, **66**, 598–607.

130. Stanley, G.P. and Pender M.P. (1991) The pathophysiology of chronic relapsing experimental allergic encephalomyelitis in the rat. *Brain*, **114**, 1827–53.

131. Tsukada, N., Koh, C.-S., Yanagisawa, N. *et al.* (1987) A new model for multiple sclerosis: chronic experimental allergic encephalomyelitis induced by immunization with cerebral endothelial cell membrane. *Acta Neuropathol. (Berlin)*, **73**, 259–66.

132. Amor, S., Groome, N., Linington, C. *et al.* (1994) Identification of epitopes of myelin oligodendrocyte glycoprotein for the induction of EAE in SJL and Biozzi AB/H mice. *J. Immunol.*, **153**, 4349–56.

133. Johns, R.G., Kerlero de Rosbo, N., Menon, K.K. *et al.* (1995) Myelin oligodendrocyte glycoprotein induces a demyelinating encephalomyelitis resembling multiple sclerosis. *J. Immunol.*, **154**, 5536–41.

134. Raine, C.S., Traugott, U., Nussenblatt, R.B. and Stone, S.H. (1980) Optic neuritis and chronic relapsing experimental allergic encephalomyelitis: relationship to clinical course and comparison with multiple sclerosis. *Lab. Invest.*, **42**, 327–35.

135. Raine, C.S., Wisniewski, H. and Prineas, J. (1969) An ultrastructural study of experimental demyelination and remyelination. II. Chronic experimental allergic encephalomyelitis in the peripheral nervous system. *Lab. Invest.*, **21**, 316–27.

136. Prineas, J., Raine, C.S. and Wisniewski, H. (1969) An ultrastructural study of experimental demyelination and remyelination. III. Chronic experimental allergic encephalomyelitis in the central nervous system. *Lab. Invest.*, **27**,

137. Moore, G.R.W. and Raine, C.S. (1986) Leptomeningeal and adventitial gliosis as a consequence of chronic inflammation. *Neuropathol. Appl. Neurobiol.*, **12**, 371–8.

138. Moore, G.R.W., Traugott, U. and Raine, C.S. (1984) Survival of oligodendrocytes in chronic relapsing, autoimmune encephalomyelitis. *J. Neurol. Sci.*, **65**, 137–45.

139. Snyder, D.H., Hirano, A. and Raine, C.S. (1975) Fenestrated CNS blood vessels in chronic experimental allergic encephalomyelitis. *Brain Res.*, **100**, 645–9.

140. Raine, C.S., Brown, A.M. and McFarlin, D.E. (1982) Heterotopic regeneration of peripheral nerve fibres into the sub-arachnoid space. *J. Neurocytol.*, **11**, 109–18.

141. Raine, C.S. and Cross, A.H. (1989) Axonal dystrophy as a consequence of long-term demyelination. *Lab. Invest.*, **60**, 714–25.

142. Snyder, D.H., Valsamis, M.P., Stone, S.H. and Raine, C.S. (1975) Progressive and reparatory events in chronic experimental allergic encephalomyelitis. *J. Neuropathol. Exp. Neurol.*, **34**, 209–21.

143. Sobel, R.A., Blanchette, B.W., Bhan, A.K. and Colvin, R.B. (1984) The immunopathology of experimental allergic encephalomyelitis. II. Endothelial cell Ia increases prior to inflammatory cell infiltration. *J. Immunol.*, **132**, 2402–7.

144. Sobel, R.A., Natale, B.A. and Schneeberger, E.E. (1987) The immunopathology of acute experimental allergic encephalomyelitis. IV. An ultrastructural immunocytochemical study of class II major histocompatibility complex molecule (Ia) expression. *J. Neuropathol. Exp. Neurol.*, **46**, 239–49.

145. Lassmann, H., Vass, K., Brunner, Ch. and Seitelberger, F. (1986) Characterization of inflammatory infiltrates in experimental allergic encephalomyelitis. *Prog. Neuropathol.*, **6**, 33–62.

146. Raine, C.S. (1978) Pathobiology of demyelination, in *Physiology and Pathobiology of Axons* (ed. S.G. Waxman), New York, Raven, pp. 283–310.

147. Lampert, P.W. and Carpenter, S. (1965) Electron microscopic studies on the vascular permeability and the mechanisms of demyelination in experimental allergic encephalomyelitis. *J. Neuropathol. Exp. Neurol.*, **24**, 11–24.

148. Dal Canto, M., Wisniewski, H.M., Johnson, A.B., Brostoff, S.W. and Raine, C.S. (1975) Vesicular disruption of myelin in autoimmune demyelination. *J. Neurol. Sci.*, **24**, 313–19.

149. Pekovic, D., Traugott, U. and Raine, C.S. (1990) Increase in anti-astrocyte antibodies in the serum of guinea pigs during experimental autoimmune encephalomyelitis. *J. Neuroimmunol.*, **26**, 251–9.

150. Schluesener, H.J., Sobel, R.A., Linington, C. and Weiner, H.L. (1987) A monoclonal antibody against a myelin oligodendrocyte glycoprotein induces relapses and demyelination in central nervous system autoimmune disease. *J. Immunol.*, **139**, 4016–21.

151. Stone, S.H., Traugott, U. and Raine, C.S. (1983) Chronic experimental allergic encephalomyelitis in Strain 2 guinea pigs: sex dependence of clinical disease and absence of resistance to nervous system changes. *J. Neuroimmunol.*, **4**, 187–200.

152. Yednock, T.A. and Rosen, S.D. (1989) Lymphocyte homing. *Adv. Immunol.*, **44**, 313–78.

153. Cannella, B., Cross, A.H. and Raine, C.S. (1990) Upregulation and co-expression of adhesion molecules correlates with relapsing autoimmune demyelination in the central nervous system. *J. Exp. Med.*, **172**, 1521–4.

154. Cannella, B., Cross, A.H. and Raine, C.S. (1991) Adhesion-related molecules in the central nervous system: upregulation correlates with inflammatory cell influx during relapsing EAE. *Lab. Invest.*, **65**, 25–31.

155. Raine, C.S., Cannella, B., Duijvestijn, A.M. and Cross, A.H. (1990) Homing to central nervous system vasculature by antigen-specific lymphocytes. II. Lymphocyte/endothelial cell adhesion during the initial stages of autoimmune demyelination. *Lab. Invest.*, **63**, 476–89.

156. Skundric, D.S., Kim, C., Tse, H.-Y. and Raine, C.S. (1993) Homing of T cells to the central nervous system throughout the course of relapsing experimental autoimmune encephalomyelitis in Thy-1 congenic mice. *J. Neuroimmunol.*, **46**, 113–22.

157. Tabira, T. (1989) Cellular and molecular aspects of the pathomechanism and therapy of murine experimental allergic encephalomyelitis. *Crit. Rev. Neurobiol.*, **55**, 113–42.

158. Lang, W., Rodriguez, M., Lennon, V.A. and Lampert, P.W. (1984) Demyelination and remyelination in murine viral encephalomyelitis. *Ann. NY Acad. Sci.*, **436**, 98–102.

159. Rodriguez, M. and Lennon, V.A. (1990) Immunoglobulins promote remyelination in the central nervous system. *Ann. Neurol.*, **27**, 12–7.

160. Howell, M.D., Winters, S.T., Olee, T. *et al.* (1989) Vaccination against experimental allergic encephalomyelitis with T cell receptor peptides. *Science*, **246**, 668–70.

161. Sriram, S. and Steinman, L. (1983) Anti-I-A antibody suppresses active encephalomyelitis: treatment model for diseases linked to IR genes. *J. Exp. Med.*, **158**, 1362–7.

162. Sriram, S. and Roberts, C.A. (1986) Treatment of established chronic relapsing experimental allergic encephalomyelitis with anti-L3T4 antibodies. *J. Immunol.*, **136**, 4404–9.

163. Waldor, M.K., Mitchell, D., Kipps, R.J., Herzenberg, L.A. and Steinman, L. (1987) Importance of immunoglobulin isotope in therapy of experimental autoimmune encephalomyelitis with monoclonal anti-CD4 antibody. *J. Immunol.*, **139**, 3660–4.

164. Ruddle, N.H., Bergman, C.M., McGrath, M.L. *et al.* (1990) An antibody to lymphotoxin and tumor necrosis factor prevents experimental allergic encephalomyelitis. *J. Exp. Med.*, **172**, 1193–200.

165. Selmaj, K., Raine, C.S. and Cross, A, H. (1991) Anti-cytokine therapy abrogates autoimmune demyelination. *Ann. Neurol.*, **30**, 694–700.

166. Monastra, G., Cross, A.H., Bruni, A. and Raine, C.S. (1993) Phosphatidylserine, a putative inhibitor of tumor necrosis factor, prevents autoimmune demyelination. *Neurology*, **43**, 153–63.

167. Gijbels, K., Galardy, R.E. and Steinman, L. (1994) Reversal of experimental autoimmune encephalomyelitis with a hydroxamate inhibitor of matrix metalloproteases. *J. Clin. Invest.*, **94**, 2177–82.

168. Sommer, N., Löschmann, P.A., Northoff, G.H. *et al.* (1995) The antidepressant rolipram suppresses cytokine production and prevents autoimmune encephalomyelitis. *Nature Medicine*, **1**, 244–8.

169. Genain, C.P., Roberts, T., Davis, R.L. *et al.* (1995) Prevention of autoimmune demyelination in non-human primates by a cAMP-specific phosphodiesterase inhibitor. *Proc. Natl Acad. Sci. (USA)*, **92**, 3601–5.

170. Racke, M.K., Cannella, B., Albert, P. *et al.* (1992) Evidence of endogenous regulatory function of transforming growth factor β1 in experimental allergic encephalomyelitis. *Int. Immunol.*, **4**, 615–20.

171. Rott, W., Fleischer, B. and Cash, E. (1994) Interleukin-10 prevents experimental allergic encephalomyelitis in rats. *Eur. J. Immunol.*, **24**, 1434–40.

172. Racke, M.K., Bonomo, A., Scott, D.E. *et al.* (1994) Cytokine-induced immune deviation as a therapy for inflammatory autoimmune disease. *J. Exp. Med.*, **180**, 1961–6.

173. Yednock, E.A., Cannon, C., Fritz, L.C. *et al.* (1992) Prevention of experimental autoimmune encephalomyelitis by antibodies against α4β1 integrin. *Nature (Lond.)*, **356**, 63–6.

174. Welsh, C.T., Rose, J.W., Hill, K.E. and Townsend, J.J. (1993) Augmentation of adoptively transferred EAE by administration of a monoclonal antibody specific for LFA-1 alpha. *J. Neuroimmunol.*, **43**, 161–8.

175. Cannella, B., Cross, A.H. and Raine, C.S. (1993) Anti-adhesion molecule therapy in experimental autoimmune encephalomyelitis. *J. Neuroimmunol.*, **46**, 43–56.

176. Willenborg, D.O., Simmons, R.D., Tamatani, T. and Miyasaka, M. (1993) ICAM-1-dependent pathway is not critically involved in the inflammatory process of autoimmune encephalomyelitis or in cytokine-induced inflammation of the central nervous system. *J. Neuroimmunol.*, **45**, 147–54.

177. Archelos, J.J., Jung, S., Maurer, M. *et al.* (1993) Inhibition of experimental autoimmune neuritis by an antibody to the intercellular adhesion molecule ICAM-1. *Ann. Neurol.*, **34**, 145–54.

178. Stoolman, L.M. (1989) Adhesion molecules controlling lymphocyte migration. *Cell*, **56**, 907–10.

179. Gimbrone, M.A. Jr. and Bevilacqua, M.P. (1988) Vascular endothelium. Functional modulation at the blood interface, in *Endothelial Cell Biology* (eds N. Simionescu and M. Simionescu), New York, Plenum, pp. 255–73.

180. Raine, C.S. (1995) Multiple sclerosis: TNF revisited, with promise. *Nature Medicine*, **1**, 211–14.

16 THE PROPOSED VIRAL ETIOLOGY OF MULTIPLE SCLEROSIS AND RELATED DEMYELINATING DISEASES

Volker ter Meulen and Michael Katz

An infectious etiology of multiple sclerosis (MS) has been an attractive hypothesis because it fits both with a number of epidemiological observations and with pathological characteristics of this disorder. This concept was first enunciated more than a century ago and has been revived periodically ever since. Although all sorts of different microorganisms have been postulated as causative agents [1], none has thus far been identified as the culprit. Nevertheless, circumstantial evidence continues to point to the possibility of an infectious etiology of MS. Moreover, there is much information pertaining to other CNS diseases – both human and animal – indicating that viruses can induce demyelination, that they can persist for years in the CNS, and that they can be responsible for chronic diseases quite different from the better-known acute infections of the CNS [2].

In this chapter we present evidence for and against the hypothesis of viral etiology of MS. We also discuss the role of viruses in those other demyelinating diseases in which these agents do play a role. Because this subject has been reviewed extensively in the past, we have considered only the more recent findings in our attempt to analyze and interpret the mechanisms of viral etiology of demyelination.

16.1 Demyelinating diseases associated with a viral agent

Destruction of myelin with a relative sparing of axons is a distinct feature of a number of viral infections of the CNS. Although none of these disorders follows a clinical course of exacerbations and remissions or is characterized by neuropathological changes comparable to MS, they provide the best models to study the mechanisms by which viruses induce destruction of myelin in a manner so slow that the incubation period of the disease is very long.

16.1.1 VIRAL INFECTIONS OF ANIMALS

Visna infection of sheep

Clinical and neuropathological characteristics

Visna, an example of the slow virus infections, is a naturally occurring CNS disorder of sheep, characterized by an aberration of gait followed by paraplegia and eventually total paralysis. The disease can be transmitted experimentally from animal to animal. Its clinical course is variable, ranging from a slowly progressive one to one of rapid deterioration. It is devoid of classical signs of an acute virus infection. As neurological signs appear, there is an elevation of CSF protein, accompanied by a slight pleocytosis. Pathological examination reveals severe meningitis, choroiditis and intense infiltration of mononuclear cells in perivascular areas. Subventricular regions of the brain and white matter of the spinal cord are most severely affected. These changes are followed by patchy demyelination, most prominent in subependymal regions.

Pathogenesis

Visna virus is a member of the group of lentiviruses, which also includes the two human immunodeficiency viruses. The three viruses resemble one another in molecular organization, pathogenesis of the infection and interactions with host cells [3]. Visna virus contains an RNA-dependent DNA polymerase, which allows it to transfer genetic information to a DNA intermediate, or provirus. The provirus forms a plasmid in the cytoplasm of the infected cell, or is integrated into the genome of the host cell. This unusual replication cycle

Multiple Sclerosis: Clinical and pathogenetic basis. Edited by Cedric S. Raine, Henry F. McFarland and Wallace W. Tourtellotte. Published in 1997 by Chapman & Hall, London. ISBN 0 412 30890 8.

plays an important role in the development of the disease.

The main target of the virus in sheep is the monocyte/macrophage. The virus replication is coupled with the maturational stages of these cells [4]. Immature monocytes/macrophages contain only the provirus DNA, whereas mature cells synthesize viral RNA and infectious virus. Current data suggest that visna virus is transported to the CNS by infected monocytes that release the virus when they differentiate into mature macrophages. This leads to infection of microglia, the primary host cell in which the virus replicates in the CNS, as well as to a recruitment and proliferation of cytotoxic T lymphocytes. In tissue culture, these lymphocytes interact with infected macrophages, stimulating production of a variety of cytokines and a consequent enhancement of MHC class II expression of antigen-presenting cells. Presumably the same mechanisms operate within the CNS and are responsible for an intense, diffuse perivascular infiltration of the infected areas of the brain by cells among which lymphocytes and macrophages predominate. Demyelinating lesions and other forms of tissue damage may be the result of an attack by the cytotoxic T cells against virus-infected cells or of auto-antibodies that form in chronic lentiviral diseases [5].

Of particular significance in the development of disease is the humoral antiviral immune response that fails to control the infection. Effective neutralizing antibodies are found only in the minority of infected sheep and – at that – only in low titers [6]. *In vitro*, these antibodies have a low affinity for the virus and require a prolonged incubation to achieve neutralization. The neutralizing capacity of these antibodies is enhanced by the removal of sialic acid from the surface of the virus by treatment with neuraminidase. This indicates that the glycosylation pattern of glycoproteins in the viral envelope interferes with the neutralization. In addition to the relative ineffectiveness of the neutralizing antibodies, non-neutralizing antibodies actually enhance infection of the macrophages. These antibodies, produced in abundance in the infected animals, bind to the virus and provide an important second route into macrophages. This happens when the virus–antibody complex attaches to the Fc receptor on the surface of the macrophage and is taken up by endocytosis mediated by the Fc receptor [7].

In addition, a high mutation rate of lentiviruses leads to an antigenic variation of the virus, but the degree of its importance in the pathogenesis of these infections is not yet known. There is no evidence of cyclical episodes of visna and fully virulent antigenic variants have been isolated from sheep experimentally infected with plaque-purified virus. It is possible that antigenic variation is more important for the survival of the virus in nature, by allowing the development of mutants with variable tissue tropism, e.g. arthro- neuro- and pneumo-tropic viruses in sheep. Moreover, mutation and selection can lead to a change in virulence for different host species as has been shown in cross-infections by viruses derived from sheep and goats [8].

Canine distemper demyelinating encephalomyelitis

Clinical and neuropathological characteristics

Canine distemper is a widespread disease occurring naturally in dogs and other members of the canine family. The virus causing this disease belongs to the group of morbilliviruses and is related to measles and rinderpest viruses [9].

Infection of a susceptible dog with canine distemper virus (CDV) causes an acute or subacute disease. In rare instances this is followed by a demyelinating encephalomyelitis known as post distemper encephalitis or subacute diffuse sclerosing encephalitis. It is characterized by severe signs such as tremor, paralysis and convulsions, which can appear weeks or months after recovery from the acute infection [10], but can also occur without a preceding acute clinical illness. The lesions are either demyelinative or necrotic and they primarily affect white matter of the cerebellum, brain stem and spinal cord. The plaques show loss of myelin with a relative sparing of axons and presence of gitter cells. Perivascular cuffs of lymphocytes and macrophages are often found in the proximity of demyelinated plaques [11, 12]. Moreover, Cowdry type A intranuclear inclusion bodies containing nucleocapsids of distemper virus are also seen. A very rare variant of this disease can develop in aged, previously immunized dogs. It is known as 'old dog encephalitis' (ODE) or 'hard pad' disease [10].

Pathogenesis

Virological studies of brains from diseased animals have revealed CDV antigens as well as nucleocapsids characteristic of a paramyxovirus in glia and neurons [10]. Attempts to isolate infectious CDV from the brain tissue were successful only when cell cultures derived from brain were co-cultivated with indicator cells in a manner similar to that developed for subacute sclerosing panencephalitis (SSPE) [13]. Studies of pathogenesis of CDV-induced CNS disease have shown that virus antigen is present at first in macrophages and subsequently spreads to lymphocytes [10]. Viremia follows, but disappears when neutralizing antibodies are detected. At the same time, lymphocytopenia develops associated with a severely induced immunosuppression lasting 3–4 weeks. CDV reaches neuronal tissue either during the viremia or by being transported there by infected lymphocytes [14] before protective antibodies are detected. The virus probably infects oligodendroglial cells and establishes a state of persistent infection associated with virus-like structures detectable by electron microscopy, although most ultrastructural studies agree that oligodendroglial infection occurs but is very rare in natural distemper [11, 15].

Inoculation into dogs of a neurotropic CDV strain derived from a case of demyelinating distemper led to an acute or subacute encephalomyelitis [16] that allowed further pathogenetic studies. The acute form of the disease was characterized by focal demyelination without perivascular cuffing but with intranuclear inclusion bodies. The subacute disease has multifocal areas of demyelination with perivascular cuffing and viral inclusion bodies. Animals experienced a depression of the response of peripheral blood lymphocytes to mitogens, probably because these cells are infected by CDV. Antibodies to CDV and to CNS myelin are detected in the serum and CSF. The role they played in the pathogenesis of this disease remains to be determined [14, 17, 18].

This subacute demyelinating encephalomyelitis of dogs resembled SSPE morphologically, virologically and immunologically. Although CDV apparently reaches the CNS during the acute phase of canine distemper, the mechanism by which it induces demyelination in its chronic phase is far from understood. Inasmuch as the early demyelinative lesions occurred in this condition in the absence of inflammatory infiltrates, inflammation was probably not a requisite step in the induction of demyelination.

Murine coronavirus JHM infection in mice and rats

Virological and neuropathological characteristics

The JHM strain of the murine coronaviruses is a neurotropic variant of this large group of viruses infecting small rodents. These agents are enveloped RNA viruses with a surface characterized by club-shaped projections forming the so-called 'corona'. Virus is released from the infected cells by intra-cytoplasmic budding from which the particles derive an envelope from the host cell membrane [19] In mice, JHM virus induces an acute encephalomyelitis with prominent scattered demyelinated lesions [20]. The virus grows readily in neurons and oligodendrocytes and eventually kills most animals. The few survivors of acute infection develop a chronic progressive neurological disease, with the virus having established a persistent infection mainly in astrocytes. The lesions associated with this persistent infection consist of demyelinated plaques and areas infiltrated by lymphocytes and macrophages. As the disease progresses, demyelination and astrogliosis increase, whereas lymphocytic infiltration disappears. These lesions resemble somewhat the chronic plaques of MS (see Chapter 9).

JHM virus infection in weanling rats leads to an acute demyelinating panencephalitis with necrotic lesions distributed throughout most parts of the CNS [21]. Both neurons and oligodendroglia are affected. Virus particles are easily detectable by electron microscopy in both cell types. Intracellular virus-specific antigens can be detected by immunofluorescent staining. Infectious virus can be recovered from brain tissue of infected animals. In other animals, a subacute demyelinating encephalomyelitis (SDE) develops after an incubation period of 12–20 days. Brain lesions consist of a widespread loss of myelin with preservation of axons and neurons. Demyelinated plaques are distributed mostly in the deep cerebral white matter, optic chiasm, brain stem, mid-brain and spinal cord. There is perivascular cuffing by monocytes and plasma cells. However, in contrast to the acute CNS infection in SDE, virus particles and viral antigen are detectable only in oligodendroglia. Infectious virus can be isolated from the brains of these animals.

Pathogenesis

Studies in mice and rats indicate that the type of CNS disease and the nature of the lesions depend on the juxtaposition of the genetic make-up of the animal and the properties of the virus. In mice, a single gene, linked to the Svp-2 locus on chromosome 7, controls resistance to acute disease based on resistance of macrophages and neurons to infection with the JHM virus [22]. In addition, a second host gene of mice – which probably controls maturation of the antigen-presenting cells that play a role in a delayed type of hypersensitivity response – also influences development of disease [23].

Similar observations have been reported in rats. In Lewis rats, infection with JHM virus is followed by the development of a clinically apparent subacute demyelinating encephalomyelitis characterized pathologically by demyelinated plaques and perivascular cuffing. These changes are characteristic of an immunopathological reaction. In contrast, Brown Norway (BN) rats infected with JHM virus develop a clinically silent subacute demyelinating encephalomyelitis associated with the persistence of virus in the brain. This condition differs markedly from that in Lewis rats because the brain lesions are small, confined to the periventricular region, and do not enlarge as the disease progresses [24]. In Lewis rats, humoral immune response to JHM virus antigens in serum and CSF is minimal; in BN rats, it is quite pronounced [25]. In contrast, lymphocytes from infected rats respond quite strongly to JHM virus antigen in a proliferation assay in Lewis rats, but to a lesser degree in BN rats. In addition, Lewis rats develop a specific lymphocyte reaction to myelin basic protein (MBP) during the course of JHM virus infection which leads to experimental allergic encephalomyelitis (EAE) in adoptive transfer experiments [26]. This phenomenon does not develop in infected BN rats. These differences correlate with the differential susceptibility to EAE in these two rat strains. Lewis rats are very susceptible to EAE; BN rats are relatively resistant [27].

In infected mice no autoimmune reaction against brain antigens has been detected. The demyelinative lesion is associated with a virus-specific cell-mediated immune response, which can be prevented by immunosuppression [20]. Elimination of the virus from the CNS depends on the presence of both virus-specific CD4$^+$ and CD8$^+$ T lymphocytes. JHM virus-specific CD4$^+$ lymphocytes alone are able to protect mice from an otherwise lethal virus infection, but they do not prevent mononuclear cell infiltration of the CNS, or demyelination [28]. Only when such mice receive virus-specific CD8$^+$ T cells in adoptive transfer experiments is the virus removed from the CNS [29]. However, function of virus-specific CD8$^+$ T cells in the CNS requires the presence of CD4$^+$ T cells, as has been demonstrated by treatment of the infected animals with both anti-CD4 and anti-CD8 monoclonal antibodies [30].

Besides the genetic make-up of the host and the immune responses that underlie the pathogenesis of this infection, the biological properties of the virus play an important role in determining which one of the different possible disorders of the CNS develops. There are experimentally developed variants of JHM that infect preferentially glia, or neurons, or lack any neurotropism [31, 32]. Infection of animals with each of these variants has demonstrated that the intensity of demyelination varies directly with the increasing ability of the virus to replicate in the CNS and to infect large numbers of oligodendroglia. Moreover, it has been shown by a comparison of JHM variants that the surface proteins of the virus are major determinants of the pathogenic properties of the virus. A change in the S proteins of murine coronaviruses can lead to reduced neurovirulence, to a change in cell tropism, and to an increase in its demyelinative potential [33–35].

Among the neurological diseases associated with JHM infection, a relapsing subacute demyelinating encephalomyelitis in rats is particularly important as a possible experimental model of MS [36]. Most Lewis rats infected with JHM virus recover from their initial encephalomyelitis and remain healthy. However, weeks to months later, a few develop a CNS disease very similar to the original one. The course of this disease parallels to some extent chronic EAE or Theiler's virus infection in mice (Chapter 15). Brains of affected animals have fresh and old demyelinating lesions and astrocytes contain virus antigen. Although the mechanism of this subacute demyelinating encephalomyelitis with a remitting and relapsing course is not known, one can assume that it results from an interaction between viral and host factors. In particular, because animals infected with JHM virus develop a cell-mediated autoimmune reaction against MBP, it is likely that this has pathogenetic importance in the development of this subacute encephalitis.

Theiler's mouse encephalomyelitis viruses (TMEV)

Clinical, neuropathological and virological characteristics

TMEV are a group of mouse enteroviruses whose usual range of infectivity is limited to the gut. Rarely, they can also invade the CNS and cause an acute inflammation of the anterior horn cells, with a resultant flaccid paralysis that resembles poliomyelitis. In mice, experimental acute infection of the CNS follows within 20 days of intracerebral inoculation of either infected brain homogenates, or infected intestinal contents. Some animals survive the acute infection – even as virus persists in the CNS – recover from the paralysis and develop spastic paresis, urinary incontinence and priapism. This disease is characterized by demyelination with the preservation of axons, a picture resembling to some extent the plaques of MS. These pathologic characteristics make TMEV infection of mice a possible model of MS, for the following reasons: (a) pathological abnormalities are initially limited to the CNS, (b) demyelination, mediated by the immune system, follows after a prolonged incubation period, (c) infection is latent and persistent and (d) there are periods of remyelination and recurrences of demyelination [37, 38].

TMEV belong to the family of picornaviridae. All strains are cross-neutralized by polyclonal serum and are therefore considered members of one group. They are divided into two subgroups on the basis of their biological characteristics, persistent, or avirulent strains (TO, BeAn, and DA) and highly virulent strains (GDVII and FA). The former cause a chronic CNS disease, the latter a rapidly fatal acute encephalitis. The genomes of both subgroups have been sequenced. They show substantial genomic and protein homology [39]. Because of the differential biological properties of the strains, it has been possible to generate chimeric viruses that contain genomic mixtures of different strains or to isolate mutants that have reverted to an avirulent phenotype. Using these viruses it has been possible to map the regions of the genome associated with neurovirulence and persistence. It is the region coding for the capsid proteins that has the greatest influence on the phenotype of the new strains and helps to determine the nature of the infection and the disease that results [40–42]. In fact, a single amino acid change of the capsid protein VP2 determines the persistence of a chimeric Theiler's virus [43].

Pathogenesis

As is true for other viral infections, severity of the disease depends on both the strain of the virus and the genetics of the host. In addition, animal age at time of infection is also an important factor in the development of the chronic demyelinating disease.

The virus enters the CNS mainly along axons, or through endothelial cells across the blood–brain barrier [44]. In the CNS, neurons, glia and macrophage-like cells become infected and support replication of virus. Rapid destruction of infected cells – especially neurons – causes acute disease. In the chronic form of the disease, virus persists in the oligodendroglia, astrocytes and macrophage-like cells. Infectious virus has been isolated from demyelinated lesions [38, 45]. The mechanism of persistence remains unknown. Some data indicate that there is blocking of RNA replication at the level of minus RNA synthesis which may be initiated and maintained by interferon [46]. Other studies using Theiler's virus DA strain infection in inbred 129 Sv mice whose receptors for interferon α, β or γ had been inactivated by homologous recombination revealed a disease pattern supporting the hypothesis that the interferon gene is involved in the resistance or susceptibility to Theiler's virus persistence [47]. Another mechanism of persistence may be related to the generation of antigenic variants which occur *in vitro* in the presence of antibody relatively easily. Perhaps this also happens *in vivo* and allows the development of neutralization escape mutants [48].

Susceptibility of mice to demyelinating disease initiated by TMEV is dependent on MHC and non-MHC genes. In the MHC genes, the region maps to the class I locus H-2D, whereas the relevant non-MHC genes have been identified on chromosomes 3 and 6 [49, 50]. Although a precise pathogenetic role for the MHC association is not known, it is reasonable to assume that the H-2D gene is involved in the presentation of viral antigens to MHC class I restricted CD8$^+$ cytotoxic T cells. If this were true and the antigen presentation were therefore impaired in mice susceptible to chronic demyelinating disease, infected cells would not be destroyed and virus would persist and eventually cause the disease. This hypothesis is supported by experimental evidence. If CD8$^+$ T cells are depleted *in vivo* by specific monoclonal antibodies, virus clearance during acute infection is delayed and the proportion of animals that develops demyelinating disease increases [51]. It is apparent, therefore, that virus-specific CD8$^+$ T cells are not essential for recovery from acute infection. In contrast, depletion of CD4$^+$ T cells leads to an overwhelming acute and lethal infection of the CNS [52]. Death can be prevented by the administration of neutralizing antibodies against TMEV. This suggests that CD4$^+$ T cells play an important helper role in the synthesis of anti-viral antibodies by B lymphocytes. Little else is known about the activity of CD4$^+$ T cells in this infection except that if their function is suppressed in infected mice shortly before onset of clinical signs, there is a reduction in the incidence of demyelinating disease. It is likely therefore that these T cells directly damage infected glial cells; they may also take part in a delayed-type hypersensitivity reaction (DTH) detectable only in mouse strains in which the virus causes disease. No autoimmune CD4$^+$ T cells have been found in diseased animals [53], but antibodies to myelin [38, 54] and proteolipid protein [55], have been detected. Whether these autoantibodies influence the course of the disease is unknown.

TMEV infection in mice is a reasonable experimental model for certain aspects of human MS because its demyelination and remyelination resemble remissions and exacerbations of MS. However, persistence of an infectious virus, its ready isolation from brain and absence of autoimmune CD4$^+$ T cells, are major differences between this mouse model and human MS.

16.1.2 HUMAN VIRAL INFECTIONS

Subacute sclerosing panencephalitis (SSPE)

Clinical, neuropathological and virological characteristics

SSPE is a rare, slowly evolving disease of the CNS, primarily of children and young adults [56]. Clinically, the condition begins with subtle intellectual deterioration, gradual appearance of incoordination and other motor abnormalities followed by myoclonic jerks, coma and death. The course of the disease varies from months to years. Patients with SSPE have exceptionally high antibody titers – in the serum and CSF – to all measles virus structural proteins except one. The exception is the membrane (M) protein. This immune response is unique and stands in contrast to host response in all other diseases associated with measles virus. CSF of SSPE patients has an abnormally high concentration of IgG, but its content of all other proteins is normal. IgG exhibits restricted banding on electrophoresis, indicative of specific oligoclonal population of measles antibodies. This implies that these antibodies are produced within the CNS by sensitized lymphocytes that have invaded this compartment and is a reflection of a hyperimmune state.

The characteristic lesions in the CNS are perivascular cuffing with lymphocytes and plasma cells, and a diffuse infiltration by these cells of the gray and white matter. The most striking feature is an enormous increase in hypertrophic astrocytes, which form a dense network of fibers throughout the CNS. There is extensive demyelination. A few neurons and many glia contain intranuclear Cowdry type A and B inclusion bodies, which are positive for measles virus-specific antigens in an immunofluorescence test. Electron microscopy reveals these inclusion bodies to contain nucleocapsids resembling those of a paramyxovirus. Measles antigen is present not only in the cells with intranuclear inclusion bodies but also in others – neurons and oligodendroglia – that have a normal morphology, where it is found in cytoplasm. No viruses, viral budding, or giant cells have been seen. Absence of such 'classic' cytopathic effects of measles virus suggests that in the CNS measles virus replicates in a manner different from that in other organs. Indeed, all attempts to isolate infectious virus from brain tissue of SSPE patients failed until brain cells grown in culture were co-cultivated or fused with continuous cell lines susceptible to measles virus. The virus isolates obtained (referred to as SSPE viruses), were subsequently compared with the known strains of measles viruses but no major genetic or functional differences between them have been found [56].

Pathogenesis

SSPE develops as a consequence of infection with measles virus. This conclusion is based on the aforementioned facts: detection of paramyxovirus structures and measles virus antigen in brain tissue, occasional isolation of virus – albeit by indirect means – from brain tissue, and the hyperimmune response of the host to this virus. Because measles is a common infection and SSPE is quite rare, it must be assumed that some additional factors are required for SSPE to develop. These could be related to the host or to the agent. Among other factors, the young age of the patient at the time of the initial infection with measles and rural residence – allowing perhaps for a co-infection with a zoonotic agent – have been suggested. Whatever the factors, it is obvious that during the initial infection, virus must escape the host's immunological defense mechanisms during acute measles and somehow persist until – after a long incubation period – the neurological disease develops. An explanation of what these factors are is not at hand and various hypotheses relating to the pathogenesis of SSPE have been proposed [56].

During acute measles, the virus interacts with the host's immune system. A direct cytopathic effect has been demonstrated in the thymus and lymph nodes which exhibit giant cells [57]. There is also a functional corollary in the anergy to the tuberculin test that measles induces. Ordinarily, the host recovers from acute measles infection and gains life-long immunity. However, measles in children with T cell deficiency – congenitally acquired or iatrogenic – is often accompanied by fatal complications, including CNS infections. On the other hand, children with agammaglobulinemia have the same pattern of recovery as do normal children. One must conclude that an intact cell-mediated immune system is necessary for a complete recovery from acute measles, whereas humoral immune response plays no significant role in recovery.

Recent studies have concentrated on the analysis of virus–host cell interactions within SSPE brain tissue. They have revealed that gene expression of measles virus is restricted at several stages, as follows. The viral envelope proteins are markedly underexpressed or absent in infected brain cells [58]. Transcriptional efficiency of the corresponding mRNAs is reduced, leading to a steep expression gradient for virus-specific monocistronic transcripts with an increased rate of bicistronic transcripts in some cases [59–61]. *In vitro* translation experiments with mRNA directly isolated from brain tissue, or with a synthetic transcript obtained from isolated genes, revealed that at least some of these mRNAs are biologically inactive or that they direct synthesis of truncated proteins [62, 63]. Sequence analysis of the isolated mRNAs has demonstrated that stop codons leading to premature termination of translation have been introduced into the corresponding genes by non-silent mutations [64]. In addition, extensive sequence analysis performed on measles virus genes cloned directly from brain tissue of patients with SSPE, or measles inclusion body encephalitis, or from persistently infected cell lines, has revealed a biased hypermutation which led to an exchange of up to 50% of the C residues to U. This was particularly prominent in the M gene [65, 66]. These hypermutations have been linked to the action of a cellular duplex RNA dependent adenosine deaminase (DRADA) activity [67], which has been found in nuclear and cytoplasmic extracts of human neural cells [68]. It is suggestive that a selective advantage for the virus spread in the CNS seems to be associated with the abrogation of M protein function since a prevalence of one of five mutated M genes was found in different brain regions of SSPE patients [69].

These studies demonstrate that measles virus replication in the CNS tissue is defective because of an altered transcription and translation, especially that concerning the viral envelope genes. Thus, when there is no synthesis of measles virus envelope proteins, no virus particles can be formed and cell fusion does not take place. Furthermore, these findings show that infected cells escape immune recognition and elimination, because host antibodies do not encounter envelope proteins in their membranes and fail to recognize that they are infected. However, as internal viral proteins are expressed, functionally unimpaired measles virus infection is maintained by an intact replicative complex consisting of viral RNA, the nucleocapsid-, phospho- and large proteins. This complex probably spreads to neighboring cells by axonal transport through synaptic clefts. Still unexplained is why virus-specific T cells do not destroy infected brain cells, even as they recognize viral nucleocapsid protein present [70].

Although molecular characterization of the mechanism of measles virus persistence in SSPE has shed light on certain aspects of the pathogenesis of this disease, several unresolved problems remain. In particular, it is not known how and when measles virus enters the CNS, what factors determine the long incubation period between the primary measles infection and SSPE, and what ultimately triggers the disease process. The answers to these questions hold clues not only to the pathogenesis of SSPE but also to that of other persistent viral infections.

Progressive multifocal leukoencephalopathy (PML)

Clinical and neuropathological characteristics

PML is an uncommon subacute demyelinating disease. It has a myriad of different neurological symptoms depending on the location of the CNS lesions [71]. Such signs as ataxia, paralysis, intellectual deterioration and sensory abnormalities are progressive and usually lead to death within one year. PML occurs in conditions associated with defective cellular immunity. These include malignancies, especially lymphomas, chronic leukemias and other tumors of the reticuloendothelial system, granulomatous inflammation, diabetes mellitus and treatment with immunosuppressive drugs. PML has been reported in 3–5% of patients with AIDS [72]. There are a few cases on record without any apparent predisposing condition.

The neuropathological changes consist of non-inflammatory multifocal demyelinated lesions associated with a human papovavirus. Plaques are found scattered throughout the white matter, and there is loss of oligodendroglia and myelin. Oligodendroglia in the periphery of the plaques are often enlarged and contain intranuclear inclusion bodies filled with papovavirus particles. Immunofluorescent staining of frozen sections demonstrates papovavirus antigen in the nuclei of cells within and around the lesions. There are also multinucleated astrocytes with abnormal mitotic figures and bizarre chromatin patterns. To some extent, these cell formations resemble neoplasia.

Pathogenesis

Two strains of papovavirus, JC virus and SV40/PML virus, have been recovered from brains of patients with PML. Overwhelming evidence points to the JC human papovavirus as the principal cause of PML [73]. JC virus is widespread in human populations. It causes mainly a subclinical infection. Sero-epidemiological studies have shown that about 65% of a sample population acquire antibodies to JC virus by the age of 14. This proportion rises only slightly to 70–80% in older age groups. Thus, subclinical JC infection apparently takes place mostly during childhood and the virus is readily transmitted, but its source is unknown.

It is of interest that JC virus is detectable in the urine of women during pregnancy, but it could not be isolated from the placenta, or from the urine of the neonate [74]. These data permit an inference that blunting of the immune response in pregnancy facilitates replication of the previously dormant JC virus. In situ hybridization has detected JC viral DNA in kidney tissue of patients with PML and in individuals who did not have PML. Virus was most concentrated in epithelial cells of the distal tubules. This suggests that the kidney is the locus of persistent JC virus [75].

The full pathogenic potential of this highly prevalent virus is not known. Thus far, the only disease attributable to the JC virus is PML. In PML, the number of viral particles in the brain is large. Estimates by electron microscopy and biochemical analysis indicate that there are approximately 10^{10} virus particles per gram of brain tissue where lesions occur [76]. Oligodendrocytes appear to be the main target cells in this CNS infection. Viral antigen, detectable by immunofluorescent staining, is concentrated mainly within the nuclei of oligodendroglia, but only rarely in astrocytes. Oligodendroglia probably represent a permissive cell population that allows virus replication. In contrast, giant astrocytes are probably non-permissive and instead of supporting growth of the virus, become transformed. Indeed, such a differential response was shown in vitro when human fetal glia and astrocytes in culture were infected with the papovavirus SV40. The glia became lysed, but the astrocytes underwent transformation [77]. Moreover, intracerebral inoculation of JC virus to experimental animals produces brain tumors such as medulloblastomas, glioblastomas, ependymomas and pineocytomas [78]. This is consistent with the clinical findings of brain tumors in a few patients with PML. Efforts to identify an association of JC virus with human brain tumors such as astrocytoma, meningioma or glioblastoma by Southern blot analysis or PCR have thus far not shown incriminating virus-specific DNA sequences.

No information about the origin of the infection in PML is available but it is conceivable that either the virus persists after primary infection and becomes activated when the immune system is impaired, or patients who develop PML may be the seronegative minority who acquire the infection during the period of immunodeficiency. In addition, JCV has been found in lymphocytes which might carry virus to the brain once activated [79].

However, acquisition of immunodeficiency alone, with the consequent exacerbation of the persistent JC virus, may not be the entire explanation of the pathogenesis of PML. With the 70–80% prevalence of antibodies to the JC virus in the population at large and the frequency of acquired immunosuppression also being high, it is difficult to explain why PML is so rare.

The difficulties of growing JC virus under laboratory conditions and failure to transmit PML by inoculation of JC virus or SV40 PML virus to various laboratory animals, has limited study of the pathogenesis of this disease. Recently an oligodendrocyte-specific expression of JC viral constructs in transgenic mice was accomplished that led to dysmyelination [80]. The data suggest that JC virus T antigens arrest the maturation of oligodendrocytes at an early stage of development. JC virus, therefore, not only destroys infected oligodendroglia as in PML, but must also be considered a potential contributor to demyelination by mechanisms other than cell lysis.

HTLV-I associated myelopathy/tropical spastic paraparesis

A neurological disease of uncertain etiology, which has borne many names in the past, has recently been termed HTLV-I associated myelopathy (HAM)/tropical spastic paraparesis (TSP). Its prevalence is limited mainly to certain tropical regions.

TSP was first described in Jamaica in 1956 and was followed by reports from Martinique, Colombia, Peru, the Seychelles, and various parts of Africa and India [81]. An apparently similar condition was reported in Japan as 'chronic myelopathy' [82]. Except for the tropical climate of most of the areas where the disease was reported, no common factors that would explain the geographic distribution of this condition have been identified. Ultimately it was shown that both diseases were associated with the human T cell leukemia virus type I (HTLV-I) [83, 84] and that they were essentially the same disorder [85]. These findings bear an important relevance to MS, because patients afflicted with TSP resemble a subgroup of MS patients with chronic progressive myelopathy.

Clinical and neuropathological characteristics

The onset of HAM/TSP is gradual in most patients, but some present with an acute episode resembling transverse myelitis [86]. In the usual case, paraparesis is asymmetric. Other symptoms include weakness of legs, back pain, dysesthesias and paresthesias. Dysfunction of sphincters and impotence are common. Progression is slow, the early deficits remaining stable for periods of years. Physical examination is consistent with asymmetric paraparesis, or even paraplegia, accompanied by increased deep tendon reflexes and extensor plantar responses. There is no sensory deficit and no intellectual deterioration. Except for a few reported cases in which retrobulbar neuropathy and deafness were noted, cranial nerves have not been affected. Rarely, cerebellar signs have been seen. Occasionally, patients with HAM/TSP also have sicca syndrome, rheumatoid-like arthropathy or a lymphocytic alveolitis.

The main histopathological feature is a chronic progressive inflammatory process involving both gray and white matter of the spinal cord, with the inflammatory changes consisting of perivascular cuffing by lymphocytes, plasma cells and histiocytes as well as parenchymal infiltrates [87]. New lesions with little parenchymal damage comprise mainly lymphocytes of the CD4+ lineage and monocytes. Older lesions, showing diffuse gliosis, characteristically contain lipid-rich macrophages and CD8+ lymphocytes in the parenchyma and perivascular spaces. CD4+ lymphocytes and monocytes are relatively few within these lesions [87–89]. As the disease progresses, there is fibroblastic thickening of the meninges, astrocytic gliosis and degeneration of long tracts. These changes are mainly found in the spinal cord, but are seen also in the midbrain, cerebellum and even the cerebrum. Distinct plaques characteristic of MS have not been described, but loss of myelin with some preservation of axons has been observed. It must be noted that, similar to what is seen in MS, the neuropathological lesions depend on the duration of the disease. If the clinical history dates back only a few years, inflammatory changes coexist with degeneration. If the disease has lasted four or more years, there are fewer inflammatory cells and their numbers continue to decrease, whereas degenerative changes increase. In patients who survive HAM/TSP 10 years or longer, the white matter presents a picture of uniform degeneration with a virtual absence of the inflammatory cells [90].

Viral pathogenesis

Genetically, HTLV-I is closely related to the animal leukemia viruses. Moreover, it contains the three characteristic genes of the retroviruses that encode for the core protein Gag, the polymerase Pol and the envelope protein Env, as well as two additional genes *Tax* and *Rex*, which are important for viral transcription. *Tax* stimulates the production of new viral RNA and *Rex* controls the splicing of viral mRNA. *In vivo*, the target cells for HTLV-I infection are CD4+ lymphocytes which in the adult T cell leukemia (ATLL) are transformed. Although the mechanism of this transformation is not known, ATLL results from the malignant proliferation of one or a few cell clones. The sites of provirus integration in the host cell genome are random, indicating that the juxtaposition of the provirus with an oncogene is not required. The transactivator protein Tax of the virus does play an important role in oncogenesis, because it can act on any region of the genome [91].

There are three important modes of transmission of HTLV-I:

1. Perinatal and neonatal infection from a seropositive mother, with breast feeding being an important factor [92–94].
2. Direct transmission, particularly by male-to-female during sexual intercourse [92].
3. Transmission by infected blood in a transfusion or through the sharing of needles by drug addicts [95].

In all instances, virus is transmitted predominantly by infected cells, because cell-free virus is rare and not very infectious.

After exposure to HTLV-I, the patient usually develops antibodies that recognize the viral proteins. The diagnosis depends on the detection of these antibodies in an immunofluorescence test, ELISA or Western blot. In addition, in about 50% of infected persons, antibody to the Tax protein is also detectable. Rare individuals who lack the characteristic immune response carry HTLV-I nucleic acid or have antibodies to Tax protein only. The significance of this variation remains obscure. Patients with HAM/TSP usually have higher antiviral titers than do the healthy carriers. However, no significant correlation has been observed between the duration of illness and titers of anti-HTLV-I antibodies. The CSF profile in HAM/TSP resembles that in MS. Most patients have a moderate pleocytosis in the spinal fluid. There is a moderate increase of protein in about half of the patients and the elevated IgG – determined by isoelectric focusing – is of oligoclonal origin [85, 96].

The pathogenesis of HAM/TSP is still uncertain. There is no evidence from molecular biological analysis of the viruses isolated from ATLL and HAM/TSP patients that they have any determinants of neurotropism. HTLV-I sequence analyses of PBMC of HAM/TSP patients have shown a pattern of polyclonal integration. ATLL patients, by contrast, have an oligoclonal or monoclonal pattern. Moreover, HAM/TSP patients have a much larger population of infected cells and a stronger antiviral immune response than HTLV-I carriers, suggesting a failure of the immune system to contain the spread of the virus. Because spinal cord lesions are associated with invading inflammatory cells – including macrophages and T cells – and there is up-regulation of MHC and cytokine molecules, it is likely that the pathogenesis of the CNS lesion is based on an immunologic host reponse [89, 97]. This hypothesis is consistent with the activated T cell state and increased levels of interleukin 2 receptor (IL-2R) on lymphocytes as well as presence of soluble IL-2R in the serum of these patients. This is probably related to the phenomenon of spontaneous lymphoproliferation in vitro [98]. Moreover, T cell receptor Vβ gene sequences from lymphocytes in spinal cord lesions reveal unique and restricted CDR3 motifs, similar to those described in T cells from brain lesions of MS patients and rats with EAE [99]. Additional evidence is based on the isolation of a large number of cytotoxic T lymphocytes recognizing HTLV-I Tax proteins from PBMC of HAM/TSP patients. This finding supports the notion that these CD8+ lymphocytes are involved in immune-mediated destruction of the nerve cells [100–102]. However, the target for these CTLs is currently unknown since it has not been possible to isolate or convincingly demonstrate the presence of HTLV-I antigen or mRNA in diseased CNS cells, even though proviral DNA can be detected by the polymerase chain reaction (PCR) [103, 104]. The only current evidence of the presence of virus has been derived from in situ hybridization using an HTLV-I Tax RNA probe capable of detecting viral RNA in sections of spinal cord and cerebellum. It is significant that it was detected in cells carrying astrocyte markers, but not cells in perivascular inflammatory areas [105]. This identification of HTLV-I RNA in the white matter of HAM/TSP patients corresponds to the histopathological changes and therefore suggests that in addition to tissue damage by immune mechanisms, there is demyelination induced directly by the virus itself.

Recently, a potentially useful model of the disease was produced after inoculation of neonatal rats with human lymphoid cells persistently infected with HTLV-I [106]. After 16 months, the rats developed spastic paraparesis and urinary incontinence. They exhibited lesions in the CNS characteristic of HAM/TSP in a distribution corresponding to human disease. This model may aid researchers and clinicians in understanding the disease process involved in HAM/TSP.

Parainfectious encephalomyelitis

Clinical and neuropathological characteristics

Parainfectious encephalomyelitis occurs as a complication of an acute virus infection. It is a demyelinating condition most frequently associated with measles virus, varicella-zoster virus, influenza virus and respiratory tract infections of unspecified, probably viral, cause. It has also been reported after vaccinations against smallpox and rabies.

Parainfectious encephalomyelitis in association with measles is a good example of this condition. It can occur shortly before, during, or after clinical measles. Its incidence has been estimated as 0.5 per 1000 reported cases of measles and its case fatality rate as 20% [107]. The neuropathological changes seen depend on the stage of the disease during which the patient died. An acute form, or necrotizing hemorrhagic encephalitis, is characterized by necrotic lesions, infiltration by neutrophilic polymorphonuclear leukocytes, and fibrinoid degeneration of blood vessel walls. A more common variety is not as destructive and is less acute. In such cases there is marked perivenular mononuclear infiltration associated with focal demyelination.

Pathogenesis

Although there is a direct association of various forms of demyelinative encephalomyelitides with viral infection, pathogenesis of these diseases remains substantially unknown. The virus responsible for the acute infection usually cannot be isolated from brain tissue by standard direct methods of virus isolation. Even when a virus is isolated, its origin can remain controversial. For example, in parainfectious measles encephalomyelitis, virus was reported to be isolated from the CSF and from the brain [108]. However, the possibility that it was derived from infected lymphocytes could not be excluded. Moreover, some patients in the past considered to have 'post-infectious encephalitis' may in fact have had progressive encephalomyelitis now recognized as 'measles inclusion body encephalitis', usually seen in immunodeficient patients [109].

In parainfectious measles encephalomyelitis, all attempts to demonstrate measles virus footprints in various tissues obtained post mortem have failed [110]. This supports the hypothesis that the development of measles encephalomyelitis is not the consequence of viral replication in CNS tissue, but rather a result of a host response through an immune process. There is much indirect evidence in support of this conclusion. Measles virus encephalitis usually has an abrupt onset and a monophasic course. A large proportion of patients show spontaneous suppressor cell activity, elevation of C-reactive proteins, high serum IgG levels and a lymphocyte proliferative response in the presence of myelin basic protein [111, 112], in a manner analogous to what happens in experimental allergic encephalomyelitis (EAE.) Moreover, IgE is persistently elevated and soluble IL-2 receptor is reduced compared to patients with uncomplicated measles [113, 114]. Finally, the histological findings resemble those of EAE. Because measles virus has lymphoid tissue tropism and a profound effect on immune regulation [115], it is assumed that this interaction leads to an inappropriate immune response to host own tissue, even though there is no direct viral infection of neural cells. Patients may experience an autoimmune disease, because measles virus has abrogated immune tolerance to autoantigens.

On the other hand, functional analysis of T lymphocytes cloned from the CSF of one case of measles encephalitis has demonstrated measles-specific CD8+ T lymphocytes that reacted specifically in a cytotoxic lymphocyte (CTL) assay with target cells infected with autologous measles virus [116]. These data indicate that cells in inflammatory exudates in cases of measles encephalitis have a high degree of measles virus antigen specificity. Whether these cells recognize brain cells infected with virus or react with autoantigens because of molecular mimicry is unknown [117].

16.2 Evidence for a possible viral etiology in MS

16.2.1 EPIDEMIOLOGICAL STUDIES

The major support for a possible viral etiology in MS derives from epidemiological studies that implicate environmental factors encountered years prior to disease onset. The data consist mainly of curves of age-specific onset, geographic distribution of the disease, studies of migration and familial clustering. An analysis of this information has led to the hypothesis that an infectious agent to which an MS patient is exposed at or shortly after puberty is responsible for the disease. Although this point of view has been widely accepted, it has also been challenged.

16.2.2 EVIDENCE BASED ON SEROLOGIC STUDIES

The search for a viral etiologic agent in MS has also taken an indirect route. Sera and CSF of patients have been examined for virus-specific antibodies and compared with those of control populations. Thus Adams and Imagawa [118] and others [107] were the first to suggest that measles virus is such an agent in MS. These authors assessed measles-neutralizing, complement-fixing and hemagglutination-inhibiting antibodies in serum and CSF specimens. They found slightly higher titers in patients with MS than in controls. These early observations were followed by numerous reports from other groups, which basically confirmed the original observations, although there were a few negative reports (reviewed by Norrby [119]. Further studies indicated that measles antibodies were not the only ones elevated in MS. Higher antibody titers against such viruses as mumps, parainfluenza 1, influenza C, herpes simplex, varicella-zoster, rubella, vaccinia, Epstein–Barr and paramyxovirus SV5, were also noted (for reviews see [119, 120]). In addition, there were studies that showed high antibody titers to more than one virus and to bacterial antigens [121–123]. However, these findings were not uniformly accepted, because others did not find differences in antibody titers to various viruses in MS and control patients (for reviews see [119, 124]).

It is important to determine what the antibodies in the CSF represent. They may be simply a 'spill-over' of circulating serum antibodies whenever the titer is high. They may be a consequence of a damaged blood–brain barrier, or they may be produced locally within the CNS as a consequence of invasion by lymphocytes. It is possible to determine which of these mechanisms is responsible in any particular case. Serological testing of paired serum and CSF samples from MS patients and controls permits a comparison of the two titers in relation to various viral antigens, total CSF protein and IgG content. The last is analyzed for its heterogeneity. Antibodies to heterogeneous clones are likely to have been transferred directly from the serum. Those of restricted heterogeneity – the oligoclonal antibodies – are likely to have been produced locally in the CNS [125]. Oligoclonal IgG bands in the CSF are not uniquely confined to MS patients. They have been demonstrated in CSF and serum specimens from control patients with different neurological diseases, with and without demyelination, infectious or non-infectious [126, 127].

A comparative analysis of the origin of antibodies was first applied to patients with SSPE. It demonstrated local production of measles antibodies within the CNS [128]. The same type of studies showed that in MS patients there is local production of antibodies against measles, rubella, mumps, herpes simplex and parainfluenza type 1 viruses (for reviews see [119, 127]). These results were not as consistent as those in SSPE. Although measles virus antibodies were found in the majority of studied cases, antibodies to other viruses were also detected, but less frequently.

Retroviruses were also suggested as possible etiologic agents in MS, because in an ELISA or Western blot analysis, antibodies reactive with Gag proteins of HTLV-I were demonstrated in specimens from MS patients in Sweden, in Key West, Florida, USA, and in Japan [129–131]. Since these findings have not been confirmed by many other investigators [132–136], the significance of the original findings has been dismissed.

Although presence of IgG antiviral antibodies of a restricted heterogeneity – and therefore produced locally – in the CSF has been considered evidence supporting a viral etiology of MS (reviewed by Johnson [1]), quantitative analysis casts a substantial doubt on this conclusion. When oligoclonal IgG of MS patients was analyzed by preparatory electrophoresis in agarose gel and by the imprint immunofixation method [123, 126, 137–140], only a small fraction of the total was found to have virus-specific activity. This is in dramatic contrast to what is found, for example, in SSPE or neurosyphilis [141, 142], in which the majority of the oligoclonal bands contain antibodies specific for the causative agent. Without an identified specificity of these antibodies for a particular agent, their importance cannot be assessed and the assignment of an etiologic role to a particular agent is impossible. It is more likely that the immune response detectable in the CSF of MS patients represents a non-specific polyclonal activation of B lymphocytes by mitogens or lymphokines.

16.2.3   VIRUS ISOLATION ATTEMPTS AND THE SEARCH FOR VIRUS STRUCTURES IN CNS TISSUE

During the past half century there have been claims of the isolation of a virus from tissues of MS patients. In parallel with these reports, transmission of MS to primates and smaller animals has also been reported. None of these reports has withstood the test of time. It is likely that at least in some of the cases these putative isolations merely reflected the presence of endogenous viruses.

Although most of the reported agents have been discounted from consideration in the analysis of the etiology and pathogenesis of MS a few remain candidate viruses (Table 16.1). One of these is measles, a highly infectious virus. Before the development of a measles vaccine, measles infected most people, the only exceptions being those who lived in ecological isolation. The virus can establish persistence, both in tissue culture and *in vivo*, as is the case in SSPE. By analogy, therefore, it has also been sought in patients with MS. Cytoplasmic tubular structures, resembling measles nucleocapsids, were claimed to have been found in astrocytes of one MS patient. Explant of this patient's brain tissue developed a cytopathic effect, which could be prevented by pretreatment with anti-measles serum [149]. This work has not been confirmed.

Using the technique of *in situ* hybridization, measles virus-specific RNA has been detected in scattered cells in brain tissue, not only of MS patients, but also of controls who did not have MS [150]. Support for this observation came from a different study in which single-stranded 35S-labeled RNA probes prepared against measles virus genomic RNA sequences revealed measles virus genes of nucleocapsid protein, phosphoprotein and fusion protein in foci of hybridization, equally in some MS brains as well as non-MS controls [151]. An inescapable conclusion from these studies is that measles virus can persist in human brain, but that it is not necessarily etiologically linked to MS. Moreover, other investigators failed to detect any measles virus genetic information in MS brains [164–166].

Organs other than brain have also been sampled in MS patients and screened for the presence of measles virus. Measles virus antigen has been detected in the jejunal tissue in 23 of 24 MS patients [167]. In a later study of the same group of patients, a paramyxovirus – presumably measles – was recovered, by co-cultivation or cell-fusion technique, from jejunal biopsy specimens of several MS cases; there was a similar subsequent report from Japan [168, 169]. Both groups used immunofluorescence techniques to detect measles virus antigen in the jejunal tissue, as well as hemadsorption and electron microscopy for the detection of paramyxovirus structures. Attempts by other laboratories to confirm

Table 16.1   Summary of reports suggesting in viral causality of MS

Virus	Evidence of association	Reference
Rabies virus	Isolation from blood and CSF of two MS patients	Margulis et al., 1946 [143]
Herpes simplex virus	Isolation in TC from MS brain homogenate Increased CSF antibody titers	Gudnadottir et al., 1964 [144] Norrby, 1978 [119]
Scrapie agent	Development of scrapie in sheep after i.c. inoculation of MS brain	Field et al., 1962 [145] Palsson, et al., 1965 [146]
Parainfluenza virus 1	Isolation in TC after cell fusion of brain cells from two MS patients	ter Meulen et al., 1972 [147]
Multiple sclerosis associated agent	Decrease of blood polymorphonuclear cells in mice following inoculation of MS brain	Carp et al., 1972 [148]
Measles virus (MV)	Development of MV-CPE in TC after inoculation of MS brain homogenate	Field et al., 1972 [149]
	MV-RNA detected by in situ hybridization in brain tissue	Haase et al., 1981 [150] Cosby et al., 1989 [151]
	Increased intrathecal MV antibody synthesis Impaired MV-CTL response	Reviewed by Norrby, 1978 [119] Jacobson et al., 1985 [152]
Bone marrow agent	Development of CPE in TC after inoculation of MS bone marrow cells	Mitchell et al., 1978 [153]
Cytomegalovirus	Isolation from a chimpanzee inoculated with MS brain cells	Wrobleska et al., 1979 [154]
Coronavirus	Isolation from mice inoculated with MS brain homogenate	Burks et al., 1980 [155]
IM virus (SMON-like agent)	Development of CPE in TC after CSF inoculation	Melnick et al., 1982, 1984 [156, 157]
Tick-borne encephalitis virus	Isolation from mice inoculated with MS blood	Vagabov et al., 1982 [158]
Retrovirus	Antibodies in CSF and serum from MS patients	Koprowski et al., 1985 [129] Ohta et al., 1986 [130]
	Detection of HTLV sequences in CSF cells and PBLs of MS patients	Koprowski et al., 1985 [129] Reddy et al., 1989 [159] Greenberg et al., 1989 [160]
	EBV activation of retroviral-like particles in a MS leptomeningeal cell line	Sommerlund et al., 1993 [161]
	Herpes simplex virus transactivation of retrovirus	Perron et al., 1993 [162]
Human herpes virus 6	Detection of DNA and antigen in MS tissue	Challoner et al., 1995 [163]

Modified from Johnson, 1985 [1].

these findings failed [170, 171]. The question of isolation of measles virus from the duodenal mucosa remains moot.

Coronavirus has also been isolated from two brain specimens of MS patients [155]. A molecular biological and immunological analysis has demonstrated that these isolates were unlike the human coronaviruses, but were related to murine coronaviruses [172, 173]. Because the isolation procedure applied included passages of MS brains through mice, it is possible that the two MS isolates were derived from mice latently infected with murine coronaviruses. However, RNA and viral antigen of the human coronavirus SD and a mouse adapted strain OC43 have been detected in MS brain tissue [174]. Moreover, inoculation of coronavirus SD into primate brain resulted in demyelination [175]. The assessment of these reports must await an independent confirmation.

Retroviruses have also been considered as possible etiological agents of MS. This postulation was based initially on the finding of antibodies to HTLV-I virus in MS patients. It has been extended by the report of the finding of sequences related to HTLV-I by in situ hybridization in CSF lymphocytes from a few MS patients, but not from the controls [129]. Subsequently, the same group reported HTLV-I sequences in peripheral blood mononuclear cells in six MS patients and in one out of 20 normal individuals identified by the technique of gene amplification [159]. A similar observation was made by another group using the same technique [160]. In their study, six of 21 MS patients revealed HTLV-I sequences in genomic DNA from peripheral blood mononuclear cells, whereas all samples from 35 normal individuals were negative. Other investigators failed to confirm these results. In those studies, the HTLV-I sequences were not detectable in peripheral blood mononuclear cells of MS patients or in DNA extracted from an MS brain by the same technique as originally described (176–181). Although these negative reports do not support the view that such a virus is HTLV-I, they do not exclude the possibility of a retrovirus being involved in MS. This concept is supported by the results of the experiments in which an EBV infection has led to the activation of retroviral-like particles in a cell line from a patient with a progressive form of MS[161]. Similarly, in another experiment herpes simplex virus has enhanced retroviral expression in a leptomeningeal cell line from an MS patient[162]. Reactivation of retroviruses by a superinfection with another virus apparently is a common phenomenon, because it has also been observed with members of the herpes virus group or hepatitis B virus in HIV infection[182]. Therefore, the possibility that a transactivation of a persistent retrovirus infection in brain tissue by a second virus may result in an aberrant immune reaction as seen in MS, cannot be excluded.

The most recent potential viral candidate as an etiological agent in MS is the human herpes virus 6 (HHV-6), which was detected in MS brain tissue by the representational difference analysis (RDA)[163]. This method of detection is based on successive routes of subtractive hybridization and PCR amplification, enriched for DNA sequences present in DNA preparations from MS and control brains. By this method non-human DNA in MS brain can be isolated and identified by sequence analysis. Examination of 86 brain specimens revealed the presence of HHV-6 DNA sequences in about 70% of both MS cases and controls. However, monoclonal antibodies against HHV-6 virion protein 101K and DNA binding protein p41 detected HHV-6 only in brain tissue of MS patients and not the controls. In the MS brains, nuclear staining was claimed in oligodendrocytes around the MS plaques more frequently than in the uninvolved white matter, whereas a prominent cytoplasmic staining appeared in the neurons in gray matter adjacent to the plaques. However, neurons expressing HHV-6 were also found in certain controls. Although these observations have not been confirmed independently, a high prevalence rate of HHV-6 infection in infants is compatible with the epidemiology of MS. Moreover, cases of fatal encephalitis caused by HHV-6 have been seen in AIDS patients and in those immunosuppressed for bone marrow transplantation[183–185]. Furthermore, higher titers of HHV-6 antibodies have been reported in MS patients than in the controls[186, 187]. Although this study awaits confirmation, the molecular biological approach applied in this investigation has proven to be very powerful and promising.

Although attempts to isolate, or to identify a causative agent in MS have been many and none has resulted yet in a convincing, reproducible conclusion, a viral etiology remains a plausible concept. It is supported by epidemiological and immunological findings. Thus, it is possible that a viral infection in childhood leads to persistence of the agent and that a host response becomes non-beneficial and results in MS. This reasoning is based on indirect evidence but should not be dismissed, because it has acted, and it continues to act, as an irrepressible stimulus to further studies of viral etiology.

16.3   Mechanisms of virus-induced demyelination

Focal demyelination without axonal damage, but with variable degrees of perivascular inflammation is a hallmark of MS (Chapters 9 and 15). These lesions can result from damage to oligodendroglia, the myelin producing cells, or the myelin sheath itself. Therefore, the mechanisms by which a virus, or viruses, can play a pathogenic role that results in demyelination in MS can be quite varied.

Direct infection of oligodendroglia takes place in man in PML and in JHM virus infection in mice and rats. In both cases, viral replication causes destruction of the target cell, which is followed by primary demyelination. Whereas in PML, lesions develop without an inflammatory reaction, in JHM virus infection the CNS lesions are accompanied by inflammation. However, most virus-induced demyelinating diseases appear to involve immune-mediated reactions as, for example, suggested in Theiler's virus infection in mice, in visna, or in chronic demyelination associated with murine neurotropic hepatitis virus. Demyelination in these instances can occur secondarily as a pathological process related to immune reactivity against viral proteins present in the membrane of the infected cell.

It has been shown that in the course of replication of most enveloped viruses, virus-specific structural proteins are inserted into the cell membrane of the host cell. Such cells can be lysed as a consequence of an antiviral humoral or cell-mediated immune response. This is a well-established mechanism of great importance in overcoming and controlling an acute viral infection. This mechanism can also operate in chronic CNS diseases and can result in the destruction of brain cells that are persistently infected with a virus, even as viral replication alone does not kill the cells. In such cases, immunosuppression can be expected to attenuate or prevent the lesions, as is the case in visna infection of sheep[188] and in Theiler's virus infection of mice[189, 190].

Another possible mechanism of virus-induced demyelination is the phenomenon of a 'non specific bystander' effect resulting from the reaction of lymphocytes or macrophages with heterologous antigens[191]. In such a situation, oligodendrocytes or myelin sheaths can be injured by lymphokines or proteases released by the activated macrophages, or the immune cells. Such cells have been detected in the CNS lesions in MS as well as in experimental animal preparations [192–195]. Moreover, tumor necrosis factor – which is secreted by the macrophages – has been shown to produce demyelination in experimental animals [196, 197]. Macrophages also release proteolytic enzymes, which can contribute to the breakdown of myelin. This mechanism of viral stimulation of immunocompetent cells which then non-specifically attack the myelin sheath could explain demyelination in the number of infections with diverse viruses. However, there is one mitigating factor in the acceptance of this hypothesis. In known situations, the delayed hypersensitivity reaction is non-specific and therefore one would expect a generalized effect, rather than specific damage to myelin, unless oligodendroglia are particularly vulnerable. This seems not to be the case because in most animal and human inflammatory diseases of the CNS there is no demyelination [198].

Demyelination might also develop as a consequence of virus-induced autoimmune reaction against brain antigens. There is indirect evidence supporting this postulate in parainfectious encephalomyelitis in man and in experimental encephalitis in animals. In these conditions, virus-specific CD4$^+$ lymphocytes proliferate in the presence of MBP [26, 112, 199]. These activated T lymphocytes induce EAE in adoptive transfer experiments in rats. These observations have raised the question as to how viruses break immune tolerance and force the host to mount a strong cell-mediated immune response to brain antigens. Although the answer is still wanting, there are a number of possible explanations.

First, as the virus replicates it might incorporate host antigens into its envelope and then insert, modify, or expose cellular antigens on the cell surface. These newly exposed antigens may be recognized and treated by the host as if they were foreign [200]. Although there has been no proof of this hypothesis, it is biologically plausible as the basis for the development of autoimmune reactions [201].

Secondly, the virus might interact with the immune regulatory system by destroying some populations of lymphocytes or stimulating the generation of auto-reactive lymphocyte clones. Many viruses are lympho-tropic, and Epstein–Barr virus (which infects and transforms human B lymphocytes, rendering them immortal) is a prime example. In vitro, under certain conditions, such immortal cells secrete autoantibodies that react with cellular constituents [202]. In animal models infected with murine JHM coronavirus or neurotropic measles virus, lymphocytes do not contain virus. However, measles virus infection in man depresses host cell immune functions such as responsiveness to antigens and as a clinical complication sometimes leads

to an exacerbation of tuberculosis [203]. It is possible therefore that the proliferative response of T cells to MBP in acute measles encephalitis is the result of such an interaction. In this context, it is of interest that transgenic mice express constitutively the T cell receptor for the encephalitogenic MBP epitope. These animals develop EAE only if they are exposed to a non-sterile environment but fail to do so if they are kept under sterile conditions [204]. It is most likely that an infection contributes to the autoimmune reaction – this may reflect what happens in humans who go on to develop MS.

A third possibility is that molecular mimicry might induce an immune response against certain viral antigens that cross-react with normal host cell components. Computer analysis of a variety of viral sequences has revealed that several viruses contain a part of the sequence of human MBP in their genome [205]. Rabbits immunized with a synthetic peptide containing sequences of the hepatitis B virus polymerase developed EAE lesions and generated humoral and cell-mediated immune response to myelin and to hepatitis B polymerase [117]. There is also evidence of molecular mimicry in cross-reaction of antibodies against proteins of herpes simplex and of measles virus with human intermediate filaments [206]. Similar cross-reactivity between a monoclonal antibody to VP1 protein of Theiler's murine encephalomyelitis virus and oligodendrocytes was demonstrated when these antibodies were administered to animals and caused demyelination [207]. These and other examples of molecular mimicry have lent support to the notion that immunological recognition of viral peptides of sufficient structural similarity to the immunodominant MBP peptide may lead to clonal extension of MBP-reactive T cells in MS. Viruses such as herpes simplex or Epstein–Barr, which are known to cause latent or persistent infections, may under specific conditions lead to a chronic antigenic stimulation of autoreactive T cell clones [208]. One of these immunodominant MBP regions – (84–102) which may be a genetic marker for susceptibility to MS and is predominantly found in subjects carrying HLA-DR2 – has sequence homology to many viruses [209, 210]. Peptides were synthesized according to these sequence homologies based on motifs required for MHC class II binding and TCR recognition and tested for the ability to activate human MBP-specific T cell clones of MS patients [211]. Those derived from one bacterium and from herpes simplex, adeno-, papilloma-, influenza- and EB viruses effectively activated T cell clones. These findings further support the hypothesis that viruses are involved in initiating an autoimmune process in MS. Nevertheless, because of the diverse nature of these peptides, it is rather unlikely that a single agent causes MS. It may well be that the steps leading to MS follow an identical pattern, but that they are initiated by a variety of agents. This concept is in congruity with the clinical and epidemiological data.

The last postulated mechanism for the development of a non-beneficial immune reaction in the course of a CNS viral infection is induction by the virus of class II antigens on brain cells and the consequent host response, such as a delayed type hypersensitivity (DTH) reaction, in the genetically susceptible host. It has been established that major histocompatibility (MHC) antigens are expressed only at low levels if – at all – on most of the cells in the CNS [212]. However, a number of glial cells can be induced by treatment with interferon gamma *in vitro* to express MHC antigens [213]. This induction also occurs *in vivo* as a result of an inflammatory reaction, presumably due to the release of interferon gamma by infiltrating T cells [214]. However, mystery still surrounds a possible event that could initiate such a reaction in the CNS. Without MHC antigens, T cells would have difficulty in recognizing the antigen, becoming activated and releasing lymphokines. Therefore, it is more likely that in a viral infection of CNS other mechanisms operate to induce MHC antigen expression, enabling the T lymphocyte to find its target cell.

Exposure of astrocytes in culture to JHM or measles virus leads directly to the expression of MHC class II antigens. It can be further enhanced by the addition of tumor necrosis factor [215, 216]. Moreover, astrocytes expressing class II antigen can present MBP to CD4$^+$ T cells [217]. Thus, a viral infection can create a situation in which cells that previously were not recognizable by the host immune system because of a lack of appropriate restriction elements now interact with and perhaps even present antigen to autoreactive T cells. Once this has occurred, subsequent induction of MHC antigens can be mediated by the products of activated T cells. This mechanism might play a role in the animal models in which these two viruses induce an autoimmune response to MBP.

The development of autoimmune reactions as a consequence of a viral infection is a likely pathogenetic basis of a number of subacute and chronic disease of animals and man. At the time of writing, no specific defect responsible for autoimmune disorders in general can be identified. It is probable that such disorders develop in a variety of ways as a result of a number of different virus-induced changes, each one a relatively common event.

16.4 Conclusion

The etiology and pathogenesis of MS remain an enigma. Circumstantial evidence suggests that a viral infection during childhood, coupled with an immune response by the host, induces MS, which develops after a long incubation period. Knowledge derived from other demyelinating diseases has provided guidelines to the means by which viruses can induce a chronic neurological disease, but there is insufficient information about the pathogenetic process. What needs to be understood is the individual steps that lead to the demyelination and the nature of the virus–host relationship that allows the agent to persist. In addition, an analysis of the mechanisms of aberrant immune reaction in relation to virus infection may provide clues to the pathogenesis of multiple sclerosis. It is important to learn more about the routes of communication between the CNS and the immune system and the variety of ways in which an immune response affects the outcome of a viral infection of the CNS.

References

1. Johnson, R.T. (1985) Viral aspects of multiple sclerosis, in *Handbook of Clinical Neurology, 3* (revised series) (ed. J.C. Koetsier), vol. 47: *Demyelinating Diseases*, Amsterdam, Elsevier, pp. 319–36.
2. ter Meulen, V. and Hall, W.W. (1978) Slow virus infections of the nervous system: virological, immunological and pathogenetic considerations. *J. Gen. Virol.*, 41, 1–25.
3. Narayan, O. and Clements, J.E. (1989) Biology and pathogenesis of lentiviruses. *J. Gen. Virol.*, 70, 1617–39.
4. Zink, M.C. and Narayan, O. (1989) Lentivirus-induced interferon inhibits maturation and proliferation of monocytes and restricts the replication of caprine arthritis-encephalitis virus. *J. Virol.*, 63, 2578–84.
5. Stricker, R.B., McHugh, T.M., Moody, D.J. *et al.* (1987) An AIDS-related cytotoxic autoantibody reacts with a specific antigen on stimulated CD4 + T cells. *Nature*, 327, 710–13.
6. Clements, J.E., Gdovin, S.L., Montelaro, R.C. and Narayan, O. (1988) Antigenic variation in lentiviral diseases. *Ann. Rev. Immunol.*, 6, 139–59.
7. Jolly, P.E., Huso, D.L., Sheffer, D. and Narayan, O. (1989) Modulation of lentivirus replication by antibodies: FC portion of immunoglobulin molecule is essential for enhancement of binding, internalization and neutralization of visna virus in macrophages. *J. Virol.*, 63, 1811–13.
8. Zink, M.C. (1992) The pathogenesis of lentiviral disease in sheep and goats. *Semin. Virol.*, 3, 147–55.
9. Kingsbury, D.W., Bratt, M.A., Choppin, P.W. *et al.* (1978) Paramyxoviridae. *Intervirology*, 10, 137–52.
10. Appel, M.J. (1969) Pathogenesis of canine distemper. *Am. J. Vet. Res.*, 30, 1167–82.
11. Wisniewsky, H.M., Raine C.S. and Kay W.J. (1972) Observations on viral demyelinating encephalomyelitis: canine distemper. *Lab. Invest.*, 26, 589–99.
12. Raine, C.S. (1976) On the development of lesions in natural canine distemper encephalomyelitis. *J. Neurol. Sci.*, 301, 13–28.
13. Imagawa, D.T., Howard, E.B., van Pelt, L.F. *et al.* (1980) Isolation of canine distemper virus from dogs with chronic neurological diseases (40877). *Proc. Soc. Exp. Biol. Med.*, 164, 355–62.
14. Summers, B.A., Whitaker, J.N. and Appel, M.J.G. (1987) Demyelinating canine distemper encephalomyelitis: measurement of myelin basic protein in cerebrospinal fluid. *J. Neuroimmunol.*, 14, 227–33.
15. Zurbriggen, A., Graber, H.U., Wagner, A. and Vandevelde, M. (1995) Canine distemper virus persistence in the nervous system is associated with non-cytolytic and selective virus spread. *J. Virol.*, 69, 1678–86.
16. McCullough, B., Krakowka, S. and Koestner, A. (1974) Experimental canine distemper virus-induced lymphoid depletion. *Am. J. Pathol.*, 74, 155–66.
17. Johnson, G.C., Fenner, W.R. and Krakowka, S. (1988) Production of immunoglobulin G and increased antiviral antibody in cerebrospinal fluid of dogs with delayed-onset canine distemper viral encephalitis. *J. Neuroimmunol.*, 17, 237–51.
18. Vandevelde, M. and Zurbriggen, A. (1995) The neurobiology of canine distemper virus infection. *Vet. Microbiol.*, 44, 271–80.
19. Spaan, W., Cavanagh, D. and Horzinek, M.C. (1988) Coronaviruses: structure and genome expression. *J. Gen. Virol.*, 69, 2939–52.
20. Kyuwa, S. and Stohlman, S.A. (1990) Pathogenesis of a neurotropic murine coronavirus, strain JHM in the central nervous system of mice. *Semin. Virol.*, 1, 273–80.

21. Nagashima, K., Wege, H., Meyermann, R. and ter Meulen, V. (1979) Corona virus induced subacute demyelinating encephalomyelitis in rats. A morphological analysis. *Acta Neuropathol.*, **44**, 63–70.

22. Knobler, R.L., Taylor, B.A., Wooddell, M.K., Beamer, W.G. and Oldstone, M.B.A. (1984) Host genetic control of mouse hepatitis virus type-4 (JHM strain) replication. II. The gene locus for susceptibility is linked to the Svp-2 locus on mouse chromosome 7. *Exp. Clin. Immunogenet.*, **1**, 217–22.

23. Stohlman, S.A., Matsushima, G.K., Casteel, N. and Frelinger, J.A. (1985) The defect in delayed-type hypersensitivity of young adult SJL mice is due to a lack of functional antigen-presenting cells. *Eur. J. Immunol.*, **15**, 913–16.

24. Watanabe, R., Wege, H. and ter Meulen, V. (1987) Comparative analysis of coronavirus JHM-induced demyelinating encephalomyelitis in Lewis and Brown Norway rats. *Lab. Invest.*, **57**, 375–84.

25. Dörries, R., Watanabe, R., Wege, H. and ter Meulen, V. (1987) Analysis of the intrathecal humoral immune response in Brown Norway (BN) rats, infected with the murine coronavirus JHM. *J. Neuroimmunol.*, **14**, 305–16.

26. Watanabe, R., Wege, H. and ter Meulen, V. (1983) Adoptive transfer of EAE-like lesions by BMP stimulated lymphocytes from rats with coronavirus-induced demyelinating encephalomyelitis. *Nature*, **305**, 150–3.

27. Günther, E., Odenthal, H. and Wechsler, W. (1978) Association between susceptibility to experimental allergic encephalomyelitis and the major histocompatibility system in congenic rat strains. *Clin. Exp. Immunol.*, **32**, 429.

28. Erlich, S.S., Matsushima, G.K. and Stohlman, S.A. (1989) Studies on the mechanism of protection from acute viral encephalomyelitis by delayed-type hypersensitivity inducer T cell clones. *J. Neurol. Sci.*, **90**, 203–16.

29. Sussman, M.A., Shubin, R.A., Kyuwa, S. and Stohlman, S.A. (1989) T-cell-mediated clearance of mouse hepatitis virus strain JHM from the central nervous system. *J. Virol.*, **63**, 3051–6.

30. Williamson, J.S.P. and Stohlman, S.A. (1990) Effective clearance of mouse hepatitis virus from the central nervous system requires both CD4$^+$ and CD8$^+$ T cells. *J. Virol.*, **64**, 4589–92.

31. Wege, H., Koga, M., Watanabe, R., Nagashima, K. and ter Meulen, V. (1983) Neurovirulence of murine coronavirus JHM temperature-sensitive mutants in rats. *Infect. Immun.*, **39**, 1316–24.

32. Goto, N., Tsutsumi, Y., Sato, A. and Fujiwara, K. (1987) Neuropathogenicity of mutant strains of mouse hepatitis virus, JHM. *Jpn. J. Vet. Sci.*, **49**, 779–86.

33. Fleming, J.O., Trousdale, M.D., Bradbury, J., Stohlman, S.A. and Weiner, L.P. (1987) Experimental demyelination induced by coronavirus JHM (MHV-4): molecular identification of a viral determinant of paralytic disease. *Microb. Pathogen.*, **3**, 9–20.

34. Dalziel, R.G., Lampert, P.W., Talbot, P.J. and Buchmeier, M.J. (1986) Site specific alteration of murine hepatitis virus type-4 (MHV-4) peplomer glycoprotein E2 results in reduced neurovirulence. *J. Virol.*, **59**, 463–71.

35. Wege, H., Winter, J. and Meyermann, R. (1988) The peplomer protein E2 of coronavirus JHM as a determinant of neurovirulence: definition of critical epitopes by variant analysis. *J. Gen. Virol.*, **69**, 87–98.

36. Wege, H., Watanabe, R. and ter Meulen, V. (1984) Relapsing subacute demyelinating encephalomyelitis in rats during the course of coronavirus JHM infection. *J. Neuroimmunol.*, **6**, 325–36.

37. Rodriguez, M., Oleszak, E. and Leibowitz, J. (1987) Theiler's murine encephalomyelitis: a model of demyelination and persistence of virus. *Crit. Rev. Immunol.*, **7**, 325–65.

38. Welsh, C.J.R., Blakemore, W.F., Tonks, P., Borrow, P. and Nash, A.A. (1989) Theiler's murine encephalomyelitis virus infection in mice: a persistent viral infection of the central nervous system which induces demyelination, in *Immune Responses, Virus Infections and Disease* (eds N.J. Dimmock and P.D. Minor), Oxford, IRL Press, pp. 125–47.

39. Pevear, D.C., Borkowski, J., Calenhoff, M. *et al.* (1988) Insights into Theiler's virus neurovirulence based on a genomic comparison of the neurovirulent GDVII and less virulent BeAn strains. *Virology*, **165**, 253–9.

40. Calenhoff, M.A., Faaberg, K.S. and Lipton, H.L. (1990) Genomic regions of neurovirulence and attenuation in Theiler's murine encephalomyelitis virus. *Proc. Natl Acad. Sci. USA*, **87**, 978–82.

41. Zurbriggen, A., Hogle, J.M. and Fujinami, R.S. (1989) Alteration of amino acid 101 within capsid protein VP-1 changes the pathogenicity of Theiler's murine encephalomyelitis virus. *J. Exp. Med.*, **170**, 2037–49.

42. McAllister, A., Tarrgy, F., Aubert, C. and Brahic, M. (1990) Genetic mapping of the ability of Theiler's virus to persist and demyelinate. *J. Virol.*, **64**, 4252–7.

43. Jarousse, M., Grant, R.A., Hugle, J.M. *et al.* (1994) In fact a single amino acid change of the capsid protein VP2 determines persistence of a chimeric Theiler's virus. *J. Virol.*, **68**, 3364–8.

44. Zurbriggen, A. and Fujinami, R.S. (1988) Theiler's virus infection in nude mice: viral RNA in vascular endothelial cells. *J. Virol.*, **62**, 3589–96.

45. Cash, E., Chamorro, M. and Brahic, M. (1985) Theiler's virus RNA and protein synthesis in the CNS of demyelinating mice. *Virology*, **144**, 290–4.

46. Roos, R.P., Richards, O.C., Green, J. and Ehrenfeld, E. (1982) Characterisation of a cell culture persistently infected with the DA strain of Theiler's murine encephalomyelitis virus. *J. Virol.*, **43**, 1118–22.

47. Fiette, L., Aubert, C., Müller, U. *et al.* (1995) Theiler's virus infection of 129Sv mice that lack the interferon α/β or interferon γ receptors. *J. Exp. Med.*, **181**, 2069–76.

48. Nash, A. (1991) Virological and pathological processes involved in Theiler's virus infection of the CNS. *Semin. Neurosci.*, **3**, 109–16.

49. Melvold, R.W., Jokinen, D.M., Miller, S.D., Dal Canto, M.C. and Lipton, H.L. (1990) Identification of a locus on chromosome 3 involved in differential susceptibility to Theiler's murine encephalomyelitis virus-induced demyelinating diseases. *J. Virol.*, **64**, 686–90.

50. Clatch, R.J., Melvold, R.W., Miller, S.D. and Lipton, H.L. (1985) Theiler's murine encephalomyelitis virus (TMEV)-induced demyelinating disease in mice is influenced by the H-2D region: correlation with TMEV-specific delayed type hypersensitivity. *J. Immunol.*, **135**, 1408–14.

51. Borrow, P., Tonks, P., Welsh, C.J.R. and Nash, A.A. (1992) The role of CD8$^+$ T cells in the acute and chronic phases of Theiler's virus-induced disease in mice. *J. Gen. Virol.*, **73**, 1861–5.

52. Welsh, C.J.R., Tonks, P., Nash, A.A. and Blakemore, W.F. (1987) The effect of L3T4 T cell depletion on the pathogenesis of Theiler's murine encephalomyelitis virus infection in CBA mice. *J. Gen. Virol.*, **68**, 1659–67.

53. Miller, S.D., Gerety, S.J., Kennedy, M.K. *et al.* (1990) Class II-restricted responses in Theiler's murine encephalomyelitis virus (TMEV)-induced demyelinating disease. III. Failure of neuroantigen-specific immune tolerance to affect the clinical course of demyelination. *J. Neuroimmunol.*, **26**, 9–23.

54. Rauch, H.C., Montgomery, I.N., Hirman, C.L., Harb, W. and Benjamins, J.A. (1987) Chronic Theiler's virus infection in mice: appearance of myelin basic protein in the cerebrospinal fluid and serum antibody directed against myelin basic protein. *J. Neuroimmunol.*, **14**, 35–48.

55. Fujinami, R.S., Zurbriggen, A. and Powell, H.C. (1988) Monoclonal antibody defines determinant between Theiler's virus and lipid-like structures. *J. Neuroimmunol.*, **20**, 25–32.

56. ter Meulen, V., Stephenson, J.R. and Kreth, H.W. (1983) Subacute sclerosing panencephalitis, in *Comprehensive Virology* (eds H. Fraenkel-Conrat and R.R. Wagner), New York, Plenum Press, pp. 105–59.

57. White, R.G. and Boyd, J.F. (1973) The effect of measles on the thymus and other lymphoid tissues. *Clin. Exp. Immunol.*, **13**, 343–57.

58. Liebert, U.G., Baczko, K., Budka, H. and ter Meulen, V. (1986) Restricted expression of measles virus proteins in brains from cases of subacute sclerosing panencephalitis. *J. Gen. Virol.*, **67**, 2435–44.

59. Cattaneo, R., Rebmann, G., Baczko, K., ter Meulen, V. and Billeter, M.A. (1987) Unbalanced levels of measles virus transcripts in diseased human brains. *Virology*, **160**, 523–6.

60. Cattaneo, R., Rebmann, G., Schmid, A. *et al.* (1987) Altered transcription of a defective measles virus genome derived from a diseased human brain. *EMBO J.*, **6**, 681–8.

61. Baczko, K., Liebert, U.G., Billeter, M.A. *et al.* (1986) Expression of defective measles virus genes in brain tissues of patients with subacute sclerosing panencephalitis. *J. Virol.*, **59**, 472–8.

62. Cattaneo, R., Schmid, A., Billeter, M.A. Sheppard, R.D. and Udem, S.A. (1988) Multiple viral mutations rather than host factors cause defective measles virus gene expression in a subacute sclerosing panencephalitis cell line. *J. Virol.*, **62**, 1388–97.

63. Cattaneo, R., Schmid, A., Spielhofer, P. *et al.* (1989) Mutated and hypermutated genes of persistent measles viruses which caused lethal human brain diseases. *Virology*, **173**, 415–25.

64. Cattaneo, R., Schmid, A., Rebmann, G. *et al.* (1986) Accumulated measles virus mutations in a case of subacute sclerosing panencephalitis: interrupted matrix protein reading frame and transcription alteration. *Virology*, **154**, 97–107.

65. Cattaneo, R., Schmid, A., Eschle, D. *et al.* (1988) Biased hypermutation and other genetic changes in defective measles virus in human brain infections. *Cell*, **55**, 255–65.

66. Schneider-Schaulies, S. and ter Meulen V. (1992) Molecular aspects of measles virus-induced central nervous system diseases, in *Molecular Neurovirology* (ed. R.P. Roos), Totowa, NJ, Humana Press, pp. 419–48.

67. Billeter, M.A., Cattaneo, R., Spielhofer, P. *et al.* (1994) Generation and properties of measles virus mutations typically associated with subacute sclerosing panencephalitis. *Ann. NY Acad. Sci.*, **724**, 367–77.

68. Ecker, A., ter Meulen, V., Baczko, K. and Schneider-Schaulies, S. (1995) Measles virus-specific dsRNAs are targets for unwinding/modifying activity in neural cells in vitro. *J. Neurovirol.*, **1**, 92–100.

69. Baczko, K., Lampe, J., Liebert, U.G. *et al.* (1993) Clonal expansion of hypermutated measles virus in a SSPE brain. *Virology*, **197**, 188–95.

70. Bankamp, B., Brinckmann, U.G., Reich, A. *et al.* (1991) Measles virus nucleocapsid protein protects rats from measles encephalitis. *J. Virol.*, **65**, 1695–700.

71. Johnson, R.T., Narayan, O., Weiner, C.P. and Greenlee, J.E. (1977) Progressive multifocal leukoencephalopathy, in *Slow Virus Infections of the CNS* (eds V. ter Meulen and M. Katz), New York, Springer Verlag.

72. Berger, J.R., Kaszovitz, B., Post, M.J.D. and Dickinson, G. (1987) Progressive multifocal leukoencephalopathy associated with human immunodeficiency virus-infection – a review of the literature with a report of 16 cases. *Ann. Intern. Med.*, **107**, 78–87.

73. Padgett, B.L. and Walker, D.L. (1976) New human papoviruses. *Progr. Med. Virol.*, **22**, 1–35.

74. Coleman, D.V., Daniel, R.A., Gardener, S.D., Field, A.M. and Gibson, P.E. (1977) Polyomavirus in urine during pregnancy. *Lancet*, **ii**, 709–10.

75. Dörries, K. and ter Meulen, V. (1983) Progressive multifocal leucoencephalopathy: detection of papovavirus JC in kidney tissue. *J. Med. Virol.*, **11**, 307–17.

76. Dörries, K., Johnson, R.T. and ter Meulen, V. (1978) Detection of polyomavirus DNA in PML-brain tissue by *in situ* hybridization. *J. Gen. Virol.*, **41**, 49–57.

77. Shein, H.M. (1967) Transformation of astrocytes and destruction of spongioblasts induced by simian tumor virus SV40 in cultures of human fetal neuroglia. *J. Neuropathol. Exp. Neurol.*, **26**, 60–76.

78. Padgett, B.L., Walker, D.L. and ZuRhein, G.M. (1977) Differential neuronegenicity of strains of JC virus, a human polyoma virus in newborn Syrian hamsters. *Cancer Res.*, **37**, 718–20.

79. Major, O.E., Amemiya, K., Tornatore, C.S., Houff, S.A. and Berger, J.R. (1992) Pathogenesis and molecular biology of progressive multifocal leukoencephalopathy, the JC virus induced demyelinating disease of the human brain. *Clin. Microbiol. Rev.*, **5**, 49–73.

80. Small, J.A., Scangos, G.A., Cork, L., Jay, G. and Khoury, G. (1986) The early region of human papovavirus JC induces dysmyelination in transgenic mice. *Cell*, **46**, 13–18.

81. Román, G.C. (1988) The neuroepidemiology of tropical spastic paraparesis. *Ann. Neurol.*, **23** (Suppl.), 113–20.

82. Osame, M., Arima, H. and Norimatsu, K. (1975) Epidemiostatistical studies of muscular atrophy in Southern Kyushu. *Jpn J. Med.*, **14**, 230–1.

83. Osame, M., Usuku, K., Izumo, S. *et al.* (1986) HTLV-I associated myelopathy, a new clinical entity, *Lancet*, **ii**, 1031–2.

84. Gessain, A., Barin, F., Vernant, J.C. *et al.* (1985) Antibodies to human T-lymphotropic virus type-I in patients with tropical spastic paraparesis. *Lancet*, **ii**, 407–10.

85. Nakagawa, N., Izumo, S., Ijichi, S. *et al.* (1995) HTLV-I-associated myelopathy: analysis of 213 patients based on clinical features and laboratory findings. *J. Neurol.*, **1**, 50–61.

86. Román, G.C., Spencer, P.S. and Schoenberg, B.S. (1987) Tropical spastic paraparesis in the Seychelles islands: a clinical and case-control neuro-epidemiologic study. *Neurology*, **37**, 1323–8.

87. Moore, G.R.W., Traugot U., Scheinberg, L.C. and Raine C.S. (1989). Tropical spastic paraparesis: a model of virus-induced; cytotoxic T cell-mediated demyelination. *Ann. Neurol.*, **26**, 523–300.

88. Iwasaki, Y. (1990) Pathology of chronic myelopathy associated with HTLV-1 infection (HAM/TSP). *J. Neurol. Sci.*, **96**, 103–23.

89. Wu, E., Dickson, D.W., Jacobson, S. and Raine, C.S. (1993) Neuroaxonal dystrophy in tropical spastic paraparesis/HTLV-I associated myelopathy. *Acta Neuropathol.*, **86**, 224–35.

90. Iwasaki, Y. (1993) Human T cell leukemia virus type I infection and chronic myelopathy. *Brain Pathol.*, **3** (1), 1–10.

91. Feuer, G. and Chen, I.S.Y. (1992) Mechanisms of human T-cell leukemia virus-induced leukemogenesis. *Biochim. Biophys. Acta*, **1114**, 223–33.

92. Kajiyama, W., Kashiwagi, S., Hayashi, J. *et al.* (1986) Intrafamilial clustering of anti-ATLA-positive persons. *Am. J. Epidemiol*, **124**, 800–6.

93. Kajiyama, W., Kashiwagi, S., Ikematsu, H. *et al.* (1986) Intrafamilial transmission of adult T cell leukemia virus. *J. Infect. Dis.*, **154**, 851–7.

94. Ando, Y., Nakano, S. and Saito, K. (1987) Transmission of adult T cell leukemia retrovirus (HTLV-I) from mother to child: comparison of bottle-with breast-fed babies. *Jpn J. Cancer Res. (Gann.)*, **78**, 322–4.

95. Osame, M., Izumo, S., Igata, A. *et al.* (1986) Blood transfusion and HTLV-I associated myelopathy. *Lancet*, **ii**, 104–5.

96. Osame, M., Matsumoto, M. and Usuku, K. (1987) Chronic progressive myelopathy associated with elevated antibodies to HTLV-I and adult T cell leukemia-like cells. *Ann. Neurol.*, **21**, 117–22.

97. Umehara, F., Izumo, S., Ronquillo, A.T. *et al.* (1994) Cytokine expression in the spinal cord lesions in HTLV-I associated myelopathy. *J. Neuropathol. Exp. Neurol.*, **53**, 72–7.

98. Tendler, C.L., Greenberg, S.J., Blattner, W.A. *et al.* (1990) Transactivation of interleukin 2 and its recepter induces immune activation in human T-cell lymphotropic virus type I-associated myelopathy: pathogenic implications and a rationale for immunotherapy. *Proc. Natl Acad. Sci. USA*, **87**, 5218–22.

99. Hara, H., Morita, M., Iwaki, T. *et al.* (1994) Detection of human T lymphotrophic virus type I (HTLV-I) proviral DNA and analysis of T cell receptor Vß CDR3 sequences in spinal cord lesions of HTLV-I-associated myelopathy/tropical spastic paraparesis. *J. Exp. Med.*, **180**, 831–9.

100. Jacobson, S., Shida, H., McFarlin, D.E., Fauci, A.S. and Koenig, S. (1990) Circulating CD8$^+$ cytotoxic T-lymphocytes specific for HTLV-I pX in patients with HTLV-I associated neurological disease. *Nature*, **348**, 245–8.

101. Wucherpfennig, K.W., Hollsberg, P., Richardson, J.H., Benjamin, D. and Hafler, D.A. (1992) T-cell activation by autologous human T-cell leukemia virus type I-infected T-cell clones. *Proc. Natl Acad. Sci. USA*, **89**, 2110–14.

102. Elovaara, I., Koenig, S., Brewah, A.Y. *et al.* (1993) High human T-cell lymphotropic virus type 1 (HTLV-1) specific precursor cytotoxic T-lymphocyte frequencies in patients with HTLV-1 associated neurological disease. *J. Exp. Med.*, **177**, 1567–73.

103. Bhigjee, A.I., Wiley, C.A., Wachsman, W. *et al.* (1991) HTLV-I associated myelopathy: clinicopathologic correlation with localization of provirus to the spinal cord. *Neurology*, **41**, 1990–2.

104. Kira, J., Itoyama, Y., Koyanagi, Y. *et al.* (1992) Presence of HTLV-I proviral DNA in central nervous system of patients with HTLV-I associated myelopathy. *Ann. Neurol.*, **31**, 39–45.

105. Lehky, T.J., Fox, C.H., Koenig, S. *et al.* (1995) Detection of human T-lymphotropic virus type I (HTLV-I) Tax RNA in the central nervous system of HTLV-I-associated myelopathy/tropical spastic paraparesis patients by in situ hybridization. *Ann. Neurol.*, **37**, 167–75.

106. Ishiguro, N., Abe, M., Seto, K. *et al.* (1992) A rat model of HTLV-1 infection. Humoral antibody response, provirus integration and HAM/TSP-like myelopathy in seronegative HTLV-1 carrier rats. *J. Exp. Med.*, **176**, 981–9.

107. Johnson, R.T. (1975) The possible viral etiology of multiple sclerosis, in *Advances in Neurology* (ed. W.J. Friedlander), New York, Raven Press.

108. Purdham, D.R. and Beatty, P.F. (1974) A case of acute measles meningoencephalitis with virus isolation. *J. Clin. Pathol.*, **27**, 994–6.

109. ter Meulen, V., Müller, D., Käckell, Y., Katz, M. and Meyermann, R. (1972) Isolation of infectious measles virus in measles encephalitis. *Lancet*, **ii**, 1172–5.

110. Gendelman, H.E., Wolinsky, J.S., Johnson, R.T. *et al.* (1984) Measles encephalomyelitis: lack of evidence of viral invasion of the central nervous system and quantitative study of the nature of demyelination. *Ann. Neurol.*, **15**, 353–60.

111. Griffin, D.E., Hirsch, R.L., Johnson, R.T. *et al.* (1983) Changes in serum C-reactive protein during complicated and uncomplicated measles virus infection. *Infect. Immun.*, **41**, 861–4.

112. Johnson, R.T., Griffin, D.E., Hirsch, R.L. (1984) Measles encephalomyelitis: clinical and immunological studies. *N. Engl. J. Med.*, **310**, 137–41.

113. Griffin, D.E., Cooper, S.J., Hirsch, R.L. *et al.* (1985) Changes in plasma IgE levels during complicated and uncomplicated measles virus infections. *J. Allergy Clin. Immunol.*, **76**, 206–13.

114. Griffin, D.E., Ward, B.J., Jouregui, E., Johnson, R.T. and Vaisberg, A. (1989) Immune activation during measles. *N. Engl. J. Med.*, **320**, 1667–72.

115. Hirsch, R.L., Griffin, D.E., Johnson, R.T. *et al.* (1984) Cellular immune responses during complicated and uncomplicated measles virus infections of man. *Clin. Immunol. Immunopathol.*, **31**, 1–12.

116. Fleischer, B. and Kreth, H.W. (1983) Clonal expansion and functional analysis of virus-specific T lymphocytes from cerebrospinal fluid in measles encephalitis. *Human Immunol.*, **7**, 239–48.

117. Fujinami, R.S. and Oldstone, M.B.A. (1985) Amino acid homology between the encephalitogenic site of myelin basic protein and virus: mechanism for autoimmunity. *Science*, **230**, 1043–5.

118. Adams, J.M. and Imagawa, D.T. (1962) Measles antibodies in multiple sclerosis. *Proc. Soc. Exp. Biol. Med.*, **111**, 562–6.

119. Norrby, E. (1978) Viral antibodies in multiple sclerosis, in *Progress in Medical Virology* (ed. J.L. Melnich), Basle, S. Karger.

120. Goswami, K.K.A., Randall, R.E., Lange, L.S. and Russell, W.C. (1987) Antibodies against the paramyxovirus SV5 in the cerebrospinal fluids of some multiple sclerosis patients. *Nature*, **327**, 244–7.

121. Salmi, A., Viljanen, M. and Reunanen, M. (1981) Intrathecal synthesis of antibodies to diphtheria and tetanus toxoids in multiple sclerosis patients. *J. Neuroimmunol.*, **1**, 333–41.

122. Salmi, A., Reunanen, M., Ilonen, J. and Panelius, M. (1983) Intrathecal antibody synthesis to virus antigens in multiple sclerosis. *Clin. Exp. Immunol.*, **52**, 241–9.

123. Vartdal, F., Vandvik, B. and Norrby, E. (1980) Viral and bacterial antibody responses in multiple sclerosis. *Ann. Neurol.*, **8**, 248–55.

124. Vandvik, B. and Norrby, E. (1989) Paramyxovirus SV5 and multiple sclerosis *Nature*, **338**, 769–71.

125. Poser, C.M., Paty, D.W. and Scheinberg, L. (1983) New diagnostic criteria for multiple sclerosis: guidelines for research protocols. *Ann. Neurol.*, **13**, 227–31.

126. Nordal, H.J., Vandvik, B. and Norrby, E. (1978) Demonstration of oligoclonal virus-specific antibodies in serum and cerebrospinal fluid by imprint electroimmunofixation. *Scand. J. Immunol.*, **7**, 381–8.

127. Nordal, H.J., Vandvik, B. and Norrby, E. (1979) Oligoclonal virus antibodies in healthy and neurological patients, in *Humoral Immunity in Neurological Diseases* (eds D. Karcher, A. Lowenthal and A.D. Strosberg), New York, Plenum Press, pp. 249–302.

128. Salmi, A.A., Norrby, E. and Panelius, M. (1972) Identification of different virus-specific antibodies in the serum and cerebrospinal fluid from patient with subacute sclerosing panencephalitis and multiple sclerosis. *Infect. Immun.*, **6**, 248–54.

129. Koprowski, H., DeFreitas, E.C., Harper, M.E. *et al.* (1985) Multiple sclerosis and human T cell lymphotropic retroviruses. *Nature*, **318**, 154–60.

130. Ohta, M., Ohta, K., Mori, F., Nishitani, H. and Saida, T. (1986) Sera from

patients with multiple sclerosis react with human T cell lymphotropic virus gag proteins but not env proteins – Western blotting analysis. *J. Immunol.*, **137** (11), 3440–3.

131. DeFreitas, E., Saida, T. and Iwasaki, Y. (1987) Association of human T lymphotropic viruses in chronic neurological disease. *Ann. Neurol.*, **21**, 215–16.

132. Madden, D.L., Mundon, F.K., Fucillo, D.A. *et al.* (1988) Antibody to human and simian retroviruses HTLV-I, HTLV-II, HIV, STLV-III, and SRV-I not increased in patients with multiple sclerosis. *Ann Neurol.*, **23**, 171–3.

133. Rice, G.P.A., Armstrong, M.A., Bulman, D.E., Paty, D.W. and Ebers, G.C. (1986) Absence of antibody to HTLV-I and II in sera of Canadian patients with multiple sclerosis and chronic myelopathy. *Ann. Neurol.*, **20**, 533–4.

134. DeRossi, A., Gallo, P., Tavolato, B., Callegaro, L. and Chieco-Bianchi, L. (1986) Search for HTLV-I and LAV/HTLV-III antibodies in serum and CSF of multiple sclerosis patients. *Acta Neurol. Scand.*, **74**, 161–4.

135. Karpas, A., Kämpf, U., Siden, A., Koch, M. and Poser, S. (1986) Lack of evidence for involvement of known human retroviruses in multiple sclerosis. *Nature*, **322**, 177–8.

136. Hauser, S.L., Aubert, C., Burks, J.S. *et al.* (1986) Analysis of human T-lymphotropic virus sequences in multiple sclerosis tissue. *Nature*, **322**, 176–7.

137. Norrby, E. and Vandvik, B. (1975) Relationship between measles virus-specific antibody activities and oligoclonal IgG in the central nervous system of patients with subacute sclerosing panencephalitis and multiple sclerosis. *Med. Microbiol. Immunol.*, **162**, 63–72.

138. Rostrom, B., Link, H., Laurenzi, M.A. *et al.* (1981) Viral antibody activity of oligoclonal and polyclonal immunoglobulins synthesized within the central nervous system in multiple sclerosis. *Ann. Neurol.*, **9**, 569–74.

139. Sandberg-Wollheim, M., Vandvik, B., Nadj, C. and Norrby, E. (1987) The intrathecal immune response in the early stage of multiple sclerosis. *J. Neurol. Sci.*, **81**, 45–53.

140. Nordal, H.J., Vandvik, B. and Norrby, E. (1978) Multiple sclerosis: local synthesis of electrophoretically restricted measles, rubella, mumps and herpes simplex virus antibodies in the central nervous system. *Scand. J. Immunol.*, **7**, 473–9.

141. Vandvik, B. and Norrby, E. (1973) Oligoclonal IgG antibody response in the central nervous system to different measles virus antigen in subacute sclerosing panencephalitis. *Proc. Natl. Acad. Sci. USA*, **70**, 1060–3.

142. Miller, J.R., Burke, A.M. and Bever, C.T. (1982) Occurrence of oligoclonal bands in multiple sclerosis and other CNS disease. *Ann. Neurol.*, **36**, 311–16.

143. Margulis, M.S., Soloviev, V.D. and Shubladze, A.K. (1946) Aetiology and pathogenesis of acute sporadic disseminated encephalomyelitis and multiple sclerosis. *J. Neurol. Neurosurg. Psychiatry*, **9**, 63–74.

144. Gudnadottir, M., Helgadottir, H., Bjarnason, O. and Jonsdottir, K. (1964) Virus isolated from the brain of a patient with multiple sclerosis. *Exp. Neurol.*, **9**, 85–95.

145. Field, E.J., Miller, H. and Russell, D.S. (1962) Observation on glial inclusion bodies in case of acute disseminated sclerosis. *J. Clin. Pathol.*, **15**, 278–84.

146. Palsson, P.A., Pattison, I.H. and Field, E. (1965) Transmission experiments with multiple sclerosis, in *Slow, Latent and Temperate Virus Infections* (eds D.C. Gajdusek, C.J. Cibbs Jr and M. Alpers), Washington DC, US GPO, pp. 49–54.

147. ter Meulen, V., Koprowski, H., Iwasaki, Y., Käckell, Y.M. and Müller, D. (1972) Fusion of cultured multiple-sclerosis brain cells with indicator cells: presence of nucleocapsids and virion and isolation of parainfluenza-type virus. *Lancet*, i, 1–5.

148. Carp, R.I., Licursi, P.C., Merz, P.A. and Merz, G.S. (1972) Decreased percentages of polymorphonuclear neutrophils in mouse peripheral blood after inoculation with material from multiple sclerosis patients. *J. Exp. Med.*, **136**, 618–29.

149. Field, E.J., Cowshall, S., Narang, H.K. and Bell, T.M. (1972) Viruses in multiple sclerosis? *Lancet*, ii, 280–1.

150. Haase, A.T., Ventura, P., Gibbs, C.J. Jr and Tourtellotte, W.W. (1981) Measles virus nucleotides sequences – detection by hybridization *in situ*. *Science*, **212**, 672–5.

151. Cosby, S.L., McQuaid, S., Taylor, M.J. *et al.* (1989) Examination of eight cases of multiple sclerosis and 56 neurological and non-neurological controls for genomic sequences of measles virus, canine distemper virus, simian virus 5 and rubella virus. *J. Gen. Virol.*, **70**, 2027–36.

152. Jacobson, S.J., Flerlage, M.L. and McFarland, H.F. (1985) Impaired measles virus-specific cytotoxic T cell response in multiple sclerosis. *J. Exp. Med.*, **162**, 839–50.

153. Mitchell, D.N., Porterfield, J.S., Micheletti, R. *et al.* (1978) Isolation of an infectious agent from bone-marrows of patients with multiple sclerosis. *Lancet*, ii, 387–91.

154. Wrobleska, Z., Gilden, D., Devlin, M. *et al.* (1979) Cytomegalovirus isolation from a chimpanzee with acute demyelinating disease after inoculation of multiple sclerosis brain cells. *Infect. Immun.*, **25**, 1008–15.

155. Burks, J.S., Devald, B.L., Jankovsky, L.D. and Gerdes, J.C. (1980) Two coronaviruses isolated from central nervous system tissue of two multiple sclerosis patients. *Science*, **209**, 933–4.

156. Melnick, J.L., Seidel, E., Inoue, Y.K. and Nishibe, Y. (1982) Isolation of virus from the spinal fluid of three patients with multiple sclerosis and one with amyotrophic lateral sclerosis. *Lancet*, i, 830–3.

157. Melnick, J.L., Wang, S.-S., Seidel, E. *et al.* (1984) Characterization of IM virus, which is frequently isolated from cerebrospinal fluid of patients with multiple sclerosis and other chronic diseases of the central nervous system. *J. Virol.*, **52**, 739–44.

158. Vagabov, R.M.A., Skortsoa, T.M., Gofman, Y.P. and Barinsky, I. F. (1982) Isolation of the tick-borne encephalitis virus from a patient with multiple sclerosis. *Acta Virol.*, **20**, 403.

159. Reddy, E.P., Sandberg-Wollheim, M., Mettus, R.V. *et al.* (1989) Amplification and molecular cloning of HTLV-I sequences from DNA of multiple sclerosis patients. *Science*, **243**, 529–33.

160. Greenberg, S.J., Ehrlich, G.D., Abbott, M.A. *et al.* (1989) Detection of sequences homologous to human retroviral DNA in multiple sclerosis by gene amplification. *Proc. Natl Acad. Sci. USA*, **86**, 2878–82.

161. Sommerlund, M., Pallesen, G., Moller-Larsen, A., Hansen, H.J. and Haahr, S. (1993) Retrovirus-like particles in an Epstein–Barr virus producing cell line derived from a patient with chronic progressive myelopathy. *Acta Neurol. Scand.*, **87**, 71–6.

162. Perron, H., Suh, M., Lalande, B. *et al.* (1993) Herpes simplex virus ICP0 and ICP4 immediate early proteins strongly enhance expression of a retrovirus harboured by a leptomeningeal cell line from a patient with multiple sclerosis. *J. Gen. Virol.*, **74**, 65–72.

163. Challoner, P.B., Smith, K.T., Parker, J.D. *et al.* (1995) Plaque-associated expression of human herpesvirus 6 in multiple sclerosis. *Proc. Natl Acad. Sci. USA*, **92**, 7440–4.

164. Stevens, J.G., Bastone, V.B., Ellison, G.W. and Myers, L.W. (1980) No measles virus genetic information detected in multiple sclerosis-derived brains. *Ann. Neurol.*, **8**, 625–37.

165. Hall, W.W. and Choppin, P.W. (1982) Failure to detect measles virus proteins in brain tissue of patients with multiple sclerosis. *Lancet*, i, 957.

166. Godec, M.S., Asher, D.M., Murray, R.S. *et al.* (1992) Absence of measles, mumps and rubella viral genomic sequences from multiple sclerosis brain tissue by polymerase chain reaction. *Ann. Neurol.*, **32**, 401–4.

167. Pertschuk, L.P., Cook, A.W. and Gupta, J. (1976) Measles antigen in multiple sclerosis: identification in the jejunum by immunofluorescence. *Life Sci.*, **19**, 1603–8.

168. Prasad, I., Pertschuk, L.P., Broome, J.D., Gupta, J. and Cook, A.W. (1977) Recovery of paramyxovirus from the jejunum of patient with multiple sclerosis. *Lancet*, i, 1117–19.

169. Ebina, T., Tsukamoto, T., Suzuki, H. *et al.* (1979) Measles virus in jejunum of patients with multiple sclerosis. *Lancet*, i, 99.

170. Kingston, D., Shiner, M., Lange, L.S., Mertin, J. and Meade, C. (1977) Measles antigen in jejunal mucosa in multiple sclerosis. *Lancet*, i, 1313.

171. Woyciechowska, J.L., Madden, D.L. and Sever, J.L. (1977) Absence of measles-virus antigen in the jejunum of multiple sclerosis patients. *Lancet*, ii, 1046–9.

172. Fleming, J.O. El Zaatari, F.A.K., Gilmore, W. *et al.* (1988) Antigenic assessment of coronaviruses isolated from patients with multiple sclerosis. *Arch. Neurol.*, **45**, 629–33.

173. Weiss, S.R. (1983) Coronaviruses SD and SK share extensive nucleotide homology with murine coronaviruses MHV-A59 more than that shared between human and murine coronaviruses. *Virology*, **126**, 669–77.

174. Murray, R.S., Brown, B., Brain, D. and Cabirac, G.F. (1992) Detection of coronavirus RNA and antigen in multiple sclerosis brain. *Ann. Neurol.*, **31**, 525–33.

175. Murray, R.S., Cai, G.-Y., Hoel, K. *et al.* (1992) Coronavirus infects and causes demyelination in primate central nervous system. *Virology*, **188**, 274–84.

176. Bangham, C.R.M., Nightingale, S., Cruickshank, J.K. and Daenke, S. (1989) PCR analysis of DNA from multiple sclerosis patients for the presence of HTLV-I. *Science*, **246**, 821–4.

177. Richardson, J.H., Wucherpfennig, K.W., Endo, N. *et al.* (1989) PCR analysis of DNA from multiple sclerosis patients for the presence of HTLV-I. *Science*, **246**, 821–4.

178. Chen, I.S.Y., Haislip, A.M., Myers, L.W. *et al.* (1990) Failure to detect human T cell leukemia virus-related sequences in multiple sclerosis blood. *Arch. Neurol.*, **47**, 1064–5.

179. Oksenberg, J.R., Mantegazza, R., Sakai, K., Bernard, C.C.A. and Steinman, L. (1990) HTLV-I sequences are not detected in peripheral blood genomic DNA or in brain cDNA of multiple sclerosis patients. *Ann. Neurol.*, **28**, 574–7.

180. Perl, A., Nagy, K., Pazmany, T. *et al.* (1990) No evidence for human T cell leukemia virus type I or human T cell leukemia virus type II infection in patients with multiple sclerosis. *Arch. Neurol.*, **47**, 1061–3.

181. Jocher, R., Rethwilm, A., Kappos, L. and ter Meulen, V. (1990) Search for retroviral sequences in peripheral blood mononuclear cells and brain tissue of multiple sclerosis patients. *J. Neurol.*, **237/6**, 352–5.

182. Chinnadurai, G. (1991) Modulation of HIV-enhancer activity by heterologous agents: a minireview. *Gene*, **101**, 165–70.

183. Knox, K.K. and Carrigan, D.R. (1994) Disseminated active HHV-6 infections in patients with AIDS. *Lancet*, **343**, 577–8.

184. Knox, K.K. and Carrigan, D.R. (1995) Active human herpesvirus (HHV-6) infection of the central nervous system in patients with AIDS. *J. Acquir. Immune Defic. Syndr. Hum. Retrovirol.*, **9**, 69–73.

185. Drobyski, W.R., Knox, K.K., Majewski, D. and Carrigan, D.R. (1994) Brief report: fatal encephalitis due to variant B human herpesvirus-6 infection in a bone marrow-transplant recipient. *N. Engl. J. Med.*, **330** (19), 1356–60.

186. Sola, P., Merelli, E., Marasca, R. *et al.* (1993) Human herpesvirus 6 and multiple sclerosis: survey of anti-HHV-6 antibodies by immunofluorescence analysis and of viral sequences by polymerase chain reaction. *J. Neurol. Neurosurg. Psychiatry*, **56** (8), 917–19.

187. Wilborn, F., Schmidt, C.A., Brinkmann, V. *et al.* (1994) A potential role for human herpesvirus type 6 in nervous system disease. *J. Neuroimmunol.*, **49**, 213–14.

188. Nathanson, N., Panitch, H., Palson, P.A., Petursson, G. and Georgsson, G. (1976) Pathogenesis of visna II. Effect of immunosuppression upon early central nervous system lesions. *Lab. Invest.*, **35**, 444–51.

189. Lipton, H.L. and Dal Canto, M.C. (1976) Theiler's virus-induced demyelination: prevention by immunosuppression. *Science*, **192**, 62–4.

190. Ross, R.P., Firestone, S., Willmann, R., Variakojis, D. and Arnason, B.G.W. (1982) The effect of short-term and chronic immunosuppression on Theiler's virus demyelination. *J. Neuroimmunol.*, **2**, 223–34.

191. Wisniewsky, H.M. and Bloom, B.R. (1975) Primary demyelination as a nonspecific consequence of a cell-mediated immune reaction. *J. Exp. Med.*, **141**, 346–59.

192. Prineas, J.W. (1985) The neuropathology of multiple sclerosis, in *Handbook of Clinical Neurology, 3* (revised series) (ed. J.C. Koetsier), vol. 47: *Demyelinating Diseases*, Amsterdamy, Elsevier, 213–57.

193. Goldstein, J.L., Anderson, R.G.W. and Brown, M.S. (1979) Coated pits, coated vesicles, and receptor-mediated endocytosis. *Nature*, **279**, 679–85.

194. Raine, C.S., Barnett, L.B., Brown, A. *et al.* (1980) Neuropathology of experimental allergic encephalomyelitis in inbred strains of mice. *Lab. Invest.*, **43**, 150–7.

195. Fleury, H.J.A., Sheppard, R.D., Burnstein, M.B. *et al.* (1980) Further ultrastructural observations of virus morphogenesis and myelin pathology in JHM virus encephalomyelitis. *Neuropathol. Appl. Neurobiol.*, **6**, 165–79.

196. Selmaj, K.W. and Raine, C.S. (1988) Tumor necrosis factor mediates myelin and oligodendrocyte damage in vitro. *Ann. Neurol.*, **23**, 339–46.

197. Brosnan, C.F., Selmaj, K. and Raine, C.S. (1988) Hypothesis: a role of tumor necrosis factor in immune-mediated demyelination and its relevance to multiple sclerosis. *J. Neuroimmunol.*, **18**, 87–94.

198. Lampert, P.W. and Rodriguez, M. (1984) Virus induced demyelination, in *Concepts in viral Pathogenesis* (ed. A.L. Notkins and M.B.A. Oldstone) New York, Springer Verlag, pp. 260–8.

199. Liebert, U.G., Linington, C. and ter Meulen, V. (1988) Induction of autoimmune reactions to myelin basic protein in measles virus encephalitis in Lewis rats. *J. Neuroimmunol.*, **17**, 103–18.

200. Hirsch, M.S. and Proffett, M.R. (1975) Autoimmunity in viral infection, in *Viral Immunology and Immunopathology* (ed. A.L. Notkins), New York, Academic Press, p. 419.

201. Notkins, A.L., Onodera, T. and Prabhakar, H. (1984) Virus induced autoimmunity, in *Concepts in Viral Pathogenesis* (eds A.L. Notkins and M.B.A. Oldstone), New York, Springer Verlag, pp. 210–15.

202. Rosen, A., Gergely, P., Jondal, M., Klein, G. and Britton, S. (1977) Polyclonal Ig production after Epstein–Barr virus infection of human lymphocytes *in vitro*. *Nature*, **267**, 5254.

203. Cherry, J.D. (1981) Measles, in *Textbook of Pediatric Infectious Diseases*, vol. II (eds R.D. Feigin and J.D. Cherry), Philadelphia, W.B. Saunders, pp. 1210–30.

204. Goverman, J., Woods, A., Larson, L. *et al.* (1993) Transgenic mice that express a myelin basic protein specific T cell receptor develop spontaneous autoimmunity. *Cell*, **72**, 551–60.

205. Jahnke, U., Fischer, E.H. and Alvord, E.C. (1985) Sequence homology between certain viral proteins and proteins related to encephalomyelitis and neuritis. *Science*, **229**, 282–4.

206. Fujinami, R.S., Oldstone, M.B., Wroblewska, Z., Frankel, M.E. and Koprowski, H. (1983) Molecular mimicry in virus infection. Cross reaction of measles virus phosphoprotein of herpes simplex virus protein with human intermediate filaments. *Proc. Natl Acad. Sci USA*, **80**, 2346–50.

207. Yamada, M., Zurbriggen, A. and Fujinami, R.S. (1990) Monoclonal antibody to Theiler's murine encephalomyelitis virus defines a determinant on myelin and oligodendrocytes and augments demyelination in experimental allergic encephalomyelitis. *J. Exp. Med.*, **171**, 1893–907.

208. Allegretta, M., Nicklas, J.A., Sriram, S. and Albertini, R.J. (1990) T cells responsive to myelin basic protein in patients with multiple sclerosis. *Science*, **247**, 718–21.

209. Pette, M., Fujita, K., Wilkinson, D. *et al.* (1990) Myelin autoreactivity in multiple sclerosis: recognition of myelin basic protein in the context of HLA-DR2 products by T lymphocytes of multiple sclerosis patients and healthy donors. *Proc. Natl Acad. Sci. USA*, **87**, 7968–72.

210. Souberbielle, B.E., Kemp, G. and Russell, W.C. (1991) Viral homologies with myelin basic protein. *Immunol. Today*, **12**, 464–5.

211. Wucherpfennig, K.W. and Strominger, J.L. (1995) Molecular mimicry in T cell-mediated autoimmunity: viral peptides activate human T cell clones specific for myelin basic protein. *Cell*, **80**, 695–705.

212. Hart, D.N.J. and Fabre, J.W. (1981) Demonstration and characterisation of Ia-positive dendritic cells in the institial tissues of rat heart and other tissues but not brain. *J. Exp. Med.*, **154**, 347–61.

213. Wong, G.H.W., Bartlett, P.F., Clark-Lewis, I. *et al.* (1985) Interferon gamma induces the expression of H-2n Ia antigens on brain cells. *J. Neuroimmunol.*, **7**, 255–78.

214. Merrill, J.E. (1987) Macroglia, neural cells responsive to lymphokines and growth factors. *Immunology Today*, **8**, 146–50.

215. Massa, P.T., Dörries, R. and ter Meulen, V. (1986) Viral particles induce Ia antigen expression on astrocytes. *Nature*, **320**, 543–6.

216. Massa, P.T., Schimpl, A., Wecker, E. and ter Meulen, V. (1987) Tumor necrosis factor amplifies measles virus-mediated Ia induction on astrocytes. *Proc. Natl. Acad. Sci. USA*, **84**, 7242–5.

217. Fontana, A., Fierz, W. and Wekerle, H. (1984) Astrocytes present myelin basic protein to encephalitogenic T-cell lines. *Nature*, **307**, 273–6.

PART THREE

TREATMENT: ETIOPATHOGENETIC

17 CURRENT DISEASE-MODIFYING THERAPIES IN MULTIPLE SCLEROSIS

Donald E. Goodkin

Multiple sclerosis (MS) is the most common cause of non-traumatic neurological disability affecting young adults in the northern hemisphere. Although the etiology of MS remains unknown, recent technological advances in immunology, molecular biology and neuroimaging have improved our understanding of the pathogenesis of this disorder. Improvements in disease-modifying therapies have accompanied these recent advances. In this chapter we review the results of clinical trials of disease-modifying therapies that have progressed beyond the pilot phase of investigation. A review of the historical background, possible mechanisms of action, clinical experience and current applications in clinical practice are presented for each therapy.

17.1 Glucocorticosteroids and adrenocorticotropic hormone

17.1.1 BACKGROUND

Glucocorticosteroids are the most commonly used treatment for exacerbations of MS. Although the precise manner by which glucocorticosteroids exert their beneficial effect in MS remains unknown, possible mechanisms of action include a reduction of focal defects in the blood–brain barrier [1–3], a reduction of focal brain edema [3], an improvement in axonal conduction [4], a reduction in intrathecal immunoglobulin G synthesis [5], and immunosuppression resulting from blockade of cytokine gene expression [6].

17.1.2 CLINICAL EXPERIENCE

Glucocorticosteroids and adrenocorticotropic hormone for acute exacerbations of multiple sclerosis

The first clinical trials to suggest that glucocorticosteroids and corticotropin had clinical efficacy in the treatment of MS exacerbations were reported in 1951 and 1952 [7, 8]. These trials and other open uncontrolled trials of that era led to the sporadic use of these therapies in clinical practice. The subsequent publication of the 'Cooperative study in the evaluation of therapy in multiple sclerosis: ACTH vs. placebo' [9] further encouraged the use of corticotropin for MS exacerbations. Patients in this multicenter, double-blind study were randomly assigned to receive corticotropin gel, 40 units intramuscularly twice a day for 7 days, 20 units intramuscularly twice a day for 4 days, and 20 units intramuscularly each day for 3 days, or matched placebo within 8 weeks of an exacerbation. Considerably more patients treated with corticotropin (65%) than those receiving placebo (47%) had improvement in Kurtzke disability status scale (DSS) scores 4 weeks after initiating therapy [10]. The duration of these benefits was not determined, since the patients were not observed for longer than 4 weeks. This study significantly influenced neurological practice by establishing ACTH as an accepted treatment for MS exacerbations. The lessons learned from this clinical trial also served to improve the design of subsequent multiple sclerosis clinical trials [11].

Corticotropin remained the preferred treatment for MS exacerbations until 1985. That year it was reported that patients treated with 1 gram of intravenous (IV) methylprednisolone (MP) for 7 days were clinically more improved than patients treated with 60 units of intramuscular corticotropin tapered by 20 units each week for 3 weeks, but the treatment benefit disappeared 3 months after therapy was initiated [12]. Other investigators observed similar clinical improvements for 4–12 weeks with either a shorter course of IV methylprednisolone sodium succinate (1 gram IV daily for 3 days) or the corticotropin protocol used in the cooperative study (80 units for 7 days, 40 units for 4 days, and 20 units for 3 days) [13]. Although clinical benefits appeared to be equal in these treatment groups, fewer adverse effects were observed with IV methylprednisolone. Similar benefits have resulted from alternative protocols of IV

Multiple Sclerosis: Clinical and pathogenetic basis. Edited by Cedric S. Raine, Henry F. McFarland and Wallace W. Tourtellotte. Published in 1997 by Chapman & Hall, London. ISBN 0 412 30890 8.

methylprednisolone administered in other double-blind, placebo-controlled, randomized clinical trials [14, 15]. The doses used in these treatment protocols ranged from 15 mg/kg body weight for 3 days tapered over 15 days, to 500 mg daily for 5 days. The administration of methylprednisolone, 500 mg/day IV for 5 days, has also been reported to reduce spasticity in chronic progressive MS patients when compared to saline placebo [16]. This benefit was only evident for 4 weeks after initiating therapy. These studies encouraged the clinical use of high dose pulses of IV MP for the treatment of MS exacerbations. Further support for this treatment was provided by the observation that high dose IV MP reduced intrathecal immunoglobulin production [1, 16], plaque edema and gadolinium enhancement evidenced by serial CT and MRI scans [2, 3]. These effects were less evident with lower doses of corticosteroids [2]. Although there is presently no agreement regarding the optimal dose or duration of IV MP therapy for MS exacerbations, most neurologists currently administer between 500 and 1000 mg of IV methylprednisolone daily for 3–7 days, followed by an oral prednisone taper from 60 mg for 10–21 days. This treatment can be administered safely on an outpatient basis unless neurological or underlying medical conditions warrant admission to a hospital. This dose range of IV methylprednisolone is generally well tolerated, but insomnia, restlessness, euphoria, hypomania and weight gain can be problematic [17]. A recent double-blind pilot study of methylprednisolone for the treatment of acute exacerbations found similar efficacy and adverse events with five daily methylprednisolone doses (500 mg) whether administered orally or intravenously [18]. Oral as compared to intravenous administration of medication is easier and less costly. If confirmed, this study will be instrumental in changing practice patterns for the treatment of acute exacerbations of multiple sclerosis.

Corticosteroids and ACTH for long-term management of multiple sclerosis

Although steroids are widely used to manage acute attacks in patients with MS, their role in the long-term disease management has not been rigorously investigated. It has been said that chronic daily use of corticosteroids does not significantly slow progression of disability [19]. In 1961 the use of prednisolone (10–15 mg per day orally) was compared with that of aspirin (6 g per day orally) and placebo in 86 patients observed for 18 months [20]. The trial was randomized, and patients were matched for disability, age, course and disease duration. No difference was seen between treatment groups by measures of disability, exacerbation rate, or patient self-assessment at 6 or 18 months. In 1967 the results of the long-term treatment of MS with corticotropin were reported [21]. In this random-

ized, controlled, but unblinded study, 181 patients were treated with corticotropin (15–25 units intramuscularly daily; dose was adjusted according to 'facial mooning just evident') and compared with 169 patients who were treated with placebo. Patients were examined each 3 months for 16 months. The authors found no benefits in the corticotropin-treated group.

These limited data do not support chronic use of corticotropin or oral prednisone in patients with multiple sclerosis. However, the value of maintenance pulses of intravenous methylprednisolone as a disease-modifying therapy is currently unknown. The following observations support the rationale for an ongoing study to examine this question:

1. serial MRI studies have shown that new lesions are less likely to develop in patients with relapsing MS during the 6-month period after a single course of IV MP therapy than during the 6-month period before initiating that therapy [22]; and
2. steroid treatment may delay the onset of MS in patients with isolated optic neuritis [23].

A study designed to compare the relative clinical efficacy of bimonthly, low dose (10 mg) and high dose (500 mg) intravenous pulses of methylprednisolone in patients with relapsing progressive multiple sclerosis is ongoing. The primary measure of clinical efficacy for this study is the proportion of patients in each treatment group experiencing sustained treatment failure as measured by a composite outcome consisting of validated tests of ambulation and upper extremity function [24]. The results from this study are expected in 1997.

The use of glucocorticosteroids and ACTH in the treatment of optic neuritis

The first double-blind, placebo-controlled, prospective study of corticotropin in optic neuritis was reported in 1966 [25]. The authors found that the corticotropin-treated group recovered vision faster, but at one year the visual acuities of the two groups were not significantly different [25, 26]. Similar results were reported for optic neuritis patients treated with retrobulbar injection of triamcinolone [27]. There have been no double-blind controlled studies of oral prednisone for this condition. Despite the lack of evidence of long-term benefits with these treatments, 59% of ophthalmologists and 81% of neurologists prior to 1992 were reported to use oral prednisone for the treatment of optic neuritis [28].

This treatment practice was challenged by the results of the Optic Neuritis Treatment Trial reported in 1992 [29]. In this study patients were randomized to one of three treatment regimens: oral prednisone, 1 mg per kg daily for 14 days; IV methylprednisolone, 250 mg every 6 hours for 3 days, followed by oral prednisone,

1 mg per kg daily for 11 days; or oral placebo for 14 days. The first two regimens were followed by a short oral taper consisting of 20 mg on day 15 and 10 mg on days 16 and 18. This study was designed specifically to determine whether corticosteroids produce a benefit in visual function in either the short or long term – that is, 2 years – in patients with acute idiopathic optic neuritis. In this regard the results of the study showed that, compared to placebo, IV MP accelerated visual recovery but did not improve visual outcome after one year, oral prednisone did not improve visual outcome at any time, and more patients who received oral prednisone experienced recurrent ON than patients who received IV methylprednisolone. Although the impact of this trial on clinical practice has not yet been formally assessed it is reasonable to predict that IV methylprednisolone will replace the use of oral prednisone for the treatment of acute optic neuritis that is associated with impairment of visual acuity.

Optic neuritis is frequently the first manifestation of MS [30]. For this reason the study group of the Optic Neuritis Treatment Trial has subsequently determined the proportion of patients in each treatment arm who during the 24-month trial period were diagnosed with clinically definite MS [31]. Patients receiving IV MP experienced a reduced incidence of clinically definite MS during the two-year study period [23]. Although design limitations have been discussed [32], the results of this study have the potential to change the routine clinical treatment of isolated acute optic neuritis. Should we extrapolate these observations to patients with isolated idiopathic acute myelopathy or isolated idiopathic brain stem dysfunction? This seems premature even though both of these conditions, particularly when associated with an abnormal MRI, have been shown to be associated with an increased risk of MS subsequently developing [33, 34]. Further studies that examine the role of IV methylprednisolone therapy in patients with isolated optic neuritis, myelopathy and brain stem signs are needed.

17.2 Immunosuppressive therapies

The use of immunosuppressant therapies in multiple sclerosis has been based on the hypothesis that the clinical manifestations are attributable to self-directed immunity. Although not proved, this hypothesis is supported by the following empirical evidence derived from MS patients and animal models of the disease.

1. Similarities between MS and animal models of chronic relapsing experimental allergic encephalomyelitis (EAE) [35].
2. Elevated intrathecal oligoclonal immunoglobulin production [36].
3. A characteristic distribution of cytokines and T cell subsets within acute and chronic MS plaques [37].
4. An association of disease frequency with specific HLA-DR haplotypes in several different ethnic groups and an MS susceptibility locus linked to the T cell receptor beta chain complex [38].
5. Diminished suppressor cell number and function and possible correlation of these abnormalities with disease activity [39].
6. Clinical worsening seen with the administration of interferon gamma [40].
7. Transient benefit seen with immunosuppressive therapy [41].

17.2.1   AZATHIOPRINE

Background

Azathioprine is a purine analog designed as a 'pro drug' to permit the slow liberation of the active metabolites 6-mercaptopurine and 6-thioinosinic acid into tissues. Because the maximal *in vivo* immunosuppressive effect requires 3–6 months of daily use, azathioprine is frequently combined with more rapidly acting corticosteroids. The precise mechanism of action is uncertain. Several studies have shown that it suppresses cell-mediated hypersensitivity reactions and produces alterations in antibody production [42].

Clinical experience

In all, 21 clinical trials of azathioprine use in multiple sclerosis have been published since the initial report in 1969 by Tucker and Kapphahn [43]. Seven of these trials were controlled and involved either exacerbating or chronic progressive MS patients [44–50]. A meta-analysis of these seven studies demonstrates a small but significant benefit for azathioprine [51]. The relative probability of remaining exacerbation-free for three years while taking azathioprine compared to placebo was 1.97 [51]. This benefit compares favorably with the reduction in exacerbation rate reported with interferon beta-1b (IFNb) in relapsing-remitting MS [52]. However, azathioprine, like interferon beta-1b, offers only a modest degree of protection against progression of disability. This modest benefit is of questionable significance and requires 2–3 years before becoming evident.

Toxicity with azathioprine is common but cessation of therapy is necessary in less than 10% of MS patients. The incidence of malignancy associated with azathioprine therapy in patients with multiple sclerosis is uncommon and cessation of therapy is usually a result of drug-related fever, rash, or gastrointestinal intolerance [53–55].

The slight but consistent reduction in relapse rate with limited toxicity and the availability of the drug have helped to establish azathioprine as one of the most commonly used immunosuppressant therapies in MS. The drug is administered daily using oral doses of 1.5–2.5 mg per kg of body weight. In 1987, azathioprine was used as a standard treatment in some European MS treatment centers [56]. It is anticipated that the use of azathioprine will decline as newer treatment options become increasingly available.

17.2.2 COPOLYMER 1

Background

Although the antigens responsible for inducing the production of autoreactive T cells in MS remain unidentified, experimental allergic encephalomyelitis (the animal model for MS) can be induced by immunization using myelin basic protein. It was therefore theorized that a polypeptide of similar structure might inhibit the immune response to myelin basic protein, and thus block its encephalitogenic action. In 1967, work began at The Weizmann Institute on a series of seven synthetic polypeptides which were created specifically to mimic myelin basic protein. One of these, copolymer 1 (COP 1), was created by random polymerization of L-alanine, L-glutamic acid, L-lysine, and L-tyrosine in the ratio of 6.0 to 1.9 to 4.7 to 1.0.

Copolymer 1 is not encephalitogenic and suppresses experimental allergic encephalomyelitis in rabbits, guinea pigs, mice and non-human primates without evident toxicity [57]. This drug also suppresses *in vitro* proliferative responses and IL-2 production in human myelin basic protein specific T cell lines with several HLA-DR restrictions and epitope specificities [58] and inhibits IFN gamma synthesis of MBP specific to TH1 cell lines [59]. Despite these observations, the mechanism(s) by which copolymer 1 might be therapeutic in patients with multiple sclerosis or in suppressing EAE remain poorly understood. Although copolymer 1 binds avidly to class II major histocompatibility complex molecules on living antigen-presenting cells [60] and cross-reactivity between copolymer 1 and myelin basic protein has been demonstrated in human T cell lines [58], cross-reactivity between copolymer 1 and immunizing species of MBP used in EAE models (i.e. guinea pig, bovine or human MBP) does not appear to be strictly required for clinical or histological disease suppression [61]. Induction of antigen-specific suppressor cells has been hypothesized to be a possible mechanism of action. Whether copolymer 1 is capable of producing myelin basic protein T cell deletion in the manner demonstrated with high dose antigen therapy in EAE MBP-reactive T cell lines [62] has not yet been rigorously investigated.

Clinical experience

In the first study of copolymer 1, 48 patients with relapsing-remitting disease were randomly assigned to receive daily subcutaneous injections of active drug (20 mg) or saline placebo for 2 years [63]. Injections were well tolerated, although the majority of patients receiving copolymer 1 reported local irritation at injection sites. Patients treated with copolymer 1 had lower annual exacerbation rates (0.6) than placebo-treated patients (2.7). In addition, those patients with minor disability at study entry (e.g. DSS scores = 0–2) had less progression of disability during treatment. No benefit was seen for patients whose DSS score was greater than 2 at study entry. This suggested that the benefit of copolymer 1 is restricted to a subset of patients with relapsing multiple sclerosis who have minimal neurologic impairment. A subsequent study in which no benefit was observed when copolymer 1 was administered to 106 patients with chronic progressive multiple sclerosis indirectly supported this hypothesis [64].

The results of a pivotal phase III multicenter clinical trial of copolymer 1 in patients with relapsing-remitting MS was reported in July 1995 [65]. This study, begun in October 1991 at 11 universities in the United States, was supported by Teva Pharmaceuticals Ltd, the United States Food and Drug Administration Orphan Drug Program, and the National Multiple Sclerosis Society. Two hundred and fifty-one ambulatory relapsing-remitting patients who experienced at least two exacerbations prior to enrolment in this double-blind study were randomly assigned to receive 20 mg of daily subcutaneous copolymer 1 or placebo for 2 years [65]. The primary outcome measure for this study was the difference in exacerbation rates between the treatment groups. The final 2-year relapse rate was 1.19 ± 0.13 for patients receiving copolymer 1 and 1.68 ± 0.13 for patients receiving placebo, a 29% reduction favoring copolymer 1 ($P = 0.007$). Significantly more patients receiving copolymer 1 were improved and more receiving placebo worsened ($P = 0.037$) as measured by a change of one step (≥ 0.5 points) in the Kurtzke Expanded Disability Status Scale (EDSS) [66]. No treatment group differences were observed for time to first exacerbation, mean change in ambulation index score [67], or proportion of progression-free patients after 24 months. The treatment was well tolerated although mild injection site reactions were noted. A transient self-limited systemic reaction consisting of chest tightness with palpitations, anxiety, or dyspnea lasting from 30 seconds to 30 minutes was observed in 15.2% of actively treated and 3.2% of placebo-treated patients.

In January 1993 the United States Public Health Service Food and Drug Administration approved a multiple year open-label study to assess the safety of copolymer 1 (Lemmon Pharmacal Co., Sellersville, PA, and Teva Pharmaceutical Ind., Jerusalem, Israel) for relapsing multiple sclerosis[68]. In this context, a maximum of 1000 patients will be permitted to purchase copolymer 1 (approximately $7300.00 per year at time of writing) and receive supervised therapy at designated treatment centers. It is expected that copolymer 1 will be approved by the FDA for use in relapsing multiple sclerosis in 1996.

17.2.3   2-CHLORODEOXYADENOSINE

Background

2-Chlorodeoxyadenosine (Cladribine) is an antilymphocyte agent that mimics the accumulation of deoxynucleotides in adenosine deaminase deficiency[69, 70]. This drug is reported to cause the death of lymphocytes by apoptosis and has relatively low toxicity toward other tissues. Unlike most other antilymphocyte drugs, it is equally effective against resting and dividing cells[71]. The decision to explore the use of 2-chlorodeoxyadenosine in chronic multiple sclerosis was based upon the observation that the drug demonstrated prolonged lymphopenia and otherwise acceptable toxicity in the treatment of hairy cell leukemia and lymphomas and autoimmune hemolytic anemia[72–74].

Clinical experience

In 1994, the results of a double-blind clinical trial comparing 2-chlorodeoxyadenosine and placebo were reported. Fifty-one patients with clinically definite or laboratory-supported definite[31] chronic progressive MS were randomized to receive either 0.1 mg 2-chlorodeoxyadenosine per kg of body weight, or placebo daily for one week each month for four months[71]. Although this study was designed originally to include a 2-year treatment phase, a planned interval analysis at 1 year demonstrated a therapeutic benefit in patients receiving active treatment. Thirty per cent (7/23) of the placebo and 4% (1/24) of the actively treated patients experienced worsening as measured by a change of one or more points on the EDSS ($P < 0.02$)[66]. Statistically significant active treatment group benefits in mean paired difference (placebo minus 2-chlorodeoxyadenosine) in total T2-weighted lesion volumes and proportion of patients with gadolinium-enhancing volumes also were observed at one year.

2-Chlorodeoxyadenosine was generally well tolerated, although seven patients developed clinically significant thrombocytopenia. One 40-year-old woman died of fulminant hepatitis B eight days after her initial 2-chlorodeoxyadenosine infusion. It seems unlikely that this complication was treatment-induced because fulminant hepatitis has not been observed in more than 5000 patients receiving Cladribine for leukemia or lymphoma. A separate report suggested that 2-chlorodeoxyadenosine induced axonal peripheral polyneuropathy in 6 patients under treatment for refractory acute leukemia[75]. These patients received 19–21 mg of 2-chlorodeoxyadenosine daily for 5 consecutive days, a total dose that is similar to that administered to patients with multiple sclerosis over 4 months.

The encouraging results of this preliminary study prompted the investigators to initiate a second double-blind, placebo-controlled trial of 2-chlorodeoxyadenosine administered subcutaneously at a dose of 0.07 mg per kg of body weight daily for 5 days each month for 6 months to 50 patients with relapsing multiple sclerosis. Outcome measures in this study include frequency and severity of exacerbations, change in EDSS and the neurological rating scale (NRS) scores[76], and change in number and volume of T2-, and gadolinium-enhanced T1-weighted monthly MRI lesions. The results of this phase II study are anticipated in late 1997. The clinical significance of 2-chlorodeoxyadenosine-induced toxicity requires further study. A phase III study of this promising therapy will ultimately be required to determine 2-chlorodeoxyadenosine's role in the treatment of patients with multiple sclerosis.

17.2.4   CYCLOPHOSPHAMIDE

Background

Cyclophosphamide (CTX) is an alkylating agent with both cytotoxic and immunosuppressive effects. Monthly IV cyclophosphamide administration in doses ranging from 1000 to 2000 mg per m^{-2} body surface results in a pronounced reduction of the number of T helper or inducer cells and a less striking decrease in suppressor or cytotoxic cells in patients with MS[77]. Monthly pulses of intravenous cyclophosphamide for 1 year induced reductions in the numbers of suppressor or cytotoxic cells, natural killer cells and antibody-dependent cellular cytotoxicity functions lasting from one to two months. In addition, reduced B cell numbers in these patients recovered in 2–4 months, whereas the recovery of helper cell subsets and total T cell numbers, helper/suppressor ratio and proliferative responses to mitogens took more than 4 months[78]. Others have found that the decrease in helper cell subset populations can still be demonstrated as long as 13.5 years after IV cyclophosphamide therapy (8 grams in 20 days)[79].

Clinical experience

In 1983 the results of a randomized, unblinded trial comparing (a) intravenous cyclophosphamide and corticotropin, (b) corticotropin alone and (c) oral cyclophosphamide, corticotropin and plasma exchange in 58 patients with chronic progressive MS were reported[67]. A statistically significant reduction in the proportion of patients experiencing clinical progression was seen after 12 months in those receiving cyclophosphamide and corticotropin. Of the cyclophosphamide–corticotropin-treated group, 80% were stabilized or had improved DSS scores[10] at 12 months compared with 20% of the group receiving only corticotropin for 21 days. Although the benefits were no longer evident two years after therapy was initiated, this study appeared to offer a promising treatment option for patients with chronic progressive MS. Neurologists began to use this drug shortly after this publication appeared.

Other investigators began to explore the possibility that booster injections of cyclophosphamide might prolong the clinical benefits reported with cyclophosphamide induction. In one study[80], patients with chronic progressive MS were randomly assigned to bimonthly cyclophosphamide booster injections (700 mg per m^{-2}) or no further cyclophosphamide treatment following completion of the Hauser[67] induction regimen. A trend was observed favoring the patients treated with booster injections, but this trend did not reach statistical significance. A subsequent report by the Northeast Cooperative Multiple Sclerosis Treatment Group suggested that bimonthly boosters were associated with prolonged clinical stability of chronic progressive MS patients[81]. Of the patients initially treated with induction and subsequently treated with bimonthly cyclophosphamide boosters, 38% were stable or improved compared with 24% of the patients who received only induction therapy. These findings encouraged the use of cyclophosphamide induction and subsequent bimonthly cyclophosphamide boosters in clinical practice.

In a placebo-controlled, single-blind study of intravenous cyclophosphamide therapy, 22 patients with MS received intravenous cyclophosphamide without corticosteroids or corticotropin, and 20 control patients received intravenous folic acid[82]. Twelve months after treatment, 64% of the cyclophosphamide- and 70% of the placebo-treated patients showed evidence of stable or improved functional status as measured by DSS scores[10]. The absence of any notable benefit found in this single-blind, placebo-controlled trial, as well as the toxicity that occurred in similarly treated patients in clinical practice, began to dampen initial enthusiasm for the use of cyclophosphamide in patients with chronic progressive MS. Support for this therapy eroded further after the report of the Canadian Cooperative Multiple Sclerosis Study Group Trial of plasmapheresis and cyclophosphamide in MS[83]. This multicentered, single-blind, randomized trial also failed to detect any important difference in treatment benefit in patients treated with IV cyclophosphamide and oral prednisone; daily oral cyclophosphamide, alternate-day prednisone and weekly plasma exchange; and placebo medications and sham plasma exchange. The reasons for inconsistent results when using IV cyclophosphamide for patients with chronic progressive MS are not entirely clear but have been attributed to differences in drug doses, patient selection, and criteria used to define clinical deterioration[84, 85]. The final report from the Northeast Cooperative Multiple Sclerosis Treatment Group suggests that benefits observed with cyclophosphamide treatment may be restricted to patients younger than 40 years and those with a secondary progressive as opposed to a primary progressive clinical course since disease onset[83].

In summary, clinical benefits observed with cyclophosphamide therapy are generally marginal and toxicity, including nausea, vomiting, alopecia and potential sterility, are frequently problematic. The benefits appear to be restricted to patients with MS who are younger than 40 years with secondary progressive disease. At present most neurologists agree that cyclophosphamide has little benefit and significant toxicity in patients older than 40 with a progressive course since disease onset.

17.2.5 CYCLOSPORINE

Background

Cyclosporine (UK, cyclosporin) is a cyclic undecapeptide that was initially isolated from two soil fungi and recognized as an antifungal metabolite. This drug has proved effective in preventing host vs graft and graft vs host responses when used alone or in combination with conventional agents, and it has been reported to be useful in treating a variety of putative autoimmune diseases in man[86]. Interest in using this drug for human neurologic diseases, including multiple sclerosis, quickly followed these initial reports.

Much work has been done in the attempt to clarify cyclosporine's mechanism of action. Many of its *in vitro* effects can be explained by the observed inhibition of the production of a number of lymphokines, including interleukin 2 (IL-2), interleukin 3, migration inhibitory factor and gamma interferon[87]. Reduced levels of IL-2 messenger RNA inhibit IL-2 production[88], and the same mechanism appears to inhibit other lymphokines[89]. However, cyclosporine appears to spare T lymphocytes that secrete a soluble factor which is critical for the expansion of nonspecific suppressor T cells. It appears possible that this T cell subpopulation belongs to the CD4$^+$CD45R$^+$ subset of T cells known as suppressor inducers[90].

Clinical experience

Three major studies have assessed the efficacy of cyclosporine in MS. The first[91] reported the results of a double-blind, controlled trial of 194 patients with clinically definite active relapsing MS: 98 were randomized to treatment with cyclosporine (5 mg kg^{-1} per day), and 96 underwent treatment with azathioprine (2.5 mg kg^{-1} per day). Eighty-five patients in the cyclosporine group and 82 in the azathioprine group completed a treatment period of 24–32 months as stipulated by the study protocol. No significant changes were detected in EDSS, frequency of relapse, or overall treatment efficacy as assessed by patients and investigators at the end of the trial. Overall, only minor deterioration occurred in both groups during the trial. The incidence of the following side-effects – hypertrichosis, gingival hyperplasia, paresthesias, elevated serum creatinine, and elevated blood pressure – was more than twice as common in the cyclosporine as the azathioprine group. The authors concluded that cyclosporine as a single agent was not acceptable as the drug of final choice for the long-term immunosuppressive treatment of relapsing multiple sclerosis.

The second study was a double-blind, placebo-controlled trial with patients enrolled at centers in London (n = 44) and Amsterdam (n = 38)[92]. Participants in this study had either relapsing or chronic progressive clinically definite multiple sclerosis. The patients were begun on daily cyclosporine 10 mg per kg of body weight for 2 months, which was thereafter adjusted to minimize toxicity for the final 22 months of observation. The mean daily maintenance dose differed at the two sites (London, 7.2 mg kg^{-1} and Amsterdam, 5.0 mg kg^{-1}). A variety of outcome measures including the EDSS were used. Investigators in Amsterdam concluded that no beneficial effects were seen and that side-effects from cyclosporine presented a major problem[93]. However, the investigators at the London site reported separately a statistically significant early benefit for the patients treated with cyclosporine at that site. These patients had fewer relapses and a longer interval to first relapse on treatment over the 2-year study and better overall functional assessments for the first 6 months of treatment[94].

The most recent study was a multicenter effort undertaken in the United States[95]. In this study, clinically definite moderately disabled (EDSS 3–7) multiple sclerosis patients were randomized to receive cyclosporine (n = 273) or placebo (n = 274) for at least 2 years. The dosage was adjusted for toxicity, resulting in trough whole-blood levels from 310 to 430 mg ml^{-1}. The mean worsening in EDSS score for cyclosporine-treated patient (0.39 ± 1.07 points) was significantly less (P = 0.002) than for placebo-treated patients (0.65 ± 1.08). Three primary efficacy criteria were used in this study: time to becoming wheelchair-bound, time to sustained progression of disability, and a composite score of activities of daily living. Cyclosporine treatment delayed patients' ultimate confinement to wheelchair (P = 0.038), but statistically significant effects were not observed for the other criteria. It is difficult to compare directly this study with the German multicenter study[91], since whole-blood trough levels and types of MS patients treated differed significantly.

Cyclosporine treatment did have a favorable effect on several secondary measures of disease outcome. A large and differential withdrawal rate (cyclosporine = 44%, placebo = 32%) complicated the analysis but did not appear to explain the observed effect of cyclosporine in delaying time to wheelchair confinement. Nephrotoxicity and hypertension were common and accounted for most of the excess loss of patients in the cyclosporine arm of the study. The authors concluded that cyclosporine was associated with a modest benefit in the chronic progressive MS patients in the study, but these benefits were not evident until 18–24 months after initiating therapy. This delay in measurable benefit and the high incidence of toxicity create practical limitations for using this drug, particularly for patients who are experiencing rapid functional deterioration.

17.2.6 METHOTREXATE

Background

Low dose (7.5 mg) weekly oral methotrexate (MTX) has been shown to be a relatively nontoxic, effective treatment for rheumatoid arthritis (RA)[96–101]. MS clinical investigators originally considered MTX to be a potential treatment for MS because of some similarities in the immune alterations and relapsing clinical courses seen in RA and MS patients. The immunological similarities which were appreciated included a reduced number of suppressor–inducer cells and an increased ratio of helper–inducer to suppressor–inducer cells in blood[102, 103]. Additionally, MTX was shown to inhibit the development of experimental allergic encephalomyelitis[104].

The mechanisms responsible for the therapeutic efficacy of MTX in autoimmune disease are unknown, but several known effects of MTX are potentially therapeutic when considered in the context of the present understanding of the immunopathogenesis of these diseases. These activities can be categorized as follows.

1. **Immunosuppressive activity.** An immunosuppressive effect of MTX is supported by the following observations: (a) significant decreases in immunoglobulin (Ig) M-rheumatoid factor levels have been observed in RA patients who improved clinically during MTX therapy[105]; (b) serial assessments of T cell subsets

in RA patients treated with weekly, low dose, oral MTX have demonstrated a significant increase in suppressor–effector $(CD8^+CD11^+)$ cell numbers and a trend for increases in suppressor–inducer $(CD4^+2H4^+)$ cells that paralleled clinical improvement[106]; and (c) peripheral blood lymphocytes from RA patients receiving MTX that are grown in low folate culture conditions show *in vitro* proliferation indices that are lower than those from normal individuals and from RA patients not being treated with MTX[107].

2. **Anti-inflammatory activity.** An anti-inflammatory effect of MTX has long been inferred from the observation that clinical manifestations of RA improve within a few weeks after initiating therapy and worsen just as quickly after the drug is discontinued[108]. The following *in vitro* observations also support an anti-inflammatory activity for MTX: (a) synthesis of the pro-inflammatory leukotriene B_4 by peripheral blood neutrophils from MTX-treated RA patients is suppressed[109]; and (b) the functional activity of IL-1 is decreased by MTX *in vitro*. This may be on the basis of binding of IL-1 to MTX by virtue of a 60% sequence homology between IL-1β and dihydrofolate reductase[110], or inhibition of IL-1β binding to IL-1 receptors on target cells[111].

3. **Immunoregulation.** MTX may also have significant immunoregulatory activities mediated by its antagonistic effect on histamine receptors located on cytotoxic T cells. It has been demonstrated that histamine binds to H_2 receptors on cytotoxic T cells thereby stimulating production of interferon gamma, which has been shown to up-regulate MHC class II expression on immunoactive cells[112]. Histamine-2 receptor antagonists (H$_2$RA) have been used with some success in the treatment of psoriasis[113] and pilot studies with H$_2$RA are already under way in MS.

Clinical experience

There have been three published studies examining the toxicity and clinical efficacy of MTX in patients with multiple sclerosis. In the first pilot study, oral MTX (2.5 mg per day) and oral 6-mercaptopurine (75 mg per day) were administered to MS patients in alternating 3-month cycles for 10–24 months[113]. Although the study was randomized and blinded, the patient groups and outcome measures were poorly defined. Additionally, disease durations in the treatment groups were dissimilar. Thus, even though no therapeutic efficacy was evident, design limitations made the results of this study difficult to interpret. In the second pilot study 45 patients with relapsing or chronic progressive multiple sclerosis were randomly assigned to receive one 2.5 mg

tablet of methotrexate every 12 hours for three consecutive doses each week for one year[114]. A marginally significant ($P = 0.05$) difference in the mean number of exacerbations favoring active treatment was seen in relapsing patients. However, no treatment group differences in progression of DSS scores was noted in relapsing or chronic progressive patients.

In the third study 60 patients with clinically definite chronic progressive multiple sclerosis, ages 21–60 years, with EDSS scores 3.0–6.5, were randomly assigned to receive 7.5 mg of oral methotrexate or placebo one day each week for 2 years[115]. The primary outcome measure for this phase II study was rate of sustained 'treatment failure' in the MTX and PLC arms of the study. As defined prior to study onset, patients could meet treatment failure requirements for the composite outcome variable in any of the following ways: (1) worsening of the entry EDSS score[66] by ≥ 1.0 point for patients with an entry score of 3.0–5.0 or by ≥ 0.5 for those patients with entry EDSS score of 5.5 to 6.5; (2) worsening of the entry ambulation index (AI)[67] score of 2–6 by ≥ 1.0 point; or (3, 4) worsening of $\geq 20\%$ from baseline value on best performance of two successive box and block (BBT) or 9-hole peg test (9HPT)[116] scores obtained with either hand. Thus the composite outcome measure was 'disjunctive'[24] in that worsening of the designated amount on any of its components was taken to indicate treatment failure. Changes on any of the components of this composite outcome measure had to be sustained for 2 or more months to be designated as treatment failure.

A significant treatment effect was measured using the composite outcome. Sustained treatment failure was experienced by 51.6% of patients treated with MTX and 82.8% of patients treated with placebo ($P = 0.011$). Individually, EDSS, 9HPT and BBT components of the composite outcome measure also favored MTX therapy. This effect was strongest for the 9HPT ($P = 0.007$), and was seen to a lesser extent by the BBT ($P = 0.068$), and the EDSS ($P = 0.205$). Sustained treatment failure as defined by change in AI did not differ between the groups. For the 19 patients who met criteria for treatment failure with the 9HPT, the median change in time from baseline 9HPT performance was 17.7 seconds and the median percentage change from baseline was 45.7%. A significant treatment effect favoring methotrexate was also seen as measured by neuropsychological measures of information processing speed (<0.025), confrontational naming ($P < 0.05$) and prose recall ($P < 0.05$)[117] and change in T2-weighted total lesion area as annual MRI score (Goodkin *et al.*, *Neurology*, in press). Adverse experiences were mild and no patient discontinued therapy as a direct result of therapy.

Methotrexate appears to offer a new, relatively well tolerated treatment option for patients with chronic progressive multiple sclerosis. Its benefit appears to be most evident on tests of upper extremity function and preliminary data suggest that patients who experience gradual progression of disability following initial relapses (secondary-progressive multiple sclerosis) are more likely to experience a therapeutic response than patients with insidiously progressive disability from disease onset (primary-progressive multiple sclerosis).

17.2.7 PLASMA EXCHANGE

Background

Although it is generally accepted that multiple sclerosis is predominantly a cell-mediated inflammatory disorder, a role for autoantibodies or other proteinaceous substances in its pathogenesis has not been entirely excluded. This possibility, and the acknowledged effectiveness of plasma exchange in autoantibody- or immune-mediated disorders such as myasthenia gravis and Guillain–Barré syndrome, fostered an interest in plasma exchange as a possible therapy for patients with multiple sclerosis.

Clinical experience

The first double-blind controlled trial of plasma exchange in patients with multiple sclerosis appeared in 1985 [118]. Fifty-four patients with chronic progressive multiple sclerosis were randomized to receive active or sham plasma exchange. Patients receiving active plasma exchange had 5% of their body weight exchanged per week for 20 weeks. All study participants received 1 mg of oral prednisone per kg of body weight every other day tapered after 15 weeks, and oral cyclophosphamide 1.5 mg kg^{-1} daily during the 20-week treatment course. A significant difference in stabilization rates as measured by Kurtzke DSS scores favoring the active plasma exchange was seen after 20 weeks. A second uncontrolled study of 200 patients with chronic progressive multiple sclerosis demonstrated an 83% stabilization or improvement rate as measured by change in Kurtzke DSS scores [119]. The clinical significance of this finding is difficult to interpret in the absence of a control group.

Initial enthusiasm for the use of plasma exchange as a potential therapy for chronic progressive multiple sclerosis was considerably reduced by the findings of the Canadian Cooperative Multiple Sclerosis Study Group [120]. These investigators reported no notable difference in treatment failure rates in patients treated with either: (a) oral prednisone plus 1 gram of intravenous cyclophosphamide every other day until the blood leukocyte count was less than 4500 per μl, or a total dose of 9 grams was administered; (b) daily oral cyclophosphamide, 1.5–2.0 mg kg^{-1}, plus alternate-day oral prednisone and weekly plasma exchange; or (c)

placebo tablets combined with sham plasma exchange. A clinical trial comparing only plasma exchange and placebo treatment for patients with chronic progressive multiple sclerosis has never been performed. At present, there are no convincing data to support the use of plasma exchange in patients with chronic progressive multiple sclerosis.

The role of plasma exchange in the management of severe acute relapses of multiple sclerosis has also received attention [121, 122]. These studies suggest a possible role for plasma exchange when administered alone or co-administered with corticotropin and oral cyclophosphamide in patients with MS-related exacerbations. A phase III study will be required to define properly the role of plasma exchange as a potential treatment option for MS-related exacerbations.

17.2.8 TOTAL LYMPHOID IRRADIATION

Background

Total lymphoid irradiation was initially developed to treat Hodgkin's disease. Shortly thereafter it was used in the treatment of rheumatoid arthritis. The rationale for its use includes: (a) its ability to induce a long-lasting suppression of T cell immune responses in animals receiving skin grafts and bone marrow transplant [123], and (b) the absence of observed long-term sequelae, including hematological malignancies [124]. The beneficial effects seen with total lymphoid irradiation in patients with rheumatoid arthritis [125] resulted in its application to patients with multiple sclerosis. Lymphopenia after total lymphoid irradiation is in general global and non-selective. However, a relatively greater susceptibility of CD4$^+$ T cells combined with the generation of nonspecific suppressor cells appears to be partly responsible for the increased functional suppression observed *in vitro* after total lymphoid irradiation [126]. This restoration of functional suppression is hypothesized to down-regulate the autoimmune response and lead to stabilization of disease activity in patients with multiple sclerosis [127].

Clinical experience

Interferon-β (IFNβ)

Natural fibroblast IFNβ was originally administered intrathecally to 20 MS patients in a randomized, placebo-controlled but unblinded pilot study [148]. The intrathecal route was chosen because it was uncertain whether IFNβ would cross the blood–brain barrier. Fewer exacerbations were experienced by the actively treated patients, and this encouraging result was subsequently confirmed in a randomized double-blind trial [149].

Interferon beta-1b (IFNβ 1b)

Two identical placebo-controlled phase III clinical trials of subcutaneously administered IFNβ-1b conducted simultaneously in the United States and Canada have also documented treatment benefits in actively treated ambulatory relapsing-remitting MS patients [135, 136]. Three-hundred and seventy-two independently ambulatory subjects were recruited, each patient having experienced at least two medically documented acute exacerbations during the 2 years before enrolment. Participants were assigned randomly to one of three treatment groups: (a) placebo, (b) low-dose IFNβ-1b (1.6 million IU) or (c) high-dose IFNβ-1b (8.0 MIU). Each treatment was self-administered subcutaneously every other day for 2–3 years. Treatment groups were well matched for various demographic and disease characteristics. Primary end points were exacerbation rate and the proportion of patients remaining free from exacerbations. Exacerbations were defined as 'the appearance of a new symptom or worsening of an old symptom, attributable to MS; accompanied by an appropriate new neurological abnormality; lasting at least 24 hours in the absence of fever; and preceded by stability or improvement for at least 30 days'. The high-dose group experienced a 34% reduction in annual on-study exacerbation rate compared with the placebo-treated patients during the first 2 years of the study. The proportion of patients who were exacerbation free 2 years after initiating therapy was also significantly greater in the high-dose IFNβ-1b-treated group. Approximately 25% of the patients in this study experienced sustained progression of disability during 3 years of clinical follow-up, but the proportions of patients experiencing sustained progression of disability did not differ significantly between the treatment groups [150]. Neutralizing antibodies to IFNβ-1b were detected at some time during the study in 11% of the placebo-treated patients, 47% of the low-dose drug group, and 45% of the high-dose group. Injection site reactions occurred in 85% and flu-like symptoms or fever occurred in more than 59% of the patients receiving high-dose therapy. Preliminary data suggest that the appearance of neutralizing antibodies is associated with a loss of treatment effect (e.g. reduction in relapse rate) after 18 months on therapy.

This study is the first phase III clinical trial to show convincingly an active treatment-related difference in serial MRI activity [136]. The placebo group showed a 17.1% increase in mean lesion area over 3 years vs. a 6.2% decrease in the high-dosage interferon group ($P = 0.002$). Subgroup analysis of 52 patients who underwent serial MRI examinations every 6 weeks for 2 years demonstrated a 75% reduction in the rate of new lesion formation in the high-dose treatment group compared to placebo. These MRI results, as well as the size and multicenter design, distinguish this study from other clinical trials which, in the absence of serial MRI monitoring, have also demonstrated similar reductions in exacerbation rates [51, 63]. The MRI data, used as a surrogate outcome measure in this trial, were pivotal in the deliberations of the United States Public Health Service Food and Drug Administration (FDA) that ultimately led to the expedited approval of interferon beta-1b for use in ambulatory relapsing-remitting MS patients in the United States. FDA approval for marketing the drug was contingent upon documentation of additional clinical data supporting the drug's efficacy 'within a reasonable amount of time'. So far, there are still no convincing clinical data to support the notion that the reduction in new MRI activity observed in MS patients treated with interferon beta-1b translates into a reduction in measurable progression of sustained disability. Nonetheless, interferon beta-1b has gained widespread acceptance as a treatment to reduce the frequency and severity of exacerbations in patients with actively relapsing-remitting MS.

Interferon beta-1a (IFNβ-1a)

The results of a double-blind placebo-controlled phase III clinical trial of IFNβ-1a were reported in March 1996 [151]. Three hundred and one ambulatory patients with relapsing-remitting clinically definite multiple sclerosis [31], ages 18–55 years, with EDSS scores 1.0–3.5. were enrolled in this multicenter trial and randomly assigned to receive 6.0 million IU of intramuscular interferon beta-1a or placebo each week for 2 years. All patients had experienced two or more medically documented exacerbations during the 2 years prior to study entry. The primary outcome measure of clinical efficacy was time to sustained progression of one or more EDSS points for at least 6 months. There was a significant treatment benefit favoring active therapy, as measured by the primary outcome measure ($P = 0.02$). Treatment benefits favouring active therapy were also seen at the conclusion of the 2-year treatment phase for the following secondary outcome measures: (a) proportions of patients with sustained progression of 1 or more EDSS points at 6, 12, 18 and 24 months; (b) the relative risk of having three or more exacerbations, defined as new or worsening neurologic symptoms for at least 48 hours that were verified by the study examining physician ($P = 0.01$); (c) the number and volume of new T1-weighted gadolinium-enhanced lesions detected on serial yearly brain MRI scans ($P = 0.02$); and (d) the percentage change in T2-weighted lesion volume at 1 year ($P = 0.02$). Drug-related toxicity was mild. In contrast to the experience reported with interferon beta-1b [135], (a) injection site reactions were uncommon, (b) elevation of serum aspartate aminotransferase or alanine aminotransferase, and menstrual disorders were seen in less than 10% of the actively treated patients, and (c) the incidence of serum antibodies against interferon beta-1a was 14% at 1 year and 22% at 2 years.

Comparison of IFNβ-1b and IFNβ-1a

Both IFNβ-1b and IFNβ-1a reduce annual exacerbation rate by approximately one-third. IFNβ-1a significantly slowed the accumulation of neurologic impairment, and a similar trend was evident in patients treated with IFNβ-1b. Some patients may find IFNβ-1a more appealing than IFNβ1b because it is easily administered by intramuscular injection once every week instead of by subcutaneous injection every other day. Additionally, painful and pruritic injection-site reactions are less commonly experienced by patients treated with IFNβ-1a. There are concerns regarding the loss of clinical efficacy in patients who form neutralizing antibodies to IFNβ-1b. Neutralizing antibodies to IFNβ-1b were observed in 45% of patients treated with 8.0 MIU for 2 years [135]. Neutralizing antibodies were also observed in 24% of patients treated with IFNβ-1a for 2 years [151]. Sufficient data have not been collected to determine the clinical significance of neutralizing antibodies to IFNβ-1a, and it is not known whether neutralizing antibodies to IFNβ-1b will degrade treatment efficacy with IFNβ-1a. Additional studies are needed to determine if there is clinically significant cross-reactivity between neutralizing antibodies to IFNβ-1b and IFNβ-1a, and to determine the optimal doses and routes of administration for these new treatment options.

Indications for use and cessation of IFNβ-1b and IFNβ-1a therapy

The Quality Standards Subcommittee of the American Academy of Neurology has issued a practice advisory to assist physicians who are evaluating patients with multiple sclerosis for treatment with interferon beta-1b [152]. This practice advisory is also appropriate for IFNβ-1a. The subcommittee recommendations for initiating and discontinuing therapy are as follows:

A. There is evidence from randomized, controlled clinical trials and expert consensus that interferon beta-1b may be helpful for relapsing-remitting patients who:

1. Have clinically definite MS [31].
2. Are aged 18–50 years.
3. Are ambulatory with EDSS scores less than 6.0 (no unilateral or bilateral constant assistance required).
4. Have had at least two acute exacerbations during the previous 2 years, consisting of the appearance of new symptoms or worsening of old symptoms lasting at least 24 hours in the absence of fever, and preceded by stability or improvement for at least 30 days.

B. There is no evidence from randomized, controlled clinical trials but expert consensus suggests that interferon beta-1b may be helpful for relapsing-remitting patients who:

1. Are older than 50 years.
2. Have EDSS scores ≥ 6.0 (at least unilateral constant assistance required).
3. Have relapsing-progressive disease and also meet criteria A.1 and A.4 above.

C. There is no evidence from randomized, controlled clinical trials nor expert consensus to support therapy with interferon beta-1b in patients with MS who:

1. Have a chronic progressive course from disease onset (primary-progressive multiple sclerosis).

D. Expert consensus suggests that interferon beta-1b should not be given to patients in whom:

1. Concurrent illness is likely to alter compliance or substantially reduce life expectancy, e.g., dementia, alcoholism, malignancy, or other chronic illness.
2. Pregnancy is planned or occurs.

E. For those patients who have been started on interferon beta-1b, expert consensus suggests that the following criteria should be considered for cessation of therapy:

1. Steady progression of disability for 6 months.
2. Treatment with at least three courses of corticotropin or corticosteroids during a 1-year period was required despite interferon beta-1b therapy.
3. Severe depression or suicidal ideation while on interferon beta-1b.
4. Consistent noncompliance in taking the medication as prescribed by the physician.
5. Severe drug toxicity.
6. Planned pregnancy or becoming pregnant.

One might consider adding a seventh recommendation for cessation of interferon beta-1b:

7. An annual exacerbation rate during interferon beta-1b therapy that exceeds the annual exacerbation rate during the year prior to initiating therapy.

Interferon alpha (IFN-α)

The first double-blind, placebo-controlled, crossover study of natural interferon alpha in patients with multiple sclerosis was reported in 1984[153]. Twenty-four patients with two or more exacerbations during the 2 years prior to study entry were randomly assigned to receive daily intramuscular injections of natural human interferon alpha (5 million IU) or placebo for 6 months. After a 6-month washout period the alternate treatment was given for 6 months, followed by a second washout. Exacerbation rates were reduced during interferon alpha and placebo phases compared with pre-study rates. A formal assessment of patient and physician blinding was not performed. However, patients who received interferon alpha after placebo improved significantly more than those who received it before placebo, and the investigators concluded that the patients were able to deduce which course of treatment they had been given. This suggested that the blind had not been effective and that a 'learning effect' could account for the benefits seen with active therapy. A subsequent double-blind, three-arm trial of natural interferon alpha, transfer factor and placebo in 182 relapsing and chronic progressive MS patients failed to detect any treatment group differences in relapse rates or progression of disability[154].

The first double-blind, placebo-controlled trial of recombinant interferon alpha-2 in patients with multiple sclerosis was reported in 1986[155]. In this study 98 clinically definite MS patients with two or more exacerbations during the 2-year period prior to study entry were randomized to receive 2 million IU of recombinant INF-α-2 subcutaneously three times each week for up to 52 weeks. During the trial, exacerbation rates and progression of disability were similar in patients treated with active drug or placebo.

A more recent double-blind placebo-controlled pilot trial with higher doses of recombinant interferon alpha-2a reported evidence of clinical efficacy[156]. Twenty clinically definite MS patients with two or more relapses in the preceding 2 years and EDSS scores less than 6.5 were randomly assigned to receive 9 million IU of INF-α-2a or placebo injected intramuscularly every other day for 6 months. This treatment was tolerated without serious side-effects and actively treated patients had a reduced on-study mean exacerbation rate and unenhanced brain MRI activity compared to placebo-treated patients. In addition, decreased *in vitro* peripheral blood lymphocyte interferon gamma production and increased percentage of suppressor–effector T cell subsets in cerebrospinal fluid were found in patients receiving active therapy. These encouraging results with higher doses of intramuscular INF-α-2a warrant further study in the context of a carefully designed phase III clinical trial.

17.3   Summary

Although the cause of multiple sclerosis remains unknown and a cure unavailable, the disease is no longer considered untreatable. Treatment effects have been demonstrated for several immunosuppressant and immune modulating drugs. Acute relapses are currently most widely treated with 3–5-day intravenous pulses of 500–1000 mg methylprednisolone followed by a tapering course of oral prednisone. Ambulatory relapsing patients are most widely treated with alternate-day subcutaneous injections of interferon beta-1b or weekly intramuscular injections of interferon beta-1a. It is anticipated that copolymer 1 will soon be approved for the treatment of ambulatory relapsing patients. The optimal treatment for non-ambulatory relapsing patients remains uncertain, although it has been suggested that interferon beta-1b and beta 1a may have a role in their management. Although not approved for use in multiple sclerosis, methotrexate is the least toxic widely available treatment option for ambulatory patients with chronic progressive disease. 2-Chlorodeoxyadenosine is a promising new treatment for patients with chronic progressive disease but additional experience will be necessary to define its role. It is increasingly apparent that patients with secondary progressive multiple sclerosis may be more responsive to global immunosuppression than patients whose disease is progressive from onset. There is still no treatment that convincingly alters the progression of disability in patients with primary progressive disease. New promising therapies for chronic progressive MS[71, 115] and biological products[157] potentially capable of enhancing the effects of interferon beta-1b in relapsing MS patients are setting the stage for additional significant therapeutic advances in MS.

References

1. Troiano, R., Hafstein, M., Ruderman, M., Dowling, P. and Cook, S. (1984) Effect of high dose intravenous steroid administration on contrast-enhancing computed tomographic scan lesion in multiple sclerosis. *Ann. Neurol.*, 15, 257–63.
2. Troiano, R., Hafstein, M., Zito, G. *et al.* (1985) The effect of oral corticosteroid dosage on CT-enhancing multiple sclerosis plaques. *J. Neurol. Sci.*, 70, 67–72.
3. Barkoff, F., Hommes, O.R., Scheltens, P. and Valk, J. (1991) Quantitative MRI changes in gadolinium-DPTA enhancement after high-dose intravenous methylprednisolone in multiple sclerosis. *Neurology*, 41, 1219–22.
4. Smith, T., Seeberg, I. and Sjo, O. (1986) Evoked potentials in multiple sclerosis before and after high dose methylprednisolone infusion. *Eur. Neurol.*, 25, 67–73.
5. Troiano, R., Cook, S.D. and Dowling, P.C. (1987) Steroid therapy in multiple sclerosis: point of view. *Arch. Neurol.*, 44, 803–7.
6. Almawi, W.Y., Sewell, K.L., Hadro, E.T. *et al.* (1990) Mode of action of the glucocorticosteroids as immunosuppressive agents, in *Molecular and Cellular Biology of Cytokines*, New York: Wiley-Liss, pp. 321–6.
7. Glaser, G.H., Randt, C.T., Hoefer, P.F.A., Merritt, H.H. and Traiger, C.H. (1950) The influence of adrenocorticotropic hormone (ACTH) on central nervous system and neuromuscular functions. *Trans. Am. Neurol. Assoc.*, 75, 98–104.

8. Jonsson, B., von Reis, G. and Sahlgren, E. (1951) Experience of ACTH and cortisone treatment in some organic neurological cases. *Acta Psychiatr. Neurol. Scand.*, Suppl. 74, pp. 60–3.

9. Rose, A.S., Kuzma, J.W., Kurtzke, J.F. *et al.* (1970) Cooperative study in the evaluation of therapy in multiple sclerosis: ACTH vs placebo. *Neurology*, **20** (part II), 1–59.

10. Kurtzke, J.F. (1955) A new scale for evaluating disability in multiple sclerosis. *Neurology*, **5**, 580–3.

11. Schumacher, G.A., Beebe, G., Kibler, R.E. *et al.* (1965) Problems of experimental trials of therapy in multiple sclerosis: report by the panel on evaluation of experimental trials of therapy in multiple sclerosis. *Ann. NY Acad. Sci.*, **122**, 552–68.

12. Barnes, M.P., Bateman, D.E., Clelenad, P.G. *et al.* (1985) Intravenous (IV) methylprednisolone for multiple sclerosis in relapse. *J. Neurol. Neurosurg. Psychiatry*, **48**, 157–9.

13. Thompson, A.J., Kennard, C., Swash, M. *et al.* (1989) Relative efficacy of IV methylprednisolone and ACTH in the treatment of acute relapses in multiple sclerosis. *Neurology*, **39**, 969–71.

14. Durelli, L., Cocito, D., Riccio, A. *et al.* (1986) High-dose intravenous methylprednisolone in the treatment of multiple sclerosis: clinical-immunologic correlations. *Neurology*, **36**, 238–43.

15. Milligan, N.M., Newcombe, R. and Compston, D.A. (1987) A double-blind controlled trial of high dose methylprednisolone in patients with multiple sclerosis. 1. Clinical effects. *J. Neurol, Neurosurg. Psychiatry*, 50, 511–16.

16. Trotter, J.L. and Garvey, W.F. (1980) Prolonged effects of large-dose methylprednisolone infusion in multiple sclerosis. *Neurology*, **30**, 702–8.

17. Myers, L. (1992) Treatment of multiple sclerosis with ACTH and corticosteroids, in *Treatment of Multiple Sclerosis: Trial Design, Results and Future Perspectives* (eds R.A. Rudick and D.E. Goodkin), New York, Springer-Verlag.

18. Alam, S.M., Kyriakides, T., Lawden, M. and Newman, P.K. (1993) Methylprednisolone in multiple sclerosis: a comparison of oral with intravenous therapy at equivalent high dose. *Neurol. Neurosurg. Psychiatry*, **56**, 1219–20.

19. Fog, T. (1965) The long-term treatment of multiple sclerosis with corticoids. *Acta Neurol. Scand.*, **41** (13, Suppl.), 473–84.

20. Miller, H., Newell, D.J. and Ridley, A. (1961) Multiple sclerosis. Treatment of exacerbations with corticotrophins (ACTH). *Lancet*, ii, 1120–2.

21. Millar, J.H.D., Vas, C.J., Naronha, M.J. *et al.* (1967) Long-term treatment of multiple sclerosis with corticotropin. *Lancet*, ii, 429–31.

22. Smith, M.E., Stone, L.A., Albert, P.S. *et al.* (1993) Clinical worsening in multiple sclerosis is associated with increased frequency and area of gadopentetate dimeglumine-enhancing magnetic resonance imaging lesions. *Ann. Neurol.*, **33**(5), 480–7.

23. Beck, R.W., Cleary, P.A., Trobe, J.D. *et al.* (1993) The effect of corticosteroids for acute optic neuritis on the subsequent development of multiple sclerosis. *N. Engl. J. Med.*, **329**, 1764–9.

24. Goodkin, D.E., Rudick, R.A., Vanderbrug-Medendorp, S. *et al.* (1992) Low-dose (7.5 mg) oral methotrexate (MTX) for chronic progressive multiple sclerosis: design of a randomized placebo-controlled trial with sample size benefits from composite outcome variable. Preliminary data on toxicity. *Online J. Curr. Clin. Trials* [serial online], 25 Sept. 1992 (Doc. No. 19), 7723 words, 89 paragraphs.

25. Rawson, M.D., Liversedge, L.A., Goldfarb, G. and McGill, B.A. (1966) Treatment of acute retrobulbar neuritis with corticotrophin. *Lancet*, ii, 1044–6.

26. Rawson, M.D., and Liversedge, L.A. (1969) Treatment of retrobulbar neuritis with corticotrophin. *Lancet*, ii, 222.

27. Gould, E.S., Bird, A.C., Leaver, P.K. and McDonald, W.I. (1977) Treatment of optic neuritis by retrobulbar injection of triamcinolone. *Br. Med. J.*, i, 1495–7.

28. Beck, R.W. and the Optic Neuritis Study Group (1992) Corticosteroid treatment of optic neuritis: a need to change treatment practices. *Neurology*, **42**, 1133–5.

29. Beck, R.W., Cleary, P.A., Anderson, M.A. *et al.* (1992) A randomized, controlled trial of corticosteroids in the treatment of acute optic neuritis. *N. Engl. J. Med.*, **326**, 581–8.

30. Ebers, G.C. (1985) Optic neuritis and multiple sclerosis. *Arch. Neurol.*, **42**, 702–4.

31. Poser, C.M., Paty, D.W., Scheinberg, L. *et al.* (1983) New diagnostic criteria for multiple sclerosis: guidelines for research protocols. *Ann. Neurol.*, **13**, 227–31.

32. Silberberg, D.H. (1993) Corticosteroids and optic neuritis. *N. Engl. J. Med.*, **329**, 1808–10.

33. Miller, D.H., Ormerod, I.E.C., Rudge, P. *et al.* (1989) Early risk of multiple sclerosis following isolated acute syndromes of the brainstem and spinal cord. *Ann. Neurol.*, **26**, 635–9.

34. Miller, D.H., McDonald, W.I., Blumhardt, L.D. *et al.* (1987) Magnetic resonance imaging in isolated noncompressive spinal cord syndromes. *Ann. Neurol.*, **22**, 714–23.

35. Lassman, H. (1983) *Comparative Neuropathology of Chronic Experimental Allergic Encephalomyelitis and Multiple Sclerosis*, Berlin, Springer-Verlag.

36. Walsh, M. and Tourtellotte, W. (1983) The cerebrospinal fluid in multiple sclerosis, in *Multiple sclerosis: Pathology, Diagnosis and Management* (eds J. Hallpike, C. Adams and W. Tourtellotte), London, Chapman & Hall, pp. 275–358.

37. Hofman, F.M., vonHanwehr, R.I., Dinarello, C.A. *et al.* (1986) Immuno-regulatory molecules and IL2 receptors identified in multiple sclerosis brain. *J. Immunol.*, **136**, 3239–5.

38. Seboun, E., Robinson, M., Doolittle, T. *et al.* (1989) A susceptibility locus for multiple sclerosis is linked to the T cell beta chain complex. *Cell*, **57**, 1095–100.

39. Morimoto, C., Hafler, D.A., Weiner, H.L. (1988) Selective loss of suppressor inducer T cell subset in progressive multiple sclerosis: analysis with anti-2H4 monoclonal antibody. *N. Engl. J. Med.*, **316**, 67–72.

40. Panitch, H.S., Hirsch, R.L., Schindler, J. and Johnson, K.P. (1987) Treatment of multiple sclerosis with gamma interferon: exacerbations associated with activation of the immune system. *Neurology*, **37**, 1097–102.

41. Rudick, R.A. and Goodkin, D.E. (eds) (1992) *Treatment of Multiple Sclerosis: Trial Design, Results, and Future Perspectives*, New York, Springer Verlag.

42. Goodkin, D.E., Rudick, R.A. and Ransohoff R.M. (1992) Treatment of multiple sclerosis: current status. Part 1. Clinical trials of experimental therapies. *Clevel. Clin. J. Med.*, **59**, 63–74.

43. Tucker, W.G. and Kapphahn, K.H. (1969) A preliminary evaluation of azathioprine (Imuran) in the treatment of multiple sclerosis. *Henry Ford Hosp. Med. J.*, **17** (2), 89–91.

44. Swinburn, W.R. and Liversedge, L.A. (1973) Long-term treatment of multiple sclerosis with azathioprine. *J. Neurol. Neurosurg. Psychiatry*, **36**, 124–6.

45. Ghezzi, A., Di Falco, M., Locatelli, C. *et al.* (1989) Clinical controlled trial of azathioprine in multiple sclerosis, in *Recent Advances in Multiple Sclerosis Therapy* (eds D.R. Gonsette and P. Delmotte), Amsterdam, Elsevier.

46. Mertin, J., Rudge, P., Kremer, M. *et al.* (1982) Double-blind controlled trial of immunosuppression in the treatment of multiple sclerosis: final report. *Lancet*, ii, 351–4.

47. British and Dutch Multiple Sclerosis Azathioprine Trial Group (1988) Double-masked trial of azathioprine in multiple sclerosis. *Lancet*, ii, 179–83.

48. Milanese, C., La Mantia, L., Salmaggi, A. *et al.* (1988) Double blind controlled randomized study on azathioprine efficacy in multiple sclerosis; preliminary results. *Ital. J. Neurol. Sci.*, **9**, 53–7.

49. Goodkin, D.E., Bailly, R.C., Teetzen, M.L. *et al.* The efficacy of azathioprine in relapsing-remitting multiple sclerosis. *Neurology*, **41**, 20–5.

50. Ellison, G.W., Myers, L.W., Mickey, M.R. *et al.* (1989) A placebo controlled, randomized, double-masked, variable dosage, clinical trial of azathioprine with and without methylprednisolone in multiple sclerosis. *Neurology*, **39**, 1018–26.

51. Yudkin, P.L., Ellison, G.W., Ghezzi, A. *et al.* (1991) Overview of azathioprine treatment in multiple sclerosis. *Lancet*, **338**, 1051–5.

52. INFB Multiple Sclerosis Study Group (1993) Interferon beta-1b is effective in relapsing-remitting multiple sclerosis. I: Clinical results of a multicenter, randomized, double-blind, placebo-controlled trial. *Neurology*, **43**, 655–61.

53. Hughes, R.A.C. (1992) Treatment of multiple sclerosis with azathioprine, in *Treatment of Multiple Sclerosis: Trial Design, Results and Future Perspective* (eds R.A. Rudick and D.E. Goodkin) London, Springer-Verlag.

54. Kinlen, L.J. (1985) Incidence of cancer in rheumatoid arthritis and other disorders after immunosuppressive treatment. *Am. J. Med.*, **78** (Suppl. 1A), 44–9.

55. Goodkin, D.E., Daughtry, M.M. and VanderBrug-Medendorp, S. (1992) The incidence of malignancy following cyclophosphamide (CTX) or azathioprine (AZA) treatment of multiple sclerosis (MS). *Ann. Neurol.*, **32**, 257.

56. Lhermitte, F., Marteau, R. and de Saxce, H. (1987) Treatment of progressive and severe forms of multiple sclerosis using a combination of antilymphocyte serum, azathioprine and prednisone. Clinical and biological results. Comparison with a control group treated with azathioprine and prednisone only: 4-year follow-up. *Rev. Neurol. (Paris)*, **143**, 98–107.

57. Arnon, R. and Teitelbaum, D. (1980) Desensitization of experimental allergic encephalomyelitis with synthetic peptide analogue, in *The Suppression of Experimental Allergic Encephalomyelitis and Multiple Sclerosis* (eds A.N. Davison and M.L. Cuzner), New York, Academic Press, pp. 105–17.

58. Teitelbaum, D., Milo, R., Arnon, R. and Sela, M. (1992) Synthetic copolymer 1 inhibits human T-cell lines specific for myelin basic protein. *Proc. Natl Acad. Sci.*, **89**, 137–41.

59. Milo, R. and Panitch, H. (1994) Additive effects of COP-1 and IFN-beta on immune responses to myelin basic protein. *Neurology*, **44** (Suppl. 2), A212.

60. Fridkis-Hareli, M., Teitelbaum, D., Gurevich, E. *et al.* (1994) Direct binding of myelin basic protein and synthetic copolymer 1 to class II major histocompatibility complex molecules on living antigen-presenting cells – specificity and promiscuity. *Proc. Natl Acad. Sci.*, **91**, 4872–6.

61. Lisak, T.P., Zweiman, B., Blanchard, N. *et al.* (1983) Effective treatment with copolymer 1 on the *in vivo* and *in vitro* manifestations of experimental allergic encephalomyelitis. *J. Neuroimmunol.*, **62**, 281–93.

62. Critchfield, J.M., Racke, M.K., Zuniga-Plucker, J.C. *et al.* (1994) T cell deletion in high antigen dose therapy of autoimmune encephalomyelitis. *Science*, **263**, 1139–42.

63. Bornstein, M., Miller, A., Slagle, S. *et al.* (1987) A pilot trial of COP 1 in exacerbating remitting multiple sclerosis. *N. Engl. J. Med.*, **317**, 408–14.

64. Bornstein, M.B., Miller, A., Slagle, S. *et al.* (1991) A placebo controlled, double-blind, randomized, two-center, pilot trial of copolymer 1 in chronic progressive multiple sclerosis. *Neurology*, **41**, 533–9.

65. Johnson, K.P., Brooks, B.R., Cohen, J.A. *et al.* (1995) Copolymer 1 reduces relapse rate and improves disability in relapsing-remitting multiple sclerosis: results of a phase III multicenter, double-blind, placebo-controlled trial. *Neurology*, **45**, 1268–76.

66. Kurtzke, J.F. (1983) Rating neurologic impairment in multiple sclerosis: an expanded disability status scale (EDSS). *Neurology*, **33**, 1444–52.

67. Hauser, S.L., Dawson, D.M., Lehrich, J.R. *et al.* (1983) Intensive immunosuppression in progressive multiple sclerosis: a randomized, three-arm study of high-dose cyclophosphamide, plasma exchange, and ACTH. *N. Engl. J. Med.*, **308**, 173–80.

68. National Multiple Sclerosis Society (1993). Open study of copolymer for multiple sclerosis News no. RMP 1–93, 15 January.

69. Carson, D.A., Wasson, D.B., Taetle, R. and Yu, A. (1983) Specific toxicity of 2-chlorodeoxyadenosine toward resting and proliferating human lymphocytes. *Blood*, **62**, 737–43.

70. Carson, D.A., Wasson, D.B. and Beutler, E. (1984) Antileukemic and immunosuppressive activity of 2-chloro-2'-deoxyadenosine. *Proc. Natl Acad. Sci. USA*, **81**, 2232–6.

71. Sipe, J.C., Romine, J.S., Koziol, J.A. *et al.* (1994) Cladribine in treatment of chronic progressive multiple sclerosis. *Lancet*, **344**, 9–13.

72. Piro, L.D. (1992) 2-Chlorodeoxyadenosine treatment of lymphoid malignancies. *Blood*, **79**, 843–5.

73. Beutler, E., Piro, L.D., Saven, A. *et al.* (1991) 2-chlorodeoxyadenosine (2-CdA): a potent chemotherapuetic and immunosuppression nucleoside. *Leuk. Lymphoma*, **5**, 1–8.

74. Beutler, E. (1992) Cladribine (2-chlorodeoxyadenosine). *Lancet*, **340**, 952–6.

75. Wong, E.T., Vahdat, L., Tunkel, R.S. *et al.* (1994) Severe motor weakness from high-dose 2-chorodeoxyadenosine. *Ann. Neurol.*, **36**, 293.

76. Sipe, J.C., Knobler, R.L., Braheny, S.L. *et al.* A neurologic rating scale (NRS) for use in multiple sclerosis. *Neurology*, **34**, 1368–72.

77. Moody, D.J., Fahey, J.L., Grable, E. *et al.* (1987) Administration of monthly pulses of cyclophosphamide in multiple sclerosis patients: effects of long-term treatment on immunologic parameters. *J. Neuroimmunol.*, **14**, 161–73.

78. Moody, D.J., Fahey, J.L., Grable, E. *et al.* (1987) Administration of monthly pulses of cyclophosphamide in multiple sclerosis patients: delayed recovery of several immune parameters following discontinuation of long-term cyclophosphamide treatment. *J. Neuroimmunol.*, **14**, 175–82.

79. Uitehaag, B.M.J., Nillesen, W.M. and Hommes, O.R. (1989) Long-lasting effects of cyclophosphamide on lymphocytes in peripheral blood and spinal fluid. *Acta Neurol. Scand.*, **79**, 12–17.

80. Goodkin, D., Plencner, S., Palmer-Saxerud, J. *et al.* (1987) Cyclophosphamide in chronic progressive multiple sclerosis: maintenance vs non-maintenance therapy. *Arch. Neurol.*, **44**(8), 823–7.

81. Weiner, H.L., Mackin, G.A., Orav, J.A. *et al.* (1993) Intermittent cyclophosphamide pulse therapy in progressive multiple sclerosis: final report of the Northeast Cooperative Multiple Sclerosis Treatment Group. *Neurology*, **43**, 910–18.

82. Likosky, W.H., Fireman, B., Elmore, R. *et al.* (1991) Intense immunosuppression in chronic progressive multiple sclerosis: the Kaiser study. *J. Neurol. Neurosurg. Psychiatry*, **54**, 1055–60.

83. The Canadian Cooperative Multiple Sclerosis Study Group (1991) The Canadian cooperative trial of cyclophosphamide and plasma exchange in multiple sclerosis. *Lancet*, **337**, 441–6.

84. Noseworthy, J.A., Vandervoort, M.K., Penman, M. *et al.* (1991) Cyclophosphamide and plasma exchange in multiple sclerosis [Letter]. *Lancet*, **337**, 1540–1.

85. Weiner, H.L., Hauser, S.L., Dawson, D.M. *et al.* (1991) Cyclophosphamide and plasma exchange in multiple sclerosis [Letter]. *Lancet*, **337**, 1033–4.

86. Bach, J.F. (1989) Cyclosporine in autoimmune diseases. *Transplant. Proc.*, **21**, 97–113.

87. Reem, G.H., Cook, L.A. and Vilck, J. (1983) Gamma interferon synthesis by human thymocytes and T lymphocytes by cyclosporine A. *Science*, **221**, 63–5.

88. Elliott, J.F., Lin, Y., Mitzel, S.B. *et al.* (1984) Induction of interleukin 2 messenger RNA inhibited by cyclosporin A. *Science*, **226**, 1439–41.

89. Colombani, P.M. and Hess, A.D. (1987) T-lymphocyte inhibition by cyclosporine. Potential mechanisms. *Biochem. Pharmacol.*, **36**, 3789–93.

90. Rich, S., Caprina, M.R. and Arthelger, C. (1984) Suppressor T cell growth and differentiation: identification of a cofactor required from suppressor T cell function and distinct from interleukin 2. *J. Exp. Med.*, **159**, 1473–90.

91. Kappos, L., Patzold, U., Poser, S. *et al.* (1988) Cyclosporine versus azathioprine in the long-term treatment of multiple sclerosis – results of the German Multicenter Study. *Ann. Neurol.*, **23**, 56–63.

92. Rudge, P., Koetsier, J.C., Mertin, J. *et al.* (1989) Randomized double-blind controlled trial of cyclosporin in multiple sclerosis. *J. Neurol. Neurosurg. Psychiatry*, **52**, 559–65.

93. Beyer, J.O.M. (1987) Second International Congress on Cyclosporine, Washington DC, USA, November 4–7, 1987 (Abstract). University of Texas Health Science Center, Organ Transplantation Center/The Division of Continuing Education.

94. Rudge, P., Koetsier, J.C., Mertin, J. *et al.* (1989) Randomized double-blind controlled trial of cyclosporin in multiple sclerosis. *J. Neurol. Neurosurg. Psychiatry*, **52**, 559–65.

95. The Multiple Sclerosis Study Group (1990) Efficacy and toxicity of cyclosporine in chronic progressive multiple sclerosis: a randomized, double-blind, placebo-controlled clinical trial. *Ann. Neurol.*, **27**, 591–605.

96. Weinblatt, M.E., Weissman, B.N., Holdsworth, D.E. *et al.* (1992) Long-term prospective study of methotrexate in the treatment of rheumatoid arthritis. 84-month update. *Arth. Rheum.*, **35**, 129–37.

97. Kremer, J.M. and Lee, J.K. (1988) A long-term prospective study of the use of methotrexate in rheumatoid arthritis. Update after a mean of fifty-three months. *Arth. Rheum.*, **31**(5), 577–84.

98. Furst, D.F. and Kremer, J.M. (1988) Methotrexate in rheumatoid arthritis. *Arth. Rheum.*, **31**, 305–14.

99. Rau, R., Herborn, G., Karger, T. and Werdier, D. (1991) Retardation of radiologic progression in rheumatoid arthritis with methotrexate therapy. *Arth. Rheum.*, **34**, 1236–44.

100. Rustin, G.J.S., Rustin, F., Dent, J. *et al.* (1983) No increase in second tumors after methotrexate chemotherapy for gestational trophoblastic tumors. *N. Engl. J. Med.*, **308**, 473–6.

101. Zatarain, E., Williams, C. and Fries, J.F. (1988) Comparison of adverse reactions of methotrexate and other disease modifying agents. *Arth. Rheum.*, **31** (Suppl.), D84.

102. Reynolds, W.J., Perra, M., Yoon, S.J. and Klein, N.M. (1985) Evaluation of clinical and prognostic significance of T-cell regulatory subsets in rheumatoid arthritis. *J. Rheumatol.*, **12**, 49–56.

103. Goto, M., Miyamoto, T., Nishioka, K. and Uchida, S. (1987) T cytotoxic and helper cells are markedly increased and T suppressor and inducer cells are markedly decreased in rheumatoid synovial fluids. *Arth. Rheum.*, **30**, 737–43.

104. Lisak, R.P., Heinz, R.G., Keis, M.W. and Alvord, E.C. (1970) Dissociation of antibody production from disease suppression in the inhibition of allergic encephalomyelitis by myelin basic protein. *J. Immunol.*, **104**, 1435–46.

105. Alarcon, G.S., Schrohenloher, R.E., Bartolucci, A.A. *et al.* (1990) Suppression of rheumatoid factor production by methotrexate in patients with rheumatoid arthritis. Evidence for differential influences of therapy and clinical status on IgM and IgA rheumatoid factor expression. *Arth. Rheum.*, **33**, 1156–61.

106. Calabrese, L.H., Taylor, J.V., Wilke, W.S., Segal, A.M. and Clough, J.D. (1988) Methotrexate (MTX) immunoregulatory T-cell subsets and rheumatoid arthritis: is MTX an immunomodulator? *Arths. Rheum.*, **31** (Suppl. 1) C20.

107. Hine, R.J., Everson, M.P., Hardon, J.M. *et al.* (1990) Methotrexate therapy in rheumatoid arthritis patients diminishes lectin-induced mononuclear cell proliferation. *Rheumatol. Int.*, **10**, 165–9.

108. Weinblatt, M.E., Coblyn, J.S., Fox, D.A. *et al.* (1985) Efficacy of low-dose methotrexate in rheumatoid arthritis. *N. Engl. J. Med.*, **312**, 818–22.

109. Sperling, R.I., Benincaso, A.I., Anderson, R.J. *et al.* (1992) Acute and chronic suppression of leukotriene B_4 synthesis ex vivo in neutrophils from patients with rheumatoid arthritis beginning treatment with methotrexate. *Arth. Rheum.*, **35**, 376–84.

110. Segal, R., Yaron, M. and Tartakovsky, B. (1990) Methotrexate: mechanism of action in rheumatoid arthritis. *Semin. Arth. Rheum.*, **20**, 190–200.

111. Brody, M., Bohm, I. and Bauer, R. (1993) Mechanism of action of methotrexate: experimental evidence that methotrexate blocks the binding of interleukin 1B to the interleukin 1 receptor on target cells. *Eur. J. Clin. Chem. Clin. Biochem.*, **31**, 667–74.

112. Nielsen, H.J. and Hammer, J.H. (1992) Possible role of histamine in pathogenesis of autoimmune diseases: implications for immunotherapy with histamine-2 receptor antagonists. *Med. Hypoth.*, **39**, 349–55.

113. Neumann, J.W. and Ziegler, D.K. (1972) Therapeutic trial of immunosuppressive agents in multiple sclerosis. *Neurology*, **22** (12), 1268–71.

114. Currier, R.D., Haerer, A.F. and Maydrech, E.F. (1993) Low dose oral methotrexate treatment of multiple sclerosis: a pilot study. *J. Neurol. Neurosurg. Psychiatry*, **56** (11), 1217–18.

115. Goodkin, D.E., Rudick, R.A., Vanderbrug Medendrop, S. *et al.* (1995) Low-dose (7.5 mg) oral methotrexate is effective in reducing the rate of progression of neurological impairment in patients with chronic progressive multiple sclerosis. *Ann. Neurol.*, **37**, 30–40.

116. Fisher, R.A. (1922) On the interpretation of the chi-square from contingency tables and the calculation of P. *J. R. Statist. Soc.*, **85**, 87–94.

117. Fischer, J.S., Goodkin, D.E., Rudick, R.A. *et al.* (1994) Low-dose (7.5 mg) oral methotrexate improves neuropsychological function in patients with chronic progressive multiple sclerosis. *Ann. Neurol.*, **36**, 289.

118. Khatri, B.O., McQuillen, M.P., Harrington, G.J. *et al.* (1985) Chronic progressive multiple sclerosis; double blind controlled trial of plasmapheresis in patients taking immunosuppressive drugs. *Neurology*, **35**, 312–19.

119. Khatri, B.O., McQuillen, M.P., Hoffman, R.G. *et al.* (1991) Plasmapheresis in chronic progressive MS: a long term study. *Neurology*, **41**, 409–14.

120. The Canadian Cooperative Multiple Sclerosis Study Group (1991) The Canadian cooperative trial of cyclophosphamide and plasma exchange in multiple sclerosis. *Lancet*, **337**, 441–6.

121. Weiner, H.L., Dau, P.C., Khatri, B.O. *et al.* (1989) Double-blind study of true vs sham plasma exchange in patients treated with immunosuppression for acute attacks of multiple sclerosis. *Neurology*, **39**, 1143–9.

122. Rodriguez, M., Cairns, W.E., Bartleson, J.D. *et al.* (1993) Plasmapheresis in acute episodes of fulminant CNS inflammatory demyelination. *Neurology*, **43**, 1100–4.

123. Slavin, S.B., Reitz, C.P., Bieber, H.S. *et al.* (1978) Transplantation tolerance in adult rats using total lymphoid irradiation; permanent survival of skin, heart and marrow allografts. *J. Exp. Med.*, **147**, 700–7.

124. Svaifler, N.J. (1987) Fractionated total lymphoid irradiation; a promising new treatment for rheumatoid arthritis? Yes, no, maybe. *Arth. Rheum.*, **30**, 109–14.

125. Field, E.D.S., Strober, R.T., Hoppe, A. *et al.* (1983) Sustained improvement of intractable rheumatoid arthritis after total lymphoid irradiation. *Arth. Rheum.*, **26**, 937–46.

126. Strober, S., Kotzin, B., Field, E. *et al.* (1986) Treatment of autoimmune disease with total lymphoid irradiation: cellular humoral mechanisms. *Ann. NY Acad. Sci.*, **475**, 285–95.

127. Weiner, H.L. and Hafler, D.A. (1988) Immunotherapy of multiple sclerosis. *Ann. Neurol.*, **23**, 211–22.

128. Cook, S.D., Troiano, R., Zito, G. *et al.* (1986) Effect of total lymphoid irradiation in chronic progressive multiple sclerosis. *Lancet*, **i**, 1405–11.

129. Cook, S.D., Devereux, C. and Troiano, R. (1990) The treatment of patients with chronic progressive multiple sclerosis with total lymphoid irradiation, in *Handbook of Multiple Sclerosis* (ed. S.D. Cook), New York, Marcel Dekker, pp. 402–23.

130. Cook, S.D., Devereux, C., Troiano, R. *et al.* (1995) Combination total lymphoid irradiation and low dose corticosteroid therapy for progressive multiple sclerosis. *Acta Neurol. Scand.*, **91** (1), 22–7.

131. Isaac, A. and Lindenmann, J. (1957) Virus interference I. The interferon. *Proc. R. Soc. Lond. [Biol.]*, **147**, 258–73.

132. Stiehm, E.R., Kronenberg, L.H., Rosenblatt, H.M. *et al.* (1982) Interferon: immunobiology and clinical significance. *Ann. Intern. Med.*, **96**, 80–93.

133. Merigan, T.C., Rand, K.H., Polland, R.B. *et al.* (1978) Human leukocyte interferon for the treatment of herpes zoster in patients with cancer. *N. Engl. J. Med.*, **298**, 981–7.

134. Neighbor, P.A. and Bloom, B.R. (1979) Absence of virus-induced lymphocyte suppression and interferon production in multiple sclerosis. *Proc. Natl Acad. Sci. USA*, **76**, 476–80.

135. The IFNB Multiple Sclerosis Study Group (1993) Interferon beta-1b is effective in relapsing-remitting multiple sclerosis. I. Clinical results of a multicenter, randomized, double-blind, placebo-controlled trial. *Neurology*, **43**, 655–61.

136. Paty, D.W., Li, D.K.B., the UBC MS/MRI Study Group and the IFNB Multiple Sclerosis Study Group (1993) Interferon beta 1-b is effective in relapsing-remitting multiple sclerosis. II. MRI analysis results of a multicenter, randomized, double-blind, placebo-controlled trial. *Neurology*, **43**, 662–7.

137. Thompson, M.R. Zhang, Z., Fournier, A. *et al.* (1985) Characterization of human beta-interferon-binding sites on human cells. *J. Biol. Chem.*, **260**, 563–7.

138. Noronha, A., Toskas, A. and Jensen, M.A. (1992) Contrasting effects of alpha, beta and gamma-interferons on nonspecific suppressor function in multiple sclerosis. *Ann. Neurol.*, **31**, 103–6.

139. Steinman, L. (1993) Autoimmune disease. *Scientific American*, **269**, 106–15.

140. Mark, D., Drummond, R., Creasey, A. *et al.* (1984) A synthetic mutant of interferon beta for clinical trial, in *Proceedings of the International Symposium on Interferons* (ed. T. Kishida), Japan, pp. 167–72.

141. Borden, E.C., Hogan, T.F. and Voelkel, J. (1982) Comparative antiproliferative activity *in vitro* of natural interferons alfa and beta for diploid and transformed human cells. *Cancer Res.*, **42**, 4948–53.

142. Herberman, R.R., Ortaldo, J.R. and Bonnard, G.D. (1979) Augmentation by interferon of human natural and antibody-dependent cell-mediated cytotoxicity. *Nature*, **277**, 221–3.

143. Huang, K.Y., Donahoe, R.M., Gordon, F.B. *et al.* (1971) Enhancement of phagocytosis by interferon-containing preparations. *Infect. Immun.*, **4**, 581–8.

144. Giacomini, P., Aguzzi, A., Pestka, S. *et al.* (1984) Modulation of recombinant DNA leukocyte (alfa) and fibroblast (beta) interferons of the expression and shedding of HLA- and tumor-associated antigens by human melanoma cells. *J. Immunol.*, **133**, 1649–55.

147. Noronha, A., Toscas, A. and Jensen, M.A. (1990) Interferon beta augments suppressor cell function in multiple sclerosis. *Ann. Neurol.*, **27**, 207–10.

148. Jacobs, L., O'Malley, J., Freeman, A. *et al.* (1981) Intrathecal interferon reduces exacerbations of multiple sclerosis. *Science*, **214**, 1026–8.

149. Jacobs, L., Salazar, A.M., Herndon, R. *et al.* (1987) Intrathecally administered natural human fibroblast interferon reduces exacerbations of multiple sclerosis. Results of a multicenter, double-blind study. *Arch. Neurol.*, **44**, 589–95.

149a. Goodkin, D.E. (1996) Interferon beta treatment for multiple sclerosis: persisting questions. *Mult. Scler.*, **1**, 321–4.

150. Department of Health and Human Services Public Health Service Food and Drug Administration. (1993) Peripheral and Central Nervous System Drugs Advisory Committee Meeting No. 35. Friday, 19 March 1993. Food and Drug Administration Freedom of Information Staff. HFI-35, Room 12a–16, Fishers Lane, Rockville, Maryland. Transcript pp. 44–53.

151. Jacobs, L.D., Cookfair, D.L., Rudick, R.A. *et al.* and The Multiple Sclerosis Research Group (MSCRG) (1996) Intramuscular interferon beta-1a for disease progression in exacerbating-remitting multiple sclerosis. *Ann. Neurol.*, **39**, 285–94.

152. Practice Advisory on Selection of Patients with Multiple Sclerosis for Treatment with Betaseron (1944) *Neurology*, **44**, 1537–40.

153. Knobler, R.L., Pantich, H.S., Braheny, S.L. *et al.* (1984) Systemic alpha-interferon therapy of multiple sclerosis. *Neurology*, **34**, 1273–9.

154. Austims Research Group (1989) Interferon-α and transfer factor in the treatment of multiple sclerosis: a double-blind, placebo-controlled trial. *J. Neurol. Neurosurg. Psychiatry*, **52**, 566–74.

155. Camenga, D.L., Johnson, K.P., Alter, M. *et al.* (1986) Systemic recombinant α-2 interferon therapy in relapsing multiple sclerosis. *Arch. Neurol.*, **46**, 1239–46.

156. Durelli, L., Bongioanni, M.R., Cavallo, R. *et al.* (1994) Chronic systemic high-dose recombinant interferon alfa-2a reduces exacerbation rate, MRI signs of disease activity, and lymphocyte interferon gamma production in relapsing-remitting multiple sclerosis. *Neurology*, **44**, 406–13.

157. Dinarello, C.A., Gelfand, J.A. and Wolff, S.M. (1993) Anticytokine strategies in the treatment of systemic inflammatory response syndrome. *J. Am. Med. Assoc.*, **269**, 1829–35.

18 AN INVESTIGATIONAL APPROACH TO DISEASE THERAPY IN MULTIPLE SCLEROSIS

Celia F. Brosnan, Michael K. Racke and Krzysztof Selmaj

Research into the etiology and pathogenesis of multiple sclerosis (MS) has led to the development of a number of model systems that provide an opportunity for defining not only the potential mechanisms involved in disease progression but also an opportunity to test the efficacy of various therapeutic strategies. These model systems include the induction of experimental autoimmune encephalomyelitis (EAE) in various species using central nervous system (CNS) myelin antigens; viral-induced models of inflammatory demyelination such as follow infection with Theiler's murine encephalomyelitis virus (TMEV); induced demyelination of CNS axons by agents such as lysophosphatidyl choline or ethidium bromide; and various myelin-deficient mutants of mice and rats. Each of these model systems has features that make them particularly suitable for testing various aspects of the pathogenesis of the inflammatory demyelinating lesion. EAE permits an analysis of factors that contribute to the development of autoimmune diseases in the CNS, viral models permit an analysis of inflammatory immune responses in the CNS that are not autoimmune-mediated, and the induction of various demyelinated lesions permits analysis of the efficacy of repair paradigms. In this chapter we review some of the experimental approaches that are being tested in these various model systems, with the long-term goal that they will provide new approaches to therapeutic intervention in patients with MS.

18.1 Therapy directed at the trimolecular complex

The activation of an immune response requires interaction between the antigen, the receptor on the immunocompetent cell (lymphocytes), and an accessory cell that functions to process and present antigen to the lymphocyte (antigen-presenting cell, APC) (Figure 18.1). In antigen responses that involve T lymphocytes bearing the $\alpha\beta$ T cell receptor (TCR), the APC express on the cell surface either class I or class II molecules of the major histocompatibility complex (MHC, the equivalent of HLA antigens in humans). This combination of antigen, T cell receptor (TCR) and major histocompatibility complex (MHC) is known as the trimolecular complex[1,2]. The interaction of these three elements, assisted by involvement of the CD4 or CD8 co-receptors, represents the initial phase of lymphocyte activation (signal 1). To achieve complete activation a second signal (signal 2) is required that is provided by engagement of costimulatory molecules on lymphocytes and APC (Figure 18.1). In this section we will explore the various avenues of approach that have been tested to block the first signal of lymphocyte activation; the therapeutic potential of interfering with the second signal of lymphocyte activation will be discussed below in the section on costimulatory molecules.

18.1.1 BLOCKADE OF ANTIGEN PRESENTATION

Antigen is presented to the lymphocyte in the context of either class I or class II MHC molecules. MHC molecules are highly polymorphic and different allelic forms have distinct peptide binding specificities. Several lines of evidence support the conclusion that class II MHC molecules play an important role in the inflammatory demyelinating diseases. Genetic analysis of components of the MHC in patients with MS has demonstrated associations with specific MHC class II molecules that vary between different ethnic

Multiple Sclerosis: Clinical and pathogenetic basis. Edited by Cedric S. Raine, Henry F. McFarland and Wallace W. Tourtellotte. Published in 1997 by Chapman & Hall, London. ISBN 0 412 30890 8.

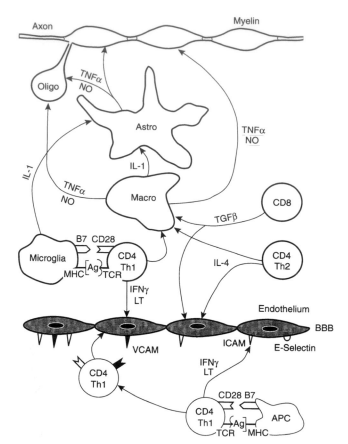

Figure 18.1 Diagrammatic representation of potential sites of therapeutic intervention in multiple sclerosis.

had no effect [7, 8]. The successful use of these antibodies in various models of EAE then led to the development of chimeric antibodies that utilized the Fab sequences of murine monoclonal antibodies directed against human HLA DR, and the Fc fragments of human IgG, with the hope that these chimeric antibodies would be less antigenic and permit the use of repeated application in patients. Using chimeric antibodies directed against CD4, a trial in MS has recently been completed. In this trial it was observed that the number of CD4+ cells decreased significantly after treatment and that repeated treatments could be employed without any serious side-effects [9]. Although no clinical efficacy was noted, the results of these trials are encouraging in that they show that chimeric antibodies can be successfully used in patients without generating any untoward side-effects and thus pave the way for the potential use of antibodies directed against other components of the immune response, as a means of therapeutic intervention in patients with MS. With respect to class II MHC molecules, current studies in the field are directed at making this mode of therapy more selective by raising antibodies to disease-specific alleles of the MHC.

18.1.2   INHIBITORY PROTEINS AND PEPTIDES

MHC class II molecules bind peptides derived from processed antigen for presentation to T cells [10]. These antigenic peptides have residues that interact with the MHC and residues that interact with the TCR. Studies in various model systems have shown that peptides can be generated that compete or inhibit binding of the native peptide to MHC class II molecules and that these peptides can block sensitization to the encephalitogenic epitopes. Several approaches are currently under investigation to use this strategy to block autoimmune diseases such as EAE. They include antigens that are structurally related to pathogenic antigens, such as MBP, as well as unrelated peptides.

The term inhibitory proteins has been proposed for compounds that compete with putative myelin antigens for binding to the MHC. The major candidate for use in this context is the synthetic basic random polymer called copolymer 1 (COP 1) that was designed as a non-encephalitogenic analogue of myelin basic protein [11]. Following the effective demonstration of its usefulness in the treatment of EAE in various animal model systems, it has now progressed through phase III trials in patients with MS, with efficacy noted in patients in the early stages of the relapsing-remitting form of the disease. The outcome of these trials and the current status of research in this area is reviewed in the previous chapter.

Several studies have now shown that minor substitutions in the amino acid sequence of a peptide can

groups [3, 4]. In caucasians, particular associations, albeit incomplete, have been identified with certain alleles of HLA DR and DQ, and sequencing data have identified amino acid residues of the antigen-binding domain that show both positive and negative associations with disease activity. An important role for class II MHC molecules in MS would be consistent with disease induction in EAE, in which it has been shown that effector mechanisms involve activation of T cells of the CD4 subtype via antigen complexed to MHC class II molecules, with different epitopes of myelin antigens being encephalitogenic in different strains of animals [5, 6]. Using EAE as the model system, two modes of intervention in the antigen presentation pathway have been tested: the use of antibodies directed against MHC class II molecules, and the use of peptides that compete with antigen for binding to the MHC molecule, rendering the T cell unresponsive on engagement.

In both EAE and the non-obese diabetic mouse, antibodies to class II MHC have been shown to block disease expression. Furthermore, in EAE specificity for this reaction has been demonstrated in that antibodies directed against Ia (the equivalent of HLA in humans) prevented EAE, whereas antibodies directed against Ij generate analogues that bind to the MHC with equal or greater affinity than the native antigen and which lead to inhibition of disease [12–16]. Similarly, unrelated peptides that bind to the same MHC class II molecules have also been found to inhibit disease induction [17]. Although it has been assumed that the mechanism involved consists of successful competition with the native peptide for binding to MHC class II, more recent studies have suggested that mechanisms distinct from MHC blockade may be activated [18]. Of interest here is the observation that activation of antigen-specific T cells by peptides that contain substitutions in the MHC binding domains that lead to changes in the affinity of the peptide for the MHC results in changes in the cytokine profile of the responding T cell, and that it is this change that modulates disease expression. A similar phenomenon has been noted in animals in which tolerance has been induced by administration of antigen by routes other than by subcutaneous sensitization in complete adjuvant. For example, oral administration of MBP has been shown to block sensitization for EAE through the induction of T cells that produce the cytokine transforming growth factor beta (TGFβ), a cytokine that has been shown to have immunosuppressive properties, rather than production of the proinflammatory cytokines interleukin 2, tumor necrosis factor beta and interferon gamma (IL-2, TNFβ, IFN-γ) (see below and [19, 20]). These, and similar observations in other models of induced tolerance, have led to the interesting hypothesis that these different modalities of immunotherapy may activate common final pathways that involve differences in the cytokine profiles of the T cells responding to the antigen. If this is indeed the case, then it may be possible to circumvent the need to define the specific antigen involved if these common final pathways can be induced by other non-antigen specific procedures. This is discussed further in the section below on enhancement of regulatory processes. Clearly, such an approach is particularly appealing in presumptive autoimmune diseases of man such as MS, in which not only is the sensitizing antigen not known, but in which other antigens are likely to be involved as the disease progresses, as has been demonstrated in shifts in the immunodominant epitopes involved at varying stages of EAE, a phenomenon known as determinant spreading.

Interestingly, a recent study has also shown that MBP-peptide analogues can reverse established disease. In these animals, the inflammatory infiltrates regressed and the heterogeneous infiltrate disappeared from the brain. Additional studies showed that this effect of the peptide could be reversed by treatment with antibodies to interleukin 4 (IL-4), thus confirming the central role of cytokines in disease expression (see below) [16]. These results also confirm the observation that determining changes in the nature of the cytokines induced

by the peptide analogue may be the most reliable method available for assessing the potential therapeutic benefits that might accrue to any given peptide analogue [21].

18.1.3 THERAPIES DIRECTED AT THE T CELL RECEPTOR

Antigen presented in the context of MHC is recognized by the TCR on lymphocytes. The TCR consists of a heterodimer with most T cells expressing a TCR comprised of one alpha and one beta chain [22]. A minor population of T cells express one gamma and one delta chain [23]. The unique characteristics of different TCRs are formed by rearrangement of the V, D, J and C region genes, with the antigen-binding site located at the junction between the V, D and J regions, an area known as the complementary defining region 2 and 3 (CDR2 and CDR3).

Analysis of TCR usage in animals sensitized to develop EAE using MBP as the antigen demonstrated the surprising finding that T cells responding to the immunodominant encephalitogenic peptide used a restricted set of V region genes. In PJ/J mice responding to MBP peptide 1–11, TCR Vβ8.2 was found to predominate, whereas in SJL/J mice (which do not contain a Vβ8.2 gene) responses to MBP peptide 89–101 were dominated by Vβ17 and Vβ4 [24]. With respect to the alpha chain, in PL/J mice Vα4.3 was most frequently used, whereas in B10.PL mice Vα2 and Vα4 were used equally. In Lewis rats, a similar prevalence of Vβ8.2 usage was found even though MBP peptide 68–88 is the dominant epitope for T cells using Vβ8.2 in these animals [25, 26]. These observations led to the development of the V region hypothesis in which it was proposed that specific V region genes were associated with the encephalitogenic potential of MBP-sensitized T cells [27, 28].

Following on from these studies, it was then shown that vaccination with these V region genes, or peptides associated with the CDR2 or CDR3 region of the TCR, could protect animals against EAE [29–34]. These observations have led to an intense study of TCR expression in T cell lines and clones established from MS patients responding to peptides of MBP, as well as analysis of TCR usage in MS lesions. Several excellent reviews of the current status of information in this field have recently been published and are further reviewed in Chapter 14. In some studies restricted usage of V region genes has been noted in peripheral blood T cell lines cultured with MBP. In particular, Vβ5.2 and Vβ6.1 were found to be over-represented in peripheral blood T cell lines reactive to MBP when these cells were derived from MS patients, whereas in MBP-reactive T cells obtained from normal healthy controls, over-expression of Vβ7 and Vβ14 was observed [35]. These findings were of interest in that a similar over-representation of Vβ5.2 and Vβ6.1 has been found in MS lesions [36]. In MBP-reactive T cell clones from DR2⁺ patients, over-expression of Vβ17 was noted in response to the 84–102 epitope, whereas T cells reactive to the 149–170 epitope over-expressed Vβ12 [37]. Several other studies, however, have failed to find evidence of restricted V region usage in either MS patients or animals sensitized to develop EAE, particularly when other myelin antigens such as proteolipid protein were examined [38–40]. Nevertheless, it remains possible that within any given patient the V region genes or the CDR2 and CDR3 regions forming the TCR may be skewed and thus may be amenable to modulation by TCR vaccination therapy in a manner similar to that found in animals [38, 41].

An alternative approach has been to use whole T cells in a vaccination paradigm. In studies in EAE, the specific questions that are being investigated in various animal models include the requirement for antigen specificity, the role of lymphocyte activation markers, and the best method for treating the cells to augment immunogenicity. The results of these studies have shown that successful vaccination against EAE can be achieved using activated antigen-specific T cells that have been subjected to hydrostatic pressure and/or procedures that result in cross-linking of cell surface molecules, such as formaldehydes or photo-activated chemical cross-linkers [41–45]. To extend these kinds of studies to the patient population, however, it will be necessary to define the specific antigen involved. As noted earlier, this may be difficult in chronic diseases of long duration in which many different antigens and/or epitopes of specific antigens appear to come into play at varying times in the disease process.

An alternative approach has been to select for activated cells in either the CSF or the peripheral blood without knowledge of their antigen specificity, in the assumption that these activated cells represent potential effector cells in the disease process [46, 47]. Experiments designed to test this approach in animals sensitized with MBP showed that a combination of T cell mitogens and growth factors was the most effective way to isolate antigen-specific T cells.

Several studies are currently ongoing using MBP-reactive or non-specifically activated T cell clones isolated from the CSF or peripheral blood as vaccines tailored to each patient, as well as peptides associated with specific regions of the TCR, as discussed above [48–50]. In all these approaches to T cell vaccination, experiments that have attempted to define the underlying mechanisms involved have strongly implicated the establishment of immunoregulatory circuits that result in suppression or depletion of antigen-specific T cells by CD4⁺ or CD8⁺ anti-clonotypic T cells [50, 51], indicating the presence of a network of interacting cells that might be amenable to modulation and the re-establishment of tolerance to autoantigens.

It should be noted here that an additional mechanism for targeting activated T cells has been the use of a toxin–IL-2 conjugate which, in interaction with the high-affinity IL-2 receptor, leads to death of the activated cells. This mode of therapy is currently in clinical trials in patients with rheumatoid arthritis and has shown efficacy in animals with EAE [52].

18.2 Inhibition of inflammatory events

In both EAE and several viral models of inflammatory demyelination, CD4⁺, TH1-type T lymphocyte responses have been implicated in the disease pathogenesis. TH1 cells are characterized by the production of the cytokines IL-2, lymphotoxin (tumor necrosis factor beta, TNFβ) and IFN-γ (Figure 18.1). The release of IL-2 leads to the influx and activation of T cells in the lesion and to up-regulation of TNFβ, a cytokine that has been shown to be cytotoxic for different cell types, including oligodendrocytes [53]. IFN-γ leads to the production of an inflammatory response, principally through the activation of class II MHC molecules and through the activating effects of this cytokine on cells of the monocyte/macrophage series. Following immune activation, macrophages produce the proinflammatory cytokines interleukin-1 (IL-1) and tumor necrosis factor alpha (TNFα), reactive oxygen, and possibly reactive nitrogen intermediates, prostaglandins and components of the complement cascade. In addition, TH1 cytokines provide help for the production of opsonizing antibodies that interact with the Fc receptor on phagocytic cells. All of these factors have been shown to be present in the MS lesion, particularly in acute or chronic active lesions, strongly implicating a role for these factors in lesion formation and chronicity.

18.2.1 INHIBITION OF PROINFLAMMATORY CYTOKINES

In several studies, the EAE model has been used to test the effect of neutralizing or down-regulating the proinflammatory cytokines TNFα, TNFβ and IL-1 on disease presentation in vivo. The most extensive and successful studies have examined the role of the TNF family of proteins. To neutralize TNF activity a number of regimens have been used with polyclonal and monoclonal anti-TNF antibodies, soluble TNF receptors, and with other natural and pharmacological TNF inhibitors.

The effect of an anti-TNF polyclonal antibody was investigated with a form of EAE in SJL/J mice induced by adoptive transfer of myelin basic protein-sensitized T lymphocytes [54]. None of the animals treated with anti-TNF antibody developed clinical EAE while receiving antibody treatment. Five to seven days after treatment ceased, however, all anti-TNF-treated mice became clinically ill. Examination of CNS tissue derived from control EAE animals, treated with phosphate buffered saline or anti-Freund's adjuvant antibodies, showed pathological features typical of EAE. However, CNS tissues sampled from animals during anti-TNF treatment demonstrated neither inflammation nor demyelination. Examination of CNS tissue from anti-TNF-treated mice in which treatment had been discontinued revealed inflammation and demyelination typical of adoptively transferred EAE. To investigate the mechanism of action of anti-TNF treatment in the prevention of EAE, the effect of anti-TNF antibody on encephalitogenic T lymphocytes was assessed. Neither preincubation with anti-TNF antibody nor anti-Freund's adjuvant antibody inhibited the induction of EAE in syngeneic recipients. Furthermore, the proliferative response to MBP by MBP-specific lymphocytes was not diminished by concurrent incubation with anti-TNF antibody. In addition, serial transfer experiments using spleen cells recovered from the anti-TNF-treated animals demonstrated that these cells retained the ability to transfer EAE. Spleen cells from anti-TNF-treated animals did not produce TNFα on stimulation with MBP or con A, whereas spleen cells recovered from anti-adjuvant-treated control animals produced TNF in response to these reagents. These results indicated that anti-TNF treatment of recipient animals was capable of eliminating the production of TNF by their spleen cells and thus might act by interfering with the effector phase of the disease. In another study, a hamster monoclonal antibody to TNF was applied in the passive-transfer model of EAE[55]. This antibody neutralized both TNFα and LTα. Application of this antibody prior to the expected development of EAE significantly diminished or prevented disease expression. Contrary to the studies with the polyclonal antibody, administration of hamster monoclonal antibody had long-lasting effects and the treated animals did not develop EAE during the 5-month follow-up period. Interestingly, when anti-TNF antibody was tested in the actively induced model of EAE, no inhibition of disease expression was noted[56]. However, in this model system, when TNF activity was neutralized by treatment with the soluble type I TNF receptor, significant inhibition of EAE was observed[57].

Natural TNF inhibitory proteins were originally discovered in human urine and serum[58]. Sequence analysis and immuno-cross reactivity revealed that TNF inhibitory proteins were soluble forms of truncated fragments of the extracellular domains for both the 55 kD and 75 kD TNFα receptors[59]. It is believed that TNF inhibitory proteins control TNFα activity that, under conditions of excess TNF production, can medi-

ate profound pathological changes. Soluble TNF receptors have many advantages over the use of anti-TNF antibodies. They are of autologous origin and may, therefore, be non-immunogenic, a serious problem in the use of passive-antibody therapy. Additionally, the low molecular weight of soluble TNF receptors may facilitate their transfer across the blood–brain barrier. The effect of the type 1 (p-55, type β) soluble TNF receptor was investigated in the passive transfer model of EAE in SJL/J mice[60]. In a series of experiments, none of the sTNF-R1-treated animals developed EAE. Furthermore, no apparent relapses were observed in the sTNF-R1-treated animals, whereas the control animals exhibited a 70% frequency for at least one clinical relapse. Thus these data resemble more closely the results obtained with the monoclonal anti-TNF since the effect of treatment was long-lived. CNS tissues from the sTNF-R1-treated animals demonstrated no pathological changes, or only an occasional inflammatory cell in the subependymal area. No demyelination was observed.

The results with the various anti-TNF treatment modalities suggest that this treatment interferes with homing of inflammatory cells to the CNS. TNFα is know to activate endothelial cells and induce or up-regulate the expression of leukocyte-adhesion molecules[61]. Treatment with the monoclonal anti-TNF antibody has been shown to markedly reduce or prevent the up-regulation of VCAM-1 expression in EAE and leukocyte infiltration was found to be 15-fold lower in the anti-TNF-treated animals than in control animals[62]. An alternative explanation is that anti-TNF treatment inhibits the activation of endogenous T cells or monocytes in animals sensitized to develop EAE. TNFα has been shown to augment the proliferation of stimulated T cells and enhance the generation of cytotoxic T cells[63]. In addition, TNF activates macrophages to express toxic factors such as reactive oxygen and nitrogen intermediates (see below). Inhibition of immune activation in the recipient animals after the transfer of sensitized T cells may, therefore, contribute to the prevention of EAE. Preliminary data have shown diminished non-antigen-specific T cell responses in the animals treated with the sTNF-R1, particularly for the con A responses, which requires the presence of APC (a source of TNFα), and also to a lesser extent lymphocyte proliferation induced by anti-CD3 responses. In contrast, soluble TNF-R1 did not affect the MBP-specific response, consistent with the results obtained with anti-TNF antibody treatment, nor did it affect the distribution of CD4 and CD8 cells in most experiments, although enhanced CD4 expression was noted in some[64]. Using the dimeric polyethylene glycol-linked form of the sTNF-R1 it was possible to lower the minimal effective dose to 1 mg/kg in mice[65], a dose level that would be feasible for human trials. Taken together, the results with both anti-TNF antibodies and the sTNF-R1 demonstrate that these treatment protocols affect the development of EAE at a step subsequent to generation of autoimmune cells, a situation relevant to MS where the putative autoimmune reactive cells have been generated before clinical presentation.

The promising results obtained with these anti-TNF therapies have prompted further investigations of pharmacological TNF inhibitors that could be tested in MS. Following experiments that showed that the phospholipid of the cell membrane, phosphatidyl serine, is capable of reducing lipopolysaccharide-induced TNFα production, phosphatidyl serine has been tested in EAE. In the passive-transfer model of EAE in mice, 20% of the animals treated with phosphatidyl serine displayed only mild clinical signs, had minimal pathology and failed to relapse [66]. More recent studies have tested a selective inhibitor of phosphodiesterase type IV, rolipram, in EAE in the Lewis rat [67]. Rolipram inhibits TNF production by LPS-stimulated human mononuclear cells and reduces the endothelial cell monolayer permeability induced by TNF. Phosphodiesterase type IV is predominantly expressed in lymphoid tissues and in the CNS. When rolipram was administered to Lewis rats before the onset of EAE, it completely prevented the disease. When given on the first day of clinical signs only moderate progression of the disease was observed whereas the control animals were all severely affected. Further studies have now shown that rolipram also confers significant and sustained protection against EAE in non-human primates in a disease model in which severe pathology has been noted in the spinal cord [68]. Other phosphodiesterase type IV inhibitors, such as pentoxifylline, are currently under study in various models of EAE. Another selective inhibitor of TNF is thalidomide, degrading TNFα mRNA without affecting the stability of mRNA for other cytokines [69]. Thalidomide is currently the drug of choice in the treatment of erythema nodosum leprosum, an acute inflammatory condition occurring in leprosy patients where TNF has been shown to be a major mediator [70].

Although the TNF family of cytokines seems to occupy a central role in inflammatory events in autoimmune conditions, the complex interaction between TNF and other cytokines has long been recognized. With regard to autoimmune demyelination, special attention has been paid to IL-1. This cytokine is also strongly proinflammatory and has been documented in both EAE and MS lesions [71] and has been shown to enhance adoptively transferred EAE [72]. Studies with the soluble IL-1 receptor have been shown to reduce both the severity and duration of EAE [73]. Although the recent disappointing results of a trial using this inhibitor in patients with rheumatoid arthritis diminishes enthusiasm for a similar trial in patients with MS, it is important to remember that this family of cytokines and receptors

shows complex interactions and combined therapy with different components of this system, perhaps in combination with TNF inhibitors, may prove to be more effective than single components used alone [74].

18.2.2   INHIBITION OF ADHESION EVENTS

As noted above, one of the primary effects of the proinflammatory cytokines is to induce changes in the property of the endothelial cell that promotes the adhesion and migration of recruited inflammatory cells across the vascular endothelium (Figure 18.1). The role of these induced adhesion molecules in the development of EAE has been the subject of several studies [61, 62, 75–84]. The expression of adhesion molecules such as intercellular adhesion molecule-1 (ICAM-1) and vascular cell adhesion molecule 1 (VCAM-1) during exacerbations in EAE implicates these molecules in disease pathogenesis [79, 84]. In normal brain, few endothelial cells express detectable ICAM-1, whereas ICAM-1 is present on both inflammatory cells and endothelium of lesion-associated blood vessels in EAE.

These observations led to the hypothesis that administration of antibodies directed against either ICAM-1, or its ligand lymphocyte function-associated antigen-1 (LFA-1), might inhibit EAE. The studies so far have produced conflicting results. Administration of anti-LFA-1 antibody clearly exacerbated disease in one study of murine EAE [78], while its effect in worsening disease was less clear in another study using much lower doses of the antibody [79]. Studies using anti-ICAM-1 antibody did not have an effect on adoptively transferred EAE in the Lewis rat, yet did inhibit disease induced by immunization with encephalitogen [80]. In murine EAE, anti-ICAM-1 antibody treatment resulted in a modest delay (5 days) in disease onset [81]. None of these studies specifically addressed the possible role of adhesion-related molecule costimulation as an explanation for the conflicting results.

Studies performed by Racke and colleagues suggest that some of the conflicting results may be due to differences in the dosage of antibody used [82]. Administration of either anti-LFA-1 or anti-ICAM-1 antibodies at lower dosages (0.2–0.4 mg per mouse per day) for days 4–10 following injection of encephalitogenic T cells at day 0 resulted in a marked enhancement of clinical disease. Increasing the dose of antibody (0.8–1.0 mg per mouse per day) resulted in a delay in the onset of disease. At the highest dose (1.0 mg per mouse per day), the combination of anti-LFA-1 and anti-ICAM-1 antibodies markedly inhibited the clinical expression of disease for 40 days following the transfer of encephalitogenic T cells. These results demonstrate that the dose of antibody directed against an accessory molecule is critical in determining whether clinical disease is suppressed or accentuated.

However, the above results do not directly address the costimulatory role of the LFA-1/ICAM-1 pathway. Prior work had demonstrated that stimulation of MBP-specific lymph node cells by anti-CD3 alone, although able to stimulate T cell proliferation, was unable to confer encephalitogenicity on the activated cells [83]. Recent experiments have shown that using anti-CD3 and anti-CD4 antibodies in the presence of APC can successfully activate encephalitogenic T cells, suggesting that APC are providing additional costimulation. In the absence of APC, additional costimulation provided through either LFA-1 or ICAM-1 resulted in the activation of encephalitogenic T cells and the successful transfer of EAE [82].

Recent studies demonstrated that anti-VLA-4 administration can prevent the clinical development of EAE [84]. Baron and colleagues also demonstrated the importance of VLA-4 expression on T cells in order to gain access to the CNS [81]. Clearly, studies such as those described above have provided important insights into the role of accessory molecules during the activation of encephalitogenic T cells and on their role *in vivo*. Understanding the diverse functions of these receptor–ligand pairs in an autoimmune disease such as EAE may eventually provide therapeutic strategies for human demyelinating disease.

18.2.3 INHIBITION OF PRODUCTS OF ACTIVATED MACROPHAGES

In addition to the pivotal role of T cells in disease induction, it is now well recognized that other factors may play an important role in lesion development. They include antibodies released by B cells present in the CNS, and factors produced by activated macrophages [85–98]. With respect to antibodies, it has now been shown in various models of EAE that if these antibodies are directed against components of the myelin sheath they may, in conjunction with effector cells and/or complement, lead to enhancement of the demyelinating process and oligodendrocyte depletion in the lesion [86, 88, 89]. With respect to macrophages, in addition to the role of proinflammatory cytokines such as TNF and IL-1 discussed above, activated macrophages produce a number of factors that could contribute to lesion development (Figure 18.1). They include proteolytic enzymes, prostaglandins, complement factors, phospholipases and reactive nitrogen and oxygen intermediates [90–92]. Many of these factors have been shown to play a role in the pathogenesis of EAE, and possibly MS; at the present time, however, experimental therapeutic intervention is principally focused on inhibiting the effects of reactive nitrogen and oxygen intermediates. In inflammatory conditions the activation of the inducible form of nitric oxide synthase (iNOS) would be expected to lead to the production of high levels of nitric oxide (NO) over extended periods of time. Furthermore, a major determinant of the fate of NO is the concentration of superoxide, since the reaction of NO with O_2 is faster than the dismutation of O_2, and peroxynitrite generates hydroxyl radical-like species more reactive than NO, but with a shorter half-life [93]. Several groups have now demonstrated NO production through an iNOS pathway in various models of CNS inflammation [93–96]. These reactive nitrogen intermediates are potentially neurotoxic for many cells within the CNS and may, therefore, play a pathogenetic role in experimental autoimmune inflammatory diseases of the CNS. Oligodendrocytes are vulnerable to cytokine-mediated toxicity, and recently Merrill and colleagues have implicated NO in this process [97]. In addition, release of NO in the CNS is likely to affect the blood–brain barrier and increased vasodilatation could contribute to edema. Conversely, reactive nitrogen intermediates may play a beneficial role in some disorders. For example, the suppressive effect of activated macrophages on the proliferative response of lymphocytes has been attributed in part to NO. NO has also been shown to inhibit the adhesion and aggregation of platelets, and the adhesion of leukocytes to activated endothelium (reviewed in [98]). Interestingly, however, in MS lesions iNOS-like reactivity has been identified principally in reactive astrocytes rather than macrophages or microglia [98, 99] consistent with the results obtained with human glial cells in culture [100].

To test for a role for NO in CNS inflammation, the effect of NOS inhibitors on disease expression has been tested in murine or rodent models of EAE [101, 102]. Interestingly, although quite striking beneficial effects were noted in the murine model of EAE [101], NO inhibitors had more complex effects in various rat models of the primary demyelinating diseases [102]. That there are species differences in the both the response to NO and in the cell types that can be induced by cytokines to express NOS has now been well demonstrated, but clearly more experimentation is needed before this mode of therapy can be considered for trials in patients. An important thrust of current research in this field is to define inhibitors that will be selective for the inducible form of NOS, leaving the constitutive and endothelial forms of NOS unaffected.

Another group of inflammatory mediators that is generating considerable interest is the group of factors known as chemokines. Chemokines are low molecular weight soluble factors released following activation by cytokines or trauma that regulate the influx, and perhaps activation, of specific subsets of inflammatory cells to sites of tissue damage. In the central nervous system, both invading inflammatory cells as well as central nervous system glial cells may be potent sources of these factors in the injured CNS (for review see [103]). The fact that chemokines may represent a promising target for future therapeutic intervention has been supported by the observation that in the mouse model of EAE, antibodies against one of these chemokines, macrophage inflammatory protein 1α, was able significantly to protect animals against disease [104].

18.3 Enhancement of regulatory mechanisms

Several studies have now shown clearly that in patients with MS there is a dysregulation of the immune system. In particular, studies have focused on the possibility that immunoregulatory circuits may be impaired, permitting either the emergence of autoimmune reactions and/or bias towards proinflammatory events. Several laboratories, therefore, are currently investigating ways in which the cytokine profile of the immune response can be modulated away from a predominantly proinflammatory TH1-type of response, and how immunoregulatory circuits might be enhanced and tolerance to self antigens re-established. As noted above, the results of these studies have indicated that the nature of the cytokines produced during activation of the immune system determines the nature of the immune response that is generated. Modulating these events by either the administration of specific cytokines to sensitized animals, or by activating the lymphocytes in such a way that specific cytokines are induced, has shown particular promise as a means for regulating disease expression in animals with EAE.

18.3.1 CYTOKINE–CYTOKINE INTERACTIONS

In many of the therapeutic approaches employed for EAE described in this chapter, precise knowledge of the TCR and encephalitogenic epitopes involved was necessary for their implementation. Implicit in these approaches is that the acquisition of similar information about TCR usage and target antigens in human disorders such as MS would provide the rationale for such experimental therapies in humans. In this section an alternative approach will be explored, in which the knowledge of TCR and antigen is not essential. Because many suspected autoimmune diseases, including MS, are of a relapsing and remitting nature, the role of endogenously secreted cytokines as a way to manipulate disease in EAE has been examined by several groups (Figure 18.1).

One such cytokine is transforming growth factor beta (TGFβ), which belongs to a family of peptides with pleiotropic effects [105]. Many of these effects include those which may be inhibitory to an immune response, including inhibition of T cell activation and proliferation, down-regulation of IFN-γ-induced class II MHC expression, and decrease in the generation of cytotoxic lymphocytes. Because of these many immunosuppressive properties, several groups have examined the effects of TGFβ in several autoimmune disease models. In the EAE model, disease induced both by multiple injections of mouse spinal cord homogenate or by injection of activated MBP-specific T cells was inhibited by the administration of TGFβ [106–108]. Importantly, TGFβ administration after established disease was able to suppress further clinical relapses [108, 109]. In addition, systemic TGFβ administration also suppressed the development of experimental arthritis, indicating that the regulatory phenomena observed were not specific for the CNS [107, 110].

Several studies have also examined the role of endogenous TGFβ secretion in the EAE model [111–113]. Karpus and Swanborg demonstrated that TGFβ is secreted by splenocytes from Lewis rats that have recovered from EAE [111], while others have shown that administration of antiserum or antibodies to TGFβ enhances disease severity [112, 113]. These findings are of interest in MS as well. TGFβ has been shown to be secreted by peripheral blood lymphocytes isolated from MS patients either when in remission or while symptoms were resolving [114, 115]. Studies such as those outlined above have led to a phase I clinical trial utilizing TGFβ-2 in chronic progressive MS [116].

It is also interesting to note that TGFβ may play an important role in the suppression of EAE observed after the induction of oral tolerance (see below and [117]). Following the feeding of myelin antigens, increased secretion of both TGFβ and IL-4 was noted in the CNS of animals, as well as diminished clinical disease.

The enhancement of IL-4 in the CNS of animals protected from EAE relates to another strategy for modifying autoimmune disease, that of immune deviation. Immune deviation was originally defined as the induction of a T cell-dependent antibody response in the absence of delayed type hypersensitivity (DTH, [118]). More recently, the concept of TH1 and TH2 lymphocyte subpopulations which interact and cross-regulate each other has evolved [119, 120]. TH1 cells, which secret IL-2, IFN-γ, and TNFβ, play a major role in DTH, while TH2 cells are involved in humoral responses by secreting IL-4, IL-5 and IL-10. As noted earlier it is important to note that EAE appears to be mediated by TH1-like cells [121].

Therefore, one approach to the immunotherapy of inflammatory autoimmune disease might involve the deviation of an immune response from one dominated by TH1 cytokines to one where a TH2 response predominates. Several studies have addressed this issue in the EAE model. Racke and colleagues have demonstrated that induction of a TH2-like MBP-specific response in the periphery results in the suppression of clinical disease and a reduction in CNS demyelination [122]. In addition, cytokine production in the target organ, the CNS, was also examined. Interestingly, the improved clinical and histological course correlated with a reduction in TNFα expression in the CNS. Studies by Kuchroo and associates demonstrated that administration of anti-B7–1 antibody suppressed EAE through an effect dependent on IL-4[123]. They further showed that injection of TH2 PLP-specific clones would suppress the development of clinical signs of disease after immunization with an encephalitogenic PLP peptide.

Other strategies that have been used to treat EAE may also modulate lymphocyte subpopulations. Massacesi and colleagues demonstrated that feeding of retinoids suppressed EAE[124]. It was later demonstrated that the presence of retinoids may actually enhance development of a TH2 population of MBP-reactive T cells[125]. Suppression of EAE using phosphodiesterase inhibitors such as pentoxifylline[126] and rolipram[66] may also exert part of their effect by manipulating the balance between TH1 and TH2 lymphocytes. The ability to generate TH2 populations which can ameliorate disease, even in the presence of pathogenic TH1 cells, raises the possibility that therapeutic strategies designed to augment TH2 activity may have efficacy in many autoimmune diseases mediated by TH1 cells, including MS.

18.3.2 COSTIMULATORY MOLECULES

The activation and differentiation of T cells require both antigen/MHC recognition and costimulatory signals[127]. The signal conferred by the TCR determines the antigen-specificity of the response. The second signal, termed costimulation, is provided by accessory molecules on the antigen-presenting cell (APC) and appears to be necessary for functional T cell activation (Figure 18.1). There are several receptor–ligand pairs which can provide this costimulation. We will initially focus on the interaction of the B7 family of cell surface molecules with its receptors on T cells, CD28 and CTLA4[128]. We will then discuss other receptor–ligand pairs and their role in costimulation.

At least two members of the B7 family of CD28 ligands have been defined, B7–1 (CD80) and B7–2 (CD86)[128, 129]. These molecules, although only having modest homology, are each able to provide costimulation to T cells for proliferation and IL-2 production. It is probably for this reason that a mouse genetically deficient for CD80 (B7–1) was essentially immunocompetent[130]. On the other hand, T cells from a mouse deficient for CD28 could not produce IL-2 after stimulation with the mitogenic lectin Con A, suggesting that costimulation through this molecule is critical for IL-2 production[131]. In addition, it is likely that there is at least a third member of the B7 family capable of providing a signal to T cells through CD28 and/or CTLA-4[132].

B7–1 (CD80) and B7–2 (CD86) may be expressed differentially on various APC and their kinetics of expression and binding also differ[133]. B7–2 is expressed by monocytes constitutively, while B7–1 can be induced on these APC with IFN-γ. B7 is expressed on B cell populations after an activation stimulus; B7–2 is expressed within 6 hours while B7–1 expression peaks after 48 hours[134].

Much has been learned about the counter-receptors for CD28 and CTLA-4 with a soluble fusion protein, CTLA-4Ig, which can prevent the interaction between B7 and CD28[135]. Administration of CTLA-4Ig prevented rat cardiac allograft rejection[136] and pancreatic islet cell xenograft rejection in mice[137]. In both instances, the mechanism of suppression appeared to involve the induction of Ag-specific tolerance. These studies demonstrate the importance of B7:CD28/CTLA-4 costimulation during T cell activation that is responsible for graft rejection.

The costimulation provided by B7 also appears to be important for the development of autoimmunity. Treatment of mice susceptible for murine lupus with CTLA-4Ig resulted in amelioration of disease[138]. Perrin and colleagues have also examined the role of the B7:CD28/CTLA-4 interaction in the induction of EAE[139]. In the adoptive transfer model of EAE, CTLA-4Ig was able to inhibit the proliferation and IL-2 production of MBP-specific lymph node cells during activation in vitro, resulting in reduced clinical disease upon subsequent transfer. Thus, B7-mediated costimulation was found to be an important factor in determining encephalitogenicity. It is important to note, however, that once activated autoreactive cells had been injected into naive recipients, CTLA-4Ig intervention did not alter the course of disease.

In the active model of EAE, several intriguing observations have been made. Cross and associates have demonstrated that, in a model using a variant of CTLA-4Ig called CTLA-4Fc, that disease induced by immunization with myelin and pertussis toxin injection can be dramatically inhibited[140]. On the other hand, in a model using a two-immunization schedule without pertussis, disease was actually enhanced following administration of multiple doses of CTLA-4Ig, yet was inhibited with one injection 48 hours after the initial antigenic challenge[141]. Interestingly, there is a precedent for these paradoxical results. Transgenic mice that expressed a soluble form of murine CTLA-4 demonstrated an enhanced expansion of antigen-specific CD4+ T cells[142]. In that report, mice receiving two immunizations separated by one week developed the most dramatic expansion of antigen-reactive cells, which is reminiscent of the two-immunization EAE protocol described above, that resulted in enhanced disease.

Initial studies indicated that CTLA-4 provided a costimulatory signal in conjunction with CD28[143].

Recent evidence suggests that the signaling through the CTLA-4 molecule may actually mediate a negative regulatory function. In CD28-deficient mice, costimulation provided by B7$^+$ APC did not transduce a positive signal[144]. In addition, constitutive expression of B7–1 on mature B cells resulted in depressed antibody responses to T cell-dependent hapten–protein conjugates, suggesting that B7–1 may contribute to feedback inhibition of T cell-dependent immune responses *in vivo* [145].

Recently, Kuchroo and associates showed that B7–1 and B7–2 provide costimulation resulting in the differentiation of T cells into either the TH1 or TH2 lymphocyte phenotype [123]. TH1 cells, which secrete IFN-γ, IL-2 and TNFβ, developed following B7–1 costimulation, while TH2 cells, which secrete IL-4, IL-5 and IL-6, develop preferentially following B7–2 costimulation [123, 146]. Because encephalitogenic T cells are of the TH1 phenotype, administration of anti-B7–1 antibodies resulted in the suppression of actively induced EAE, while anti-B7–2 antibodies had no effect. The effect of anti-B7–1 antibody was abrogated by the administration of anti-IL-4, suggesting that IL-4 secretion may be important in the clinical signs of disease. Similarly, Racke and colleagues have demonstrated that one injection of anti-B7–1 dramatically inhibits disease, while one injection of anti-B7–2 exacerbates disease [141]. In addition, giving both antibodies also resulted in disease suppression. In the Lewis rat, administration of CTLA-4Ig suppressed both the clinical and pathological expression of EAE and inhibited TH1-type cytokine expression whilst sparing TH2 cytokines [146]. Interestingly, in the non-obese diabetic mouse the effect of these treatment protocols were reversed, with anti-B7–1 exacerbating disease and anti-B7–2 blocking the development of diabetes [147]. Thus, the role of the B7 family of costimulatory molecules in animal models of autoimmune disease appears to be quite complicated.

The ability of mice deficient in CD28 to generate a cytotoxic T cell response and a delayed type hypersensitivity response indicates that there is a physiologic role for costimulatory pathways that do not involve CD28 [131]. Multiple T cell costimulatory molecules have been described, including interactions between CD2 and LFA-3, LFA-1 and ICAM-1, and very late antigen-4 (VLA-4) VCAM-1 [148]. These interactions are important both for their role in leukocyte adhesion and tissue infiltration as well as their role in costimulation. The adhesion molecule pathways are of interest in a number of human inflammatory disorders, including multiple sclerosis [76].

18.3.3   ACTIVATION OF REGULATORY CELLS

In addition to the cross-regulatory pathways involved in TH1 and TH2 responses, activation of CD4$^+$ lymphocytes is known to be regulated by CD8$^+$ suppressor and/or cytotoxic lymphocytes and activated macrophages (Figure 18.1). Although the exact mechanisms involved in these suppressor activities remain controversial, several studies have indicated that these pathways are altered in patients with MS, resulting in a loss of normal regulatory mechanisms. This has led to attempts to enhance suppressor cell circuits. At the present time, interest in this area has focused on either the use of suppressor cytokines such as IFN-β and IFN-τ [151], or administration of drugs that regulate the β-adrenergic receptor [149–152]. Of these, the work with IFN-β has progressed the furthest and a discussion of the possible modes of action of this cytokine can be found in the preceding chapter and in reference [152].

18.3.4   TOLERANCE INDUCTION AND PROGRAMMED CELL DEATH

For autoimmune diseases believed to be mediated by T cells, a fundamental issue is what mechanisms are available to re-establish tolerance to an autoantigen. In this section, some of the many mechanisms which have been used to establish tolerance in experimental animal models will be examined.

T cells stimulated with antigen can either become activated and proliferate, become anergic, or undergo antigen-induced programmed cell death (PCD, [153]). The morphologic expression of apoptosis or PCD is characterized by fragmentation of the nuclear chromatin due to activation of an endogenous nuclease, nuclear collapse, cell shrinkage and blebbing of the plasma membrane [154]. It has been demonstrated that growth lymphokines such as IL-2 are one of the crucial determinants for a T cell to undergo PCD [155]. T cells that are progressing through the cell cycle under the influence of IL-2 are highly susceptible to PCD induced by high doses of antigen, whereas resting cells are not. This serves as a feedback mechanism, termed propriocidal regulation, that limits T cell proliferation and lymphokine production during an immune response [155]. A critical requirement for death induction is repeated antigen encounter at close intervals so that T cells become activated, undergo cell cycle progression, and then again become strongly engaged through the T cell receptor. Mature T lymphocytes that undergo apoptosis following TCR stimulation may involve several mechanisms, including the Fas antigen, IFN-γ, growth lymphokines, TNFα and cytolytic mechanisms [156, 157].

Because it was already known that high doses of antigen can paradoxically suppress immune responses in adult animals [155, 158, 159], it was possible that such a mechanism could be used to induce antigen-specific tolerance in an experimental autoimmune disorder such as experimental allergic encephalomyelitis (EAE). Actually, the idea of using an encephalitogen as a form of treatment for EAE is a relatively old, well-described phenomenon [158, 159]. Levine and colleagues first demonstrated that intravenous administration of encephalitogen could inhibit the passive transfer of encephalomyelitis [158]. Over the years, many other investigators demonstrated that delivery of myelin basic protein (MBP) in many different forms and by different routes could suppress and even treat EAE [160–162]. Lisak and coworkers were able to show that pretreatment of guinea pigs with MBP in incomplete adjuvant resulted in suppression of disease and the *in vitro* proliferative response to MBP [159]. However, in these early works, the mechanisms for the suppression of disease were not well delineated.

More recent work in the EAE model has suggested several possibilities for the mechanism of disease suppression and tolerance induction. Gaur and colleagues suggested that amelioration of EAE by synthetic peptides of MBP was due to peptide-induced anergy of the autoreactive T cells [163]. Studies by Critchfield and coworkers demonstrated that high dose antigen therapy resulted in the elimination of the MBP-specific, autoreactive T cells [155]. Thus, increasing the antigenic stimulation of encephalitogenic T cells by the intravenous administration of MBP could attenuate the immune response and the clinical signs of EAE.

Interestingly, PCD may also play an important role in the relapsing and remitting disease course observed in EAE. Pender and associates have observed that during the normal course of EAE in the rat, apoptosis of T cells in the central nervous system occurs [164]. They speculated that this loss of autoreactive T cells in the central nervous system could be a possible explanation for the decrease in inflammation and subsequent acquisition of tolerance observed in EAE.

Finally, the use of autoantigens as a therapy in multiple sclerosis needs to be discussed. Several trials of MBP administration were conducted during the 1970s as a treatment for multiple sclerosis [165, 166]. No clear beneficial treatment effects were observed in most patients; however a few did show improvement. More recently, studies have focused on the use of oral administration of MBP as a means to establish tolerance to autoantigens. In EAE, oral tolerance induced by feeding MBP has been shown to be an effective means of modulating disease expression. Depending on the amount of antigen encountered by the mucosal immune system several different mechanisms of tolerance induction have been observed, with low doses favoring active suppression and higher doses favoring anergy [19, 167]. The mechanisms involved include a switch in the cytokine profile of the responding cell to cells producing TGFβ or the TH2 cytokines IL-4 and IL-10, or clonal

deletion of antigen-reactive T cells. Additional studies suggested that, at least in some of these models, specificity for the antigen fed to the animals was not critical to the success of the suppressive regimen as long as the regulatory cells involved were targeted to the CNS, leading to the release of regulatory cytokines at the site of inflammation. The success obtained with this mode of therapy in experimental animals has led to the initiation of a trial in patients with MS, using myelin derived from bovine brain, as well as in patients with rheumatoid arthritis, uveitis and juvenile diabetes, using antigens known to be involved in the induction of autoimmune animal models of these diseases. In patients with MS, a pilot trial has been completed in which no deleterious side-effects were noted and in which a benefit to a small subgroup of patients may have been observed. A phase III multicenter trial is currently ongoing [20].

It is likely that the examination of high dose antigen therapy, or other antigen-specific therapies such as oral tolerance or altered peptide ligands, will eventually determine whether an immune response to these autoantigens is a critical factor in inflammatory diseases such as MS.

18.4 Enhancement of repair processes

Chronic MS plaques are characterized by demyelination, gliotic scar formation and loss of oligodendrocytes. However, during the initial stages of lesion formation, several studies have shown that oligodendrocytes may display proliferative and remyelinative activity, which, in view of their eventual loss, are probably transient events (reviewed in Chapters 9 and 15). Nevertheless, these observations have given rise to the hope that repair processes can be enhanced and thus lead to sustained recovery of function. The factors that lead to oligodendrocyte loss in the lesion are not known but may reflect immune-mediated damage or the lack of necessary growth and/or differentiation factors needed to sustain repopulation and remyelination of the lesion. Therefore, attempts to enhance remyelination within the lesion have focused on the replacement of oligodendrocytes by engraftment or by provision of oligodendrocyte growth and differentiation factors. An important advance in the progress of these studies has been the characterization of the steps involved in oligodendrocyte development and differentiation, and the growth factors involved at each stage of this process [168–173]. This has permitted the expansion in culture of relatively large numbers of specific populations of oligodendrocytes and selection of potentially relevant growth and/or differentiation factors that can be tested for remyelinating activity *in vivo*.

18.4.1 ENGRAFTMENT OF OLIGODENDROCYTES

To test whether transplantation of oligodendrocytes can lead to remyelination and restoration of function, several studies have examined transplantation into either myelin deficient (md) animals or lesions demyelinated by agents such as lysolecithin or ethidium bromide and in which normal repair activity has been blocked by radiation. An important consideration in the design of these experiments has been the question of which cells are the most appropriate for transplantation: stem cells (progenitors) or differentiated oligodendrocytes [174–176]. Potentially stem cells possess several properties that might be expected to be more appropriate for transplantation. These include their rapid rates of division, the relative lack of elaborate cell processes that could impede migration in the tissues and their undifferentiated state that should lead to remyelination following the same steps that occur during development. Several studies have now successfully demonstrated that transfer of CNS grafts or oligodendrocytes into these various model systems can lead to significant myelination/remyelination and some recovery of function [177–184]. Grafts containing relatively pure populations of glial cells appear to be well tolerated whereas grafts that contain endothelial cells and/or other vascular bed contaminants are rapidly rejected. These studies suggest, therefore, that suspensions of pure populations of progenitor cells may be the donor material of choice for transplantation. These experiments have clearly shown that potentially adequate numbers of progenitor cells can be generated *in vitro* using specific growth factors and that these cells, when transplanted *in vivo*, possess the capacity to remyelinate CNS lesions. However, when long-term cultures of progenitor cells are used, fewer of the axons show evidence of remyelination and many of the transplanted cells do not always differentiate into myelinating cells and continue to proliferate in the lesion [181].

Interestingly, studies in lesions that remyelinate have indicated that adult oligodendrocytes also possess significant reparative properties [182]. Although mature, differentiated oligodendrocytes do not normally divide in adult tissues, several groups have now shown convincingly that oligodendrocytes can be reactivated to proliferate in areas adjacent to certain types of lesions (see Chapter 15 for review). Results in culture support these observations and further suggest that this reactivation is accompanied by partial dedifferentiation to a cell type that has greater proliferative and remyelinating activity in culture than adult progenitor cells isolated from the same source [171, 174]. Thus, both mature and precursor populations of oligodendrocytes may be suitable for transplantation into lesioned areas of the brain, and future experiments will need to determine which cell population preferentially leads to long-term

establishment of myelin and restoration of secure conduction. With respect to repair of the chronic MS lesions, it will also be important to study the effect of astrocytic scar tissue on the transplanted oligodendrocytes. Astrocytes are known to produce growth factors that are required for oligodendrocyte development and differentiation and co-transplantation of type I astrocytes has been shown to facilitate remyelination in glial-free areas of demyelination induced by ethidium bromide [178, 185, 186]. How the development of an astrocytic scar alters the production of these growth factors and changes the microenvironment of the CNS is not known at the present time.

18.4.2 GROWTH FACTOR REPLACEMENT THERAPY

An alternative strategy to transplantation is the use of growth factors known to promote oligodendrocyte proliferation and differentiation [187]. As noted above, the role of specific growth factors in oligodendrocyte proliferation, differentiation and myelination has now been relatively well defined, and although some controversies still remain, a role for insulin-like growth factors 1 and 2 (IGF-1, IGF-2), platelet-derived growth factor (PDGF), basic fibroblast growth factor (bFGF) interleukin-6, neurotrophin-3 and ciliary neurotrophic factor (CNTF) in various steps in these pathways has been well established [168–173]. Although studies testing the effects of these factors in various demyelinating model systems are not as well advanced as those involving the transplantation of oligodendrocytes, preliminary results with IGF-1 in EAE are encouraging and further suggest that systemic delivery may be as efficacious as intra-cerebral delivery [188]. However, since this may not be true for all of the possible growth factors involved, others are working on the potential use of viral vectors for delivery of these factors to the CNS. IGF-1, as well as brain-derived neurotrophic factor, is currently in phase III and phase I/II trials respectively in patients with MS [189].

18.5 Conclusions

In this review we have touched on some of the therapeutic approaches that are being tested for efficacy in the primary demyelinating disorders. The various animal models currently available for studying inflammatory demyelinating conditions have led to a wealth of experimental strategies for affecting disease expression in patients. Many of them have been developed using the knowledge gained from studies on the animal model EAE, and as such they principally involve mechanisms related to T cell-mediated pathogenesis. Pathological analysis of MS tissue strongly implicates a role for T lymphocytes and macrophages in disease expression and, as noted earlier, many of the factors associated with cell-mediated inflammatory responses have been detected in acute and chronic active MS lesions. However, not all investigators concur in this analysis and a principal role for antibodies and activated macrophages cannot be ruled out at the present time. Nevertheless, the demonstrable effects of injecting regulatory cytokines such as IFN-β and proinflammatory cytokines such as IFN-γ on disease expression in patients with MS suggest that treatment modalities directed at cytokine activity are likely to have an effect and thus considerable interest is directed at the use of other regulatory cytokines such as TGFβ, and inhibitors of proinflammatory cytokines such as members of the TNF family. Many of these, and other procedures, discussed above have performed well in animal experimentation and have moved rapidly into the clinical arena, with completion of phase I clinical trails showing no significant toxic or untoward side-effects. Given the widespread acceptance of standardized protocols for clinical trials, and the recognition of the kind of data needed to support claims of efficacy, it is to be expected that useful and interpretable data will be obtained for most of these therapeutic regimens relatively efficiently. The results are eagerly anticipated.

ACKNOWLEDGMENT

Supported in part by NIH grants NS 11920 and NS31919. M.K.R. is a Harry Weaver Neuroscience Scholar of the National Multiple Sclerosis Society and K.S. is a recipient of a Fogarty US–Poland Science program award, FIC-246/HHSp-105.

References

1. Lanzavecchia, A. (1993) Identifying strategies for immune intervention. *Science*, **260**, 937–44.
2. Gaur, A. and Fathman, G.C. (1994) Immunotherapeutic strategies directed at the trimolecular complex. *Adv. Immunol.*, **26**, 219–65.
3. Sadovnick, A.D. and Ebers G.C. (1995) Genetics of multiple sclerosis. *Neurol. Clin.*, **13**, 99–118.
4. Ebers, G.C., Sadovnick, A.D. and Risch, N.J. (1995) A genetic basis for familial aggregation in multiple sclerosis. Canadian Collaborative Study. *Nature*, **377**, 150–1.
5. Zamvil, S.S. and Steinman, L. (1990) The T lymphocyte in experimental allergic encephalomyelitis. *Ann. Rev. Immunol.*, **8**, 579–621.
6. Miller, S.D. and Karpus, W.J. (1994) The immunopathogenesis and regulation of T-cell-mediated demyelinating diseases. *Immunol. Today*, **15**, 356–61.
7. Sriram, S. and Steinman, L. (1983) Anti-I-A antibody suppresses active encephalomyelitis: treatment model for disease linked IR genes. *J. Exp. Med.*, **158**, 1362–8.
8. Steinman, L. (1995) Escape from 'horror autotoxicus': pathogenesis and treatment of autoimmune disease. *Cell*, **80**, 7–10.
9. Lindsey J.W., Hodgkinson, S., Mehta, R., Mitchell, D. *et al.* (1994) Repeated treatment with chimeric anti-CD4 antibody in multiple sclerosis. *Ann. Neurol.*, **36**, 183–9.
10. Buus, S., Sette, A. and Grey, H.M. (1987) The interaction between protein-derived immunological peptides and Ia. *Immunol. Rev.*, **98**, 115–41.
11. Teitelbaum, D., Webb, C., Meshorer, A., Arnon, R. and Sela, M. (1972) Protection against experimental allergic encephalomyelitis. *Nature*, **240**, 564–6.
12. Smilek, D.E., Wraith, D.C., Hodginson, D. *et al.* (1991) A single amino acid change in a myelin basic protein peptide confers the capacity to prevent rather than induce experimental autoimmune encephalomyelitis. *Proc. Natl Acad. Sci. (USA)*, **88**, 9633–7.
13. Sakai, K., Zamvil, S.S., Mitchell, D.J. *et al.* (1989) Prevention of experimental encephalomyelitis with peptides that block interaction of T cells with major histocompatibility complex proteins. *Proc. Natl Acad. Sci. (USA)*, **86**, 9470–4.
14. Lamont, A.G., Sette, A., Fujima, R. *et al.* (1990) Inhibition of experimental autoimmune encephalomyelitis induction in SJL/J mice by using a peptide with high affinity for I-A^s molecules. *J. Immunol.*, **145**, 1687–93.
15. Gautam, A.M. and Glynn, P. (1990) Competition between foreign and self proteins in antigen presentation: ovalbumin can inhibit activation of myelin basic protein-specific T cells. *J. Immunol.*, **144**, 1177–80.
16. Brocke, S., Gijbels, K., Allegretta, M. *et al.* (1996) Treatment of experimental encephalomyelitis with a peptide analogue of myelin basic protein. *Nature*, **379**, 343–6.
17. Gautam, A.M., Pearson, C., Sinha, A.A. *et al.* (1992) Inhibition of experimental autoimmune encephalomyelitis by non-immunogenic non-self peptide that binds to I-A^{u1}. *J. Immunol.*, **148**, 3049–54.
18. Karin, N., Mitchell, D.J., Brocke, S., Ling, N. and Steinman, L. (1994) Reversal of experimental autoimmune encephalomyelitis by a soluble peptide variant of a myelin basic protein epitope: T cell receptor antagonism and reduction of interferon gamma and tumor necrosis factor alpha production. *J. Exp. Med.*, **180**, 2227–37.
19. Ridgway, W., Weiner, H.L. and Fathman, G.C. (1994) Regulation of autoimmune responses. *Curr. Opin. Immunol.*, **6**, 946–55.
20. Weiner, H.L., Hohol, M.J., Khoury, S.J., Dawson, D.M. and Hafler, D.A. (1995) Therapy for multiple sclerosis. *Neurol. Clin.*, **13**, 173–96.
21. Karin, N., Mitchell, D.J., Brocke, S., Ling, N. and Steinman, L. (1994) Reversal of experimental autoimmune encephalomyelitis by a soluble peptide variant of a myelin basic protein epitope: T cell receptor antagonism and reduction of interferon-gamma and tumor necrosis factor alpha production. *J. Exp. Med.*, **180**, 2227–37.
22. Davis, M.M. and Bjorkman, P.J. (1988) T-cell antigen receptor genes and T-cell recognition. *Nature*, **334**, 395–402.
23. Brenner, M.B., Strominger, J.L. and Krangel, M.S. (1988) The γδ T cell receptor. *Adv. Immunol.*, **43**, 133–92.
24. Urban, J.L., Kumar, V., Kono, D.H. *et al.* (1988) Restricted use of T cell receptor V genes in murine autoimmune encephalomyelitis raises possibilities for antibody therapy. *Cell*, **54**, 577–92.
25. Burns, F.R., Li, X., Shen, N. *et al.* (1989) Both rat and mouse T cell receptor specific for the encephalitogenic determinant of myelin basic protein use similar Vα and Vβ chain genes even though the major histocompatibility complex and encephalitogenic determinants being recognized are different. *J. Exp. Med.*, **169**, 27–39.
26. Chluba, J., Steeg, C., Becker, A., Wekerle, H. and Epplen, J.T. (1989) T cell receptor β chain usage in myelin basic protein-specific rat T lymphocytes. *Eur. J. Immunol.*, **19**, 279–84.
27. Heber-Katz, E. (1991) The autoimmune receptor in experimental disease. *Immunol. Series*, **55**, 155–69.
28. Wilson, D.B., Steinman, L. and Gold, D.P. (1993) The V-region disease hypothesis: new evidence suggests it is possibly wrong. *Immunol. Today*, **14**, 376–80.
29. Vandenbark, A.A., Hashim, G.A. and Offner, H. (1989) Immunization with a synthetic T cell receptor V-region peptide protects against experimental autoimmune encephalomyelitis. *Nature*, **342**, 541–50.
30. Brostoff, S.W. (1995) T cell receptor peptide vaccines as immunotherapy. *Agents Actions*, **47**, 53–8.
31. Vaniene, M., Gold, D.P., Clenik, B. *et al.* (1992) Common sequence on distinct Vβ genes defines a protective idiotope in experimental encephalomyelitis. *J. Neurosci. Res.*, **31**, 413–20.
32. Offner, H., Hashim, G.A. and Vandenbark, A.A. (1991) T cell receptor peptide therapy triggers autoregulation of experimental encephalomyelitis. *Science*, **251**, 430–2.
33. Hashim, G.A., Vandenbark, A.A., Galang, A.B. *et al.* (1990) Antibodies specific for a Vβ8 T cell receptor peptide suppress experimental autoimmune encephalomyelitis. *J. Immunol.*, **144**, 4621–7.
34. Offner, H., Hashim, G.A., Chou, Y.K., Bourdette, D. and Vandenbark, A.A. (1993) Prevention, suppression and treatment of experimental autoimmune encephalomyelitis with a synthetic T cell receptor V region peptide, in *Molecular Mechanisms of Immunological Self-Recognition* (eds F.W. Alt and M.G. Vogel), New York, Academic Press, pp. 199–230.
35. Kotzin, B.L., Karuturi, S., Chou, Y.K. *et al.* (1991) Preferential T cell receptor Vβ gene usage in myelin basic protein reactive T cell clones from patients with multiple sclerosis. *Proc. Natl Acad. Sci. (USA)*, **88**, 9161–5.
36. Oksenberg, J.R., Stuart, S., Begovitch, A.B. *et al.* (1990) Limited heterogeneity of rearranged T cell receptor Valpha transcripts in brain lesions of multiple sclerosis. *Nature*, **345**, 344–6.
37. Wucherpfennig, K.W., Ota, K., Endo, N. *et al.* (1990) Shared human T cell receptor Vβ usage to immunodominant regions of myelin basic protein. *Science*, **248**, 1016–9.

38. Ben-Nun, A., Liblau, R.S., Cohen, L. *et al.* D., (1991) Restricted T-cell receptor Vβ gene usage by myelin basic protein-specific T-cell clones in multiple sclerosis: predominant genes vary in individuals. *Proc. Natl Acad. Sci. (USA)*, **88**, 2466–70.

39. Martin, R., Utz, U., Coligan, J.E. *et al.* (1992) Diversity and fine specificity and T-cell receptor usage of the human CD4+ cell response specific for the immunodominant myelin basic protein peptide 87–106. *J. Immunol.*, **148**, 1359–66.

40. Hafler, D.A., Saadeh, M.G., Kuchroo, V.K., Milford, E. and Steinman, L. (1996) TCR usage in human and experimental demyelinating disease. *Immunol. Today*, **17**, 152–9.

41. Vandevyer, C., Mertens, N., van der Elsen, P. *et al.* (1995) Clonal expansion of MBP-reactive T cells in patients with multiple sclerosis: restricted T cell receptor V gene rearrangements and CDR3 sequence. *Eur. J. Immunol.*, **25**, 958–68.

42. Ben-Nun, A., Wekerle, H. and Cohen, I.R. (1981) Vaccination against autoimmune encephalomyelitis with T-lymphocyte line cells reactive against myelin basic protein. *Nature*, **292**, 60–1.

43. Lider, O., Karin, N., Shinitzky, M. and Cohen, I.R. (1987) Therapeutic vaccination against adjuvant arthritis using autoimmune T cells treated with hydrostatic pressure. *Proc. Natl Acad. Sci. USA*, **84**, 4577–80.

44. Lider, O., Reshefj, T., Beraud, E., Ben-Nun, A. and Cohen, I.R. (1988) Anti-idiotypic network induced by T-cell vaccination against experimental autoimmune encephalomyelitis. *Science*, **239**, 181–3.

45. Lohse, A.W., Mor, F., Karin, N. and Cohen, I.R. (1989) Control of experimental autoimmune encephalomyelitis by T cells responding to activated T cells. *Science*, **244**, 820–2.

46. Cohen, I.R. and Weiner, H.L. (1988) T cell vaccination. *Immunol. Today*, **9**, 332–5.

47. Zhang, J., Markovic-Plese, S., Lacet, B. *et al.* (1994) Increased frequency of interleukin-2-responsive T cells specific for myelin basic protein and proteolipid protein in peripheral blood and cerebrospinal fluid of patients with multiple sclerosis. *J. Exp. Med.*, **179**, 973–84.

48. Zhang, J. and Raus, J. (1994) T cell vaccination in multiple sclerosis: hopes and facts. *Acta Neurol. Belg.*, **94**, 112–15.

49. Bourdette, D.N., Whitham, R.H., Chou, Y.K. *et al.* (1994) Immunity to TCR peptides in multiple sclerosis. I. Successful immunization of patients with synthetic Vβ 5.2 and Vβ 6.1 CDR2 peptides. *J. Immunol.*, **152**, 2510–19.

50. Chou, Y.K., Morrison, W.J., Weinberg, A.D. *et al.* (1994) Immunity to TCR peptides in multiple sclerosis. II. T cell recognition of Vβ 5.2 and Vβ 6.1 CDR2 peptides. *J. Immunol.*, **152**, 2520–9.

51. Zhang, J., Medaer, R., Stinissen, P., Hafler, D.A. and Raus, J. (1993) MHC-restricted depletion of human myelin basic protein-reactive T cells by T cell vaccination. *Science*, **261**, 1451–4.

52. Ralph, P. (1993) Clinical and preclinical studies presented at the Keystone Symposium on Arthritis, Related Diseases and Cytokines. *Lymph. Cytokine Res.*, **12**, 261–3.

53. Selmaj, K.W. (1992) The role of cytokines in inflammatory conditions of the central nervous system. *Sem. Neurosci.*, **4**, 221–9.

54. Selmaj, K., Raine, C.S. and Cross, A.H. (1991) Anti-tumor necrosis factor therapy abrogates autoimmune demyelination. *Ann. Neurol.*, **30**, 694–700.

55. Ruddle, N.H., Bergaman, C.M., McGrath, M.L. *et al.* (1990) An antibody to lymphotoxin and tumor necrosis factor prevents transfer of experimental allergic encephalomyelitis. *J. Exp. Med.*, **172**, 1193–1200.

56. Teuscher, C., Hickey, W.F. and Korngold, R. (1990) An analysis of the role of tumor necrosis factor in the phenotypic expression of actively induced experimental allergic orchitis and experimental allergic encephalomyelitis. *Clin. Immunol. Immunopathol.*, **54**, 442–53.

57. Martin, D., Near, S.L., Bendele. A. and Russell, D.A. (1995) Inhibition of tumor necrosis factor is protective against neurological dysfunction after active immunization of Lewis rats with myelin basic protein. *Exp. Neurol.*, **131**, 221–8.

58. Seckinger, P., Idaaz, S. and Dayer, J-M. (1988) A human inhibitor to tumor necrosis factor. *J. Exp. Med.*, **167**, 1511–22.

59. Kohno, T., Brewer, M.T., Baker S.L. *et al.* (1990) A second tumor necrosis factor receptor gene product can shed a naturally occurring tumor necrosis factor inhibitor. *Proc. Natl Acad. Sci. (USA)*, **87**, 9331–6.

60. Selmaj, K., Papierz, W., Glabinski, A. and Kohno, T. (1995) Prevention of chronic relapsing experimental autoimmune encephalomyelitis by soluble TNF receptor 1. *J. Neuroimmunol.*, **56**, 135–41.

61. Cavender, D.E., Edelbaum, D. and Ziff, M. (1989) Endothelial cell activation by tumor necrosis factor and lymphotoxin. *Am. J. Physiol.*, **134**, 551–63.

62. Barten, D.M. and Ruddle, N.H. (1994) Vascular cell adhesion molecule-1 modulation by tumor necrosis factor in experimental allergic encephalomyelitis. *J. Neuroimmunol.*, **51**, 123–34.

63. Hackett, R.J., Davis, L.S. and Lipsky, P.E. (1988) Comparative effects of tumor necrosis factor-α and IL-1β on mitogen-induced T cell activation. *J. Immunol.*, **140**, 2639–48.

64. Brightman, B.K. and Fan, H. (1993) The CD4 surface antigen is induced and maintained on T-lymphoid cell line by tumor necrosis factor-a. *Lymph. Cytokine Res.*, **12**, 293–302.

65. Selmaj, K. and Raine, C.S. (1995) Experimental autoimmune encephalomyelitis: immunotherapy with anti-tumor necrosis factor antibodies and soluble tumor necrosis factor receptors. *Neurology*, **45**, S44–9.

66. Monastra, G., Cross, A.H., Bruni, A. and Raine, C.S. (1993) Phosphatidylserine, a putative inhibitor of tumor necrosis factor, prevents autoimmune demyelination. *Neurology*, **43**, 153–63.

67. Sommer, N., Loschmann, P-A., Northoff, G.H. *et al.* (1995) The antidepressant rolipram suppresses cytokine production and prevents autoimmune encephalomyelitis. *Nature Med.*, **1**, 244–8.

68. Genain, C.P., Roberts, T., Davis, R.L. *et al.* (1995) Prevention of autoimmune demyelination in non-human primates by a cAMP-specific phosphodiesterase inhibitor. *Proc. Natl Acad. Sci. (USA)*, **92**, 3601–5.

69. Moreira, A.L., Sampaio, E.P., Zmuidzinas, A. *et al.* (1993) Thalidomide exerts its inhibitory action on tumor necrosis factor a by enhancing mRNA degradation. *J. Exp. Med.*, **177**, 1675–80.

70. Sarno, E.N., Grau, G.E., Vieira, L.M. *et al.* (1991) Serum levels of TNF-α and IL-1β during leprosy reactional states. *Clin. Exp. Immunol.*, **84**, 103–11.

71. Bauer, J., Berkenbosch, F., Van-Dam, A.M. and Dijkstra, C.D. (1993) Demonstration of interleukin-1 beta in Lewis rat brain during experimental allergic encephalomyelitis by immunocytochemistry at the light and ultrastructural level. *J. Neuroimmunol.*, **48**, 13–21.

72. Mannie, M.D., Dinarello, C.A. and Paterson, P.Y. (1987) Interleukin 1 and myelin basic protein synergistically augment adoptive transfer activity of lymphocytes mediating experimental autoimmune encephalomyelitis in Lewis rats. *J. Immunol.*, **138**, 4229–35.

73. Jacobs, C.A., Baker, P.E., Roux, E.R. *et al.* (1991) Experimental autoimmune encephalomyelitis is exacerbated by IL-1α and suppressed by soluble IL-1 receptor. *J. Immunol.*, **146**, 2983–9.

74. Dinarello, C.A. and Thompson, R.C. (1991) Blocking IL-1: interleukin 1 receptor antagonist in vivo and in vitro. *Immunol. Today*, **12**, 404–10.

75. Cannella, B. and Raine, C.S. (1995) The adhesion molecule and cytokine profile of multiple sclerosis lesions. *Ann. Neurol.*, **37**, 424–35.

76. Wilcox, C.E., Ward, A.M.V., Evans, A. *et al.* (1990) Endothelial cell expression of the intercellular adhesion molecule-1 (ICAM-1) in the central nervous system of guinea pigs during acute and chronic relapsing experimental allergic encephalomyelitis. *J. Neuroimmunol.*, **30**, 43–51.

77. Cannella, B, Cross, A.H. and Raine, C.S. (1990) Up-regulation and coexpression of adhesion molecules correlate with relapsing autoimmune demyelination in the central nervous system. *J. Exp. Med.*, **172**, 1521–4.

78. Welsh, C.T., Rose, J.W., Hill, K.W. and Townsend, J.J. (1993) Augmentation of adoptively transferred experimental allergic encephalomyelitis by administration of a monoclonal antibody specific for LFA-1a. *J. Neuroimmunol.*, **43**, 161–8.

79. Cannella, B., Cross, A.H. and Raine, C.S. (1993) Anti-adhesion molecule therapy in experimental autoimmune encephalomyelitis. *J. Neuroimmunol.*, **46**, 43–55.

80. Archelos, J.J., Jung, S., Maurer, M. *et al.* (1993) Inhibition of experimental autoimmune encephalomyelitis by an antibody to the intercellular adhesion molecule ICAM-1. *Ann. Neurol.*, **34**, 145–54.

81. Baron, J.L., Madri, J.A., Ruddle, J.A., Hashim, G. and Janeway, C.A. Jr (1993) Surface expression of a4 integrin by CD4 T cells is required for their entry into brain parenchyma. *J. Exp. Med.*, **177**, 57–68.

82. Racke, M.K., Quigley, L. Cannella, L. Raine, C.S., McFarlin, D.E. and Scott, D.E. (unpublished observations).

83. Zhao, M.-L., Xia, J.-Q. and Fritz, R.B. (1992) Experimental allergic encephalomyelitis in susceptible and resistant strains of mice after the adoptive transfer of T cells activated by antibodies to the T cell receptor complex. *J. Neuroimmunol.*, **40**, 31–9.

84. Yednock, T.A., Cannon, C., Fritz, L.C. *et al.* (1992) Prevention of experimental autoimmune encephalomyelitis by antibodies against α4β1 integrin. *Nature*, **356**, 63–6.

85. Hartung, H.P., Jung, S., Stoll, G. *et al.* (1992) The inflammatory mediators in demyelinating disorders of the CNS and PNS (Review). *J. Neuroimmunol.*, **40**, 197–210.

86. Wekerle, H., Kojima, K., Lannes-Vieira, J., Lassmann, H. and Linington, C. (1994) Animals models (Review). *Ann. Neurol.*, **36**, S47–53.

87. Williams, K.C., Ulvestad, E. and Hickey, W.F. (1994) Immunology of multiple sclerosis. *Clin. Neurosci.*, **2**, 229–45.

88. Compston, A. (1993) Inflammation and the brain. *Mol. Chem. Neuropathol.*, **19**, 47–64.

89. Linington, C., Engelhardt, B., Kapocs, G. and Lassmann, H. (1992) Induction of persistently demyelinated lesions in the rat following the repeated adoptive transfer of encephalitogenic T cells and demyelinating antibody. *J. Neuroimmunol.*, **40**, 219–24.

90. Gijbels, K., Galardy, R.E. and Steinman, L. (1994) Reversal of experimental autoimmune encephalomyelitis with a hydroxamate inhibitor of matrix metalloproteases. *J. Clin. Invest.*, **94**, 2177–82.

91. Weber, F., Meyermann, R. and Hempel, K. (1991) Experimental allergic encephalomyelitis – prophylactic and therapeutic treatment with the cyclooxygenase inhibitor piroxicam (Feldene). *Int. Arch. Allerg. Appl. Immunol.*, **95**, 136–41.

92. Simmons, R.D., Hugh, A.R., Willenborg, D.O. and Cowden, W.B. (1992) Suppression of active but not passive autoimmune encephalomyelitis by dual cyclo-oxygenase and 5-lipoxygenase inhibition. *Acta Neurol. Scand.*, **85**, 197–9.

93. Xie, Q. and Nathan, C. (1994) The high-output nitric oxide pathway: role and regulation. *J. Leukocyte Biol.*, **56**, 576–82.

94. Lin, R.F., Lin T.-S., Tilton, R.G. and Cross, A.H. (1993) Nitric oxide localized to spinal cords of mice with experimental allergic encephalomyelitis: an electron paramagnetic resonance study. *J. Exp. Med.*, **178**, 643–8.

95. MacMicking, J.D., Willenborg, D.O., Weidemann, M.J. *et al.* (1992) Elevated secretion of reactive nitrogen and oxygen intermediates by inflammatory leukocytes in hyperacute experimental autoimmune encephalomyelitis: enhancement by the soluble products of encephalitogenic T cells. *J. Exp. Med.*, **176**, 303–7.

96. Koprowski, H., Zheng, Y.M., Heber-Katz, E. *et al.* (1993) *In vivo* expression of inducible nitric oxide synthase in experimentally induced neurologic disease. *Proc. Natl Acad. Sci. USA*, **90**, 3024–7.

97. Merrill, J.E., Ignarro, L.J., Sherman, M.P., Melinek, J. and Lane, T.E. (1993) Microglial cell cytotoxicity of oligodendrocytes is mediated through nitric oxide. *J. Immunol.*, **151**, 2132–41.

98. Brosnan, C.F., Battistini, L., Raine, C.S. *et al.* (1994) Reactive nitrogen intermediates in human neuropathology: an overview. *Dev. Neurosci.*, **16**, 152–61.

99. Bo, L., Dawson, T.M., Wesselingh, S. *et al.* (1994) Induction of nitric oxide synthase in demyelinating regions of multiple sclerosis brains. *Ann. Neurol.*, **36**, 778–86.

100. Lee, S.C., Dickson, D.W., Liu, W. and Brosnan, C.F. (1993) Induction of nitric oxide synthase activity in human astrocytes by interleukin-1β and interferon-γ. *J. Neuroimmunol.*, **46**, 19–24.

101. Cross, A.H., Misko, T.P., Lin, R.F. *et al.* (1994) Aminoguanidine, an inhibitor of inducible nitric oxide synthase, ameliorates experimental autoimmune encephlomyelitis in SJL mice. *J. Clin. Invest.*, **93**, 2684–90.

102. Zielasek, J., Jing, S., Gold, R. *et al.* (1995) Administration of nitric oxide synthase inhibitors in experimental autoimmune neuritis and experimental autoimmune encephalomyelitis. *J. Neuroimmunol.*, **58**, 81–8.

103. Glabinski, A.R., Tani, M. Aras, S. *et al.* (1995) Regulation and function of central nervous system chemokines. *Intl. J. Devl. Neurosci.*, **13**, 153–65.

104. Karpus, W.J., Lukacs, N.W., McRae, B.L. *et al.* (1995) An important role for the chemokine macrophage inflammatory protein-1α in the pathogenesis of the T cell-mediated autoimmune disease, experimental autoimmune encephalomyelitis. *J. Immunol.*, **155**, 5003–10.

105. Kehrl, J.H., Wakefield, A.L., Roberts, A.B. *et al.* (1986). Production of transforming growth factor B by human T lymphocytes and its potential role in the regulation of T cell growth. *J. Exp. Med.*, **163**, 1037–50.

106. Johns, L.D., Flanders, K.C., Ranges, G.E. and Sriram, S. (1991) Successful treatment of experimental allergic encephalomyelitis with transforming growth factor-β1. *J. Immunol.*, **147**, 1792–6.

107. Kuruvilla, A.P., Sah, R., Hochwald, G.M. *et al.* (1991) Protective effect of transforming growth factor-β1 on experimental diseases in mice. *Proc. Natl Acad. Sci. (USA)*, **88**, 2918–21.

108. Racke, M.K., Dhib-Jalbut, S., Cannella, B. *et al.* (1991) Prevention and treatment of chronic relapsing experimental allergic encephalomyelitis by transforming growth factor-β1. *J. Immunol.*, **146**, 3012–17.

109. Racke, M.K., Sriram, S., Carlino, J. *et al.* (1993) Long-term treatment of chronic relapsing experimental allergic encephalomyelitis by transforming growth factor-β2. *J. Neuroimmunol.*, **46**, 175–83.

110. Brandes, M.E., Allen, J.B., Ogawa, Y. and Wahl, S.M. (1991) Transforming growth factor-β1 suppresses acute and chronic arthritis in experimental animals. *J. Clin. Invest.*, **87**, 1108–13.

111. Karpus, W.J. and Swanborg, R.H. (1991) CD4 + suppressor cells inhibit the function of effector cells of experimental autoimmune encephalomyelitis through a mechanism involving transforming growth factor-β. *J. Immunol.*, **146**, 1163–8.

112. Racke, M.K., Cannella, B., Albert, P. *et al.* (1992) Evidence of endogenous regulatory function of transforming growth factor-β1 in experimental allergic encephalomyelitis. *Int. Immunol.*, **4**, 615–20.

113. Johns, L.D. and Sriram, S. (1993) Experimental allergic encephalomyelitis: neutralizing antibody to TGFβ1 enhances the clinical severity of the disease. *J. Neuroimmunol.*, **47**, 1–8.

114. Beck, J., Rondot, P., Jullien, P., Wietzerbin, J. and Lawrence D.A. (1991) TGF-β-like activity produced during regression of exacerbations of multiple sclerosis. *Acta Neurol. Scand.*, **84**, 452–5.

115. Correale, J., Gilmore, W., McMillan, M. *et al.* (1995) Patterns of cytokine secretion by autoreactive proteolipid protein-specific T cell clones during the course of multiple sclerosis. *J. Immunol.*, **154**, 2959–68.

116. Calabresi, P.A., Hanham, A., Carlino, J. *et al.* (1995) Report of an ongoing phase I trial of recombinant transforming growth factor-beta-2 (TGF-β2) in chronic progressive multiple sclerosis. *Neurology*, **45** (Suppl. 4), A417.

117. Chen, Y., Kuchroo, V.K., Inobe, J-I., Hafler, D.A. and Weiner, H.L. (1994) Regulatory T cell clones induced by oral tolerance and suppression of autoimmune encephalomyelitis. *Science*, **265**, 1237–40.

118. Asherson, G.L. and Stone, S.H. (1965) Selective and specific inhibition of 24 hour skin reactions in the guinea-pig. I. Immune deviation: description of the phenomenon and the effect of splenectomy. *Immunology*, **9**, 205–9.

119. Fiorentino, D.F., Bond, M.W. and Mosmann, T.R. (1989) Two types of mouse T helper cell. IV. Th2 clones secrete a factor that inhibits cytokine production by Th1 clones. *J. Exp. Med.*, **170**, 2081–95.

120. Mosmann, T.R. and Coffman, R.L. (1989) TH1 and TH2 cells: different patterns of lymphokine secretion lead to different functional properties. *Ann. Rev. Immunol.*, **7**, 145–73.

121. Ando, D.G., Clayton, J., Kono, D., Urban, J.L. and Sercarz, E.E. (1989) Encephalitogenic T cells in the B10.PL model of experimental allergic encephalomyelitis (EAE) are of the Th1 lymphokine subtype. *Cell. Immunol.*, **124**, 132–43.

122. Racke, M.K., Bonomo, A., Scott, D.E. *et al.* (1994) Cytokine-induced immune deviation as a therapy for inflammatory autoimmune disease. *J. Exp. Med.*, **180**, 1961–6.

123. Kuchroo, V.J., Das, M.P., Brown, J.A. *et al.* (1995) B7–1 and B7–2 costimulatory molecules activate differentially the Th1/Th2 developmental pathways: application to autoimmune disease therapy. *Cell*, **80**, 707–18.

124. Massacesi, L., Castigli, E., Vergelli, M. *et al.* (1991) Immunosuppressive activity of 13-cis-retinoic acid and prevention of experimental autoimmune encephalomyelitis in rats. *J. Clin. Invest.*, **88**, 1331–7.

125. Racke, M.K., Burnett, D., Pak, S-H. *et al.* (1995) Retinoid treatment of experimental allergic encephalomyelitis. IL-4 production correlates with improved disease course. *J. Immunol.*, **154**, 450–8.

126. Rott, O., Cash, E. and Fleischer, B. (1993) Phosphodiesterase inhibitor pentoxifylline, a selective suppressor of T helper type 1-but not type 2-associated lymphokine production, prevents induction of experimental autoimmune encephalomyelitis in rats. *Eur. J. Immunol.*, **23**, 1745–51.

127. Mueller, D.L., Jenkins, M.K. and Schwartz, R.H. (1989) Clonal expansion versus functional clonal inactivation: a costimulatory signaling pathway determines the outcome of T cell antigen receptor occupancy. *Annu. Rev. Immunol.*, **7**, 445–80.

128. June, C.H., Bluestone, J.A., Nadler, L.M. and Thompson, C.B. (1994) The B7 and CD28 receptor families. *Immunol. Today*, **15**, 321–31.

129. Hathcock, K.S., Laszlo, G., Dickler, H.B. *et al.* (1993) Identification of an alternative CTLA-4 ligand costimulatory for T cell activation. *Science*, **262**, 905–7.

130. Freeman, G.J., Borriello, F., Hodes, R.J. *et al.* (1993) Uncovering of functional alternative CTLA-4 counter-receptor in B7-deficient mice. *Science*, **262**, 907–9.

131. Shahinian, A., Pfeffer, K., Lee, K.P. *et al.* (1993) Differential T cell costimulatory requirements in CD28-deficient mice. *Science*, **261**, 609–12.

132. Boussiotis, V.A., Freeman, G.J., Gribben, J.G. *et al.* (1993) Activated human B lymphocytes express three CTLA-4 counter-receptors that costimulate T-cell activation. *Proc. Natl. Acad. Sci. USA*, **90**, 11059–63.

133. Linsley, P.S., Greene, J.L., Brady, W. *et al.* (1994) Human B7–1 (CD80) and B7–2 (CD86) bind with similar avidities but distinct kinetics to D28 and CTLA-4 receptors. *Immunity*, **1**, 793–801.

134. Hathcock, K.S., Laszlo, G., Pucillo, C., Linsley, P. and Hodes, R.J. (1994) Comparative analysis of B7–1 and B7–2 costimulatory ligands: expression and function. *J. Exp. Med.*, **180**, 631–40.

135. Linsley, P.S., Wallace, P.M., Johnson, J. *et al.* (1992) Immunosuppression in vivo by a soluble form of the CTLA-4 T cell activation molecule. *Science*, **257**, 792–5.

136. Lin, H., Bolling, S.F., Linsley, P.S. *et al.* (1993) Long-term acceptance of major histocompatibility complex mismatched cardiac allografts induced by CTLA4Ig plus donor-specific transfusion. *J. Exp. Med.*, **178**, 1801–6.

137. Lenschow, D.J., Zeng, Y., Thistlethwaite, J.R. *et al.* (1992) Long-term survival of xenogeneic pancreatic islet grafts induced by CTLA4Ig. *Science*, **257**, 789–92.

138. Finck, B.K., Linsley, P.S. and Wofsy, D. (1994) Treatment of murine lupus with CTLA4Ig. *Science*, **265**, 1225–7.

139. Perrin, P.J., Scott, D., Quigley, L. *et al.* (1995) Role of B7:CD28/CTLA-4 in the induction of chronic relapsing experimental allergic encephalomyelitis. *J. Immunol.*, **154**, 1481–90.

140. Cross, A.H., Girard, T.J., Giacoletto, K.S. *et al.* (1995) Long-term inhibition of murine experimental autoimmune encephalomyelitis: using CTLA-4-Fc supports a key role for CD28 costimulation. *J. Clin. Invest.*, **95**, 2783–9.

141. Racke, M.K., Scott, D.E., Quigley, L. *et al.* (1995) Distinct roles for B7–1 (CD80) and B7–2 (CD-86) in the initiation of experimental allergic encephalomyelitis. *J. Clin. Invest.*, **96**, 2195–203.

142. Ronchese, F., Hausmann, B. Hubele, S. and Lane, P. (1994) Mice transgenic for a soluble form of murine CTLA-4 show enhanced expansion of antigen-specific CD4 + T cells and defective antibody production in vivo. *J. Exp. Med.*, **179**, 809–17.

143. Linsley, P.S., Greene, J.L., Tan, P. *et al.* (1992) Coexpression and functional cooperation of CTLA-4 and CD28 on activated T lymphocytes. *J. Exp. Med.*, **176**, 1595–604.

144. Green, J.M., Noel, P.J., Sperling, A.I. *et al.* (1994) Absence of B7-dependent responses in CD28-deficient mice. *Immunity*, 1, 501–8.

145. Sethna, M.P., van Parijs, L., Sharpe, A.H., Abbas, A.K. and Freeman, G.J. (1994) A negative regulatory function of B7 revealed in B7–1 transgenic mice. *Immunity*, 1, 415–21.

146. Khoury, S.J., Akalin, E., Chandraker, A. *et al.* (1995) CD28-B7 costimulatory blockade by CTLA4Ig prevents actively induced experimental autoimmune encephalomyelitis and inhibits Th1 but spares Th2 cytokines in the central nervous system. *J. Immunol.*, 155, 4521–4.

147. Lenschow, D.J., Ho, S.C., Sattar, H. *et al.* (1995) Differential effects of anti-B7–1 and anti-B7–2 monoclonal antibody treatment on the development of diabetes in the non-obese diabetic mouse. *J. Exp. Med.*, 181, 1145–55.

148. Damle, N.K., Klussman, K., Linsley, P.S. and Aruffo, A. (1992) Differential costimulatory effects of adhesion molecules B7, ICAM-1, LFA-3, and VCAM-1 on resting and antigen-primed CD4+ T lymphocytes. *J. Immunol.*, 148, 1985–92.

149. Karaszewski, J.W., Reder, A.T., Anlar, B. and Arnason, B.G. (1993) Increased high affinity β-adrenergic receptor densities and cAMP responses of CD8 cells in multiple sclerosis. *J. Neuroimmunol.*, 43, 1–7.

150. Chelmicka-Schorr, E. and Arnason, B.G. (1994) Nervous system-immune interactions and their role in multiple sclerosis. *Ann. Neurol.*, 36, S29–32.

151. Soos, J.M., Subramanim, P.S., Hobeika, A.C., Schiffenbauer, J. and Johnson, H.M. (1995) The IFN pregnancy recognition hormone IFN-tau blocks both development and superantigen reactivation of experimental allergic encephalomyelitis without associated toxicity. *J. Immunol.*, 155, 2747–53.

152. Weinstock-Guttman, B., Ransohoff, R.M., Kinkel, R.P. and Rudick, R.A. (1995) The interferons: biological effects, mechanisms of action, and use in multiple sclerosis. *Ann. Neurol.* 37, 7–13.

153. Russell, J.H., White, C.L., Loh, D.Y. and Meleedy-Rey, P. (1991) Receptor-stimulated death pathway is opened by antigen in mature T cells. *Proc. Natl Acad. Sci. (USA)*, 88, 2151–5.

154. Cohen, J.J. (1993) Apoptosis. *Immunol. Today*, 14, 126–130.

155. Critchfield, J.M., Racke, M.K., Zuniga-Pflucker, J.C. *et al.* (1994) T cell deletion in high antigen dose therapy of autoimmune encephalomyelitis. *Science*, 263: 1139–43.

156. Webb C., Morris C. and Sprent, J. (1990) Extrathymic tolerance of mature T cells: clonal elimination as a consequence of immunity. *Cell*, 63, 1249–56.

157. Nagata, S. and Suda, T. (1995) Fas and Fas ligand: lpr and gld mutations. *Immunol. Today*, 16, 39–43.

158. Levine, S., Hoenig, E.M. and Kies, M.W. (1968) Allergic encephalomyelitis: passive transfer prevented by encephalitogen. *Science*, 161, 1155–7.

159. Lisak, R.P., Zweiman, B., Dzida, L. *et al.* (1980) *In vitro* response to basic protein in experimental allergic encephalomyelitis: effect of pretreatment with basic protein in incomplete adjuvant. *Cell. Immunol.*, 52, 443–50.

160. Miller A., Lider O. and Weiner, H.L. (1991) Antigen driven bystander suppression following oral administration of antigens. *J. Exp. Med.*, 174, 791–8.

161. Tan, L-J., Kennedy, M.K., Dal Canto, M.C. and Miller, S.D. (1991) Successful treatment of paralytic relapses in adoptive experimental autoimmune encephalomyelitis via neuroantigen-specific tolerance. *J. Immunol.*, 147, 1797–802.

162. Sharma, S.D., Nag, B., Su, X-M. *et al.* (1991) Antigen-specific therapy of experimental allergic encephalomyelitis by soluble class II major histocompatibility complex-peptide complexes. *Proc. Natl Acad. Sci. USA*, 88, 11465–9.

163. Gaur, A., Wiersm, B., Liu, A., Rothbard, J. and Fathman, G.C. (1993) Amelioration of autoimmune encephalomyelitis by myelin basic protein synthetic peptide-induced anergy. *Science*, 258, 1491–3.

164. Pender, M.P., McCombe, P.A., Yoong, G. and Nguyen, K.B. (1992) Apoptosis of αβ T lymphocytes in the nervous system in experimental autoimmune encephalomyelitis: its possible implications for recovery and acquired tolerance. *J. Autoimmun.*, 5, 401–10.

165. Romine, J.S. and Salk, J. (1983) A study of myelin basic protein as a therapeutic probe in patients with multiple sclerosis, in *Multiple Sclerosis: Pathology, Diagnosis, and Management* (eds J.F. Hallpike, C.W.M. Adams and W.W. Tourtellotte), Baltimore, MD, Williams and Wilkins, pp. 621–30.

166. Alvord, E.C. Jr, Shaw, C-M., Hruby, S. and Kies, M.W. (1979) Has myelin basic protein received a fair trial in the treatment of multiple sclerosis? *Ann. Neurol.*, 6, 461–8.

167. Chen, Y., Inobe, J-I., Marks, R. *et al.* (1995) Peripheral deletion of antigen-reactive T cells in oral tolerance. *Nature*, 376, 177–80.

168. Raff, M.C., Miller, R.H. and Noble, M. (1983) A glial progenitor cell that develops *in vitro* into an astrocyte or an oligodendrocyte depending on culture medium. *Nature*, 303, 390–6.

169. Raff, M.C., Lillien, L.E., Richardson, W.D., Burne, J.F. and Nobel, M. (1988) Platelet derived growth factor from astrocytes drives the clock that times oligodendrocyte development in culture. *Nature*, 333, 562–5.

170. Bogler, O., Wren, D., Barnett, S.C., Land, H. and Noble, M. (1990) Cooperation between two growth factors promotes extended self-renewal and inhibits differentiation of oligodendrocytes-type-2 astrocyte (O-2A) progenitor cells. *Proc. Natl Acad. Sci. (USA)*, 87, 6368–73.

171. Gard, A.L. and Pfeiffer, S.E. (1990) Two proliferative stages of the oligodendrocyte lineage (A2B5 + O4 + GalC–) under different mitogenic control. *Neuron*, 5, 615–25.

172. McKinnon, R.D., Smith, C., Behar, T., Smith, T. and Dubois-Dalcq, M. (1993) Distinct effects of bFGF and PDGF on oligodendrocyte progenitor cells. *Glia*, 7, 245–54.

173. Noble, M. (1991) Points of controversy in the O-2A lineage: clocks and type-2 astrocytes (Review). *Glia*, 4, 157–64.

174. Wood, P.M. and Mora, J. (1993) Source of remyelinating oligodendrocytes. *Adv. Neurol.*, 59, 113–23.

175. Knapp, P.E., Skoff, R.P. and Booth, C.S. (1993) Essential prerequisites for remyelination of oligodendrocytes. Division, motility, and structural rearrangement. *Adv. Neurol.*, 59, 105–12.

176. Franklin, R.J.M. and Blakemore, W.F. (1995) Glial cell transplantation and plasticity in the O-2A lineage – implications for CNS repair. *Trends Neurosci.*, 18, 151–7.

177. Blakemore, W.F. and Crang, A.J. (1988) Extensive oligodendrocyte remyelination following injection of cultured central nervous system cells demyelinating lesions in adult central nervous system. *Dev. Neurosci.*, 10, 1–11.

178. Franklin, R.J.M., Crang, A.J. and Blakemore, W.F. (1990) Transplanted type-1 astrocytes facilitate repair of demyelinating lesions by host oligodendrocytes in adult rat spinal cord. *J. Neurocytol.*, 20, 420–30.

179. Hasegawa, M. and Rosenbluth, J. (1991) Transplantation of labeled fetal spinal cord fragments into juvenile myelin-deficient rat spinal cord. *Anat. Rec.*, 229, 138–43.

180. Rosenbluth, J., Liu, Z., Guo, D. and Schiff, R. (1993) Myelin formation by mouse glia in myelin-deficient rats treated with cyclosporine. *J. Neurocytol.*, 22, 967–77.

181. Groves, A.K., Barnett, S.C., Franklin, R.J.M., Crang, A.J. *et al.* (1993) Repair of demyelinated lesions by transplantation of O-2A progenitor cells. *Nature*, 362, 453–5.

182. Ludwin, S.K. and Szuchet, S. (1993) Myelination by mature ovine oligodendrocytes in vivo and in vitro: evidence that different steps in the myelination process are independently controlled. *Glia*, 8, 219–31.

183. Warrington, A.E., Barbarese, E. and Pfeiffer, S.E. (1993) Differential myelinogenic capacity of specific developmental stages of the oligodendrocyte lineage upon transplantation into hypomyelinating hosts. *J. Neurosci. Res.*, 34, 1–13.

184. Tontsch, U., Archer, D.R., Dubois-Dalcq, M. and Duncan, I.D. (1994) Transplantation of an oligodendrocyte cell line leading to extensive myelination. *Proc. Natl. Acad. Sci. (USA)*, 91, 11616–20.

185. Mayer, M., Bogler, O. and Noble, M. (1993) The inhibition of oligodendrocytic differentiation of O-2A progenitors caused by basic fibroblast growth factor is overriden by astrocytes. *Glia*, 8, 12–19.

186. Franklin, R.J.M., Crang, A.J. and Blakemore, W.F. (1993) The role of astrocytes in the remyelination of glia-free areas of demyelination. *Adv. Neurol.*, 59, 125–33.

187. Compston, A. (1995) Brain repair (Review) *J. Int. Med.*, 237, 127–34.

188. Yao, D.L., Liu, X., Hudson, L.D. and Webster, H.D. (1995) Insulin-like growth factor I treatment reduces demeylination and up-regulates gene expression of myelin-related proteins in experimental autoimmune encephalomyelitis. *Proc. Natl Acad. Sci. (USA)*, 92, 6190–4.

189. Marshall, A. (1996) Approved or advanced experimental MS therapies. *Nature Biotech.*, 14, 812–3.

19 CONDUCT OF A CLINICAL TRIAL IN MULTIPLE SCLEROSIS

Richard A. Rudick and Diane L. Cookfair

19.1 Introduction

19.1.1 HISTORICAL PERSPECTIVE

In 1982, the Multiple Sclerosis Society of Canada and the National Multiple Sclerosis Society, United States, sponsored the first International Conference on Therapeutic Trials in Multiple Sclerosis on Grand Island, New York. As stated in the introduction to the published proceedings [1], the purpose of the conference was 'to discuss some of the problems in assessing drugs and other therapeutic modalities, particularly in terms of their efficacy in the treatment of MS'. Specific issues considered at the conference included the rationale for specific interventions; therapeutic fads and quack cures; difficulties evaluating and scoring the disease for different purposes; and obstacles to obtaining a statistically clear-cut result in any given trial. Workshops during the conference recommended a committee responsible for planning and coordinating future clinical trials (currently the Advisory Committee on Clinical Trials of New Agents in Multiple Sclerosis of the National Multiple Sclerosis Society), development of high-quality protocols for preliminary and definitive clinical trials in MS, and a conference on the role of third party payers in clinical trials. The prevailing sentiments among participants at the 1982 Grand Island conference were caution and widespread skepticism. There was great emphasis placed on difficulties inherent in clinical trials in MS, as lucidly articulated 15 years previously by Schumacher and colleagues [2]. The conference followed three years after the publication of an important paper by Brown and colleagues [3] indicating the need to refine the research question and to restrict treatment groups to homogeneous types of MS patients; the conference also coincided with the publication of a compendium of unsubstantiated therapeutic claims in MS [4], which listed in agonizing detail the myriad of claimed interventions for which no convincing data on efficacy existed. Thus the Grand Island workshop represented a watershed event in the recent history of MS therapy, representing activism and optimism in the context of widespread therapeutic nihilism and skepticism about the feasibility of clinical trials in MS.

There have been a number of critical advances since the Grand Island conference, some of which were highlighted in a historical perspective on MS clinical trials [5]. Diagnostic criteria that permitted use of MRI, multi-modality, sensory evoked potentials and CSF abnormalities were recommended for research protocols [6]; Kurtzke published his expanded disability status scale (EDSS) [7], which achieved widespread use as a single measure of MS severity; and magnetic resonance imaging was invented, applied to MS [8] and quickly established as a sensitive marker of MS lesions [9]. These key events served not only to accelerate progress in MS clinical trials, but also to create a sense of momentum in the field.

Since 1990, a number of large multi-center definitive clinical trials have been completed and their results have been published [10–12], a monograph focused exclusively on clinical trials in MS was published [13]; and the US FDA approved the use of Betascron for exacerbating (relapsing) remitting MS. In February 1994, an international workshop entitled 'Outcomes Assessment in Multiple Sclerosis Clinical Trials: A Critical Analysis', was held in Charleston, South Carolina [14]. Discussions were held on clinical assessment tools, the different stages of clinical trials, the use of MRI and immunologic markers, the optimal primary outcome measure for various types of trials, the roles of monitoring committees, the implications of interim analyses and stopping rules, the use of surrogate markers, and the process of analyzing study results.

This chapter provides additional information on these and other topics relevant to the conduct of clinical trials in MS. Its primary focus is the multi-center, double-blinded, randomized, placebo-controlled trial.

19.1.2 TYPES OF TRIALS

Clinical trials may be divided into four basic types or phases. **Phase I studies** involve the initial introduction of

Multiple Sclerosis: Clinical and pathogenetic basis. Edited by Cedric S. Raine, Henry F. McFarland and Wallace W. Tourtellotte. Published in 1997 by Chapman & Hall, London. ISBN 0 412 30890 8.

an investigational new drug into humans. While they may be conducted on healthy volunteers, they are more commonly conducted on subjects with a specific disease condition, and frequently skewed toward more severely affected cases. According to the FDA (US Food, Drug, Cosmetic Act), a phase I study generally involves no more than 20–80 subjects, and should be designed to determine the metabolism and pharmacologic action of the drug in humans, to identify potential side-effects of treatment and, if possible, to gain early evidence on effectiveness. The onset and duration of biologic effects over a range of dosing should be studied in a phase I trial, in order to provide information on toxicity at different doses and to begin to identify an optimal dosing strategy.

Phase II studies are conducted to define more narrowly the appropriate dose and dosing regimen in patients with the disease under study. In addition, they should provide some information on the clinical effectiveness of therapy versus its adverse effects, and may be used to evaluate possible endpoints for more definitive phase III studies. Phase II studies are well controlled and closely monitored, and should be conducted in no more than several hundred subjects.

According to FDA guidelines, **phase III studies** are expanded controlled and uncontrolled trials, performed after preliminary evidence for efficacy has been determined. They are intended to gather the additional information about effectiveness and safety that is needed to evaluate the overall benefit–risk relationship of the drug and to provide a basis for physician labeling. As many as several thousand subjects may be entered into a phase III study, depending on the disease and therapeutic regimen being evaluated. Therefore, an MS clinical trial generally involves multiple centers. A phase III trial is meant to be a pivotal efficacy trial. As such, it is generally placebo controlled, and should be both randomized and double blinded. Clear, objective endpoints reflecting clinical benefit should be prospectively defined, and a specific primary endpoint should be identified. Prior to the beginning of the study, a protocol should be developed that clearly establishes these endpoints, and contains a detailed statistics section. It should be demonstrated within the protocol that the sample size that is planned has sufficient power to detect the primary endpoint for the study.

Phase IV studies are conducted after FDA approval and licensure. Phase IV studies involve collecting and accumulating safety and efficacy data in the context of clinical practice.

Alternative terminology has gained favor in recent years, as discussed by Whitaker and colleagues [14] **Toxicity trials** correspond with **phase I** studies. **Exploratory or preliminary trials** correspond with small **phase II** studies. Exploratory or preliminary trials are not meant to be definitive with respect to efficacy, although they contain outcome measures designed to gain information relating to efficacy. Surrogate laboratory measures, such as MRI, may be the principal efficacy outcome measures in preliminary trials. **Definitive or critical trials** correspond with larger **phase II** studies, or with **phase III** studies. These studies are designed to provide substantial evidence of a product's safety and efficacy, and form the basis for regulatory review and approval.

19.1.3   TARGETS FOR INTERVENTIONS IN MS

The target for intervention influences not only the design of a clinical trial but also the types of problems that one will encounter while conducting such a trial. In MS the four major targets for intervention include the symptoms of MS, exacerbations, disease progression and neurologic recovery.

Symptoms

Clinical trials targeting MS symptoms are exemplified by studies of 4-aminopyridine [15, 16]; oral baclofen [17], progabide [18] or intrathecal baclofen [19] for spasticity; or amitriptyline for emotional lability [20]. Generally these trials employ specific outcome measures designed around the symptom in question. An example would be use of the Ashworth scale for spasticity [21]. In many instances widely accepted outcome measures for specific symptoms do not exist for MS symptom trials.

Symptomatic trials commonly employ cross-over designs, since therapeutic effects are expected to last only during treatment, while there are adequate blood and tissue levels of the drug. In a cross-over design, it is important that the effect of therapy is transient so that therapeutic impact of the intervention does not contaminate the group crossed from active to control therapy.

Exacerbations

Two distinct types of studies have focused on the impact of intervention on exacerbations. In the first type, interventions are tested for their ability to ameliorate the severity or duration of individual exacerbations. A double-blind, placebo-controlled randomized trial for acute exacerbations showed that ACTH was significantly better than placebo in resolving neurologic deficits at 1–3 weeks, but that the benefit had largely disappeared by four weeks [22]. Similarly, a study of acute optic neuritis showed that intravenous (IV) methylprednisolone improved the rate of recovery but not the eventual visual recovery measured at one year [23]. The second type of study uses exacerbations as the measure of disease severity in trials of disease-modifying agents. In these studies, it is common to count exacerbations and then to determine rates per unit time. Examples include azathioprine [24] and interferon beta-1b [12].

Two issues have complicated exacerbation studies. The first is the methodology for defining and grading exacerbations. Some investigators have used the Scripps Neurologic Rating Scale [25] to grade exacerbation severity [12], but it is not at all clear that this reflects the overall activity of the disease. Another problem relates to defining exacerbations. Nearly all definitions of exacerbation require the presence of new neurologic symptoms reported by the patient. This implies that the patient must be cognizant of new problems, and report them to the examiner. Thus, exacerbations can be considered a 'patient-driven' outcome. Is an exacerbation present if the clinical investigator finds that the neurologic examination is worse but the patient does not report worsening? Further, since neurologic symptoms fluctuate considerably, it is often unclear when a patient is only experiencing minor symptom fluctuations and when an exacerbation has occurred. Once an exacerbation has occurred, it is not clear when it is over, thus rendering a patient at risk of another exacerbation. The second problem inherent in both measuring exacerbations and analyzing exacerbation data is the uncertain relationship between the exacerbation frequency and subsequent disease course. Weinshenker and colleagues [26] suggested that a short inter-exacerbation interval early in the course predicted more rapid progression to EDSS 6.0, but this has not been confirmed by other investigators.

Disease progression

A key goal for disease-modifying therapies is to halt disease progression; a number of large-scale efficacy studies of disease therapy have focused on the ability of the intervention to impact favorably on progression. There is no ideal measure of disease progression, however. The Kurtzke expanded disability status scale (EDSS) [7] is a commonly used single measure that uses data from the neurologic examination to categorically rate severity in eight functional systems, and to assign a single score from 0 to 10 to disease severity. Change in EDSS over time has been commonly used as a measure of disease progression. More recently, MRI lesions have been quantified and their progression over time has been used to monitor disease worsening. At present, the impact of intervention on disease progression is considered clinically important, but the most precise methodology to measure such progression is debated.

Neurologic recovery

As strategies to enhance remyelination are applied to patients with MS, neurologic improvement will become a critically important outcome. With the exception of interventions at the time of exacerbations, no studies have attempted to achieve neurologic recovery to date.

19.2 Designing the trial

19.2.1 WRITING A PROTOCOL

Key to the success of any clinical trial is adequate pre-study planning and completion of a well-written protocol *before* the trial begins. The protocol for a phase III study must be extremely detailed. A clear, concise description of study objectives and hypotheses to be tested, outcome measures, criteria for selection of subjects and treatment regimen to be followed should be included, along with a detailed plan for statistical analyses.

19.2.2 DEFINING THE QUESTION

Once a target for intervention has been identified, the first step is to define the questions that will be asked and answered in the course of the trial. The objectives of the trial should be clearly stated. In the case of a pivotal efficacy trial, the hypotheses to be tested should be stated, and specific outcomes should be identified. While it is appropriate to include secondary outcomes that may support a broader understanding of efficacy results, it is essential that one primary outcome be chosen. The design of the study, sample-size estimates, and statistical methods chosen should reflect this primary outcome. While positive results on secondary outcomes are desirable, if there is no evidence of efficacy based on the primary outcome, the study will generally be considered negative with regard to efficacy, regardless of the secondary outcome results. Once the primary and any secondary outcomes have been identified, appropriate outcome measures must be chosen.

19.2.3 OUTCOME MEASUREMENT

Objective outcome measures must be chosen that are appropriate for testing the stated hypotheses and capable of detecting the clinical difference in treatment arms determined to be important when planning the study. Questions that should be addressed when choosing an outcome measure include:

- How feasible is the use of this measure in the population to be studied?
- How valid and reliable is the measure?
- How precise is the measure?
- How objective is the measure?

The variable course of MS has made the development of reliable, objective measurements of clinical efficacy extremely difficult. As is evident from the discussion in the preceding section, endpoints must be clearly defined, and if an outcome measure involves the use of raters (e.g. the EDSS), it may be appropriate to determine inter- and intra-rater reliability for raters who will participate in the trial prior to starting the trial in order to ensure that the endpoint has adequate reliability to achieve the goals of the study [27].

More sensitive and reliable clinical outcome measures are needed for future clinical trials for a number of reasons [28]. As partially effective therapies emerge, new trials will need to compare two active treatments. More sensitive clinical measures will reduce the necessary sample sizes, which escalate in active arm comparisons, particularly with partially effective therapy in one or more arms of the trial. Additionally, more sensitive outcome measures will allow earlier detection of treatment failure for individual subjects, minimizing the number of drop-outs from trials.

19.2.4 SELECTION OF STUDY SUBJECTS

The study protocol should clearly describe criteria for the selection of study subjects. Depending on the hypothesis to be tested, it may be appropriate to restrict the study population to a group that is homogeneous with regard to specific disease characteristics at entry, such as range of EDSS scores, recent disease activity, or MRI profile. The necessary sample size must be determined, and the availability of appropriate subjects must be assessed. The numbers of centers that will be necessary to carry out the study will depend in part on the length of trial and accrual period that is planned, as well as the number of patients available at each center.

19.2.5 STATISTICAL ISSUES

Sample size and power considerations

Establishing the appropriate sample size is critical to the success of a clinical trial. Type I and type II errors must be considered. The statistical methodology used to establish the sample size should reflect the primary outcome measure of interest and the statistical methods that will be used to analyze the primary outcome.

Statistical analysis plan

The protocol should provide a detailed plan for analysis of the primary outcome variable, some discussion of the analyses of secondary outcomes, and analyses of safety data that will be conducted during the trial, including interim efficacy analyses. Interim efficacy analyses should be conducted only in the context of safety monitoring. Endpoints to be analyzed should be specified in advance, along with the number and timing of the interim analyses that are planned. P values derived from these analyses should be adjusted for multiple

testing using appropriate methodology, such as that described by Fleming and colleagues [29], in order to avoid stopping the study prematurely as a result of a significant finding due solely to the large number of interim analyses conducted (type I error).

A specific plan detailing who will review interim efficacy analyses and under what situations a wider dissemination of information will take place (e.g. there is evidence for significant toxicity in the treatment arm of the study) should be provided in the protocol. The procedures that will be used to ensure patient safety as well as maintain the blinding necessary to protect the scientific integrity of the study should also be outlined.

Efficacy analyses

There are several factors that determine the statistical methods used to test the efficacy of a therapeutic agent within the context of a clinical trial. The statistical test(s) that are chosen should reflect the hypotheses being tested and the outcome measure(s) that will be used to define a treatment failure/success in a particular trial. Techniques should be utilized that reduce the likelihood of introducing bias into the results. The power of the statistical text should also be considered, along with the underlying assumptions that must be met in order for a particular text to be valid. In general, if the distribution of data fits a particular model (for example, it is normally distributed), the appropriate parametric test will be more powerful in its ability to detect an effect than its non-parametric equivalent. Time-to-event or survival analyses techniques such as the Kaplan–Meier method or Cox Proportional Hazards Modeling will usually be more powerful and less prone to bias than fixed-time point methods, such as pre–post differences in mean EDSS score. This is because survival analysis allows the use of data up to the point that a subject is censored, rather than eliminating that subject (and their data) from the analysis if they are lost to follow-up prior to their final evaluation. Furthermore, survival analysis allows study subjects to have variable lengths of follow-up.

It is not necessary for the principal investigator of a trial to be an expert in statistics. However, particularly for phase III trials, an expert in the statistical design of clinical trials should be involved in the planning phases of the trial in order to ensure that the study will have sufficient power and use the techniques that are most appropriate to achieve the goals of a pivotal efficacy study.

19.2.6 OTHER DESIGN ISSUES

Other important issues that must be considered during the design of the trial include the comparison group that will be used during the study, and methods of reducing both random and non-random bias.

Comparison group

Choice of comparison group will depend on the target for intervention, as well as the type of trial planned (phase I, II, or III). In a phase I trial, patients may serve as their own comparison group, comparing toxicity and biological response at varying dose levels and/or schedules within each patient. Phase I and II trials may also utilize historical controls. Phase III studies require more complicated design strategies with regard to comparison groups, since these are meant to be pivotal efficacy trials. The gold standard for phase III studies is the randomized, placebo-controlled, double-blinded study that utilizes an intent-to-treat design. Controls are usually concurrent. Occasionally, cross-over designs may be utilized, but this is only appropriate when the therapeutic agent is expected to be short-lasting in effect and the target for intervention is an acute manifestation of the disease (i.e. symptoms).

Randomization schedules should be prepared by the DCC, and patients should be randomized in a fashion that ensures the continued blinding of all clinical site personnel with regard to treatment status.

Intent-to-treat design

Patients should be followed and data analyzed according to intent-to-treat principles. This means that patients should continue to be followed and evaluated even if they discontinue treatment, and their data should be included in statistical analysis. This will minimize biases that may be introduced by excluding data on patients who discontinue treatment due to worsening status or adverse effects related to treatment. Furthermore, it will provide a more realistic picture of the true efficacy of a therapeutic regimen in the clinical setting. It is possible, for example, that a therapy is highly effective in those completing treatment, but the majority of patients will discontinue treatment prematurely due to adverse side-effects of therapy. This might not be clear from the results of a phase III trial, if patients who discontinue treatment are then dropped from the study and/or excluded from statistical analyses.

19.3   Study procedures and trial conduct

In addition to careful planning and developing a detailed written protocol prior to the start of a trial, there are other issues of a more practical nature that must be addressed to carry out the trial successfully. Key to the successful completion of a clinical trial is a strong and smoothly functioning administrative structure. The larger the trial, the greater the need for and complexity of the administrative structure that will be necessary. For this reason, we will continue to focus our discussion on the requirements of a pivotal phase III efficacy trial.

19.3.1   ADMINISTRATIVE STRUCTURE

Phase III MS clinical trials generally involve multiple clinical sites, a data coordinating center, frequently a central laboratory and/or MRI reading site, one or more sponsors, and often more than one regulatory body (e.g. the FDA and multiple institutional review boards – IRBs). Therefore, it is critical that an administrative structure be created that facilitates rapid, regular communication and problem resolution during the study in order to ensure consistency and adherence to the protocol and to regulatory requirements. Furthermore, the division of responsibilities within this structure must be spelled out in clear terms.

There is no universally accepted structure to accomplish these goals. An organizational structure that we have used in prior MS clinical trials is presented in Figure 19.1. In a multicenter, investigator-initiated trial, the administrative structure of the trial is usually organized so as to reflect the clinical and specialty centers that will participate in that trial. Two types of coordinating centers are key to the successful conduct of a multicenter trial. One is the data coordinating center (DCC), which is responsible for coordinating all data collection and data management activities associated with a trial, for ensuring the quality of the data that are entered into the database, and for analyzing all trial data. The other is the treatment coordinating center, which is responsible for coordinating treatment administration and monitoring

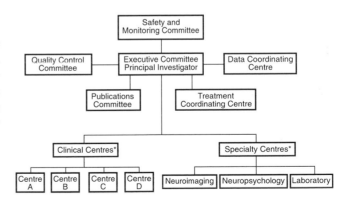

*Core staff at each clinical centre: Centre Principle Investigator, Examining MD, Treating MD, Nurse Clinician, Data Cordinator, Neuropsychologist, Neuropsychology Technician, Consulting Neurologist

Figure 19.1   Organizational structure of a phase III clinical trial. The principal components of the study and their relationships are depicted. See text for discussion of composition, roles and communication.

clinical activities during the trial. In some trials one large coordinating center may be responsible for both data and treatment coordination. It is strongly advised that the DCC be both administratively and physically separate from the sponsor(s) of the trial; furthermore, in order to successfully carry out its coordinating responsibilities, the DCC should be fiscally and physically separate from the clinical centers participating in the trial.

The full administrative structure will vary depending on the trial. The example given in Figure 19.1 illustrates the type of structure that might exist in an investigator-initiated, multicenter study sponsored by a federal agency.

19.3.2 JOB DUTIES AND COMMITTEE RESPONSIBILITIES

Each of the committees, centers and individuals involved in a clinical trial should have clearly delineated responsibilities that have been defined in advance of the study. Pre-study training sessions should be carried out for all of the various functional groups. The various duties and responsibilities of each individual and committee listed in Figure 19.1 could be described as follows.

Principal investigator

The principal investigator is responsible for the conduct of the study, chairs the executive committee, and reports to the safety and monitoring committee, regulatory agencies and the study sponsor. The principal investigator bears ultimate responsibility for adhering to the study protocol, for human subject protection, for appropriate reporting of adverse events and protocol deviations, for data quality control and for data analysis and reporting.

Executive committee

An executive committee is chaired by the study-wide principal investigator and includes the principal investigators from each site, the head of the data coordinating center and the chair of the quality control committee. The executive committee advises the principal investigator. When a multicenter study is actively involved in patient accrual and/or the treatment phase of the study, the committee should meet frequently at regularly scheduled times; weekly telephone conference calls may even be appropriate. During these meetings, the committee monitors programmatic, methodological, or policy issues that arise during the course of the trial, patient accrual by clinical site, quality control, toxicity, interim status of the blind, data analysis, study reporting and publication.

Data coordinating center

This center is responsible for administrating randomization procedures, for coordinating all data collection and data management activities for the study, for creating and maintaining the computerized database, for quality control of all data entered into the database, and for performing all statistical analyses for the clinical trial. The DCC monitors individual clinical center patient accrual, stratification across the clinical centers to ensure balance, study drop-outs and protocol deviations due to systematic errors. One hundred per cent data verification should be performed for all key variables entered into the database, including all primary and secondary outcome variables. Standardized query forms are sent to clinical centers by the DCC to resolve questions that arise during the DCC quality control process. Investigators and data coordinators are informed regularly regarding completeness, accuracy or inconsistencies in data. The DCC is responsible for semi-annual reports to the Safety and Monitoring Committee and the study sponsor. The reports must contain information about safety and compliance with the protocol. The DCC is also responsible for planned interim analyses, which are reported to the Safety and Monitoring Committee.

Quality control committee

The quality control committee, chaired by one of the clinical site principal investigators, conducts annual audits at each clinical site as well as the DCC, MRI and treatment coordinating center. The purpose of clinical center audits is to assess compliance with the study protocol, including compliance with inclusion criteria, accurate and timely completion of informed consent, patient and laboratory data, and proper maintenance of drug log books and administration records; documentation of protocol deviations and adverse reactions are also reviewed. DCC procedures for data processing, quality control, data entry and verification and other aspects of data management are reviewed during the audit of the DCC. During the audit of an MRI coordinating center, the entire MRI protocol from arrival of film and digitized data through the analytic and qualitative procedures and recording of data as well as completion of records to date and delinquent data may be reviewed. The quality control committee may arrange for outside consultants to audit specific aspects of the study as appropriate. Reports and recommendations generated from these audits are submitted to the study principal investigator and then reviewed as necessary with the entire executive committee for the purpose of timely resolution of any problems that are identified.

On-site monitoring of all data collected may also be done at regularly scheduled intervals by an organization external to the clinical trial to ensure compliance with FDA requirements for phase III clinical trials. The data from each of the clinical centers are then submitted to the DCC after on-site monitoring, where they undergo further quality control procedures before being entered into the database.

External safety and monitoring committee

This committee consists of independent authorities selected to monitor patient safety and protocol compliance during the investigation. This committee monitors statistical analysis without jeopardizing the blind. The safety and monitoring committee may visit the DCC or any of the clinical sites to assess compliance with the protocol or ensure adequate quality control. The principal investigator reports to the safety and monitoring committee. Generally, the safety and monitoring committee reports to the study's sponsor.

Publications committee

A publications committee establishes guidelines for authorship and a plan for presenting and publishing the study results. The chair of the publications committee is appointed by the study principal investigator; membership generally includes representatives from each of the clinical sites and from the DCC. This type of committee is especially important in large multicenter trials involving several co-investigators.

Specialty directors

Functional specialty groups each have a designated director. For example, these might include the examining physicians, treating physicians, neuroradiologists, neuropsychologists, data coordinators and study nurses. These groups meet as appropriate by telephone to standardize procedures and resolve common problems across clinical sites. The director of each group has regular communication as well as access to the executive committee.

Treating physicians

In an MS trial, treating physicians may register study subjects with the DCC, obtain informed consent, examine subjects at all study visits, and provide general neurologic care throughout the study, performing regularly scheduled as well as symptom-prompted neurologic examinations, and prescribing steroids and other medications as needed. The treating physicians are responsible for recording and fully documenting adverse events that occur during the course of the study.

Examining physicians

Examining physicians determine subject eligibility for the study and perform neurologic examinations at all study visits. Examining physicians from different centers should meet prior to the study for pre-study training and may meet at a designated time during the study to standardize their use of outcome measures. Examining physicians follow a very specific protocol for examinations, and they should avoid talking with their patients about symptoms or reviewing medical data, in order to maintain blinding.

Study nurses

Study nurses recruit and screen potential study participants, instruct the patients about the protocol, educate the patients about the intervention and supervise its administration, and provide easy access for the participants to the study treating physician.

Data coordinators

Data coordinators schedule all examinations, treatments and laboratory tests, may conduct structured interviews with study patients as appropriate per the protocol, arrange toxicity testing, forward laboratory and interview results to the treating physician, maintain patient data forms and files, collate clinical and laboratory records, and forward those data to the DCC.

19.3.3 PATIENT ACCRUAL

Prior to initiating the study, each site should compile a list of potential study subject candidates and pre-screen the appropriate medical records to establish those individuals most likely to meet study eligibility criteria. Each patient recruited into the study should have protocol-defined documentation of eligibility, which may also include meeting specific clinical and laboratory criteria at the time of initial screening and admission testing. Pre-screening medical records will reduce the number of patients who undergo screening and admission testing only to be found not to meet the eligibility criteria for entry into the study. If sufficient patients are not available, additional recruitment efforts, including advertising via patient newsletters and recruiting from other neurologists, should be considered.

Before conducting screening and admission tests to confirm eligibility and establish baseline data, each patient should be given a complete description of the study by a nurse or other study personnel, and an informed consent document that has been approved by the institution's IRB should be reviewed with the patient by the study center treating physician or a nurse.

Baseline testing should not take place until the patient has signed an informed consent form.

19.3.4   TREATMENT ADMINISTRATION

Following confirmation of eligibility, and patient registration and randomization, treatment administration may begin. The type of treatment and dosing regimen may vary from study to study. However, all clinical trials should have a well-defined protocol for treatment administration prior to the start of the study, and this protocol should be strictly adhered to by all sites. Protocol deviations should be recorded on appropriate case report forms. The protocol for treatment administration should describe how the drug will be administered, but also how it will be labeled and distributed. Procedures for maintenance of blinding and ensurance of patient compliance with the treatment regimen should be clearly stated. Those individuals who will be involved in treatment administration should receive appropriate training that includes procedures for reporting and handling adverse events.

19.3.5   STUDY EVALUATIONS

The patient evaluations conducted during the course of a trial are dependent on the target and type of therapeutic intervention planned. Other factors, such as dosing schedule, the length of the trial, and the resources available to carry out the trial will also have an impact in determining what evaluations will be conducted and when they will be conducted.

Patient evaluations must be planned and conducted in a manner that both ensures patient safety and answers the scientific questions that are central to the study in a cost- and time-efficient manner. Evaluations must be conducted in a manner that ensures adequate blinding and minimizes other types of bias from affecting the study. If, for example, the target for intervention is exacerbations, it may be important to schedule evaluations more frequently than if the target for intervention is sustained progression. If resources are not available to permit regularly scheduled individual patient examinations with sufficient frequency to identify all new exacerbations, the protocol for evaluations may call for weekly patient telephone interviews by a data coordinator or study nurse to identify those patients with possible exacerbations and bring them in for evaluation between their regularly scheduled evaluations to confirm that an exacerbation is taking place.

In a phase I study, where possible toxicity is not yet completely known, the focus of evaluations will be more on toxicity testing and clinical evaluation at frequent intervals to identify any possible adverse events as soon as possible. In phase II and phase III studies, the outcome measures that will be used to determine

efficacy must also be considered. The schedule for baseline and follow-up evaluations must then include not only clinical and laboratory evaluations that will be conducted, but also details for the administration of primary and secondary outcome measures.

In order to ensure that baseline and follow-up evaluations are conducted in a correct manner, it is recommended that a procedures manual that includes a specific outline of the tests, procedures and assessments that will be conducted on every patient during each week of the study be developed before the study begins. For multicenter trials, it may be helpful for the DCC to prepare an individual patient schedule at the time of registration showing the appropriate dates for each of the patient's evaluations and laboratory tests, based on the patient's date of entry into the study.

19.3.6   MANAGEMENT OF INTERCURRENT EVENTS

It is not generally adequate to state that 'standard treatment for MS symptoms will be provided during the course of the study', since treatments between sites may differ significantly without careful planning. It is considered ethically unjustifiable to withhold standard treatment but anticipated interventions should be standardized and planned to the extent possible. It is particularly important to consider whether standard therapies might alter the endpoint. For trials of disease-modifying agents this would include immunosuppressive or immunomodulatory therapy and corticosteroids. Generally, immunosuppressive or immunomodulatory therapy will be prohibited, but corticosteroid therapy for acute exacerbation will be allowed. The exact indications for corticosteroid administration and the details of corticosteroid treatment (choice of steroid, route of administration, dose, frequency and duration of treatment) should be explicitly defined, standardized across centers and recorded. Repeated courses of corticosteroids for gradual worsening should be avoided. Treatment of symptoms with drugs or rehabilitation programs should be standardized as well. The effects of intervention on outcome need to be considered. For example, antidepressant use may influence results on a self-report measure, antispastic drug use may influence results on ambulation tests, and urinary tract infection prophylaxis may influence the frequency of exacerbation.

19.3.7   MONITORING AND REPORTING ADVERSE EVENTS

Adverse events (AEs) are defined as any symptom, sign, laboratory abnormality, or negative experience of a subject participating in a clinical trial. It is the responsibility of the investigator to solicit, record and report adverse events to the study monitor, sponsor and the IRB. When planning the study, investigators should determine what adverse events should trigger cessation of therapy in individual patients and develop a protocol for monitoring and reporting all adverse events in a timely and complete manner. Specific case report forms that are consistent with FDA guidelines should be developed and used during the study. Treating physicians and other study personnel who will be involved in monitoring patient safety and completing adverse event reports should be thoroughly trained in AE monitoring and reporting procedures. In a multiple sclerosis trial, it will be important to clearly differentiate between adverse health events that are an expected part of the disease process (e.g. symptoms of an exacerbation) and events that are not necessarily associated with the disease process. AEs should be reported even if the treating physician feels that AE could not possibly be associated with treatment.

Finally, serious adverse events (i.e. those requiring hospitalization, deaths) must be reported to the FDA immediately. All investigators should be thoroughly familiar with FDA requirements regarding the reporting of serious AEs, and procedures should be in place to ensure that these requirements are met in a timely fashion throughout the study.

19.3.8   DATA MANAGEMENT

The flow of data, from collection at the clinical site through the numerous steps leading to verified data within the master database at the DCC, is shown diagrammatically in Figure 19.2. Data management is an important aspect of any clinical trial. The type and complexity of the data management system will depend on the type of trial conducted. Large multicenter phase III trials will require more complex data management systems and result in a large volume of data handling than other types of trials. Data or case report forms should be developed and pre-tested prior to the beginning of patient accrual. Similarly, data handling procedures also should be in place prior to the start of patient accrual. Procedures for handling data and quality control procedures, both on-site and at the DCC, should be well developed and documented in writing. The computerized database structure should also be described, and procedures for data entry and verification established. Data back-up systems should be in place before data entry begins.

When a package of data is first received by the DCC, the data contained in the package should be checked against the enclosed transmittal form to ensure that nothing is missing. All data forms should then be checked for missing and illegible values. If there are no errors or missing values identified, the data may be entered into the database. If errors are identified during

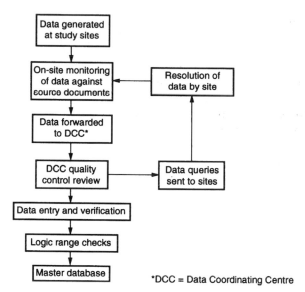

Figure 19.2   Data flow from collection at the clinical sites through to final form within the master database.

DCC review, an edit query is returned to the site for resolution. Once data have been entered into the computerized database, the accuracy of data entry must be verified. Verification using computer printouts of entered data or double entry of data is the most common method. One hundred per cent of key variables should be verified. Periodic computerized logic checks are also helpful. Questions that arise during entry should be referred to the DCC quality control reviewer for resolution.

In a double-blinded trial, the security of the database is another issue that must be considered. Steps must be taken to ensure patient confidentiality, and to maintain the blinding of clinical site personnel.

19.3.9   COMPLETING THE TRIAL

Following the completion of data collection, the activities that are carried out as part of the trial begin to change somewhat. At this point, activities at the clinical sites and treatment coordinating center are substantially reduced, and personnel needs are lessened considerably. However, the level of activity at the DCC increases considerably, and an increase in resources allocated to the DCC may be necessary.

In a multicenter study that is expected to generate more than one publication, the role of the publications committee may also become more prominent at this stage.

During the final phase of a clinical trial, the major activities that must be carried out include completion of quality control, data entry verification, statistical analyses and report preparation. In a double-blinded study, blinding should not be broken until data collection is complete, all data have been entered into the database at the DCC and the database has been locked.

During this phase-out period, activities at the clinical centers will include answering final quality control queries from the DCC and ensuring that source documentation and copies of case report forms have been stored in an organized, accessible manner. This is especially important in a phase III study, where future audits by the FDA may be expected as part of the licensing process. Finally, the clinical sites must advise patients who have participated in the trial with regard to any post-treatment activities or data collection that will take place, and answer patients' questions on the outcome of the trial as information becomes available.

19.4   Human subject protection

Human subject protection should be considered the most important aspect of any clinical trial. A 'human subject' may be defined as any individual who is or becomes a participant in research, either as a recipient of a test article or as a control subject. The human subject may have a medical condition, such as MS, or may be a healthy volunteer. The key requirements for human subject protection include:

1. review and approval of the research protocol by an institutional panel (the Institutional Review Board) to ensure that the potential risks to human subjects are minimized, and that the potential benefits justify those risks;
2. voluntary and informed participation by the human subject (informed consent);
3. mechanisms to report and monitor adverse events related to the research (adverse event monitoring);
4. confidentiality.

19.4.1   IRB APPROVAL

Institutional review boards (IRB) are regulated in the United States by the Food and Drug Administration under sections 505(i), 507(d) and 520(g) of the Federal Food, Drug, and Cosmetic Act. The functions of the IRB are to follow written procedures for conducting initial and continuing review of research and for reporting findings and actions to the investigator and institution; for determining which projects require review more often than annually, and which projects need verification from sources other than the investigators that no material changes have occurred since previous IRB review; for ensuring prompt reporting to the IRB of changes in research activity; for ensuring that changes in approved research, during the period for which IRB approval has already been given, have

not been initiated without IRB review and approval except where necessary to eliminate apparent immediate hazards to the human subjects; and for ensuring prompt reporting to the IRB of unanticipated problems involving risks to subjects or others. Additionally, the IRB must review proposed research at convened meetings at which a majority of the members of the IRB are present, including at least one member whose primary concerns are in nonscientific areas. The research proposal must receive approval of a majority of members present at the meeting. Finally, the IRB is responsible for reporting to the appropriate institutional officials and the Food and Drug Administration any serious or continuing noncompliance by investigators with the requirements and determinations of the IRB.

The IRB must have at least five members with varying backgrounds to promote complete and adequate review of research activities commonly conducted by the institution. The IRB must have adequate representation to consider issues such as community attitudes and to possess the professional competence necessary to review specific research activities. No IRB may consist entirely of men, or entirely of women, or entirely of members of one profession. Each IRB must include at least one member whose primary concerns are in nonscientific areas, such as lawyers, ethicists or members of the clergy. Each IRB must include at least one member who is not otherwise affiliated with the institution and who is not part of the immediate family of a person who is affiliated with the institution.

The criteria used to approve research include:

1. risks to the research subjects must be minimized;
2. risks to the subjects are reasonable in relation to the anticipated benefits, if any, to the subjects, and the importance of the knowledge that may be expected to result;
3. selection of subjects is equitable;
4. informed consent will be sought from each prospective subject or the subject's legally authorized representative;
5. informed consent is appropriately documented;
6. the research plan makes adequate provisions for monitoring the data collected to ensure the safety of subjects;
7. there are adequate provisions to protect the privacy of subjects and to maintain the confidentiality of data;
8. where all or some of the subjects are likely to be vulnerable to coercion or undue influence, such as persons with acute or severe physical or mental illness, or persons who are economically or educationally disadvantaged, appropriate additional safeguards have been included in the study to protect the rights and welfare of these subjects.

Clinical trials involving MS patients should be scrutinized carefully by IRBs to ensure compliance with the above criteria. Patients with MS are frequently desperate for help and vulnerable to exploitation for many reasons. They often harbor entirely unrealistic and unstated expectations or beliefs about medical interventions, including clinical trials. Furthermore, many MS patients have unrecognized cognitive impairments that complicate or even preclude adequate informed consent. In many cases IRBs do not have adequate expertise to optimally evaluate proposals for MS clinical trials, placing a heavy burden on the investigator and sponsor for adequate informed consent.

19.4.2 INFORMED CONSENT

The basic elements of informed consent include:

1. a statement that the study involves research and an explanation of the purposes of the research and expected duration of the subject's participation, a description of the procedures to be followed, and identification of any procedures that are experimental;
2. a description of any reasonably foreseeable risks or discomforts to the subject;
3. a description of any benefits to the subject or others that may reasonably be expected from the research;
4. a disclosure of appropriate alternative procedures or courses of treatment, if any, that might be advantageous to the subject;
5. a statement describing the extent, if any, to which confidentiality of records identifying the subject will be maintained and which notes the possibility that the Food and Drug Administration may inspect the records;
6. for research involving more than minimal risk, an explanation as to whether any compensation and medical treatments are available if injury occurs and, if so, what they consist of, or whether further information may be obtained;
7. an explanation of whom to contact for answers to pertinent questions about the research and research subjects' rights, and whom to contact in the event of a research-related injury to the subject;
8. a statement that participation is voluntary, that refusal to participate will involve no penalty or loss of benefits to which the subject is otherwise entitled, and that the subject may discontinue participation at any time without penalty or loss of benefits to which the subject is otherwise entitled.

Additionally, as appropriate, informed-consent documents may contain:

1. a statement that certain risks to the subject or to an embryo or fetus are unknown at present;

2. circumstances in which the subject's participation may be terminated by the investigator without the subject's consent;
3. any costs that may result to the subject as a result of participating in the research;
4. consequences of a subject's decision to withdraw from the research and procedures for orderly termination of participation by the subject;
5. a statement that significant new findings developed during the course of the research which may be related to the subject's willingness to continue will be provided;
6. the approximate number of subjects involved in the study.

A written consent form that has been approved by the IRB must be signed by the subject and the investigator. In lieu of this, the study can be presented to the subject orally and a 'short form' consent document signed. The 'short form' document must state that the above elements have been presented to the subject, and the 'short form' must be signed by a witness in addition to the investigator and subject.

Subjects should be reassured that records will be held in confidence and never released with identifying information about individual research subjects. The subject should be informed that their data forms may be released to the sponsor, IRB, or FDA without their permission.

19.5 Conclusion

The general guidelines presented herein for the conduct of a clinical trial in MS patients are meant to provide a context for the many details that need to be considered for a specific protocol. Implicit in the preceding discussion, it is now clear that well-constituted controlled clinical trials in MS populations are feasible, and that partially effective therapies can be identified.

There are presently many opportunities and challenges that face investigators in this rapidly changing field.

- What are the optimal therapeutic strategies to test at present?
- Should we combine interventions and test polypharmacy?
- What is the role of a placebo group in future MS trials?
- What is the optimal clinical outcome measure to use in future MS trials?
- What is the role of MRI in measuring therapeutic effect?
- What are the most sensitive designs for measuring therapeutic effect?

- What is the optimal administrative structure for an MS clinical trial?
- What is the role for peer-review and monitoring for drug company-sponsored trials?

There are several reports of partially effective therapies for MS patients that have been defined in careful, well-controlled clinical trials. Should the drugs with established partial efficacy be combined? If so, what would constitute the optimally informative comparison group? Since it is not possible to determine the best therapeutic strategy from our limited knowledge of disease pathogenesis or mechanisms of action of current drugs, it is not clear what intervention or combination deserves the most emphasis in subsequent trials. Nevertheless, planned clinical trials in MS should have a persuasive scientific rationale underlying the specific intervention.

Should placebo groups be included in subsequent trials? Omitting a placebo group is ethically appropriate when there is established meaningful benefit from an existing therapy. In addition, a placebo group may not be feasible if the established therapy is widely available in the community. The absence of a placebo group requires an active therapy control group, which can substantially increase the complexity, size and expense of a trial.

The optimal outcome instruments for an MS clinical trial are not established. One of the principal limitations of the EDSS is its lack of sensitivity to change, particularly in the mid and high portions of the scale. This means that the average untreated trial participant cannot be expected to change much during the 2–3-year duration of most clinical trials. This makes demonstrating a therapeutic effect impossible, unless the active treatment group improves. Development of a more sensitive and valid measure of MS disease progression would greatly facilitate progress in future trials. It is hoped that MRI may represent a more sensitive outcome measure, but the exact MRI parameter to use has not been established to date. There are currently task forces from the National Multiple Sclerosis Society to recommend optimal clinical and MRI outcome measures for future trials. It will be important to establish predictive validity for change in clinical or MRI measures seen in short-term protocols. For example, does a given amount of change in the MRI during a 2-year protocol predict the subsequent development of clinically relevant disability?

The optimal design for MS clinical trials needs to be better defined. It should be possible to improve trials by using more powerful techniques like survival analysis, which maximizes the use of all available clinical data, even when a subject discontinues treatment during the study. It may be optimal to remove patients from the study when they reach treatment failure,

thereby conserving costs and human resources. Similarly, the optimal administrative structure for an MS clinical trial needs to be defined. The model presented in this chapter has worked well in prior studies, but needs to be adapted to future circumstances and optimized.

Finally, it will be necessary to consider the various parties involved in MS clinical trials. The major sponsors for MS trials will likely be pharmaceutical and biotechnology companies. What is the optimal role for the independent investigator, who may be in the best position to define the clinical and experimental issues? What will be the role of peer-review, which has the clear potential to focus the scientific question and strengthen the protocol? What will be the optimal role for impartial oversight of the trial? These questions are central to the conduct of a clinical trial in MS patients and critical to future progress in MS experimental therapeutics.

References

1. Herndon, R.M. (1983) Proceedings of the International Conference on Therapeutic Trials in Multiple Sclerosis. *Arch. Neurol.*, **40**, 663–710.
2. Schumacher, G.A., Beebe, G., Kibler, R.E. *et al.* (1965) Problems of experimental trials of therapy in multiple sclerosis: report by the panel on evaluation of experimental trials of therapy in multiple sclerosis. *Ann. NY Acad. Sci.*, **122**, 552–68.
3. Brown, J.R., Beebe, G.W., Kurtzke, J.F. *et al.* (1979) The design of clinical studies to assess therapeutic efficacy in multiple sclerosis. *Neurology*, **29**, 1–23.
4. IFMSS (International Federation of Multiple Sclerosis Societies) (1982) *Therapeutic Claims in Multiple Sclerosis*. New York, National Multiple Sclerosis Society.
5. Ellison, G.W. (1992) Experimental therapies for multiple sclerosis: historical perspective, in *Treatment of Multiple Sclerosis: Trial Design, Results and Future Perspectives* (eds R.A. Rudick and D.E. Goodkin), London, Springer-Verlag.
6. Poser, C.M., Paty, D.W., Scheinberg, L. *et al.* (1983) New diagnostic criteria for multiple sclerosis: guidelines for research protocols. *Ann. Neurol.*, **13**, 227–31.
7. Kurtzke, J.F. (1983) Rating neurologic impairment in multiple sclerosis: an expanded disability status scale (EDSS). *Neurology*, **33**, 1444–52.
8. Li, D., Mayo, J., Fache, S. *et al.* (1984) Early experience in nuclear magnetic resonance imaging of multiple sclerosis. *Ann. NY Acad. Sci.*, **436**, 484–6.
9. Johnson, M.A., Li, D.K.B., Briant, D.J. and Payne, J.A. (1984) Magnetic resonance imaging: serial observations in multiple sclerosis. *Am. J. Neuroradiol.*, **5**, 495–9.
10. Canadian Cooperative Multiple Sclerosis Study Group (1991) The Canadian cooperative trial of cyclophosphamide and plasma exchange in progressive multiple sclerosis. *Lancet*, **337**, 441–6.
11. MS Study Group (1990) Efficacy and toxicity of cyclosporine in chronic progressive multiple sclerosis: randomized, double-blind, placebo-controlled clinical trial. *Ann. Neurol.*, **127**, 591–605.
12. IFNβ Multiple Sclerosis Study Group (1993) Interferon beta-1b is effective in relapsing-remitting multiple sclerosis. I. Clinical results of a multi-center, randomized, double-blind, placebo-controlled trial. *Neurol.*, **43**, 655–61.
13. Rudick, R.A. and Goodkin, D.E. (1992) *Treatment of Multiple Sclerosis: Trial Design, Results and Future Perspectives*. London, Springer-Verlag.
14. Whitaker, J.N., McFarland, H.F., Rudge, P. and Reingold, S.C. (1995) Outcomes assessment in multiple sclerosis clinical trials: a critical analysis. *Multiple Sclerosis*, **1**, 37–47.
15. Davis, F.A., Stefoski, D. and Rush, J. (1990) Orally administered 4-aminopyridine improves clinical signs in multiple sclerosis. *Ann. Neurol.*, **27**, 186–92.
16. Bever, C.T., Young, D., Anderson, P.A. *et al.* (1994) The effects of 4-aminopyridine in multiple sclerosis patients: results of a randomized, placebo-controlled, double-blind, concentration-controlled, crossover trial. *Neurology*, **44**, 1054–9.

17. Feldman, R.G., Kelly-Hayes, M., Conomy, J.P. and Foley, J.M. (1978) Baclofen for spasticity in multiple sclerosis. Double-blind crossover and three-year study. *Neurol.*, **28**, 1094–8.
18. Rudick, R.A., Breton, D. and Krall, R.L. (1987) The GABA-agonist progabide for spasticity in multiple sclerosis. *Arch. Neurol.*, **44**, 1033–6.
19. Penn, R.D. and Kroin, J.S. (1985) Continuous intrathecal baclofen for severe spasticity. *Lancet*, ii, 125–7.
20. Schiffer, R.B., Herndon, R.M. and Rudick, R.A. (1985) Treatment of pathologic laughing and weeping with amitriptyline. *N. Engl. J. Med.*, **312**, 1480–2.
21. Ashworth, B. (1964) Preliminary trial of carisoprodol in multiple sclerosis. *Practitioner*, **192**, 540–2.
22. Rose, A.S., Kuzma, J.W., Kurtzke, J.F. *et al.* (1970) Cooperative study in the evaluation of therapy in multiple sclerosis: ACTH vs. placebo. Final report. *Neurology*, **20**, 1–59.
23. Beck, R.W., Cleary, P.A., Anderson, M.M. *et al.* (1992) A randomized, controlled trial of corticosteroids in the treatment of acute optic neuritis. *N. Engl. J. Med.*, **326**, 581–8.
24. Yudkin, P.L., Ellison, G.W., Ghezzi, A. *et al.* (1991) Overview of azathioprine treatment in multiple sclerosis. *Lancet*, **338**, 1051–5.
25. Sipe, J.C., Knobler, R.L., Braheny, S.L. *et al.* (1984) A neurological rating scale (NRS) for use in multiple sclerosis. *Neurology*, **34**, 1368–72.
26. Weinshenker, B.G., Bass, B., Rice, G.P.A. *et al.* (1989) The natural history of multiple sclerosis: a geographically-based study. 2. Predictive value of the early clinical course. *Brain*, **112**, 1419–28.
27. Goodkin, D.E., Cookfair, D., Wende, K. *et al.* (1992) Inter- and intrarater scoring variability using grades 1.0–3.5 of the Kurtzke Expanded Disability Status Scale (EDSS). *Neurology*, **42**, 859–63.
28. Rudick, R., Antel, J., Confavreux, C. *et al.* (1996) Clinical outcomes assessment in multiple sclerosis. *Ann. Neurol.*, in press.
29. Flemming, T.R., Harrington, D.P. and O'Brien, P.C. (1984) Designs for group sequential tests. *Control Clin. Trials*, **5**, 348–61.

PART FOUR

TREATMENT: SYMPTOMATIC

20 NEUROPSYCHOLOGICAL ASPECTS OF MULTIPLE SCLEROSIS

Stephen M. Rao

20.1 Introduction and background

Neuropsychological research during the past 15 years has called attention to the cognitive deficits of patients with multiple sclerosis (MS). These studies have shown that some degree of cognitive dysfunction is present in approximately 43–65% of MS patients on formal neuropsychological testing[1–11]. Severe dementia is observed in approximately 20–30% of cognitively impaired MS patients[9]. Most studies have found a nonsignificant or weak correlation between the degree of physical disability, as measured by the Kurtzke disability status scale (DSS) or the expanded disability status scale (EDSS), and performance on neuropsychological testing[3, 9, 12, 13].

There is relatively little information regarding the natural history of dementia in MS. Clinical experience suggests that some patients demonstrate neurobehavioral changes early in the course of the disease[14–16], while others never develop such changes. Cross-sectional neuropsychological studies have generally not found a relationship between cognitive test performance and length of illness[9, 17–19]. Longitudinal studies[18–23] have also produced conflicting results, perhaps owing to numerous methodological shortcomings (i.e. small sample size, inadequate controls for practice effects, and brief retest intervals). In a recently completed longitudinal study[24], 16 of 77 MS patients (21%) experienced a deterioration on cognitive testing after a 3-year follow-up period relative to a control group.

Dementia in MS patients can have a negative impact on social functioning. MS patients with cognitive dysfunction are less likely to be in employment, require greater personal assistance and are less likely to engage in social activities than cognitively intact MS patients[12], even after controlling for severity of physical disability, disease course, presence of an affective disorder and medication usage.

This chapter is divided into three sections. The first describes the pattern of cognitive dysfunction in MS patients based on the extant neuropsychological literature. The second reviews the relationship between neuropsychological test findings and neuroimaging and electrophysiological indices of MS pathology. Finally, the third section discusses two potential applications of neuropsychological testing: as a screening instrument in the clinical setting and as an outcome measure in clinical trials.

20.2 Patterns of neuropsychological dysfunction in MS

In this section we review the literature on the most common neurobehavioral abnormalities in MS. It is important to recognize that many MS patients will have no discernible cognitive deficits on neuropsychological testing. Of those patients with cognitive dysfunction, considerable interpatient variability is observed with regard to its pattern and severity. A small percentage of patients (less than 10%) experience a significant dementia affecting multiple cognitive domains, whereas other patients experience relatively isolated cognitive deficits[9, 25]. Most of the neuropsychological investigations of MS patients are based on group studies, the conclusions from which may mask these individual differences.

20.2.1 INTELLIGENCE AND EXECUTIVE FUNCTIONS

As a group, MS patients display relatively small declines on standardized measures of intelligence[26]. On the Wechsler scales, the Performance IQ score is typically 7–10 points less than the Verbal IQ. Interpretation of the lower Performance IQ is difficult because the upper extremity motor slowing and incoordination may negatively affect these timed subtests. On more specialized measures of abstract or conceptual reasoning, such as the Category Test[3, 5, 27], Wisconsin Card Sorting

Multiple Sclerosis: Clinical and pathogenetic basis. Edited by Cedric S. Raine, Henry F. McFarland and Wallace W. Tourtellotte. Published in 1997 by Chapman & Hall, London. ISBN 0 412 30890 8.

Test [2, 5, 28], Grassi Block Substitution Test [10], Levine Concept Formation task [29], and Weigl Sorting Test [30], MS patients are frequently impaired. On the sorting tasks, MS patients make an inordinate number of perseverative responses. MS patients also have difficulty on untimed picture sequencing tasks [31] and deficient planning skills, as measured by the Tower of Hanoi [32].

20.2.2   ATTENTION AND SPEED OF INFORMATION PROCESSING

Several studies [2, 13, 33–39] have shown that MS patients are impaired on such diverse measures as the Sternberg High Speed Scanning Task, Paced Auditory Serial Addition Test (PASAT), Stroop Interference Test, Symbol Digit Modalities Test, and comparisons of simple versus complex reaction time. In each of these studies an attempt was made to separate the relative contributions of pure motor speed from decision time. Results of these studies indicate a generalized slowing of mental processing speed in MS patients.

20.2.3   MEMORY

Memory is the most extensively studied cognitive function in MS patients (for a review, see [40]. Most investigators have examined explicit (conscious) memory mechanisms with tests of primary (short-term or working), secondary (recent long-term) and tertiary (remote long-term) memory, although more recent studies have evaluated implicit (non-conscious) memory.

MS patients perform normally on measures of primary (short-term) memory capacity, such as digit span [5, 9, 30, 41, 42] and the recency effect on list learning [43]. The rate of forgetting from primary memory, as tested by the Brown–Peterson Interference task [42, 43] is also normal. More recently, investigators have begun to examine aspects of working memory, which involves both storage and processing components [44]. Two such studies [42, 45] have suggested a defect in the articulatory loop slave system in MS patients. Additionally, the studies reviewed above demonstrating a slowing of information processing speed suggest that the central executive is impaired as well. As noted above, MS patients perform poorly on tests like the PASAT [2, 36], which requires the patient to perform noncumulative mental addition of single digit numbers presented at relatively rapid rates (e.g. one digit every 2 seconds).

The majority of studies have examined secondary memory mechanisms. MS patients perform poorly on tasks which require the spontaneous and free recall of supraspan information [5, 9, 30, 35, 37, 39, 41, 45–49]. This robust finding is apparent with presentation of either verbal (stories, word lists) or nonverbal (geometric or matrix designs) information. In contrast, learning and forgetting rates are generally normal [9, 13, 42]. Recognition memory is normal or less impaired than retrieval [9, 50, 51], suggesting relatively intact encoding and storage mechanisms. Normal semantic encoding is also implied by a normal build-up and release from proactive interference on the Wickens [52] task [53, 54]. Relative to controls, MS patients are as sensitive to semantically relevant information in recalling the gist of stories [46]. Performance on measures of verbal fluency (e.g. Controlled Oral Word Association Test) is correlated with deficits on list learning tests [43], suggesting problems with semantic retrieval. Finally, MS patients perform normally on automatic memory tests (e.g. estimating the frequency of stimulus presentation), but are impaired on tests requiring effortful processing (e.g. free recall) [55]. In total, these results strongly suggest that secondary memory is impaired due to an inability to spontaneously retrieve previously learned information. In light of the working memory deficits cited above, however, one cannot rule out the possibility that MS patients experience a reduction in the speed of encoding of novel information [35].

Tertiary or remote memory has been examined in only a few studies. Beatty and colleagues [38, 39] have shown that identification of famous people or public events from several decades is impaired, although accuracy was equivalent across the decades. This finding suggests that the remote memory failure was not the result of faulty acquisition, but rather a result of retrieval failure.

Implicit memory has also been examined in MS patients [45, 56, 57]. These studies have shown that MS patients perform normally on measures of semantic and lexical priming and on tests of perceptual and motor (i.e. procedural) learning.

20.2.4   LANGUAGE

Clinical case reports would suggest that aphasia is rare in MS, occurring only when acute demyelinating lesions extend into gray matter structures of the dominant cerebral hemisphere [58–60]. This is somewhat surprising since various disconnection syndromes, such as conduction aphasia, would be expected to occur with some regularity in this white matter disease. The only report of conduction aphasia in the MS literature was by our group [61]. As expected, conduction aphasia was associated with a large white matter lesion underlying the left supramarginal gyrus.

Group neuropsychological studies indicate that while paraphasic disturbance is uncommon and repetition speech and comprehension are generally intact in MS, naming difficulties occur with some regularity [13, 30, 43, 51, 62]. It is possible that the naming deficits result from a more general breakdown in semantic retrieval processes [63].

20.2.5   VISUOSPATIAL SKILLS

Until recently, little information has been available pertaining to visuospatial perceptual skills in MS patients. Beatty *et al.* [39] observed that MS patients are impaired on Money's Road Map Test. A significant number of MS patients are impaired on the Hooper Visual Organization Test and on three of Benton's tests: Judgment of Line Orientation, Facial Recognition and Visual Form Discrimination [2]. Interpretation of these findings is difficult, since many MS patients have primary visual impairments due to optic neuritis. Neither of the above studies has ruled out primary visual loss as a possible cause of the impaired performance on visuoperceptual testing.

20.2.6   PERSONALITY

The extensive literature on affective disturbance in MS patients has been reviewed elsewhere [64–67]. Both unipolar and bipolar depression are more commonly observed in MS patients than the general population [68–73]. Less commonly, some MS patients experience apathy and euphoria [8, 74]. The presence of euphoria has been associated with cognitive deficits [75, 76]. MS patients with euphoria display behavioral symptomatology that is similar to that observed in patients with frontal lobe damage.

20.3   Clinicopathological correlations

Pathological studies indicate that virtually all definite MS patients have cerebral white matter lesions at autopsy [77–79]. Atrophy of the corpus callosum [77] and enlargement of the ventricles [78, 79] are also common. Numerous studies have examined the relationship between cognitive test performance and indices of cerebral pathology obtained during life. These indices have been derived from structural brain imaging – computed tomography (CT) and magnetic resonance imaging (MRI) – functional brain imaging – positron emission tomography (PET) and single photon emission computed tomography (SPECT) – and electrophysiological measures (long latency evoked potentials). The following section briefly summarizes the findings in this area.

20.3.1   STRUCTURAL BRAIN IMAGING

Robust correlations ($r = 0.40$–0.60) have been found between cognitive test performance and a variety of structural imaging indices, such as total cerebral lesion burden on MRI, size of the lateral and third ventricles measured from CT and MRI, and size of the corpus callosum from MRI [80–93]. These studies suggest that

there is a critical threshold for developing cognitive dysfunction, since 95% of definite MS patients have white matter hyperintensities on T2-weighted MRI scans, yet a much smaller percentage (43–65%) experience cognitive dysfunction. In a study performed at our medical center [86], 83% of MS patients with greater than 30 cm^2 of total lesion area (TLA) were cognitively impaired, whereas only 22% of patients demonstrated cognitive impairment if TLA was less than 30 cm^2, providing support for the threshold hypothesis.

As a white matter disease, one might expect to see various disconnection syndromes in MS [94]. While syndromes like conduction aphasia, alexia without agraphia, pure word deafness and callosal apraxia would be predicted to occur with regularity in MS, clinical case reports have not appeared in the literature. There is evidence, however, of impaired interhemispheric communication. MS patients experience left ear suppression in reporting consonant–vowel syllables presented in a dichotic listening paradigm [95, 96]. These studies suggest that linguistic information, which is initially processed in the right hemisphere, does not effectively cross the corpus callosum for subsequent analysis by the language-dominant left hemisphere. Using dichotic listening and a visual object naming latency task, we found that only those MS patients with corpus callosum atrophy exhibited an exaggerated right ear effect on dichotic listening and slower vocal reaction times to naming objects presented in their left visual field [97].

Attempts to relate the location of cerebral white matter lesions to specific patterns of cognitive test performance have recently been reported [98, 99]. Swirsky-Sacchetti *et al.* [98] found a significant correlation between left frontal lobe lesion area and the number of perseverative responses on the Wisconsin Card Sorting Test (WCST) based on a stepwise regression involving a total of six brain regions. This finding suggests a specific relationship between lesion location and conceptual reasoning ability. Unfortunately, these investigators also found a strong correlation with TLA, suggesting that their findings may not be specific to the frontal lobes. We [99] subdivided MS patients into three groups based on MR findings: frontal and nonfrontal groups with high TLA ($>20 \text{ cm}^2$) and an MS group with low TLA ($<20 \text{ cm}^2$). While the two high TLA groups obtained significantly lower scores on a measure of global cognitive functioning (WAIS-R verbal intelligence) relative to the low TLA group, the frontal group achieved significantly fewer categories, made more perseverative responses, and required more trials to reach the first category on the WCST than both the nonfrontal/high TLA and the low TLA groups. These results suggest that the pattern of cognitive decline in MS is also a function of the location of demyelinating lesions within the cerebral hemispheric white matter.

20.3.2 FUNCTIONAL BRAIN IMAGING

A limited number of studies have correlated cognitive test findings with functional neuroimaging. Using PET, Brooks et al. [100] measured regional cerebral oxygen utilization, oxygen extraction, blood flow and blood volume in 15 MS patients in remission. Compared to normal controls, cerebral oxygen utilization and blood flow were reduced in both white and peripheral gray matter, particularly in those MS patients with cognitive dysfunction and with cerebral atrophy on CT scan. In a SPECT study, Pozzilli et al. [101] found significant reductions in regional uptake of technetium-99m HMPAO in the frontal lobes and left temporal lobe in 17 MS patients relative to 17 controls. The reduction in the left temporal lobe was correlated with deficits in verbal fluency and verbal memory.

20.3.3 ELECTROPHYSIOLOGICAL INDICES

Event-related potentials (ERPs) have been correlated with cognitive testing in three studies. Newton et al. [102] demonstrated a high incidence of abnormal ERPs in 13 of 23 MS patients (57%), while the early components in response to auditory or visual stimuli were rarely abnormal. The correspondence between abnormal ERPs and cognitive testing (administered to a subset of 18 patients) was weak: 5 of 8 patients with intact cognitive test performance had abnormal ERPs and 4 of 10 patients with abnormal cognitive testing had normal ERPs. In contrast, Giesser et al. [103] found that the N100, P200, and P300 ERP components were longer in latency in demented versus non-demented MS patients. Increased P300 latency was particularly associated with poorer performance on neuropsychological testing. Van Dijk et al. [104] did not find abnormal N2 or P3 latencies in their MS group relative to healthy controls; it should be noted, however, that their MS group did not differ from controls on neuropsychological testing.

20.4 Applications of neuropsychological testing

In the remainder of this chapter, I will examine two potential applications of neuropsychological tests in MS: first as a screen for identifying cognitively impaired patients for clinical or research purposes, and secondly as an adjunctive outcome measure in MS clinical trials. In both situations, specific methodological and procedural issues must be addressed to obtain meaningful information from neuropsychological testing.

20.4.1 SCREENING FOR COGNITIVE DYSFUNCTION

A key question is whether neuropsychological tests should be administered to patients with MS as part of their routine clinical care. Comprehensive neuropsychological test batteries may take 2–6 hours to administer and should be interpreted by properly trained clinical neuropsychologists. Such lengthy testing is essential to address complicated questions regarding employability, competency and disability status. The length and costs of such testing dictate that the assessments be performed on the patients that will benefit the most. One criterion, of course, is the importance of the clinical question. Another important factor is identifying those patients who are most likely to be experiencing cognitive dysfunction. Self-report is unreliable, since many intact patients may report cognitive problems because of depression; alternatively, severely impaired patients minimize problems due to anosognosia (unawareness of deficit) resulting from significant brain dysfunction. Furthermore, the mental status examination performed as part of the neurological examination is frequently insensitive to mild cognitive dysfunction [3].

Consequently, there is a need for a brief cognitive screening instrument that

1. can validly discriminate cognitively impaired from cognitively intact patients;
2. can be easily administered and scored by non-neuropsychologically trained clinicians; and
3. has a standardized database with appropriate corrections for age and education to adjust for differences in premorbid ability levels.

Traditional screening instruments like the Mini-Mental State Examination (MMSE), which are useful in assessing 'cortical' dementias like Alzheimer's disease, have proved to be relatively insensitive to the cognitive deficits in MS [2, 105]. This is not surprising since MS, as noted previously, does not produce gross language disturbance or a dense amnesia, as would be observed in a cortical dementia. Instead, MS results in retrieval failure (rather than a storage problem) and impaired performance on measures of conceptual and abstract reasoning, sustained attention, information processing speed, visuospatial skills and verbal fluency, a pattern of deficits similar to that observed in other so-called 'subcortical' dementias, like Parkinson's disease, Huntington's disease and progressive supranuclear palsy.

We [2] recently constructed a brief (25 minute) screening instrument by selecting the most sensitive measures from our extended, 7-hour, experimental neuropsychological test battery. This brief battery has yielded significantly improved sensitivity and specificity relative to the MMSE. Other screening batteries have also been proposed for MS[105]. Further studies are needed to identify the optimal screening tool for MS patients.

20.4.2 COGNITIVE TESTS IN CLINICAL TRIALS

The recent FDA approval of interferon beta-1b as a treatment for relapsing-remitting MS was in part influenced by the lack of progression of MRI changes in the treatment groups[106]. While the absence of progression of MRI changes can provide highly convincing evidence that a treatment is effective in a controlled study, the practical effect of this outcome on the patients' quality of life is less well understood. In light of the studies cited above demonstrating a correlation between cognitive testing and MRI lesion load, one might reasonably expect to have observed a worsening of cognitive functions in the placebo group over the course of the study, while the treated groups would have remained cognitively stable. This hypothesis cannot be evaluated since neuropsychological measures were not included as part of this study.

Neuropsychological testing may provide the explanatory bridge between a positive MRI outcome effect and changes in social outcomes, such as employment status. The long-term natural history study cited at the beginning of this chapter suggests that changes in MRI lesion load and cognitive test performance may change in parallel. Another longitudinal study[107] administered cognitive testing and MRI scans to MS patients on a more frequent basis (e.g. every 4–6 weeks); results of this short-term natural history study suggest a relationship between the appearance of new lesions and changes in cognitive test performance.

A major methodological problem in conducting serial neuropsychological evaluations is the practice effects associated with repeated testing. These effects can occur even if the investigator uses alternate, equivalent forms of a test. In addition, we have shown that practice effects can occur even after lengthy retest intervals (three years)[108]. If the only goal of a randomized clinical trial is to identify a statistically significant difference between the treatment and placebo groups, corrections for practice effects are not necessary since both groups should experience equal amounts of change due to practice. However, if the question is to identify the number of patients within each group that have experienced cognitive deterioration over the course of the study, then it is essential that an additional control group, composed of healthy individuals, be evaluated at the same time intervals as the MS subjects. In this way, it is possible to convert the scores of all MS patients relative to the healthy control group at each testing session, thereby obtaining a true measure of deterioration free from practice effects. Of course, this assumes that the practice effects are identical in MS and healthy

populations. Our preliminary data suggest that this, in fact, is the case.

An additional concern in using cognitive testing as an outcome measure is the large number of testing variables that can be produced even with a brief (30 minute) assessment. Since virtually all cognitive variables are normally distributed, it is common to convert individual test scores to a common metric, such as a z distribution with the overall mean set to 0 and each standard deviation from the mean equal to 1. By performing this conversion of raw scores to a standardized metric, it is then possible to average scores and create an overall composite score.

20.5 Rehabilitation of cognitive disorders

As noted above, cognitive dysfunction in MS patients can have a negative impact on social functioning[12]. Very few studies, however, have attempted to evaluate potential symptomatic treatments for cognitive dysfunction. Smits et al.[109] found no effect of 4-aminopyridine, a potassium channel blocker, on neuropsychological testing. Foley et al.[110] have recently described a comprehensive psychological approach for managing the communication problems of cognitively impaired MS patients.

20.6 Conclusions

The literature reviewed above illustrates several key features of the cognitive disturbances in MS. MS patients commonly exhibit deficits on measures of effortful retrieval from secondary memory, working memory, attention and information processing speed, executive functions and visuospatial perception. In contrast, MS patients perform normally or with relatively minor impairment on tests of general intelligence, language, primary memory capacity and implicit memory. The degree and pattern of cognitive dysfunction is highly correlated with the amount and location of white matter disease within the cerebral hemispheres, as reflected by neuroimaging studies. There is now abundant evidence to suggest that cognitive dysfunction has a significant impact on the MS patient's quality of life above and beyond the physical symptoms of the disease. The observation that cognitive and physical symptoms are not correlated in MS patients suggests that one cannot predict the severity of cognitive dysfunction from the neurological examination, hence the importance of neuropsychological testing. Brief neuropsychological test batteries are needed to screen patients with cognitive dysfunction in the clinical setting. Finally, neuropsychological testing is being incorporated as an outcome measure in several ongoing clinical trials in

MS. The next few years will determine whether these secondary outcome measures provide meaningful scientific and clinical information to the MS community.

ACKNOWLEDGMENT

Preparation of this chapter was supported in part by a grant from the National Multiple Sclerosis Society (RG2605).

References

1. McIntosh-Michaelis, S.A., Roberts, M.H., Wilkinson, S.M. *et al.* (1991) The prevalence of cognitive impairment in a community survey of multiple sclerosis. *Br. J. Clin. Psychol.*, **30**, 333–48.
2. Rao, S.M., Leo, G.J., Bernardin, L. and Unverzagt, F. (1991) Cognitive dysfunction in multiple sclerosis: I. Frequency, patterns, and prediction. *Neurology*, **41**, 685–91.
3. Peyser, J.M., Edwards, K.R., Poser, C.M. and Filskov, S.B. (1980) Cognitive function in patients with multiple sclerosis. *Arch. Neurol.*, **37**, 577–9.
4. Bertrando, P., Maffei, C. and Ghezzi, A. (1983) A study of neuropsychological alterations in multiple sclerosis. *Acta Psychiatr. Belg.*, **83**, 13–21.
5. Heaton, R.K., Nelson, L.M., Thompson, D.S., Burks, J.S. and Franklin, G.M. (1985) Neuropsychological findings in relapsing-remitting and chronic-progressive multiple sclerosis. *J. Consult. Clin. Psychol.*, **53**, 103–10.
6. Lyon-Caen, O., Jouvent, R., Hauser, S. *et al.* (1986) Cognitive function in recent-onset demyelinating diseases. *Arch. Neurol.*, **43**, 1138–41.
7. Staples, D. and Lincoln, N.B. (1979) Intellectual impairment in multiple sclerosis and its relation to functional abilities. *Rheumatol. Rehabl.*, **18**, 153–60.
8. Surridge, D. (1969) An investigation into some aspects of multiple sclerosis. *Br. J. Psychiatry.*, **115**, 749–64.
9. Rao, S.M., Hammeke, T.A., McQuillen, M.P. *et al.* (1984) Memory disturbance in chronic progressive multiple sclerosis. *Arch. Neurol.*, **41**, 625–31.
10. Parsons, O.A., Stewart, K.D. and Arenberg, D. (1957) Impairment of abstracting ability in multiple sclerosis. *J. Nerv. Ment. Dis.*, **125**, 221–5.
11. De Smedt, L., Severts, M., Geutjens, J. and Medaer, R. (1984) Intellectual impairment in multiple sclerosis, in *Immunological and Clinical Aspects of Multiple Sclerosis* (eds R.F. Gonsette and P. Delmotte), Lancaster, MTP Press, pp. 342–5.
12. Rao, S.M., Leo, G.J., Ellington, L. *et al.* (1991) Cognitive dysfunction in multiple sclerosis: II. Impact on social functioning. *Neurology*, **41**, 692–6.
13. van den Burg, W., van Zomeren, A.H., Minderhoud, J.M. *et al.* (1987) Cognitive impairment in patients with multiple sclerosis and mild physical disability. *Arch. Neurol.*, **44**, 494–501.
14. Hotopf, M.H., Pollock, S. and Lishman, W.A. (1994) An unusual presentation of multiple sclerosis. *Psychol. Med.*, **24**, 525–8.
15. Young, A.C., Saunders, J. and Ponsford, J.R. (1976) Mental change as an early feature of multiple sclerosis. *J. Neurol. Neurosurg. Psychiatry*, **39**, 1008–13.
16. Bergin, J.D. (1957) Rapidly progressing dementia in disseminated sclerosis. *J. Neurol. Neurosurg. Psychiatry*, **20**, 285–92.
17. Marsh, G. (1980) Disability and intellectual function in multiple sclerosis. *J. Nerv. Ment. Dis.*, **168**, 758–62.
18. Ivnik, R.J. (1978) Neuropsychological test performance as a function of the duration of MS-related symptomatology. *J. Clin. Psychiatry*, **39**, 304–7.
19. Ivnik, R.J. (1978) Neuropsychological stability in multiple sclerosis. *J. Consult. Clin. Psychol.*, **46**, 913–23.
20. Feinstein, A., Kartsounis, L.D., Miller, D.H., Youl, B.D. and Ron, M.A. (1992) Clinically isolated lesions of the type seen in multiple sclerosis: a cognitive, psychiatric, and MRI follow up study. *J. Neurol. Neurosurg. Psychiatry*, **55**, 869–76.
21. Jennekens-Schinkel, A., Laboyrie, P.M., Lanser, J.B.K. and Van der Velde, E.A. (1990) Cognition in patients with multiple sclerosis. After four years. *J. Neurol. Sci.*, **99**, 229–47.
22. Fink, S.L. and Houser, H.B. (1966) An investigation of physical and intellectual impairment changes in multiple sclerosis. *Arch. Phys. Med. Rehab.*, **47**, 56–61.
23. Canter, A.H. (1951) Direct and indirect measures of psychological deficit in multiple sclerosis. *J. Gen. Psychol.*, **44**, 3–50.
24. Bernardin, L.J., Rao, S.M., Luchetta, T.L. *et al.* (1993) A prospective, long-term, longitudinal study of cognitive dysfunction in MS. *J. Clin. Exp. Neuropsychol.*, **15**, 17.
25. Fischer, J.S., Foley, F.W., Aikens, J.E. *et al.* (1994) What do we *really* know about cognitive dysfunction, affective disorders, and stress in multiple sclerosis? A practitioner's guide. *J. Neurol. Rehab.*, **8**, 151–64.
26. Rao, S.M. (1986) Neuropsychology of multiple sclerosis: a critical review. *J. Clin. Exp. Neuropsychol.*, **8**, 503–42.
27. Reitan, R.M., Reed, J.C. and Dyken, M. (1971) Cognitive, psychomotor, and motor correlates of multiple sclerosis. *J. Nerv. Ment. Dis.*, **153**, 218–24.
28. Rao, S.M., Hammeke, T.A. and Speech, T.J. (1987) Wisconsin Card Sorting Test performance in relapsing-remitting and chronic-progressive multiple sclerosis. *J. Consult. Clin. Psychol.*, **55**, 263–5.
29. Rao, S.M. and Hammeke, T.A. (1984) Hypothesis testing in patients with chronic progressive multiple sclerosis. *Brain Cognition*, **3**, 94–104.
30. Jambor, K.L. (1969) Cognitive functioning in multiple sclerosis. *Br. J. Psychiatry*, **115**, 765–75.
31. Beatty, W.W. and Monson, N. (1994) Picture and motor sequencing in multiple sclerosis. *J. Clin. Exp. Neuropsychol.*, **16**, 165–72.
32. Rao, S.M. and Arnett, P.A. (1995) Executive functions in multiple sclerosis. Unpublished manuscript.
33. Grigsby, J., Kaye, K. and Busenbark, D. (1994) Alphanumeric sequencing: a report on a brief measure of information processing used among persons with multiple sclerosis. *Perceptual Motor Skills.*, **78** (1), 883–7.
34. DeLuca, J., Johnson, S.K. and Natelson, B.H. (1993) Information processing efficiency in chronic fatigue syndrome and multiple sclerosis. *Arch. Neurol.*, **50**, 301–4.
35. DeLuca, J., Barbieri-Berger, S. and Johnson, S.K. (1994) The nature of memory impairments in multiple sclerosis: acquisition versus retrieval. *J. Clin. Exp. Neuropsychol.*, **16**, 183–9.
36. Litvan, I., Grafman, J., Vendrell, P. and Martinez, J.M. (1988) Slowed information processing in multiple sclerosis. *Arch. Neurol.*, **45**, 281–5.
37. Rao, S.M., St Aubin-Faubert, P. and Leo, G.J. (1989) Information processing speed in patients with multiple sclerosis. *J. Clin. Exp. Neuropsychol.*, **11**, 471–7.
38. Beatty, W.W., Goodkin, D.E., Monson, N. and Beatty, P.A. (1989) Cognitive disturbances in patients with relapsing remitting multiple sclerosis. *Arch. Neurol.*, **46**, 1113–19.
39. Beatty, W.W., Goodkin, D.E., Monson, N., Beatty, P.A. and Hertsgaard, D. (1988) Anterograde and retrograde amnesia in patients with chronic progressive multiple sclerosis. *Arch. Neurol.*, **45**, 611–19.
40. Grafman, J., Rao, S.M. and Litvan, I. (1990) Disorders of memory, in *Neurobehavioral Aspects of Multiple Sclerosis* (ed. S.M. Rao), New York, Oxford University Press, pp. 102–17.
41. Vowels, L.M. (1979) Memory impairment in multiple sclerosis, in *Brain Impairment: Proceedings of the 1978 Brain Impairment Workshop* (eds M. Molloy, G.V. Stanley and K.W. Walsh), Melbourne, University of Melbourne, pp. 10–22.
42. Litvan, I., Grafman, J., Vendrell, P. *et al.* (1988) Multiple memory deficits in patients with multiple sclerosis: exploring the working memory system. *Arch. Neurol.*, **45**, 607–10.
43. Rao, S.M., Leo, G.J. and St Aubin-Faubert, P. (1989) On the nature of memory disturbance in multiple sclerosis. *J. Clin. Exp. Neuropsychol.*, **11**, 699–712.
44. Baddeley, A. (1986) *Working Memory*. Oxford: Clarendon Press.
45. Rao, S.M., Grafman, J., DiGiulio, D. *et al.* (1993) Memory dysfunction in multiple sclerosis: its relation to working memory, semantic encoding, and implicit learning. *Neuropsychology*, **7**, 364–74.
46. Goldstein, F.C., McKendall, R.R. and Haut, M.W. (1992) Gist recall in multiple sclerosis. *Arch. Neurol.*, **49**, 1060–4.
47. Minden, S.L., Moes, E.J., Orav, J., Kaplan, E. and Reich, P. (1990) Memory impairment in multiple sclerosis. *J. Clin. Exp. Neuropsychol.*, **12**, 566–86.
48. Fischer, J.S. (1988) Using the Wechsler Memory Scale-Revised to detect and characterize memory deficits in multiple sclerosis. *Clin. Neuropsychol.*, **2**, 149–72.
49. Beatty, P.A. and Gange, J.J. (1977) Neuropsychological aspects of multiple sclerosis. *J. Nerv. Ment. Dis.*, **164**, 42–50.
50. Carroll, M., Gates, R. and Roldan, F. (1984) Memory impairment in multiple sclerosis. *Neuropsychol.*, **22**, 297–302.
51. Caine, E.D., Bamford, K.A., Schiffer, R.B., Shoulson, I. and Levy, S. (1986) A controlled neuropsychological comparison of Huntington's disease and multiple sclerosis. *Arch. Neurology*, **43**, 249–54.
52. Wickens, D.D. (1970) Encoding categories of words: an empirical approach to meaning. *Psychol. Rev.*, **77**, 1–15.
53. Rao, S.M., Bernardin, L., Ellington, L. and Leo, G.J. (1990) Memory loss in patients with multiple sclerosis: the role of semantic encoding. *J. Clin. Exp. Neuropsychol.*, **12**, 74.
54. Beatty, W.W., Goodkin, D.E., Beatty, P.A. and Monson, N. (1989) Frontal lobe dysfunction and memory impairment in patients with chronic progressive multiple sclerosis. *Brain Cognition*, **11**, 73–86.
55. Grafman, J., Rao, S.M., Bernardin, L. and Leo, G.J. (1991) Automatic memory processes in patients with multiple sclerosis. *Arch. Neurol.*, **48**, 1072–5.

56. Beatty, W.W., Goodkin, D.E., Monson, N. and Beatty, P.A. (1990) Implicit learning in patients with chronic progressive multiple sclerosis. *Int. J. Clin. Neuropsychol.*, **12**, 166–72.

57. Beatty, W.W. and Monson, N. (1990) Semantic priming in multiple sclerosis. *Bull. Psychonom. Soc.*, **28**, 397–400.

58. Achiron, A., Ziv, I., Djaldetti, R. *et al.* (1992) Aphasia in multiple sclerosis: clinical and radiologic correlations. *Neurology*, **42**, 2195–7.

59. Friedman, J.H., Brem, H. and Mayeux, R. (1983) Global aphasia in multiple sclerosis. *Ann. Neurol.*, **13**, 222–3.

60. Olmos-Lau, N., Ginsberg, M.D. and Geller, J.B. (1977) Aphasia in multiple sclerosis. *Neurology*, **27**, 623–6.

61. Arnett, P.A., Rao, S.M., Hussain, M., Swanson, S.J. and Hammeke, T.A. (1996) Conduction aphasia in multiple sclerosis: a case report with MRI findings. *Neurology* (in press).

62. Beatty, W.W. and Monson, N. (1989) Lexical processing in Parkinson's disease and multiple sclerosis. *J. Geriatr. Psychiatry Neurol.*, **2**, 145–52.

63. Beatty, W.W., Monson, N. and Goodkin, D.E. (1989) Access to semantic memory in Parkinson's disease and multiple sclerosis. *J. Geriatr. Psychiatry Neurol.*, **2**, 153–62.

64. Rao, S.M., Huber, S.J. and Bornstein, R.A. (1992) Emotional changes with multiple sclerosis and Parkinson's disease. *J. Consult. Clin. Psychol.*, **60**, 369–78.

65. Minden, S.L. and Schiffer, R.B. (1990) Affective disorders in multiple sclerosis: review and recommendations for clinical research. *Arch. Neurol.*, **47**, 98–104.

66. Ron, M.A. (1986) Multiple sclerosis: psychiatric and psychometric abnormalities. *J. Psychosom. Res.*, **30**, 3–11.

67. Devins, G.M. and Seland, T.P. (1987) Emotional impact of multiple sclerosis: recent findings and suggestions for future research. *Psychol. Bull.*, **101**, 363–75.

68. Berrios, G.E. and Quemada, J.I. (1990) Depressive illness in multiple sclerosis. Clinical and theoretical aspects of the association. *Br. J. Psychiatry*, **156**, 10–16.

69. Minden, S.L., Orav, J. and Reich, P. (1987) Depression in multiple sclerosis. *Gen. Hosp. Psychiatry*, **9**, 426–34.

70. Schiffer, R.B. (1987) The spectrum of depression in multiple sclerosis: an approach for clinical management. *Arch. Neurol.*, **44**, 596–9.

71. Joffe, R.T., Lippert, G.P., Gray, T.A. Sawa, G. and Horvath, Z. (1987) Mood disorder and multiple sclerosis. *Arch. Neurol.*, **44**, 376–8.

72. Whitlock, F.A. and Siskind, M.M. (1980) Depression as a major symptom of multiple sclerosis. *J. Neurol. Neurosurg. Psychiatry*, **43**, 861–5.

73. Schiffer, R.B. and Babigian, H.M. (1984) Behavioral disorders in multiple sclerosis, temporal lobe epilepsy and amyotrophic lateral sclerosis: an epidemiological study. *Arch. Neurol.*, **41**, 1067–9.

74. Brown, S. and Davis, T.K. (1922) The mental symptoms of multiple sclerosis. *Arch. Neurol. Psychiatry*, **7**, 629–34.

75. Rao, S.M. and Glatt, S.L. (1987) Association of euphoria and ventricular enlargement in multiple sclerosis. *Neurol.*, **37** (Suppl. 1), 181.

76. Rabins, P.V., Brooks, B.R., O'Donnell, P. *et al.* (1986) Structural brain correlates of emotional disorder in multiple sclerosis. *Brain*, **109**, 585–97.

77. Barnard, R.O. and Triggs, M. (1974) Corpus callosum in multiple sclerosis. *J. Neurol. Neurosurg. Psychiatry*, **37**, 1259–64.

78. Lumsden, C.E. (1970) The neuropathology of multiple sclerosis in *Handbook of Clinical Neurology* (eds P.J. Vinken and G.W. Bruyn), vol. 9: *Multiple Sclerosis and Other Demyelinating Diseases* New York, Elsevier, pp. 217–309.

79. Brownell, B. and Hughes, J.F. (1962) The distribution of plaques in the cerebrum in multiple sclerosis. *J. Neurol. Neurosurg. Psychiatry*, **25**, 315–20.

80. Clark, C.M., James, G., Li, D. *et al.* (1992) Ventricular size, cognitive function and depression in patients with multiple sclerosis. *Can. J. Neurol. Sci.*, **19**, 352–6.

81. Comi, G., Filippi, M., Martinelli, V. *et al.* (1993) Brain magnetic resonance imaging correlates of cognitive impairment in multiple sclerosis. *J. Neurol. Sci.*, **115**(Suppl.), S66–73.

82. Huber, S.J., Bornstein, R.A., Rammohan, K.W. *et al.* (1992) Magnetic resonance imaging correlates of neuropsychological impairment in multiple sclerosis. *J. Neuropsychiatry Clin. Neurosci.*, **4**, 152–8.

83. Maurelli, M., Marchioni, E., Cerretano, R. *et al.* (1992) Neuropsychological assessment in MS: clinical, neurophysiological and neuroradiological relationships. *Acta Neurol. Scand.*, **86**, 124–8.

84. Moller, A., Wiedemann, G., Rohde, U., Backmund, H. and Sonntag, A. (1994) Correlates of cognitive impairment and depressive mood disorder in multiple sclerosis. *Acta Psychiatr. Scand.*, **89**, 117–21.

85. Pugnetti, L., Mendozzi, L., Motta, A. *et al.* (1993) MRI and cognitive patterns in relapsing-remitting multiple sclerosis. *J. Neurol. Sci.*, **115**, Suppl. S59–65.

86. Rao, S.M., Leo, G.J., Haughton, V.M., St Aubin-Faubert, P. and Bernardin, L. (1989) Correlation of magnetic resonance imaging with neuropsychological testing in multiple sclerosis. *Neurology*, **39**, 161–6.

87. Anzola, G.P., Bevilacqua, L., Cappa, S.F. *et al.* (1990) Neuropsychological assessment in patients with relapsing-remitting multiple sclerosis and mild functional impairment: correlation with magnetic resonance imaging. *J. Neurol. Neurosurg. Psychiatry*, **53**, 142–5.

88. Callanan, M.M., Logsdail, S.J., Ron, M.A. and Warrington, E.K. (1989) Cognitive impairment in patients with clinically isolated lesions of the type seen in multiple sclerosis: a psychometric and MRI study. *Brain*, **112**, 361–74.

89. Brainin, M., Goldenberg, G., Ahlers, C *et al.* (1988) Structural brain correlates of anterograde memory deficits in multiple sclerosis. *J. Neurol.*, **235**, 362–5.

90. Reischies, F.M., Baum, K., Brau, H., Hedde, J.P. and Schwindt, G. (1988) Cerebral magnetic resonance imaging findings in multiple sclerosis: relation to disturbance of affect, drive, and cognition. *Arch. Neurol.*, **45**, 1114–16.

91. Medaer, R., Nelissen, E., Appel, B. *et al.* (1987) Magnetic resonance imaging and cognitive functioning in multiple sclerosis. *J. Neurol.*, **235**, 86–9.

92. Huber, S.J., Paulson, G.W., Shuttleworth, E.C. *et al.* (1987) Magnetic resonance imaging correlates of dementia in multiple sclerosis. *Arch. Neurol.*, **44**, 732–6.

93. Franklin, G.M., Heaton, R.K., Nelson, L.M. *et al.* (1988) Correlation of neuropsychological and MRI findings in chronic/progressive multiple sclerosis. *Neurology*, **38**, 1826–9.

94. Geschwind, N. (1965) Disconnexion syndromes in animals and man. *Brain*, **88**, 237–94.

95. Rubens, A.B., Froehling, B., Slater, G. and Anderson, D. (1985) Left ear suppression on verbal dichotic tests in patients with multiple sclerosis. *Ann. Neurol.*, **18**, 459–63.

96. Jacobson, J.T., Deppe, U. and Murray, T.J. (1983) Dichotic paradigms in multiple sclerosis. *Eye Hearing*, **4**, 311–17.

97. Rao, S.M., Bernardin, L., Leo, G.J. *et al.* (1989) Cerebral disconnection in multiple sclerosis: relationship to atrophy of the corpus callosum. *Arch. Neurol.*, **46**, 918–20.

98. Swirsky-Sacchetti, T., Mitchell, D.R., Seward, J. *et al.* (1992) Neuropsychological and structural brain lesions in multiple sclerosis: a regional analysis. *Neurology*, **42**, 1291–5.

99. Arnett, P.A., Rao, S.M., Bernardin, L. *et al.* (1994) Relationship between frontal lobe lesions and Wisconsin Card Sorting Test performance in patients with multiple sclerosis. *Neurology*, **44**, 420–5.

100. Brooks, D.J., Leenders, K.L., Head, G. *et al.* (1984) Studies on regional cerebral oxygen utilisation and cognitive function in multiple sclerosis. *J. Neurol. Neurosurg. Psychiatry*, **47**, 1182–91.

101. Pozzilli, C., Passafiume, D., Bernardi, S. *et al.* (1991) SPECT, MRI and cognitive functions in multiple sclerosis. *J. Neurol. Neurosurg. Psychiatry*, **54**, 110–15.

102. Newton, M.R., Barrett, G., Callanan, M.M. and Towell, A.D. (1989) Cognitive event-related potentials in multiple sclerosis. *Brain*, **112**, 1637–60.

103. Giesser, B.S., Schroeder, M.M., LaRocca, N.G. *et al.* (1992) Endogenous event-related potentials as indices of dementia in multiple sclerosis patients. *Electroencephalogr. Clin. Neurophysiol.*, **85**, 320–9.

104. van Dijk, J.G., Jennekens-Schinkel, A., Caekebeke, J.F. and Zwinderman, A.H. (1992) Are event-related potentials in multiple sclerosis indicative of cognitive impairment? Evoked and event-related potentials, psychometric testing and response speed: a controlled study. *J. Neurol. Sci.*, **109**, 18–24.

105. Beatty, W.W. and Goodkin, D.E. (1990) Screening for cognitive impairment in multiple sclerosis: an evaluation of the Mini-Mental State Exam. *Arch. Neurol.*, **47**, 297–301.

106. Paty, D.W., UBC MS/MRI Study Group and IFNβ Multiple Sclerosis Study Group (1993) Interferon beta-1b is effective in relapsing-remitting multiple sclerosis. II. MRI analysis results of a multicenter, randomized, double-blind, placebo-controlled trial. *Neurology*, **43**, 662–7.

107. Feinstein, A., Ron, M. and Thompson, A. (1993) A serial study of psychometric and magnetic resonance imaging changes in multiple sclerosis. *Brain*, **116**, 569–02.

108. Anderson, B.L., Rao, S.M., Bernardin, L.J. and Luchetta, T. (1996) Long term practice effects in neuropsychological testing. *Clin. Neuropsychol.* (in press).

109. Smits, R.C.F., Emmen, H.H., Bertelsmann, F.W. *et al.* (1994) The effects of 4-aminopyridine on cognitive function in patients with multiple sclerosis: a pilot study. *Neurology*, **44**, 1701–5.

110. Foley, F.W., Dince, W.M., Bedell, J.R. *et al.* (1994) Psychoremediation of communication skills for cognitively impaired persons with multiple sclerosis. *J. Neurol. Rehab.*, **8**, 165–76.

21 THE BLADDER IN MULTIPLE SCLEROSIS

C. Lowell Parsons and Mohamed Bidair

It has been estimated that as many as 90% of patients with multiple sclerosis will at some point have difficulties with lower urinary tract symptoms [1–4], and one of the more difficult management problems that may present in patients with multiple sclerosis is a neuromuscular dysfunction of the bladder. The voluminous data concerning evaluation, classification and therapy of urinary bladder dysfunction can make the treating physician thoroughly confused in setting up an optimum therapeutic management of the individual patient. Knowledge of the complex interactions among the central neuronal cells, ganglion and smooth muscle receptors is not needed, however, to treat most cases of vesical dysfunction secondary to multiple sclerosis. What follows is an overview of the neurophysiology, pharmacology and neuroanatomy of the detrusor and urethra and the classification of the bladder in pathological states. A simple method of classifying bladder dysfunction in terms of its normal function will be presented and the appropriate therapy for each condition discussed. This approach offers a practical solution to the problem of treating the majority of urological complications seen in patients with multiple sclerosis.

21.1 Motor innervation of the bladder

21.1.1 MOTOR INNERVATION

The musculature of the urinary bladder is innervated by both the parasympathetic and sympathetic divisions of the autonomic nervous system [5–7]. The parasympathetic fibres originate in the lateral horns of spinal segments S2, S3 and S4, and travel via the pelvic nerves to synapse with ganglia in and around the bladder. Postganglionic fibres are distributed in the bladder muscle on a regional basis. The bladder base (the part of the bladder below the ureteral orifices) has more innervation with cholinergic receptor sites than the bladder body (the part above the ureteral orifices), but the bladder body is more sensitive to pharmacological stimulation with cholinergic drugs [7, 8]. Figure 21.1 shows the rich motor end

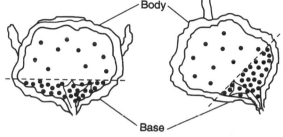

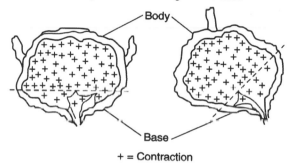

Figure 21.1 Cholinergic innervation and neuromorphology of the bladder body and bladder base.

plates in the trigone area, with the entire musculature being sensitive to cholinergic drugs.

21.1.2 SENSORY INNERVATION

Sensory afferents from the urethra and detrusor, travelling in the pelvic nerve through the sacral roots S2–S4 [9], are primarily concerned with tension. They are distributed in all areas of the detrusor [10], with the highest concentration in the trigone as is seen with motor fibres. Pain fibres from the bladder travel via the hypogastric nerves to the spinal column between T10 and L1 and ascend in the lateral spinothalamic tracts. The sensory fibres feed back to the sacral parasympathetics to form the micturition reflex arc.

Multiple Sclerosis: Clinical and pathogenetic basis. Edited by Cedric S. Raine, Henry F. McFarland and Wallace W. Tourtellotte. Published in 1997 by Chapman & Hall, London. ISBN 0 412 30890 8.

21.1.3 EXTERNAL SPHINCTER INNERVATION

The somatic innervation of the striated muscle of the genitourinary diaphragm is carried by the pudendal nerves. It has been shown experimentally that the detrusor reflex contraction is accompanied by depression of the tonic pudendal motor nerve impulses that results in relaxation of periurethral striated muscle [11]. This is important in the coordination of micturition that permits emptying of the bladder. The dyscoordinated contractions of the detrusor muscle and striated musculature that are seen in pathological states are called detrusor–sphincter dyssynergia.

21.1.4 SPINAL AND SUPRASPINAL PATHWAYS

The reader is referred to *Campbell's Urology* [12, 13] for a more detailed review of these pathways. Briefly, the descending motor pathways include the reticulospinal tracts and the corticospinal tracts with ascending proprioceptric sensory impulses located in the posterior columns. Lesions that acutely affect these tracts can lead to a temporary flaccid paralysis of the detrusor muscle. In permanent lesions, the bladder will develop a degree of hyperreflexia that corresponds to the severity of loss of corticospinal tracts. The interruption of nerve loops between the frontal lobes and the brain stem can result in hyperreflexia of the micturition reflex arc.

21.2 Physiology and pharmacology of the bladder and its outlet

The autonomic nerve endings in the bladder and its outlet are composed of both cholinergic and adrenergic fibres. Cholinergic fibres, which include all the parasympathetic post-ganglionic fibres, employ acetylcholine as the synaptic transmitter. Cholinergic receptor sites are further classified as muscarinic or nicotinic, depending on whether they are stimulated by muscarine or nicotine. The bladder smooth-muscle cells are stimulated by muscarine and are blocked by atropine-like drugs. Other neurons in the bladder and bladder neck employ the neurotransmitter norepinephrine (adrenergic) and include receptor sites that are both alpha and beta depending on their response to catecholamine stimulation. Alpha-adrenergic receptors are in the smooth musculature of the bladder, with the heaviest concentration at the bladder neck. They are stimulated by norepinephrine and cause a smooth muscle contraction Beta-adrenergic receptors occur primarily in the smooth muscle of the bladder body, are sensitive to isoproterenol, and cause a relaxation of the smooth muscle [5, 7, 14–17]. These areas of response in the bladder are illustrated in Figure 21.2.

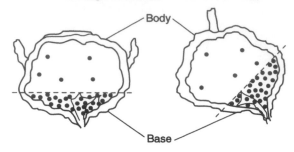

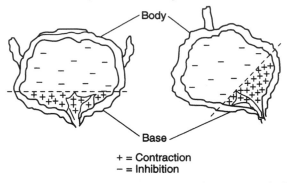

Figure 21.2 Adrenergic innervation and neuromorphology of the bladder body and bladder base.

It is theorized that beta-adrenergic neurons are active during the filling phase of the bladder and account for the increased activity in the hypogastric nerve that Edvardsen [18, 19], has observed during this phase. This beta effect may cause relaxation of the detrusor and account for the fact that while the bladder is filling no increase is seen in intravesical pressure until the bladder volume is reached.

Urinary continence is felt to depend in part on the concentration of alpha-adrenergic receptor sites in the posterior urethra and at the level of the bladder neck.

When pathological processes interrupt the normal function of the detrusor and its outlet, it is theoretically possible to restore function using pharmacological stimulation. If the bladder smooth muscle fails to permit emptying, cholinergic stimulation of ganglia and the smooth muscle may facilitate contraction. Alpha- or beta-sympathomimetic agents can potentially promote urine storage in two ways. First, they could exert a beta effect on the smooth muscle; unfortunately, no clinically useful drugs are available but L-dopa may work in such a fashion [20]. Secondly, they could be employed to produce alpha stimulation of the bladder neck. Conversely, alpha-blocking agents such as phenoxybenzamine can potentially reduce bladder outlet resistance.

Data also suggest that the sympathetic and parasympathetic systems interact since stimulation of the hypogastric nerve inhibits the parasympathetic ganglia [21]. Chromaffin cells may also be an inhibitory adrenergic link [22]. The clinical significance of these possibilities is unknown.

For an in-depth survey of the complex interactions that are seen experimentally between the neurons and ganglia of the sympathetic and parasympathetic system, the reader is referred to the review by Wein [23].

21.3 Classification

Several systems have attempted to classify neuromuscular vesical dysfunction. Probably the one most widely employed is that of McClellan as popularized by Lapides [24], where the types of dysfunction are divided into five categories according to the innervation that is impaired:

1. sensory paralytic bladder;
2. motor paralytic bladder;
3. autonomous neuropathic bladder;
4. uninhibited neuropathic bladder;
5. reflex neuropathic bladder.

More extensive reviews of various systems of classification of neuropathic bladder are offered by Kendall and Karafin [24], Bradley *et al.* [25], McGuire [12] and Wein [13].

21.3.1 CLASSIFICATION BY THE INNERVATION IMPAIRED

Sensory paralytic bladder

In sensory paralytic neuropathic bladder, sensory innervation is lost but motor function is preserved. Sensory loss may occur gradually; as it progresses, the patient voids with increasing bladder volumes that lead to detrusor hypotonia. An example of the results of cystometrics performed on this type of bladder is shown schematically in Figure 21.3. This type of bladder is not associated with multiple sclerosis but is

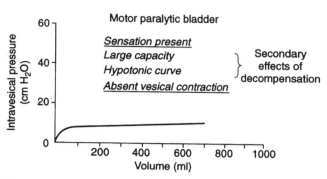

Figure 21.4 Cystometrogram performed on a patient with motor paralytic neuropathic bladder.

most commonly seen in diabetes mellitus [26], vitamin B_6 deficiency and tabes dorsalis.

Motor paralytic bladder

Individuals with motor paralytic neuropathic bladders have lost lower motor neurons, or pre- or post-ganglionic fibres but retain intact sensation and consequently present clinically in painful retention. This type of bladder is also rarely associated with multiple sclerosis and is likely to be seen in poliomyelitis, herniated discs, trauma, tumour or any central nervous system lesion that destroys the anterior motor cells or the dorsal nerve roots as they exit the spinal cord. A representative cystometrogram is shown in Figure 21.4.

Autonomous neuropathic bladder

In patients with an autonomous neuropathic bladder, the bladder has no motor or sensory innervation. Pathological processes that destroy all peripheral nerves, the cona medullaris or the S2–S4 portion of the spinal cord can lead to this type of denervation. Specific causes include trauma, tumours, herniated discs, degenerative arthritis or vascular malformations. This type of neuropathic bladder is found in a small percentage of patients with multiple sclerosis. Figure 21.5 shows a cystometrogram typical for this dysfunction.

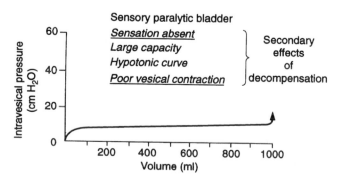

Figure 21.3 Cystometrogram performed on a patient with sensory paralytic neuropathic bladder.

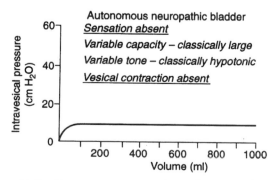

Figure 21.5 Cystometrogram performed on a patient with autonomous neuropathic bladder.

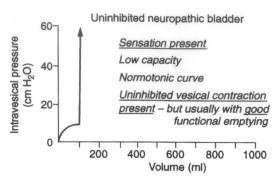

Figure 21.6 Cystometrogram performed on a patient with uninhibited neuropathic bladder.

Uninhibited neuropathic bladder

Both motor function and sensation are intact in this type of neuropathic bladder. The deficit is the partial loss of descending corticospinal tracts in the central nervous system which normally regulate the micturition reflex arc. Symptomatically the individual with this problem has detrusor instability and is unable to inhibit the voiding urge for very long. The patient will have mild urinary urgency to frank incontinence, depending on the severity of the loss. Detrusor instability is the most common type of neuromuscular dysfunction in patients with multiple sclerosis and is manifested on cystometrogram as schematically shown in Figure 21.6. Any lesion of the central nervous system interrupting the cortical spinal pathways can lead to this dysfunction, the most common causes being cerebrovascular accidents, brain tumours, degenerative arthritic problems of the spine and herniated discs.

Reflex neuropathic bladder

Reflex neuropathic bladders have an intact micturition reflex arc but have lost the ascending and descending pathways of the spinal cord above the level of the neuronal bodies at S2–S4. Destructive lesions above approximately T10 lead to this type of loss of innervation. The most common cause of this problem is trauma

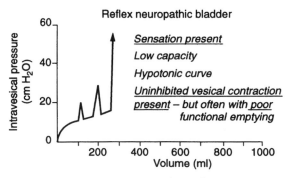

Figure 21.7 Cystometrogram performed on a patient with reflex neuropathic bladder.

followed by any pathological process that leads to a functional transection of the spinal cord, including infections (viral or bacterial), tumours, vascular accidents, herniated discs, or degenerative arthritis. Changes found on cystometrics are illustrated diagrammatically in Figure 21.7.

21.3.2   FUNCTIONAL CLASSIFICATION

Systems in which neuropathic bladders are classified by their actual supraspinal, spinal or peripheral nerve losses may be helpful in defining the active pathological process that is present but may not indicate accurately the optimum management of an individual patient's neuromuscular bladder dysfunction. The approach to actual therapy is better understood when one employs a functional classification [8]. In this system, abnormal bladder function is divided into two categories based on the bladder's function: storage of urine and emptying. Therapy is directed at restoring the lost function.

Low pressure reservoir function

Elastic properties of the bladder wall will contribute to a flat pressure response with increasing bladder volume. This results in maintenance of a low intravesical pressure. Low pressure is critical to maintaining stable renal function in that a high pressure, developed clinically in the bladder, will necessarily transmit to high pressure in the ureter and ultimately to the kidney in order for the upper tract to drain into the high pressure bladder [27, 28] This transmitted high pressure has the potential of leading to pressure atrophy of the kidneys, and it is also believed that there is increased risk of pyelonephritis and kidney loss, although this is not conclusive [29]. Since the individual with multiple sclerosis is at risk to develop elevated intravesical pressure, this is an important reason to monitor patients with some type of urodynamic assessment, primarily a cystometrogram. Therapeutic options when a high pressure system is involved will be discussed in a subsequent section [30, 31].

Failure to store

This is the type of impairment seen in an uninhibited neuropathic bladder and a reflex neuropathic bladder. The bladder acts as a reservoir in which urine is stored. The ability to store urine is not only an important function socially but it can become important medically, since a wet perineum or buttock area may lead to skin breakdown. Rarely does this type of problem lead to loss of renal parenchyma. The principal goal of management in the patient whose bladder is classified as a failure to store is to restore this function. This can be accomplished by a variety of strategies, including decreasing bladder muscle contractility or increasing bladder outlet resistance. Another clinical problem of failure to store is the risk that a bladder which develops a voiding sphincter dyssynergia may lead to a high intravesical pressure. This pressure, as noted above, can lead to pressure atrophy of the kidney. Therapy for this problem is discussed below.

Failure to empty

This is the type of impairment seen in either a motor or sensory paralytic bladder or an autonomic neuropathic bladder. Bladders that fail to empty represent a more serious health hazard than do failures to store since this dysfunction can lead to loss of kidney function. Therapy to restore the ability to empty is directed at promoting detrusor contractility and reducing bladder outlet resistance or performing intermittent catheterization.

Failure to store and empty

This is the type of impairment seen in a reflex neuropathic bladder or detrusor–sphincter dyssynergia. The combination of failure to store and failure to empty is seen in multiple sclerosis patients whose detrusor instability and poor vesical contractility produce incontinence and urinary retention. Therapy directed at improving vesical contractility and decreasing outlet resistance will often increase the patient's incontinence while attempts to diminish vesical contractility will make it impossible for the patient to void. Therapy usually involves converting the patient's bladder condition into a failure to empty and treating the dysfunction as described below.

23.4 Neuromuscular vesical dysfunction in multiple sclerosis

A variety of vesical dysfunction syndromes are seen clinically in patients with multiple sclerosis. Urinary symptoms occur as the presenting symptoms for multiple sclerosis in 0–2.3% [3, 32, 33]. Involvement of the genitourinary tract occurs in as many as 96% of individuals with multiple sclerosis [2] and may be a major source of morbidity in 54–70% of patients [1, 33–36]. The majority of patients are initially managed successfully by their neurologist but as their disease progresses, complicated management problems often require the addition of urologic care. Bladder symptoms are believed to be associated with the degree of pyramidal tract dysfunction affecting the lower limbs [32, 33, 37].

The ultimate serious complication of the involvement of the genitourinary tract in multiple sclerosis is upper urinary tract deterioration. Older studies have reported that 21–55% of patients with multiple sclerosis have upper tract deterioration [38, 39], but recent advances in the management of neuropathic bladder have drastically reduced its incidence. Later studies suggest that there is virtually no significant incidence of upper tract deterioration in multiple sclerosis [2, 40]. Detrusor hypocontractility is felt by some authors to protect the bladder and upper urinary tract [41].

Three basic patterns of dysfunction are seen in individuals with multiple sclerosis. The first is detrusor hyperreflexia secondary to impaired volitional control. This occurs when the pathway from the frontal cortex or pontine-mesencephalic reticular formation to the bladder is impaired, since this is necessary for voluntary control of micturition, and results in involuntary detrusor contraction and involuntary sphincter relaxation (which usually results in precipitous voiding) [42]. Detrusor hyperreflexia occurs in 52–78% of patients [3, 37, 43, 44].

A second pattern of vesical dysfunction noted is voiding sphincter–detrusor dyssynergia. This type of problem may be present in as many as 50% of patients [1, 42, 45] or as few as 6% [41]. However, this type of dyscoordinated voiding may be present with other bladder dysfunctions. It is felt that in order for coordinated micturition to occur there must be integrity of the pathway between the pontine-mesencephalic reticular formation and the sacral parasympathetic nucleus. Interruptions of this pathway may result in involuntary dyssynergic bladder and sphincter contractions. As with the dysfunction mentioned above, these patients will also be incontinent due to involuntary bladder contraction.

The third dysfunction that may be present is an areflexic bladder. This will usually occur later in the disease as the multiple sclerosis progresses. The incidence of areflexia varies from 0 to 40% [32, 34, 45]. A recent study using videourodynamics on 89 patients showed areflexia in only 6% but a combination of hypocontractility and hyperreflexia in 63% [41].

Although involvement of frontal lobe centers for micturition or the pontine micturition center can occur in multiple sclerosis, the most common cause of voiding dysfunction is spinal pathology [32, 46]. Due to the multiplicity of lesions that are occurring in the central nervous system, one frequently sees a combination of various types of bladder dysfunction as noted above. Patients will frequently have, for example, bladders that are areflexic but have sufficient uninhibited contractions to cause incontinence, and will also have dyssynergic voiding.

It is reported that as many as 50% of patients have complex voiding problems involving any or all of the three types of dysfunction one sees [45]. Patients with more severe dysfunctions represent a more complex management problem because they have both storage and emptying impairments. Consequently, the patient may be both wet and unable to empty the bladder.

Details on how to handle this type of dysfunction will be discussed below.

With good urodynamic evaluation and aggressive therapy and monitoring, it would appear that most of the patients remain stable for prolonged periods of time. In one study of 46 patients, only five ultimately required a Foley or condom catheter for control[45].

21.5   Evaluation

21.5.1   HISTORY AND PHYSICAL EXAMINATION

The most important objective in documenting the history of a multiple sclerosis patient with voiding problems is to obtain a careful voiding history. At this point, one should have categorized the patient's bladder dysfunction as a failure to store or a failure to empty. It is important to know if he/she has severe urinary urgency or urge incontinence, and whether or not he/she voids spontaneously or has to force the urine out. A history of bowel function is also useful in alerting the physician to problems in the sacral reflex arc. It is important to pursue any history of voiding dysfunction in terms of the following studies, since as many as 70% of patients treated solely on the basis of history and physical examination may receive inappropriate and ineffectual therapy[1].

In the neurological examination, it is worth remembering that the physician can check the patient's sacral reflexes by placing a finger in the rectum and squeezing the glans penis or the clitoris. A contraction of the perianal musculature, the bulbocavernosus reflex, indicates that the internal pudendal (somatic) nerves and the pelvic (parasympathetic) nerves are intact since both arise from the sacral roots S2, S3 and S4.

21.5.2   CYSTOMETRICS

Because diagnostic tests of detrusor function check for presence of detrusor contractions and not necessarily for the direct effects of denervation, they contribute little information that is useful in characterizing primary problems with the smooth muscle. The cystometrogram, which is a continuous recording of bladder tension during infusion at a constant rate with water or gas, is the principal method for evaluating and characterizing a neuropathic bladder[47, 48]. As the bladder is filled with fluid, the patient is asked to state when he or she first feels the urge to void (usually about 100–125 ml) but is requested to suppress the urge. During filling, intravesical pressure remains low until bladder volume is reached (350–500 ml). When the patient states that they can 'hold no more', they are asked to void and maximum detrusor pressure is noted. A schematic representation of a normal cystometrogram is shown in Figure 21.8.

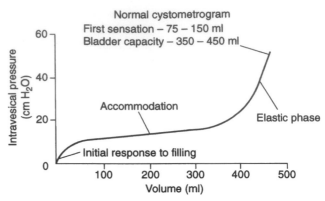

Figure 21.8   Normal cystometrogram.

Figures 21.3–21.7 are schematic representations of abnormal cystometric examinations associated with the five types of neuropathic bladder. A key point to be made concerning the normal cystometrogram, as noted in Figure 21.8, is that there is a flat pressure response curve with a normal elastic bladder wall. The bladder must have a low filling pressure in order for the upper tracts to empty at low pressure not causing pressure atrophy of the kidney. The low filling pressure is an important point to note on a normal cystometrogram.

Not only is the cystometrogram valuable initially when setting up the treatment program for the patient, it is an important monitoring aid to make sure therapy is successful. Cystometrograms can readily detect patients who have high intravesical pressure from dyssynergic voiding and who are areflexic, warranting alterations of therapies described below for control of symptoms.

21.5.3   URODYNAMICS

Urodynamic evaluation combines the cystometrogram with a simultaneous assessment of uroflow rate and anal or perineal electromyography[49, 50] to detect voiding sphincter–detrusor dyssynergia. Its routine use in patients with multiple sclerosis is probably not justified, but it may help in determining the strategy for management of patients who have multiple neurological lesions affecting the bladder, bladder neck and external sphincter.

Tracings from a normal urodynamic evaluation are depicted in Figure 21.9. Note that as the patient initiates micturition, the electrical activity of the perineal musculature subsides and uroflow begins. Voiding is initiated by relaxing the perineal musculature which then leads to a coordinated contraction of the bladder muscle. Volitional constraint of detrusor activity in a normal individual is associated with a burst of EMG activity of the external sphincter and a secondary inhibition of the contraction of the detrusor motor activity[51]. In contrast, Figure 21.10 is a study of a patient with external sphincter dyssynergia. As the

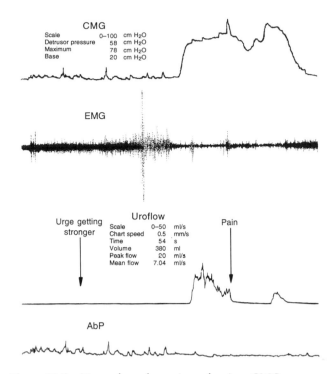

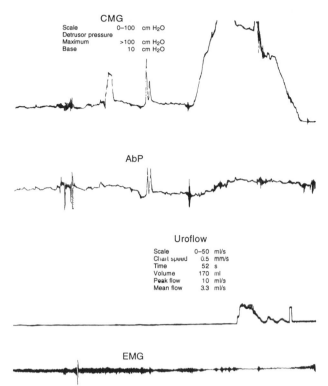

Figure 21.9   Normal urodynamic evaluation. CMG = cysto-metrogram; EMG – electromyogram (perineal musculature); AbP = abdominal pressure from intrarectal balloon.

Figure 21.11   Urodynamic evaluation performed on an individual with multiple sclerosis showing bladder neck dyssynergia.

patient's detrusor contraction begins, there is actually an augmentation of electrical activity of the sphincter and interruption of the uroflow. This is a common finding in patients with multiple sclerosis, who unfortunately may show a low intravesical pressure due to poor detrusor function. An example of a urodynamic evaluation showing bladder neck dyssynergia in a female with multiple sclerosis is seen in Figure 21.11. When the detrusor contraction begins, it generates an inordinately

high pressure for a female (over $100\,cmH_2O$). There is no decrease in perineal musculature activity and no detected urine flow. This patient was treated with phenoxybenzamine to block the alpha-adrenergic fibres of the bladder neck; she had modest improvement and remains catheter-free.

The asymptomatic patient with multiple sclerosis most likely does not need urodynamic evaluation. However, if the patient is symptomatic with frequency, urgency or incontinence, it is worthwhile obtaining this study, since they can have very complex findings [1, 45]. It has been reported that urodynamic testing in patients with multiple sclerosis will show three discrete patterns of bladder dysfunction. Pattern one is a detrusor areflexia, poor subjective sensation of the bladder and failure to relax the external sphincter and initiate voiding. This pattern is associated with the symptoms of slow urinary stream, poor voiding, urgency, incontinence and enuresis. Pattern two consists of simple bladder instability without significant residual urine and relaxation of the external sphincter at the time of voiding. Symptoms of this pattern include pressure sensation, urgency, incontinence and enuresis. The third pattern involves detrusor–sphincter dyssynergia during micturition and difficulty with volitional relaxation of the sphincter. Associated symptoms are inability to void voluntarily, pressure,

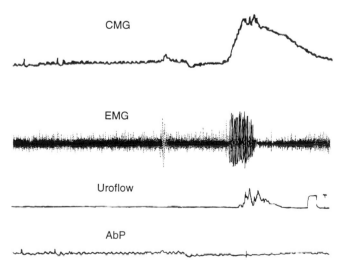

Figure 21.10   Urodynamic evaluation performed on an individual with external sphincter dyssynergia.

urgency and incontinence. Most people ultimately depend on management as described below once the type of bladder dysfunction is characterized as either failure to empty, failure to store or both.

Not all patients with neuropathic bladder secondary to multiple sclerosis will require a full urodynamic evaluation. However, there are many who may have silent problems, such as obstruction of the upper tracts, and at a minimum a cystometrogram should be performed to rule out problems with high pressure bladders. Patients who are symptomatic should have a urodynamic evaluation, for, as noted by McGuire and Savastano [45], there are many patients with complex problems and significant dysfunction of the bladder that can be corrected by understanding what is taking place.

21.5.4 VIDEOURODYNAMICS

This modality combines the use of full urodynamics described above plus simultaneous fluoroscopic evaluation of bladder filling and emptying. Videourodynamics yields more information, but is only necessary in a few patients with very difficult disorders to diagnose (e.g. detrusor internal sphincter dyssynergia). Transrectal ultrasound has also been used instead of fluoroscopy and achieves the same results [52].

21.6 Management

The most important general principle to remember in the management of urinary bladder dysfunctions is that one is ultimately attempting to preserve renal tissue. Several conditions may lead to deterioration of renal function, one of these being pyelonephritis. Bacteriuria *per se* does not always lead to involvement of the upper tracts, but persistent bacteriuria does raise the risk of renal infection especially in the presence of high intravesical pressure. These high pressures lead to hydroureteronephrosis and increased infection rates. Consequently, prevention of bacteriuria has long been important in the management of bladder dysfunction. A second condition that may result in destruction of kidneys is obstruction, since secondary hydroureteronephrosis leads to progressive renal atrophy. Poor emptying with large bladder volumes or increased thickness of the bladder wall obstructing the ureter are potential causes of hydroureteronephrosis. In addition, dyssynergic voiding, poor bladder wall compliance or chemically increased detrusor muscle tension can lead to high intravesical pressure. Pressure over $40\,cmH_2O$ means the upper tract pressure must rise to greater levels to empty. Hydronephrosis and infection, two significant causes of renal loss in MS, require one carefully to monitor the urinary system.

Optimum surveillance methods of kidney function include periodic urinalysis and urine culture to detect bacteriuria, serum blood urea nitrogen and serum creatinine (more sensitive and even better, creatinine clearance) to detect declining renal function, pyelography or renal ultrasound to exclude the presence of hydroureteronephrosis or subtle anatomic alterations of the kidneys, and regular cystometrograms.

The frequency with which the above tests should be performed depends on the clinical status of the patient. Those having no problems with infection or obstruction need urine examinations every 3–4 months initially, and at greater or lesser intervals as the need arises. Radiographic (or ultrasound) and cystometrogram (CMG) studies should be obtained annually at first and biannually if the patient is doing well.

A third goal of management in vesical dysfunction is imposed by the social concern of the patient, namely, is he or she incontinent of urine, or wet? Urinary incontinence does not necessarily cause a health problem for the patient, but can be a complicating factor in the presence of existing decubitus ulcers. For many the only problem caused by incontinence is one of social concern. If the patient requests therapy for this problem, then it must be dealt with; if he is not concerned (if he is bedridden, for example), then condom catheters or diapers may be employed.

In the management of the patient with vesical dysfunction, then, the physician should keep in mind the three management goals described above and classify all patients' bladder dysfunctions as (1) failure to store, (2) failure to empty, or (3) the combination of (1) and (2). In addition, one should generally try simple methods of treatment first, reserving irreversible procedures (e.g. surgery) for use when the simpler methods have proved unsuccessful.

21.6.1 FAILURE TO STORE

As mentioned above, the most common type of neuromuscular dysfunction seen in multiple sclerosis is the uninhibited type of neuropathic bladder (detrusor hyperreflexia) which is basically a failure to store urine. Fortunately, this type of bladder rarely leads to obstruction, infection or renal deterioration [2]. It is generally more manageable than bladders that fail to empty; the mainstay of therapy is pharmacological manipulation of the bladder.

Initial management of symptoms associated with a failure to store includes a bladder training program and perhaps fluid restriction during certain hours. The training program is begun by doing a voiding history to determine how long after drinking the patient needs to urinate and then plan for it. Patients should be training to appreciate the first vague sensation of desire to void and not to panic, which will only increase urgency. They should be cautioned that sudden changes in temperature (warm or cold), excitement, change in posture from lying to sitting or standing can bring on bladder urgency. Next the patient is instructed to schedule regular periods of voiding. An attempt should be made to empty the bladder by relaxation techniques, by the Credé maneuver, or massage of the bladder via the rectum utilizing a finger cot. The amount of time between voiding should be increased to find the maximal interval which comfortably eliminates the risk of incontinence. The bulk of drinking should be done at home or sufficiently ahead of planned outings. Voiding just before going out is also helpful.

As reviewed earlier, there are many ways pharmacologically to manipulate the bladder's ability to store urine. This may be accomplished by producing direct

Table 21.1   Effect of various drugs on detrusor activity

Promote Urine Storage	Promote Bladder Emptying
Anticholinergics	**Cholinomimetic**
Inhibit cholinergic transmission and detrusor contractions	Stimulate detrusor muscle Bethanecol chloride (Urecholine)
Propantheline bromide (Pro-Banthine)	Carbamylcholine chloride (Carbachol)
Methantheline bromide (Banthine)	Neostigmine methylsulphate[b] (Prostigmin)
Dicyclomine HCl (Bentyl)	Acetyl-β-methacholine
Atropine	
	Alphasympathetic blockade
Direct muscle relaxation	Relax vesical neck sphincter
Reduce detrusor smooth muscle tone	Phenoxybenzamine HCl (Dibenzylene)
L-Dopa	Guanethidine sulphate (Ismelin)
Oxybutynin chloride (Ditropan)	Methyldopa[c] (Aldomet)
Flavoxate HCl (Urispas)	
Imipramine[a] (Tofranil)	
Sympathomimetics	
Stimulate vesical neck sphincter	
Ephedrine sulphate (Ephedrine)	
Pseudoephedrine (Sudafed, Actifed)	
Phenylpropanolamine HCl (Propadrine)	
Imipramine[a] (Tofranil)	
Phenylephrine HCl	

[a]Prevents re-uptake of norepinephrine by nerve terminals, resulting in sympathomimetic action.
[b]Cholinesterase inhibitor.
[c]False neurotransmitter.

Adapted from W.A. Brock and G.W. Kaplan (1980) *Current Problems in Pediatrics*, **10**(8), 1–63.

effects on the musculature or indirect effects on ganglia. Table 21.1 is a list of compounds and their effects on the lower urinary tract. In practice only a few compounds have significant clinical effects which are useful. They include the anticholinergics propantheline bromide, methantheline bromide, and oxybutynin chloride, all of which aid in reducing detrusor instability and enabling the patient to have better control over his incontinence, and are a reasonable first choice in the wet patient. The proper initial doses of drug are summarized in Table 21.2. It is worthwhile to try several different compounds, for where one fails another may work. The usual doses of these drugs may be too low for some patients. Increased benefit can sometimes be seen with oxybutynin chloride in doses up to 40 mg/day or propanthelene bromide up to 180 mg/day with good tolerance. The side-effects of these drugs, which are largely caused by their anti-muscarinic effects, include dryness of salivary secretions, mydriasis, blurred vision, increased heart rate, mild drowsiness and constipation. Most of the symptoms are mild; the 'dry mouth' is the side-effect the patients most dislike. Watch for increasing difficulty with complete voiding and measure urinary residual if hesitancy and urinary tract infection occurs. The prescription of these compounds is contraindicated in glaucoma.

In the event that the anticholinergic compounds do not provide relief from symptoms, one may try tricyclic antidepressants, imipramine being quite effective. Imipramine seems to act directly on the smooth muscle of the bladder as an antispasmodic. The dose to be used is 0.5–1 mg kg^{-1} body weight. One should never exceed 1.5 mg kg^{-1} body weight per day since the drug can be quite toxic at higher levels. In general, the authors start out with the paediatric dose of 10 mg q.i.d. If this dose is ineffective, increase to full dosage. Unlike the antidepressant effects of imipramine, the bladder effects are immediate and last only as long as there is a blood level. The most frequent side-effects are produced by its anticholinergic activity and include dry mouth, constipation, blurred vision and tachycardia. Hypertensive patients should not receive these drugs since they make management of the blood pressure difficult. If they are used, the blood pressure must be monitored closely (weekly). Usage in patients with cardiovascular disease should be cautious. Incontinence at night can be controlled sometimes with intermittent self-catheterization at bedtime or intranasal vasopressin either alone or with anticholinergic drugs [53].

Increasing bladder outlet resistance

Theoretically, increasing the alpha response in the bladder neck [7, 54, 55] or urethra [56, 57] can augment continence. Practical application of this concept

Table 21.2 Basic therapy for failures to store

1. Propantheline bromide 15–30 mg q.i.d.
   [or]
   Oxybutynin chloride 5 mg t.i.d.
2. Imipramine 10–25 mg q.i.d.
3. Propantheline bromide
   [or]
   Oxybutynin *plus* imipramine

in patients with uninhibited-type neuropathic bladder has not been successful, however, but ephedrine sulphate 25 mg t.i.d. or q.i.d. may be tried.

Artificial sphincters

Multiple sclerosis patients with bladders that fail to store are not good candidates for management with artificial sphincters such as the Scott *et al.* type [58]. As a rule, these devices are employed in patients with inadequate outlet resistance, something that is rarely a problem in the type of neuropathic bladder that is seen in multiple sclerosis patients.

21.6.2 FAILURES TO EMPTY

It is when the urinary bladder fails to empty that one sees the major complications associated with destruction of renal tissue: obstruction, reflux and infection. In such cases the prime goal of therapy becomes to aid the bladder in emptying. Treatment can often be confusing unless one remembers the three goals of management, as discussed above, and these basic principles: try simple things first, tubeless drainage is usually superior to a tube, irreversible procedures such as surgery should be saved until last. The general scheme for managing the bladders that fail to empty is summarized in Table 21.3. When a method of management is initiated, it should be considered successful until infection (especially of the upper tract) or bacteriuria become uncontrollable, a high pressure bladder

Table 21.3 Basic therapy for failures to empty

1. Increase intravesical pressure
   (a) Pharmacology – bethanecol
   (b) Valsalva–Credé
2. Reduce outlet resistance – then employ Valsalva–Credé
   (a) Pharmacology – phenoxybenzamine
3. Intermittent catheterization
4. Surgery
   Resect sphincters (may reserve depending upon patient)
   Interrupt pudendal nerve
5. Permanent tube
6. Urinary diversion

occurs, hydroureteronephrosis appears, or renal function deteriorates. If these processes occur, then one proceeds to the next highest therapeutic maneuver listed in Table 21.3. The amount of residual urine, if less than normal bladder volume (400–450 ml), is not significant unless the patient is infected or shows upper tract damage (e.g. hydronephrosis). A residual urine of 250–300 ml in a dry patient with sterile urine and normal upper tracts is perfectly acceptable; an alteration in management may only make the patient worse. The first line of therapy to improve bladder emptying is increasing intravesical pressure.

Pharmacology

Of the acetylcholine-like drugs methacholine, carabachate, bethanecol chloride (Urecholine), pilocarpine, muscarine and arecoline, only bethanecol chloride exhibits any selective effect on the bladder and gastro-intestinal tract and little activity at the ganglionic level [59, 60]. However, oral administration of this drug has often not been found to be clinically useful as it can aggravate urgency and incontinence [23]. The employed doses are 25–50 mg q.i.d. orally; it should never be administered intramuscularly or intravenously since it could cause cardiac arrest.

Valsalva and Credé maneuvers

The use of Valsalva and Credé maneuvers, sometimes with massage of the bladder via the rectum, is often the simplest way to empty the bladder and should be employed first. These maneuvers are often successful in multiple sclerosis patients, especially females, since they have less resistance to urine flow at the bladder outlet.

Decreasing outlet resistance (pharmacologically)

Phenoxybenzamine is an alpha-blocking agent which, given in doses of 10 mg orally twice a day, may interfere with the tonic closure of the bladder neck [61–63]. It has limited clinical effects but it can be combined with Valsalva–Credé in a therapeutic trial to decrease bladder outlet resistance and facilitate voluntary bladder emptying. Phenoxybenzamine has many possible side-effects with which the prescribing physician should ensure familiarity. The alpha-blocker prazocin and the more selective alpha-1-blocker terazocin may be used with some improvement. One should watch for side-effects associated with possibly lowering blood pressure [46, 64]. Striated muscle relaxants (baclofen, diazepren, dantrolene) have been used but may increase general fatigue and muscle weakness [46]. Imipramine may be useful if the obstruction is primarily due to detrusor–sphincter dyssynergia [65].

Intermittent catheterization program

The single most important advance in the management of neuropathic bladders has been the development of the intermittent catheterization technique. This procedure involves catheterizing a patient at regular intervals in lieu of voiding and is extremely successful. At first look one might be repulsed by this concept but the data strongly support its success [66–68]. Approximately 50% of patients on this regimen will have sterile urine (as opposed to 0% with indwelling catheters) at any one time, with an overall infection rate of 20–30 infections for more than 1000 days of catheterization (number of patients on catheterization multiplied by days catheterized) [69]. Many of the episodes of bacteriuria can be managed with antibiotics, even with chronic suppression with low-dose antibiotic therapy when necessary. Patients with bacteriuria will often have lower titres of bacteria in their urine and the degree of pyuria is reduced. The majority of patients categorized as failures to empty are best managed with this program provided they have the motor coordination to perform it or someone else available to do it, and only when there is persistent symptomatic bacteriuria or signs of upper tract infection or deterioration should one alter management. In some MS patients managed with long-term intermittent catheterization, there is a gradual reduction of residual urine volume and catheterization may be stopped. Thus periodic review of bladder capacity and residual volume is prudent [65].

Reduction of outlet resistance surgically

The outlet resistance of the bladder can be reduced to a degree by overdilatation of the urethra or ablated surgically by destroying the bladder neck in the male [70–72]; If bladder neck resistance is reduced, the patient can then attempt Valsalva–Credé maneuvers. If this fails then external sphincterotomy can be performed [73–77], and also in the patient who has dyssynergic contraction of the external sphincter with voiding, leaving the bladder neck continent and having the patient attempt Valsalva–Credé maneuvers. Lastly, one can do a total urethral sphincterotomy in the male to render him incontinent, after which he can wear an external collecting device.

Ileal or colonic conduit diversion

Ileal or colonic conduit diversion in the earlier 1960s was felt to be the management of choice in bladders that were classified as failures to empty, but late complications of upper tract deterioration [78–81] make it essentially no better than chronic tube drainage with a suprapubic (male) or urethral (female) catheter. The decision as to whether to perform diversion or use chronic tube drainage is determined individually. The majority of patients today probably are placed on chronic tube diversion before a conduit is considered, the conduit reserved for those doing poorly on tube drainage. Multiple sclerosis patients in general tolerate bowel surgery poorly, which is another reason to avoid diversion.

21.6.3 FAILURES TO STORE AND EMPTY

As mentioned before, 50% of individuals with multiple sclerosis tend to develop a failure to store and failure to empty as their disease progresses. In general, it is this type of patient whom the author most often has referred to him by neurologists. The basic task of management is to convert the patient's bladder dysfunction from failure to store into a complete failure to empty pharmacologically and to then treat it as a failure to empty. The one situation in which the author has found it difficult to convert such cases into failures to empty is that of acute exacerbation of the multiple sclerosis; with remission, the symptoms often improve.

This presumes, of course, that the individual will have either sufficient muscular coordination to perform the intermittent catheterization necessary to treat a bladder that fails to empty or have an attendant who is capable of performing this task. In the event that neither is available, then one may be forced to treat the individual with Foley catheter drainage. As mentioned, 5–10% of patients ultimately will require this type of therapy.

21.6.4 DEVELOPMENT OF HIGH PRESSURE BLADDERS

A certain percentage of patients (30–50%) may develop high intravesical pressures for all the reasons stated above. Should this occur, patients are best treated by aggressive pharmacological manipulation to control the bladder contractions that usually lead to the high intravesical pressures. Then the patients can be treated as failures to empty. If the pharmacological manipulation fails to control the patient's high intravesical pressure, one may be forced to place an indwelling Foley catheter, which should resolve the problem.

21.7 Summary

Patients with multiple sclerosis can be difficult management problems. Initially, in the milder forms of the disease, most of the patients suffer from difficulty in controlling their detrusor reflex and they can be successfully managed with pharmacology. As the disease progresses and the neurologic deficit increases, they may develop bladders that have a dyssynergic voiding pattern or become areflexic, which results in combinations of failures to store and empty. In general, these patients are best treated with pharmacological manipulation to control the hyperreflexia and then treated as patients who fail to empty. It is recognized that a small percentage of patients, as the disease progresses, will require some type of medical therapy to stay dry and emptying may require therapy involving Foley or condom catheters. Both seem to be in a minority of the patients.

Overall, it is to be emphasized that no matter what course of therapy the patient has initially tried, as the disease progresses they may require a change in therapy even though they may be stable for many years. Careful monitoring for silent obstruction, infection or renal atrophy should be undertaken and a surveillance program of urine cultures, cystometrograms and upper tract evaluations should include IVP and ultrasound.

ACKNOWLEDGEMENTS

Figures 21.1–21.9 are reproduced from J.W. Duckett and D.M. Raezer (1976) Neuromuscular function of the lower urinary tract, in *Clinical Pediatric Urology*, vol. 1 (eds P.P. Kaelis and L.R. King), Philadelphia, Saunders, with permission.

References

1. Blaivas, J.G., Bhimani, G. and Labib, K.B. (1979) Vesicourethral dysfunction in multiple sclerosis. *J. Urol.*, **122**, 342–47.
2. Andersen, J.T. and Bradley, W.E. (1976) Bladder and urethral innervation in multiple sclerosis. *Br. J. Urol.*, **48**, 193–8.
3. Goldstein, I., Siroky, M.B., Sax, D.S. and Krane, R.J. (1982) Neurourologic abnormalities in multiple sclerosis. *J. Urol.*, **128**, 541–5.
4. Schoenberg, H.W. and Gutrich, J.M. (1980) Management of vesical dysfunction in multiple sclerosis. *Urology*, **16**, 444.
5. El-Badawi, A. and Schenk, E.A. (1966) Dual innervation of the mammalian urinary bladder: a histochemical study of the distribution of cholinergic and adrenergic nerves. *Am. J. Anat.*, **119**, 405–27.
6. El-Badawi, A. and Schenk, E.A. (1971) A new theory of the innervation of bladder musculature. II. The innervation apparatus of the ureterovesical junction. *J. Urol.*, **105**, 368–71.
7. Raezer, D.M., Wein, A.J., Jacobowitz, D. and Corriere, J.N. Jr (1973) Autonomic innervation of canine urinary bladder: cholinergic and adrenergic contributions and interaction of sympathetic and parasympathetic nervous systems in bladder function. *Urology*, **2**, 211–21.
8. Duckett, J.W. Jr and Raezer, D.M. (1976) Neuromuscular dysfunction of the lower urinary tract, in *Clinical Pediatric Urology*, vol. 1 (eds P.P. Kelalis and L.R. King), Philadelphia, W.B. Saunders pp. 401–26.
9. Fletcher, T.F. and Bradley, W.E. (1970) Vesical afferent endings in the cat. *Am. J. Anat.*, **128**, 147–58.
10. Uemura, E., Fletcher, T.F., Dirks, V.A. *et al.* (1973) Distribution of sacral afferent axons in the cat urinary bladder. *Am. J. Anat.*, **136**, 805–13.
11. Garry, R.C., Roberts, T.D.M. and Todd, J.K. (1959) Reflexes involving the external urethral sphincter in the cat. *J. Physiol.*, **149**, 653–5.
12. McGuire, E.J. (1986) Neuromuscular dysfunction of the lower urinary tract, in *Campbell's Urology*, 5th edn, vol. 1 (eds P.C. Walsh, R.F. Gittes, A.D. Perlmutter and T.A. Stamey), Philadelphia, W.B. Saunders, pp. 615–38.
13. Wein, A.J. (1992) Neuromuscular dysfunction of the lower urinary tract, in *Campbell's Urology*, 6th edn, vol. 1 (eds P.C. Walsh, A.B. Retik, T.A. Stamey and E.D. Vaughan Jr), Philadelphia, W.B. Saunders, pp. 573–642.
14. Sundin, T. and Dahlström, A. (1973) The sympathetic innervation of the urinary bladder and urethra in the normal state and after parasympathetic denervation at the spinal root level. An experimental study in cats. *Scand. J. Urol. Nephrol.*, **7**, 131–49.
15. Hamberger, B. and Norberg, K.A. (1965) Adrenergic synaptic terminals and nerve cells in bladder ganglia of the cat. *Int. J. Neuropharm.* **4**, 41–5.
16. Wakade, A.R. and Kirpekar, S.M. (1972) Sympathetic innervation of urinary bladder of the guinea pig. *Am. J. Physiol.*, **223**, 1477–80.
17. Benson, G.S., McConnel, J.A. and Wood, J.G. (1979) Adrenergic innervation of the human bladder body. *J. Urol.*, **122**, 189–91.
18. Edvardsen, P. (1967) Nervous control of urinary bladder in cats. A survey of recent experimental results and their relation to clinical problems. *Acta Neurol. Scand.*, **43**, 543–63.
19. Edvarsden, P. (1972) Neurophysiological aspects of enuresis. *Acta. Neurol. Scand.*, **48**, 222–30.
20. Benson, G., Raezer, D.M., Anderson, J.R. *et al.* (1976) The effect of L-dopa therapy on the urinary bladder. *Urology*, **7**, 24–8.
21. DeGroat, W.C. and Saum, W.R. (1971) Adrenergic inhibition in mammalian parasympathetic ganglia. *Nature (New Biol.)*, **231**, 188–9.
22. Wein, A.J., Gregory, J.G., Cromie, W.J. *et al.* (1974) Sympathetic innervation and chemical sympathectomy of canine bladder. *Urology*, **4**, 27–32.
23. Wein, A.J. (1979) Pharmacologic approaches to the management of neurogenic bladder dysfunction. *J. Cont. Ed. Urol.*, **18**, 17–34.
24. Kendall, A.R. and Karafin, L. (1974) Classification of neurogenic bladder disease. *Urol. Clin. North. Am.*, **1**, 37–44.
25. Bradley, W.E., Timm, G.W. and Scott, F.B. (1974) Innervation of the detrusor muscle and urethra. *Urol. Clin. North Am.*, **1**, 3–27.
26. Hopkins, W.F. and Pierce, J.M. Jr (1967) The neurogenic bladder in diabetes mellitus, in *Neurogenic Bladder* (ed. S. Boyarsky), Baltimore, MD, Williams and Wilkins, pp. 155–7.
27. Kondo, A. (1972) Visocoelastic properties of the bladder. PhD thesis, Faculty of Medicine, University of Sherbrooke, Sherbrooke, Quebec.
28. Kondo, A., Susset, J. and Lefaivre, J. (1972) Visocoelastic properties of bladder. I. Mechanical model and its mathematical analysis. *Invest. Urol.*, **10**, 154–63.
29. Perkash, I. and Giroux, J. (1985) Prevention, treatment, and management of urinary tract infections in neuropathic bladders. *J. Am. Paraplegia Soc.*, **8**, 15–17.
30. Coolsaet, B.L.R.A., van Venrooij, G.E.P.M. and Blok, C. (1982) Detrusor pressure versus wall stress in relation to ureterovesical resistance. *Neurourol. Urodyn.*, **1**, 105–12.
31. McGuire, E.J., Savastano, J.A. and Morrissey, S. (1983) Bladder and ureteral pressure relationships in nonhuman primates. *J. Urol.*, **130**, 374–6.
32. Betts, C.D., D'Mellow, M.T. and Fowler, C.J. (1993) Urinary symptoms and the neurological features of bladder dysfunction in multiple sclerosis. *J. Neurol. Neurosurg. Psychiatry*, **56**, 245–50.
33. Miller, H., Simpson, C.A. and Yeates, W.K. (1965) Bladder dysfunction in multiple sclerosis. *Br. Med. J.*, **1**, 1265–9.
34. Bradley, W.E., Logothetis, J.L. and Timm, G.W. (1973) Cystometric and sphincter abnormalities in multiple sclerosis. *Neurology*, **23**, 1131–9.
35. Piazza, D.H. and Diokno, A.C. (1979) Review of neurogenic bladder in multiple sclerosis. *Urology*, **14**, 33–5.
36. Summers, J.L. (1978) Neurogenic bladder in the woman with multiple sclerosis. *J. Urol.*, **120**, 555–6.
37. Awad, S.A., Gajewski, J.B., Sogbein, S.K., Murray, T.J. and Field, C.A. (1984) Relationship between neurological and urological states in patients with multiple sclerosis. *J. Urol.*, **132**, 499–502.
38. Damaski, M. and Sutcliffe-Kerr, A. (1964) Paraplegia of non-traumatic origin and disseminated (multiple) sclerosis: urinary complications, their nature and treatment. *Acta Neurol. Psychiatr. Belg.*, **64**, 495–519.
39. Samellas, W. and Rubin, B. (1965) Management of upper urinary tract complications in multiple sclerosis by means of diversion to an ileal conduit. *J. Urol.*, **93**, 548–52.
40. Phadke, J.G. (1987) Survival pattern and cause of death in patients with multiple sclerosis: results from an epidemiological survey in northeast Scotland. *J. Neurol. Neurosurg. Psychiatry*, **50**, 523–31.
41. Mayo, M.E. and Chetner, M.P. (1992) Lower urinary tract dysfunction in multiple sclerosis. *Urology*, **39**(1), 67–70.
42. Blaivas, J.G. (1980) Management of bladder dysfunction in multiple sclerosis. *Neurology*, **30**, 12–18.
43. Bradley, W.E. (1978) Urinary bladder dysfunction in multiple sclerosis. *Neurology*, **28**, 52–8.
44. Van Poppel, H., Vereecken, R.L. and Leruilte, A. (1983) Neuromuscular dysfunction of the lower urinary tract in multiple sclerosis. *Paraplegia*, **21**, 374–9.
45. McGuire, E.J. and Savastano, J.A. (1984) Urodynamic findings and long-term outcome management of patients with multiple sclerosis-induced lower urinary tract dysfunction. *J. Urol.*, **132**, 713–15.
46. Fowler, C.J., VanKerrebroeck, P.E.V., Nordenbo, A. and Van Poppel, H. (1992) Treatment of lower urinary tract dysfunction in patients with multiple sclerosis. *J. Neurol. Neurosurg. Psychiatry*, **55**, 986–9.
47. Lapides, J. (1967) Cystometry. *J. Am. Med. Assoc.*, **201**, 618–21.
48. Lapides, J. (1970) Neuromuscular vesical and ureteral dysfunction, in *Urology*, 3rd edn, vol. 2 (eds M.F. Campbell and J.H. Harrison), Philadelphia, W.B. Saunders, pp. 1343–78.
49. Scott, F.B., Quesada, E.M. and Cardus, D. (1964) Studies on the dynamics of micturition: observations on healthy men. *J. Urol.*, **92**, 455–63.
50. Scott, F.B., Quesada, E.M. and Cardus, D. (1967) The use of combined uroflowmetry, cystometry and electromyography in evaluation of neuro-

genic bladder dysfunction, in *Neurogenic Bladder*, Baltimore, MD, Williams and Wilkins, pp. 106–14.

51. Susset, J.G., Brissot, R.B. and Regnier, C.H. (1982) Stop flow technique: a way to measure detrusor strength. *J. Urol.*, **127**, 489.

52. Bidair, M., Teichman, J.M.H., Brodak, P.P. and Juma, S. (1993) Transrectal ultrasound urodynamics. *Urology*, **42**, 640–5.

53. Fowler, C.J. (1994) Bladder dysfunction in multiple sclerosis: causes and treatment. *Int. MS J.*, **1**, 91–107.

54. Awad, S.A., Bruce, A.W., Carro-Ciampi, G. *et al.* (1974) Distribution of a and β- adrenoreceptors in human urinary bladder. *Br. J. Pharmacol.*, **50**, 525–9.

55. Nergardh, A. and Boréus, L.O. (1972) Autonomic receptor function in the lower urinary tract of man and cat. *Scand. J. Urol. Nephrol.*, **6**, 32–6.

56. Tanagho, E.A., Meyers, F.H. and Smith, D.R. (1969) Urethral resistance: its components and implications. I. Smooth muscle component. *Invest. Urol.*, **7**, 136–49.

57. Diokno, A.C. and Taub, M. (1975) Ephedrine in treatment of urinary incontinence. *Urology*, **5**, 624–5.

58. Scott, F.B., Bradley, W.E. and Timm, G.W. (1973) Treatment of urinary incontinence by implantable prosthetic sphincter. *Urology*, **1**, 252–9.

59. Koelle, G.B. (1975) Anticholinesterase agents in *The Pharmacologic Basis of Therapeutics* (eds L.S. Goodman and A. Gilman), New York, Macmillan, pp. 445–66.

60. Koelle, G.B. (1975) Parasympathomimetic agents, in *The Pharmacologic Basis of Therapeutics* (eds L.S. Goodman and A. Gilman), New York, Macmillan, pp. 467–76.

61. Kleeman, F.J. (1970) The physiology of the internal urinary sphincter. *J. Urol.*, **104**, 549–54.

62. Krane, R.J. and Olsson, C.A. (1973) Phenoxybenzamine in neurogenic bladder dysfunction. I. A theory of micturition. *J. Urol.*, **110**, 650–2.

63. Awad, S.A., Downie, J.W., Lywood, D.W. *et al.* (1976) Sympathetic activity in the proximal urethra in patients with urinary obstruction. *J. Urol.*, **115**, 545–7.

64. Vereecken, R.L., Van Poppel, J., Boeckx, G. and Leruilte, A. (1988) Long term alpha-adrenergic blocking therapy in detrusor urethra dyssynergia. *Eur. Urol.*, **9**, 167–9.

65. Blaivas, J.G., Holland, N.J., Geisser, B., LaRocca, N. *et al.* (1984) Multiple sclerosis bladder. Studies and care. *Ann. NY Acad. Sci.*, **436**, 328–46.

66. Pearman, J.W. and England, E.J. (1973) *The Urological Management of the Patient Following Spinal Cord Injury*, Springfield, IL, Charles C. Thomas.

67. Donovan, W.H., Stolov, W.C., Clowers, D.E. and Clowers, M.R. (1978) Bacteriuria during intermittent catheterization following spinal cord injury. *Arch. Phys. Med. Rehab.*, **59**, 351–7.

68. Lapides, J., Diokno, A.C., Lowe, B.S. and Kalish, M.D. (1974) Follow-up on unsterile, intermittent self-catheterization. *J. Urol.*, **111**, 184–8.

69. Rhame, F.S. and Perkash, I. (1979) Urinary tract infections occurring in recent spinal cord injury patients on intermittent catheterization. *J. Urol.*, **122**, 669–73.

70. Bunce, P.L. (1967) Transurethral resection and Y-V plasty for neurogenic bladder, in *Neurogenic Bladder* (ed. S. Boyarsky), Baltimore, MD, Williams and Wilkins, pp. 196–9.

71. Comarr, A.E. (1959) The practical urological management of the patient with spinal cord injury. *Br. J. Urol.*, **31**, 1–46.

72. Turner-Warwick, R., Whiteside, C.G., Worth, P.H.L. *et al.* (1973) A urodynamic view of the clinical problems associated with bladder neck dysfunction and its treatment by endoscopic incision and transtrigonal posterior prostatectomy. *Br. J. Urol.*, **45**, 44–59.

73. Currie, R.J., Bilbisi, A.A., Schiebler, J.C. and Bunts, R.C. (1970) External sphincterotomy in paraplegics: technique and results. *J. Urol.*, **103**, 64–8.

74. Gibbon, N.O.K. (1973) Division of the external sphincter. *Br. J. Urol.*, **45**, 110–15.

75. Hackler, R.H. (1973) Spinal cord injuries: urologic care. *Urology*, **2**, 13–18.

76. Malament, M. (1972) External sphincterotomy in neurogenic bladder dysfunction. *J. Urol.*, **108**, 554–7.

77. Schellhammer, P.F., Hackler, R.H. and Bunts, R.C. (1973) External sphincterotomy: an evaluation of 150 patients with neurogenic bladder. *J. Urol.*, **110**, 199–202.

78. Gregory, J.G., Gursahani, M. and Schoenberg, H.W. (1974) Five-year radiographic review of ileal conduits. *J. Urol.*, **112**, 327–31.

79. Shapiro, S.R., Lebowitz, R. and Colodny, A.H. (1975) Fate of 90 children until ileal conduit urinary diversion a decade later: analysis of complications, pyelography, renal function and bacteriology. *J. Urol.*, **114**, 289–95.

80. Johnson, D.E. and Lamy, S.M. (1977) Complications of a single stage radical cystectomy and ileal conduit diversion: review of 241 cases. *J. Urol.*, **117**, 171–3.

81. Rabinowitz, R. and Price, S.E. Jr (1975) Ileal conduit urinary diversion in children. *J. Urol.*, **114**, 444–8.

22 SEXUAL DYSFUNCTION IN THE PATIENT WITH MULTIPLE SCLEROSIS

George S. Benson

Sexual dysfunction is a common symptom in patients with multiple sclerosis and is reported to be one of the most distressing aspects of their disease [1]. The incidence of erectile dysfunction in men has generally been reported to be in the 60–70% range, but, in the advanced stages of their disease, as many as 91% report a change in sexual function [2–4]. Some 56–72% of women with multiple sclerosis report sexual difficulties [4]. In one series, 33% of women experienced loss of orgasm, 27% loss of libido and 12% reported difficulty with sexual intercourse because of spasticity [4].

Recent advances in our understanding of the physiology of penile erection have led to new diagnostic and therapeutic approaches to patients with erectile dysfunction secondary to a variety of causes. At present, much more data exist concerning patients with erectile dysfunction from vascular or endocrinologic causes than in patients with neurologic disease. The primary reason for the relative paucity of information in patients with neurologic disease is the inability of current diagnostic studies to directly determine the integrity of the autonomic motor innervation of the penis. Little information exists concerning the anatomy and physiology of sexual function in women. There are virtually no data concerning the physiologic changes in women with multiple sclerosis which lead to sexual difficulties.

An understanding of the physiology of penile erection is important in determining appropriate clinical evaluation and therapy of impotence in men. The minimal information available concerning clitoral anatomy and function is also presented. This chapter has three major divisions: Mechanisms of penile and clitoral erection; Clinical evaluation of impotence in the patient with multiple sclerosis; and Therapy of impotence in the patient with multiple sclerosis.

22.1 Mechanisms of penile and clitoral erection

Our understanding of the physiology of penile erection has undergone major changes in the past decade. The most significant advance has been the recognition that the smooth muscle of the corpora cavernosa is of primary importance in the erectile process. Neurologic control of the cavernosal smooth muscle has been the subject of much recent research.

22.1.1 PENILE ANATOMY

Penile erectile tissue is contained within two dorsal corpora cavernosa and the single ventral corpus spongiosum which also contains the urethra (Figure 22.1). Each of the corporal bodies is surrounded by a layer of fibrous tissue (tunica albuginea). Buck's fascia lies superficial to the tunica albuginea and surrounds all three corporal bodies.

The erectile tissue of the corpora cavernosa and corpus spongiosum is comprised of cavernous spaces separated by trabeculae composed of smooth muscle, elastic fibers, collagen and fibroblasts. The surfaces of the trabeculae are lined by endothelial cells resembling those found in blood vessels [5]. Significant differences exist between the architecture of the corpora cavernosa and the corpus spongiosum. The corpus spongiosum is composed of larger cavernous spaces and smaller

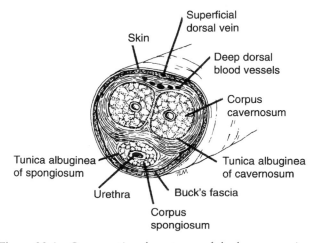

Figure 22.1 Cross-sectional anatomy of the human penis.

Multiple Sclerosis: Clinical and pathogenetic basis. Edited by Cedric S. Raine, Henry F. McFarland and Wallace W. Tourtellotte. Published in 1997 by Chapman & Hall, London. ISBN 0 412 30890 8.

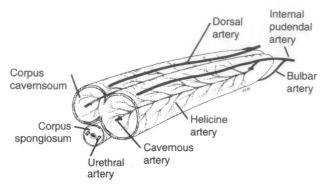

Figure 22.2 Arterial blood supply to the human penis.

trabeculae with fewer smooth muscle cells than are present in the corpora cavernosa.

The penile arterial blood supply is derived from the pudendal arteries, branches of the hypogastric arteries (Figure 22.2). The terminal portion of the pudendal artery gives off branches which supply the posterior scrotum and bulbous urethra and then divides into the dorsal and deep (central) arteries of the penis. The paired dorsal arteries course between Buck's fascia and the tunica albuginea of the corpora cavernosa. Anatomically, the primary blood supply to the erectile tissue of the corpora cavernosa is the paired deep (central) arteries. Numerous branches from the deep arteries further subdivide into helicine arteries which empty directly into the cavernous spaces [6]. In man, the paired central arteries are connected by anastomotic vessels which results in the two corpora functioning as a single unit. In addition, anastomoses between the dorsal and deep arterial systems as well as between the deep arteries and the arteries of the corpus spongiosum have been described [7–9]. The physiologic significance of these numerous anastomoses is not known.

The venous drainage of the penis is varied and complex (Figure 22.3) [6, 10]. Venules located just below the tunica albuginea drain the cavernous spaces. Venules join to form emissary veins which traverse the tunica albuginea and then drain into one of four primary venous drainage systems consisting of (1) the

superficial dorsal vein, (2) the deep dorsal vein, (3) the cavernous veins and (4) the urethral veins. The distal and mid-corpora cavernosa drain primarily by circumflex veins which enter the deep dorsal vein, while the proximal corpora cavernosa drain into the cavernous veins [11]. The superficial dorsal vein drains the penile skin while the urethral veins drain the proximal corpus spongiosum. Numerous anastomoses inter-connect all of the venous drainage systems.

The autonomic innervation of the corporal smooth muscle and its vasculature has been the subject of much recent investigation. Adrenergic nerves, whose neurotransmitter is by definition a catecholamine, are easily identified in the corpora cavernosa utilizing histo-fluorescent techniques [5]. These adrenergic fibers take a circuitous course through the trabeculae of the corpora and frequently approach the walls of the cavernous spaces. Few adrenergic fibers, however, can be identified in the corpus spongiosum. Adrenergic fibers can also be identified in the outer tunic of penile arterioles. Cholinergic nerves, whose neurotransmitter by definition is acetylcholine, are also present in the corpora cavernosa and in the outer tunic of penile arterioles, but the density of cholinergic innervation is much less than the density of the adrenergic innervation. Cholinergic nerves are sparse in the corpus spongiosum. In addition to adrenergic and cholinergic nerves, nerve fibers containing a variety of putative neurotransmitters have been identified in corporal tissue. Nerve fibers containing vasoactive intestinal polypeptide (VIP), substance P, somatostatin and neuropeptide Y (NPY) have been demonstrated with immunocytochemical and radioimmunoassay techniques [12–14]. VIP and NPY have also been colocalized in the same nerve terminals by immunocytochemistry in the corpora cavernosa of green monkeys [15]. Recently, much physiologic and pharmacologic evidence has been presented which implicates nitric oxide in the physiology of erection. Nitric oxide synthase, the enzyme that catalyzes nitric oxide production, has been identified in the pelvic plexus, cavernous nerves and their terminal endings within the corporal erectile tissue, branches of the dorsal penile nerves and nerve plexuses in the adventitia of the deep cavernosal arteries in man. In addition, these same nerves stain for reduced nicotinamide adenosine dinucleotide phosphate (NADPH) diaphorase. Since NADPH derives from nitric oxide synthase activity in neurons, this finding also supports the concept that nitric oxide is present in penile nerves [16]. The possible significance of this finding is discussed below.

22.1.2 NEUROVASCULAR ASPECTS OF ERECTION

Penile erection is a complex physiologic event under neurologic control. Erection is primarily a vascular phenomenon and results from both increased arterial

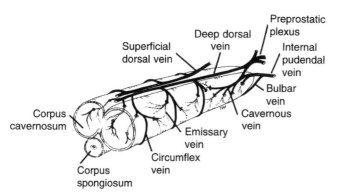

Figure 22.3 Venous drainage of the human penis.

blood flow into the corpora and 'trapping' of blood within the corpora because of increased venous resistance. The importance of increased arterial flow into the penis has been recognized for many years. The fact that in the cat aortic occlusion prevented the development of penile erection produced by sacral nerve root stimulation was observed in the 1930s and the Leriche syndrome (impotence associated with thrombotic obliteration of the aortic bifurcation) was described in the 1940s [17, 18]. Recent clinical studies utilizing color Doppler technology have reconfirmed the importance of increased arterial flow into the penis during the development of penile erection [19]. In man, erection can be produced by the infusion of saline directly into the corpora cavernosa at rates of 20–50 ml/min. Erection can be maintained at lower perfusion rates (approximately 10 ml/min) [20].

Although the necessity of obstruction of venous outflow in the production of full penile erection has been debated for years, most investigators currently believe that the development of a rigid erection does require venous blockade. Initial studies in the canine were unable to detect a pressure gradient during erection between the corpora cavernosa and the internal pudendal vein [21]. Subsequent studies in animal models, however, indicated that the production of increased venous resistance may be an important factor in the normal physiology of penile erection. In the dog, the highest pressures in the corpora cavernosa occur during intromission and coincide with the maximum electromyographic activity in the ischiocavernosus muscles [22]. The injection of lidocaine into the ischiocavernosus muscles prevents the goat, stallion and bull from achieving an erection [22, 23]. These animal data are consistent with the hypothesis that contraction of the perineal musculature results in venous obstruction and promotes erection. Electromyography of perineal musculature in man, however, reveals that erection can occur without contraction of the bulbocavernosus or deep transverse perineal musculature [24]. Conflicting data in man utilizing the ^{133}Xe washout technique have been presented; discrepancies in results are probably related to measuring ^{133}Xe washout during different phases of the erectile process [25, 26]. Recent work by Lue *et al.* performed in the dog and monkey has clarified much of our understanding of the hemodynamic aspects of erection [27, 28]. By producing erection with electrical cavernous nerve stimulation and simultaneously infusing saline directly into the corpora cavernosa, Lue demonstrated that both relaxation of the trabeculae of the corpora cavernosa and impedance of venous outflow from the penis were necessary for the development of penile erection. This obstruction to venous flow is thought to be secondary to passive obstruction of the venules draining the corpora secondary to high intracorporal pressure generated during erection.

The two primary events leading to erection, namely relaxation of the smooth muscle of the corpora cavernosa and penile arteriolar dilatation, are clearly under neurologic control. The peripheral nerve supply to the penis in man has only relatively recently been described in detail. The paired cavernosal nerves are derived from the pelvic ganglionic plexus located retroperitoneally near the rectum [29]. The pelvic plexus receives innervation from both the sympathetic and parasympathetic divisions of the autonomic nervous system (Figure 22.4). The parasympathetic component is derived from nerves whose cell bodies are located in the sacral (S2–4) spinal cord. These parasympathetic fibers unite to form the pelvic nerve which courses in the endopelvic fascia before entering the pelvic plexus. Sympathetic nerve fibers are derived from the lower thoracic and upper lumbar portion of the spinal cord and course retroperitoneally before converging into the superior hypogastric plexus, which is located inferior to the aortic bifurcation. The paired hypogastric nerves carry sympathetic fibers from the superior hypogastric plexus to the pelvic plexus. After leaving the pelvic plexus, the right and left cavernosal nerves course between the rectum and urethra, pierce the urogenital diaphragm near the urethra and enter the dorsal medial aspect of the corpora cavernosa. Other nerves leaving the pelvic plexus innervate the bladder, seminal vesicles, vasa deferentia, prostate and rectum. The sensory innervation of the penis is carried in the dorsal nerve of the

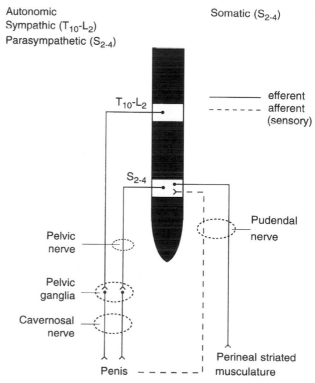

Figure 22.4 Innervation of human penis.

penis, a branch of the pudendal nerve which courses with the internal pudendal artery and vein along the lateral wall of the ischiorectal fossa.

The importance of the parasympathetic pelvic nerves has been recognized since Eckhard's demonstration that stimulation of these nerves causes erection in the dog[30]. The role of the sympathetic nervous system is less well defined. Classic experiments by Muller in the dog and Root and Bard in the cat are consistent in both findings and conclusions[31, 32]. In both the dog and cat, reflex erections secondary to genital stimulation can no longer be produced after ablation of the sacral and lower lumbar spinal cord. These animals do, however, still achieve erection when placed in proximity to an estrous female. In addition, when male cats or dogs undergo transection of the spinal cord at a low thoracic level, no erections are observed in the presence of an estrous female, but full erections can be produced by genital stimulation. Furthermore, ablation of the abdominal sympathetic nerves has no effect on erection in animals with an intact spinal cord. These data are consistent with the hypothesis that two neural pathways for the production of erection exist in these animal models: (1) a sacral parasympathetic center capable of producing penile erection secondary to either genital or psychic stimulation and (2) a lumbar sympathetic center capable of responding to psychic stimulation.

Very few similar data exist in man. Some information has been gathered from patients with spinal cord injury, although these reports are difficult to evaluate because the extent of the neurologic deficit is often difficult to document and the data have been obtained by retrospective questionnaire or interview. Two large series of patients with spinal cord injury have been studied by Bors and Comarr[33, 34]. None of the patients with complete lower motor neuron lesions (no reflex activity through the sacral cord) experienced erections secondary to genital stimulation. Twenty-four per cent of these patients, however, did experience erections secondary to psychic stimuli. In patients with complete suprasacral spinal cord injury, the ability to achieve erection from psychic or genital stimuli depended upon the level of the injury. In patients with cervical cord injury, only 4% were able to achieve erection with psychic stimuli while 91% achieved erection with genital stimulation. In patients with lumbar spinal cord lesions, 57% achieved psychogenic and 100% reflexogenic erections. These data are, in general, in agreement with the data obtained from animal models. It is clear that ablation of the abdominal sympathetic nerves has no adverse effect on penile erection in man because men undergoing extensive retroperitoneal lymph node dissection for testicular cancer experience no difficulty with erectile function[35, 36]. Although the role of the thoracolumbar sympathetic nerves in penile erection is not completely understood, the primary innervation responsible for erection in man appears to be the sacral parasympathetic system.

22.1.3 NEUROPHARMACOLOGY OF ERECTION

Recent neuropharmacologic research has not only yielded significant new information concerning the physiologic mechanisms of erection but has also resulted in innovative approaches to the treatment of erectile dysfunction. As previously discussed, electrical stimulation of pelvic parasympathetic nerves does result in penile erection; this erection is, however, not abolished by pretreatment with atropine. Penile erection, therefore, is not considered to be a cholinergically, or exclusively cholinergically, mediated event.

A major advance in our understanding of penile physiology occurred with the demonstration that the intracavernosal injection of drugs which relax corporal smooth muscle causes penile erection[37, 38]. Papaverine and phentolamine were the first such drugs described but, subsequently, the intracavernosal injection of imipramine, nitroglycerin, verapamil and prostaglandin E_1 was also shown to cause penile erection[39–42]. All of these agents cause both relaxation of the corporal smooth muscle as well as increased arterial flow into the penis. The clinical use of these drugs has proved efficacious in the therapy of erectile dysfunction, particularly in patients with neurologic disorders[41–44].

Although it is clear that relaxation of the corpora cavernosa and increased arterial inflow are of primary importance in the development of erection, the neurologic control of these processes is unclear. Specifically, the neurotransmitter(s) responsible for penile smooth muscle relaxation is not known[45]. In an attempt to explain the atropine-resistant relaxation of corporal smooth muscle, studies of a variety of putative non-adrenergic non-cholinergic neurotransmitters have been undertaken. Bradykinin, 5-hydroxytryptamine, prostaglandins and histamine do not appear to be responsible for normal penile erection[46, 47]. Because VIP has been reported to cause relaxation of corporal tissue *in vitro*, some investigators have suggested that VIP is the non-adrenergic non-cholinergic neurotransmitter responsible for penile erection. This polypeptide has been proposed to be a neurotransmitter in both vascular and non-vascular smooth muscle, and in cerebral vessels VIP is thought to act as an inhibitory cotransmitter with acetylcholine[48]. *In vivo* experiments of the effects of VIP on penile erection have yielded contradictory results. In monkeys, the intracavernosal injection of VIP has yielded conflicting results ranging from no response to full penile erection[14]. VIP may be involved with the physiology of penile erection, but its exact role is still uncertain.

The recent recognition of the importance of endothelium-derived relaxation factor (EDRF) in the physiology of vascular smooth muscle relaxation has led to new insights into the mechanisms responsible for penile erection. This endothelium-dependent relaxation is mediated by nitric oxide[49]. In strips of corporal smooth muscle from rabbit and man, nitric oxide causes relaxation which mimics electrical field stimulation. This relaxation occurs in the presence of guanethidine and atropine in the bathing medium and is therefore thought to be mediated by nonadrenergic, noncholinergic neurons[50]. Acetylcholine is also capable of causing endothelium-dependent relaxation by mechanisms which involve nitric oxide[51]. The relaxation produced by nitric oxide is mediated through increased intracellular levels of cyclic GMP. Relaxant responses to nitric oxide are enhanced by pretreating the smooth muscle strips with a cyclic GMP phosphodiesterase inhibitor. These observations support the hypothesis that stimulation of nonadrenergic, noncholinergic neurons in the corpus cavernosum increases the endogenous formation of nitric oxide in either neurons, smooth muscle, or endothelial cells. Nitric oxide then causes smooth muscle relaxation through a cyclic GMP mechanism.

The neuropharmacology of corporal smooth muscle contraction is better understood. Detumescence is thought to be caused by sympathetic nerve stimulation acting via alpha-adrenergic receptors. Stimulation of strips of corporal smooth muscle with a variety of alpha-adrenergic agonists results in contraction[5]. The most convincing evidence that the sympathetic nervous system acting through alpha-adrenergic receptors promotes penile detumescence is the fact that priapism can be treated by the intracorporal injection of alpha-adrenergic agonists such as phenylephrine[52, 53].

22.1.4 CLITORAL ANATOMY AND FUNCTION

The clitoris has not been as extensively studied as its male counterpart. Like the penis, the clitoris consists of two paired corpora cavernosa and a glans clitoris. Unlike the penis, however, the clitoris does not contain a corpus spongiosum. As in the male penis, the corpora cavernosa of the clitoris are composed of sinusoids lined by endothelial cells and smooth muscle. Histochemical studies of human clitoral erectile tissue have demonstrated vasoactive intestinal polypeptide (VIP) and neuropeptide Y (NPY) immunoreactive nerves[54].

In the canine, cavernosal nerve stimulation does result in both increased internal pudendal arterial blood flow and increased clitoral cavernosal pressure. Intracavernosal pressure increases in the clitoris are, however, much lower than those generated in the penis from cavernosal nerve stimulation; penile intracavernosal pressure increases about 15-fold and clitoral intracavernosal pressure increases only two-fold over baseline[55]. Clitoral engorgement is thought to be responsible for extrusion of the glans clitoris[56].

22.2 Clinical evaluation of impotence in the patient with multiple sclerosis

Impotence is a common complaint in the male with multiple sclerosis. Most of these patients are 20–40 years old and in some the erectile dysfunction is temporally related to the diagnosis of multiple sclerosis and not to the onset of neurologic symptoms. The psychologic impact of the diagnosis of multiple sclerosis can undoubtedly contribute to erectile difficulty. When evaluating the patient with multiple sclerosis, two facts must be kept in mind. First, the erectile dysfunction may not be the direct result of neurologic disease and, secondly, no reliable laboratory tests exist to prove that impotence is secondary to neurologic disease.

22.2.1 HISTORY AND PHYSICAL EXAMINATION

The initial evaluation of the patient with multiple sclerosis and impotence should be directed at both neurologic and non-neurologic causes of erectile dysfunction. The duration and nature of onset of impotence often aid in the differentiation of psychogenic from an organic etiology. Patients with impotence on a primarily psychogenic basis often experience an abrupt onset of symptoms. Most causes of organic impotence, however, result in a slow but progressive deterioration in erectile ability. The occurrence of morning erections and the occurrence of erections in situations apart from the usual sexual partner are important historical facts.

A history of symptoms consistent with not only neurologic but also vascular, hormonal and other systemic diseases should be obtained. Changes in libido should alert the physician to the possibility of a hormonal abnormality. Symptoms compatible with intermittent claudication should be sought. Questions related to specific diseases (atherosclerosis and diabetes mellitus), previous pelvic surgery and radiation therapy should be asked. A detailed history of bladder and bowel symptoms should be obtained, particularly in patients with multiple sclerosis. Several reports have shown a relationship between bladder dysfunction and sexual dysfunction in patients with multiple sclerosis[3, 57]. All medications taken by the patient should be noted. Many drugs, particularly those which act on the vascular or nervous systems, have been associated with erectile dysfunction. All unnecessary medication should be discontinued. Although it is reasonable to change medication and dosages in patients who require therapy for hypertension or psychiatric disease in an attempt to improve erectile function, these efforts are usually not beneficial.

A complete physical examination should be performed with emphasis on neurologic, vascular, genital and hormonal abnormalities. A neurologic examination to include perineal sensation in the area of the sacral dermatomes and the quality of rectal sphincter tone should be performed. The presence or absence of the bulbocavernosus reflex, elicited by simultaneously squeezing the glans penis and noting anal sphincter contraction, should be noted. The femoral and peripheral lower extremity arteries should be palpated and the abdomen and femoral areas examined for bruits. The prostate gland should be examined and the abdomen palpated to ascertain the presence of a distended bladder. The size and consistency of the tests should be noted. The genital area should be inspected for hygiene and the type of urinary collecting devices used if the patient is incontinent. A sensory examination of the skin of the genitalia should be performed.

22.2.2 LABORATORY EVALUATION

The laboratory evaluation of the patient with impotence, particularly the patient with multiple sclerosis, is controversial. Determination of serum testosterone is a reasonable hormonal screening study. Serum prolactin is not routinely measured unless the serum testosterone is low or the patient complains of decreased libido. A serum multiple analysis (SMAC) is helpful and serves as a screening study for diabetes, liver disease and renal function. Because of the significant incidence of urinary tract disease as well as sexual dysfunction in patients with multiple sclerosis, a urinalysis should be obtained.

22.2.3 NEUROLOGIC TESTING

When performing neurophysiologic testing on impotent patients, including the patient with multiple sclerosis, two important points need to be remembered. First, the presence of a demonstrable neurologic lesion does not necessarily indicate that the lesion is responsible for the patient's erectile dysfunction and, secondly, currently utilized neurologic studies do not directly measure the integrity of the autonomic innervation of the penis. In addition, therapeutic decisions are generally not based on the results of neurologic testing and these studies are, therefore, not routinely indicated.

The integrity of neural pathways can be ascertained by measuring evoked potentials. Both sacral evoked potentials and genitocerebral evoked potentials have been utilized in the evaluation of patients with erectile dysfunction [58, 59]. Both of these studies, however, do have significant limitations in the evaluation of impotence. The sacral evoked potential (sacral latency) is an electrophysiologic study that essentially measures the latency of the bulbocavernosus reflex. The test is performed by electrically stimulating penile skin and recording bulbocavernosus muscle activity by means of

a needle electrode. The time from stimulation to first response of the bulbocavernosus muscle is measured and termed the sacral latency. As previously discussed, penile erection is normally governed by a reflex consisting of pudendal afferent (sensory) fibers and parasympathetic efferent (motor) fibers. The sensory portion of the reflex that governs erection and the sensory portion of the reflex which is measured by sacral evoked potential testing are, therefore, identical. This portion of the reflex arc can also be evaluated by performing dorsal penile nerve conduction velocity [60]. The efferent (parasympathetic) portion of the reflex controlling erection cannot be adequately studied by means currently available. The sacral latency measures reflex activity over pudendal sensory nerves and pudendal (somatic) motor nerves. Although measurement of the sacral evoked response does provide some information concerning reflex activity through the sacral spinal cord, it does not directly test penile autonomic innervation.

Sacral-evoked response measurement has been recommended in the evaluation of impotence associated with multiple sclerosis [3]. In a comprehensive study of 41 men with multiple sclerosis, sexual dysfunction was present in 29. Eight of these 29 patients had prolonged sacral latency values. The authors concluded that abnormal sacral-evoked responses may imply neurogenic impotence. In this study the authors also observed patients with a combination of abnormal perineal electromyography, abnormal sacral latency and bladder detrusor hyperreflexia, which suggests multilevel spinal cord dysfunction.

The objective measurement of the integrity of the central nervous system as it relates to erectile function is even more limited. Genitocerebral evoked responses have been measured following electrical stimulation of the penis and recording from electroencephalographic leads on the scalp [59]. As with the sacral evoked response, an abnormal genitocerebral evoked response must be cautiously interpreted. Although an abnormal evoked response may be demonstrated, it may bear no relationship to the patient's symptom of erectile dysfunction.

Urodynamic studies designed to test bladder and urethral innervation are at times helpful in evaluating the patient with multiple sclerosis [3]. A cystometrogram that demonstrates detrusor contractions indicates that the parasympathetic motor fibers to the bladder are intact. Since bladder and penile efferent innervation originates from the same levels of the sacral spinal cord, demonstration of bladder contraction indicates that at least some reflex activity is occurring at the level of the sacral spinal cord. In addition, since patients with multiple sclerosis are at increased risk for lower urinary tract dysfunction, urodynamic testing is often beneficial in the urologic management of these patients.

22.2.4   TESTING WITH INTRACORPORAL INJECTION OF VASOACTIVE DRUG

In 1982, Virag reported that the intracorporal injection of the smooth muscle relaxant papaverine resulted in penile erection[37]. Subsequently, alpha-adrenergic blocking agents such as a phenoxybenzamine and drug combinations of papaverine and phentolamine were found to produce similar results[38]. Multiple other agents, including verapamil and imipramine, demonstrate similar effects[39]. Prostaglandin E_1 alone or in combination with other agents (papaverine and phentolamine) is currently the most widely used drug for intracorporal injection[42, 61]. Maximum erection is usually evident within 10–20 minutes.

The office use of these drugs has been advocated as a diagnostic tool in evaluating patients with erectile dysfunction. If, after the injection of vasoactive drug, the patient develops a rigid erection that lasts for more than 15 minutes, significant arterial disease or 'venous leakage' is unlikely[62]. The presence of an erection after the intracorporal injection of drug does not rule out a psychogenic or a neurogenic etiology of erectile dysfunction. In fact, patients with neurologic lesions often respond to lower doses of vasoactive drugs than do patients with impotence secondary to other etiologies[44]. If the patient does not develop an erection following the injection of vasoactive drug, no conclusion can be drawn. Either vascular disease or neurologic disease may be present. In addition, anxiety with presumably increased sympathetic nervous system activity may account for the lack of response to drug injection. In the patient with multiple sclerosis, therefore, testing with intracavernosal drugs yields little diagnostic information. Patients who desire self-intracavernosal injection as a means of therapy should undergo office testing. This will be subsequently addressed.

22.2.5   VASCULAR STUDIES

Until relatively recently, most men presenting with a complaint of erectile dysfunction, including those with overt neurologic disease, underwent evaluation of their penile arterial blood supply with Doppler penile blood pressure determinations. The central artery pressure was divided by the brachial artery pressure and the penile–brachial index determined. This non-invasive, readily available study is no longer considered to be a reliable screening study for two reasons. First, the conventional Doppler ultrasound wave is so wide that the operator cannot be sure which artery (dorsal, cavernosal, or urethral) is being evaluated. Secondly, the study is performed with the penis in the unstimulated, flaccid state and the significance of the results obtained uncertain.

Most investigators currently utilize duplex Doppler or color Doppler studies before and after the intra-cavernosal injection of vasoactive drugs. To evaluate the penile arterial blood supply, individual arteries can be visualized, their diameters measured, and arterial blood flow velocity determined. Blood flow can then be calculated utilizing the diameter and flow velocity data. Values for 'normal arterial capacity' have been set at an increase in mean arterial diameter of more than 75% of the flaccid value and a mean peak flow velocity of greater than 25 cm/second following the intracavernosal injection of vasoactive drug[63]. Questions concerning the accuracy and reliability of this study have been raised. The accuracy of the diameter measurements in these small vessels and the relationship between blood flow velocity and actual blood flow have been questioned. Normal values have not been well defined. Despite the uncertainties in interpretation of the results of duplex or color Doppler evaluation, this study is generally considered to be the screening study of choice. When an abnormal duplex or color Doppler is obtained, and when the patient is considered a candidate for a penile arterial revascularization operation, penile arteriography is performed. Arteriography, following the intracavernosal and/or intra-arterial injection of vasoactive drugs, is an anatomic study which aids in the planning of arterial reconstructive surgery[64].

Which patients with erectile dysfunction should undergo an evaluation of the penile arterial supply? Should any patient with multiple sclerosis and impotence be evaluated? In general, only patients who are considered candidates for arterial reconstructive surgery should undergo evaluation. The definition of 'suitable candidates' is totally dependent upon the urologist's opinion of which patients really benefit from penile arterial reconstruction. Reported success rates vary considerably (from 20% to 80%)[65, 66]. The best results (approximately 80%) are reported in young men with isolated vascular injury secondary to pelvic trauma, while only approximately 25% of patients with generalized atherosclerosis benefit from the procedure[66]. The efficacy of arterial reconstructive surgery is such that, in my opinion, only young patients with a history of pelvic trauma should be studied. I do not routinely perform penile arterial studies on patients with multiple sclerosis and impotence. These patients already have two significant risk factors (neurologic and psychologic) and I do not think performance of arterial studies is warranted.

The same clinical reasoning applies to the performance of studies aimed at evaluating the venous drainage. As previously discussed, penile erection is dependent not only on increased arterial perfusion and smooth muscle relaxation of the corpora cavernosa, but also on increased venous resistance and 'trapping' of blood within the cavernous spaces. The venous component of the erectile process is currently evaluated by cavernosometry and cavernosography. These studies are performed by the infusion of saline (or contrast) directly into the corpora after the intracavernosal injection of vasoactive drug [67]. The maintenance flow rate necessary to maintain high intracorporal pressure or the decay rate following discontinuation of infusion is measured. Standardized methodology for the performance of these studies and normal control data are lacking. Furthermore, the results of venous ligation surgery vary considerably; the restoration of potency has been reported to occur in 28–73% of patients [68]. As reported success rates have fallen, more extensive surgical procedures have been described. In summary, the efficacy of venous ligation surgery remains in doubt. With so many unanswered questions, I do not believe that the patient with multiple sclerosis and impotence should undergo studies to determine the presence of a 'venous leak'.

22.2.6 NOCTURNAL PENILE TUMESCENCE (NPT) TESTING

Nocturnal erections normally occur approximately five times per night and are temporally related to rapid eye movement (REM) sleep [69]. A variety of transducers and recorders have been developed to objectively measure penile tumescence and rigidity during sleep. For years, NPT testing was considered the 'gold standard' for the diagnosis of erectile dysfunction. Full, sustained erections during sleep were indicative of psychogenic impotence, while the absence of turgid nocturnal erections indicated organic impotence [70]. The value of NPT testing is currently controversial. Although in some instances men with psychogenic impotence may not experience nocturnal penile tumescence, the presence of rigid nocturnal erections strongly supports a diagnosis of psychogenic impotence. The significance of impaired or abnormal nocturnal erections is less clear. Numerous cases of patients with abnormal NPT patterns suggestive of impotence exist in which the patient reports normal coital activity [71]. Dreams with high anxiety content may not be associated with nocturnal penile tumescence at all or may cause rapid detumescence [69, 72]. Conversely, normal NPT tracings have been reported in patients with impotence secondary to hyperprolactinemia and the 'pelvic steal' syndrome [71]. NPT testing alone is not adequate to differentiate psychogenic from organic erectile dysfunction. Because of this shortcoming, NPT testing is not routinely performed in patients with multiple sclerosis and impotence.

22.3 Therapy of impotence in the patient with multiple sclerosis

No specific therapy exists which will cure erectile dysfunction secondary to multiple sclerosis. If low serum testosterone levels are documented, a serum prolactin level should be obtained and the patient treated with intramuscular injections of testosterone. If the patient's erectile dysfunction improves, therapy is continued with the realization that the response may be secondary to placebo effect. Testosterone therapy in patients with normal serum testosterone levels is no more efficacious than placebo [73]. In addition, significant side-effects can and do occur with testosterone therapy. Testosterone is contraindicated in the presence of prostate cancer and, before initiating therapy, digital rectal examination and a prostate-specific antigen (PSA) test should be performed. Despite the fact that hepatotoxicity has been markedly reduced when esterified rather than alkylated testosterone is used, evaluation of liver function studies before and periodically during therapy is prudent. Androgen therapy has been demonstrated to increase hematocrit and red blood cell volume and a serum hematocrit should be periodically determined in patients on long-term testosterone [74].

Other drugs have been advocated for the therapy of impotence. Yohimbine, in combination with testosterone, was extensively used for the treatment of impotence in the 1960s. Although initial recent studies suggested that yohimbine was effective in the therapy of erectile dysfunction, further controlled studies have shown no statistical difference between yohimbine and placebo in treating patients with organic impotence [75, 76]. In summary, if the patient with multiple sclerosis has a normal serum testosterone level, testosterone therapy is not indicated. Liberal use of psychiatric, psychologic and sex therapy experts is helpful. If these methods fail, three therapeutic options are available:

1. intracavernosal injection therapy;
2. vacuum-constriction devices;
3. penile prostheses.

Because symptoms and objective findings in patients with multiple sclerosis may change over time, initial therapy should be conservative and potentially reversible [3].

22.3.1 INTRACAVERNOSAL INJECTION THERAPY

Reports of clinical trials of intracavernosal injection therapy emerged soon after the demonstration that penile erection could be produced by injecting agents which relax corporal smooth muscle directly into the penis. Initially, papaverine alone and combinations of papaverine and phentolamine were used. Patients are taught to inject themselves and the correct dosage of drug determined in the physician's office (Figure 22.5). After the patient has mastered the technique, he is allowed to inject himself once or twice a week at home. Since the two corporal bodies are connected by vascular

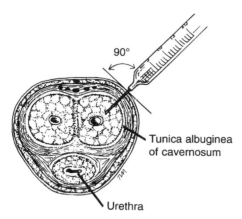

Figure 22.5 Technique of intracavernosal injection of vasoactive drugs.

spaces, the patient is required to inject the drug only into one corporal body to achieve an erection.

Significant complications, particularly with the use of papaverine alone and papaverine–phentolamine mixtures, have been reported. Both fibrotic penile lesions and penile nodules occur in a significant number of patients [77, 78]. The fibrosis may be related to the acidic pH of papaverine. In animal studies, long-term use of papaverine causes not only fibrosis in the area of injection sites, but also corporal smooth muscle hypertrophy in other areas of the penis [79]. Although hepatotoxicity is a known side-effect of papaverine use, this complication has been rarely reported in patients in self-injection programs [78].

By far the most significant complication of intracorporal injection therapy is the occurrence of priapism. Although the exact incidence is not known, it has been reported to occur in 1–4% of patients [44, 78]. Priapism tends to occur during the initial injection phase in the physician's office or when patients inject themselves with higher than the recommended dose. The treatment of choice for drug-induced priapism is the intracorporal injection of an alpha-adrenergic agonist [52, 53]. These agents cause contraction of corporal smooth muscle and detumescence in the majority of patients. Phenylephrine, norepinephrine, epinephrine and metaraminol have all been utilized [80]. Because phenylephrine possesses less beta-adrenergic activity than the other agents, it is currently the drug of choice to treat priapism [81].

PGE$_1$ does appear to have some advantages over other agents. Enzymes that metabolize PGE$_1$ are present in penile tissue, and therefore, at least theoretically, the risk of priapism is lessened [82]. Large series of patients have been reported in which the efficacy and low complication rate have been documented [42, 83]. Priapism does occur, but the frequency appears to be less than with papaverine–phentolamine mixtures.

Several points regarding self-injection therapy, particularly in patients with neurologic disease, deserve emphasis. Manual dexterity and the willingness to inject one's penis with drug are obvious prerequisites. Patients with impotence secondary to neurologic disease tend to respond to lower doses of drugs than patients whose impotence is secondary to other causes. The risk of priapism, therefore, must always be kept in mind. Although many patients initially do well on self-injection programs, only approximately 50% of those initially enrolled continue to inject themselves at one year [78]. Detailed informed consent should be obtained and the patient should be provided with readily available access to medical care should complications arise.

22.3.2 VACUUM-CONSTRICTION DEVICES

Vacuum-constriction devices have in recent years become an increasingly popular form of management of impotence secondary to many etiologies. The majority of these devices consist of a plastic cylinder placed over the penis, tubing connected to a hand-held vacuum pump which creates negative pressure within the cylinder, and elastic constriction bands which are placed around the base of the penis once an erection is obtained (Figure 22.6). High patient acceptance rates and extremely low morbidity have been reported [84]. A questionnaire survey of 1517 users of this device showed that 92% of patients obtained a satisfactory erection when using the device and 77% of patients engaged in intercourse at least every two weeks [85]. Only one case report of a significant complication has surfaced. A paraplegic patient suffered skin necrosis when the constricting band was left on the penis for a prolonged period [86]. Many patients are able to ejaculate even though the constricting band is in place. The use of the device does require some degree of manual dexterity, and some patients with multiple

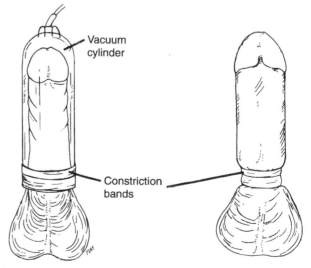

Figure 22.6 Vacuum-constriction device.

sclerosis may not be able to manage a vacuum-constriction device successfully. Patients tend to use the device with more frequency when they have a steady, supportive sexual partner.

22.3.3 PENILE PROSTHESES

Further experience is needed to define the precise roles of vacuum-constriction devices and intracorporal injection therapy, and to determine how these treatments will interface with the surgical implantation of penile prostheses. Prostheses have been a mainstay in the therapy of impotence for approximately 15 years. A variety of new devices are currently available for implantation, but the indications for insertion and surgical techniques have essentially not changed since their introduction.

The indications for penile prosthesis implantation include organic impotence and psychogenic impotence refractory to psychiatric therapy. Because symptoms, presumably including impotence, of multiple sclerosis may wax and wane, many urologists are hesitant to implant penile prostheses in this group of patients. If, for reasons such as infection and erosion, the prosthesis needs to be removed, the patient may be worse than before implantation.

A variety of penile prostheses are available. These can be grouped into semirigid prostheses, mechanically activated prostheses and inflatable prostheses [87]. The operative techniques and operative morbidity are similar. Incisions are made in each corpus and cylinders inserted bilaterally. When inflatable prostheses are placed, the pump mechanism is placed in the scrotum (Figure 22.7). Although outpatient surgery in this situation has been advocated, most urologists prefer to hospitalize patients for one or two days.

Complications of prosthetic surgery include infection, urethral or skin erosion, and device malfunction [88]. Infection and erosion nearly always necessitate device removal and malfunction of the prosthesis requires operative replacement. The device malfunction rates are predictably higher with the mechanically activated and inflatable prostheses. Despite potential problems, the majority of patients and their sexual partners are satisfied following insertion of a penile prosthesis [89, 90]. With proper patient selection and preoperative counseling, satisfaction rates with all types of prostheses are high. Unrealistic expectations, cost of the prosthesis and possibility of reoperation are all important issues to discuss in the preoperative consultation.

22.4 Conclusion

Sexual dysfunction in both men and women with multiple sclerosis is a common and distressing symptom. Progress has been made in understanding the physiology and pharmacology of penile erection in men. Clinical advances have also been made. Vacuum constriction devices, intracavernosal injection therapy and penile prostheses are all viable treatment alternatives. We know little about normal and abnormal female sexual function, and investigative efforts in this area are needed. The patient with multiple sclerosis and sexual dysfunction is a clinical challenge. The patient's physical and psychological needs should be addressed: an experienced sex therapist is often of significant benefit to these troubled patients.

References

1. Szasz, G., Paty, D., Lawton-Speert S. *et al.* (1984) A sexual functioning scale in multiple sclerosis. *Acta Neurol. Scand.*, **70**, 37–43.
2. Miller, H., Simpson, Ch. A. and Yeates, W.K. (1965) Bladder dysfunction in multiple sclerosis. *Br. Med. J.*, **i**, 1265–1269.
3. Goldstein, I., Siroky, M.B., Sax, D.S. *et al.* (1982) Neurological abnormalities in multiple sclerosis. *J. Urol.*, **128**, 541–5.
4. Lilius, H.G., Valtonen, E.J. and Wikstrom, J. (1976) Sexual problems in patients suffering from multiple sclerosis. *Scand. J. Soc. Med.*, **4**, 41–4.
5. Benson, G.S., McConnell, J.A., Lipshultz, L.I. *et al.* (1980) Neuromorphology and neuropharmacology of the human penis. *J. Clin. Invest.*, **65**, 506–13.
6. Newman, H.F. and Northup, J.D. (1981) Mechanism of human penile erection: an overview. *Urology*, **17**, 399–407.
7. Reiss, H.F., Northup, H.F. and Zorgniotti, A. (1982) Artificial erection by perfusion of penile arteries. *Urology*, **20**, 284–8.
8. Deysach, L.J. (1939) The comparative morphology of the erectile tissue of the penis with especial emphasis on the probable mechanism of erection. *Am. J. Anat.*, **64**, 111–31.
9. Wagner, G., Bro-Rasmussen, F., Willis, E.A. *et al.* (1982) New theory on the mechanism of erection involving hitherto undescribed vessels. *Lancet*, **i**, 416–18.
10. Van Arsdalen, K.N., Malloy, T.R. and Wein, A.J. (1983) Erectile physiology, dysfunction, and evaluation. I: Physiology of erection. *Monogr. Urol.*, **4**, 137.
11. Lue, T.F. and Tanagho, E.A. (1988) Hemodynamics of erection, in *Contemporary Management of Impotence and Infertility* (eds E.A. Tanagho, T.F. Lue and R.D. McClure), Baltimore, MD, Williams and Wilkins, ch. 2, pp. 28–38.

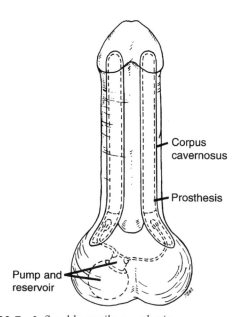

Figure 22.7 Inflatable penile prosthesis.

Corpus cavernosus

Prosthesis

Pump and reservoir

12. Polak, J.M., Gu, J., Mina, S. *et al.* (1981) Vipergic nerves in the penis. *Lancet*, ii, 217–19.
13. Gu, J., Polak, J.M., Probert, L. *et al.* (1983) Peptidergic innervation of the human male genital tract. *J. Urol.*, 130, 386–91.
14. Steers, W.D., McConnell, J.A. and Benson, G.S. (1984) Anatomical localization and some pharmacologic effects of vasoactive intestinal polypeptide in human and monkey corpus cavernosum. *J. Urol.*, 132, 1048–53.
15. Schmalbruch, H. and Wagner, G. (1989) Vasoactive intestinal polypeptide (VIP)-and neuropeptide Y (NPY)-containing nerve fibers in the penile cavernous tissue of green monkeys (Cercopithecus aethiops). *Cell Tissue Res.*, 256, 529–41.
16. Burnett, A.L., Tillman, S.L. and Chang T.S.K. (1993) Immunohistochemical localization of nitric oxide synthase in the autonomic innervation of the human penis. *J. Urol.*, 150, 73–6.
17. Semans, J.H. and Langworthy, O.R. (1939) Observations on the neurophysiology of sexual function in the male cat. *J. Urol.*, 40, 836–46.
18. Leriche, A. and Morel, A. (1948) Syndrome of thrombotic obliteration of aortic bifurcation. *Ann. Surg.*, 127, 193–206.
19. Schwartz, A.N., Wang, K.Y., Mock, L.A. *et al.* (1989) Evaluation of normal erectile function with color flow Doppler sonography. *Am. J. Roentgeol.*, 153, 1155–60.
20. Newman, H.F., Northup, J.D. and Devlin, J. (1964) Mechanism of human penile erection. *Invest. Urol.*, 1, 350–3.
21. Dorr, L.D. and Brody, M.J. (1967) Hemodynamic mechanism of erection in the canine penis. *Am. J. Physiol.*, 213, 1526–31.
22. Purohit, R.C. and Beckett, S.D. (1976) Penile pressures and muscle activity associated with erection and ejaculation in the dog. *Am. J. Physiol.*, 231, 1343–8.
23. Beckett, S.D., Hudson, R.S., Walker, D.F. *et al.* (1972) Corpus cavernosum penis pressure and extenal penile muscle activity during erection in the goat. *Biol. Reprod.*, 7, 359–64.
24. Kollberg, S., Peterson, I. and Stener, I. (1962) Preliminary results of an electromyographic study of ejaculation. *Acta Chir. Scand.*, 123, 478–83.
25. Shirai, M. and Ishii, N. (1981) Hemodynamics of erection in man. *Arch. Androl.*, 6, 27–32.
26. Wagner, G. (1981), Erection, physiology and endocrinology, in Wagner, G. and Green, R. (eds), *Impotence*. New York, Plenum Press, pp. 29–30.
27. Lue, T.F., Takamura, T., Schmidt, R.A. *et al.* (1983) Hemodynamics of erection in the monkey. *J. Urol.*, 130, 1237–41.
28. Lue, T.F., Takamura, T., Umraiya, M. *et al.* (1984) Hemodynamics of canine corpora cavernosa during erection. *Urology*, 24, 347–52.
29. Walsh, P.C. and Donker, P.J. (1982) Impotence following radical prostatectomy: insight into etiology and prevention. *J. Urol.*, 128, 492–7.
30. Eckhard, C. (1863) Untersuchungen Uber die Erection des Penis Beim Hunde: Beitrage zur Anatomie und Physiologie von C. Eckhard. *Beitr. Anat. Physiol.*, 3, 123–56.
31. Muller, L.R. (1902) Klinishe: Und experimentelle studien uber die innervation der blase, das mastdarms, und des genitalapparates. *Deutsch. Z. Nervenheilk.*, 21, 86–154.
32. Root, W.S. and Bard, D. (1947) The mediation of feline erection through sympathetic pathways with some remarks on sexual behaviour after deafferentiation of the genitalia. *Am. J. Physiol.*, 151, 80–90.
33. Bors, E. and Comarr, A.E. (1960) Neurologic disturbances of sexual function with special reference to 529 patients with spinal cord injury. *Urol. Surv.*, 10, 191–222.
34. Comarr, A.E. (1970) Sexual function among patients with spinal cord injury. *Urol. Int.*, 25, 314–68.
35. Kedia, K.R., Markland, C. and Fraley, E.E. (1975) Sexual function following high retroperitoneal lymphadenectomy. *J. Urol.*, 114, 237–9.
36. Kom, C., Mulholland, S.G. and Edson, M. (1971) Etiology of infertility after retroperitoneal lymphadenectomy. *J. Urol.*, 105, 528–30.
37. Virag, R. (1982) Intracavernous injection of papaverine for erective failure. *Lancet*, ii, 938.
38. Brindley, G.S. (1983) Cavernosal alpha blockade: a new technique for investigating and treating penile impotence. *Br. J. Psychiatry*, 143, 332–7.
39. Brindley, G.S. (1986) Pilot experiments on the actions of drugs injected into the human corpus cavernosum penis. *Br. J. Pharmacol.*, 87, 495–501.
40. Hedlund, H. and Andersson, K.E. (1985) Contraction and relaxation induced by some prostanoids in isolated human penile erectile tissue and cavernous artery. *J. Urol.*, 134, 1245–50.
41. Lue, T.F. and Tanagho, E.A. (1987) Physiology of erection and pharmacological management of impotence. *J. Urol.*, 137, 829–36.
42. Stackl, W., Hasun, R. and Marberger, M. (1988) Intracavernous injection of prostaglandin E$_1$ in impotent men. *J. Urol.*, 140, 66–8.
43. Zorgniotti, A.W. and Lefleur, R.S. (1985) Auto-injection of the corpus cavernosum with a vasoactive drug combination for vasculogenic impotence. *J. Urol.*, 133, 39–41.
44. Sidi, A.A., Cameron, J.S., Duffy, L.M. *et al.* (1986) Intracavernous drug-induced erections in management of male erectile dysfunction: experience with 100 patients. *J. Urol.*, 135, 704–6.
45. Benson, G.S. (1983) Penile erection: in search of a neurotransmitter. *World J. Urol.*, 1, 209–12.
46. Klinge, E. and Sjostrand, N.O. (1974) Contraction and relaxation of the retractor penis muscle and the penile artery of the bull. *Acta Physiol. Scand.*, 420 (Suppl.), 1–88.
47. Klinge, E. and Sjostrand, N.O. (1977) Comparative study of some isolated mammalian smooth muscle effectors of penile erection. *Acta Physiol. Scand.*, 100, 354–67.
48. Bevan, J.A., Moscowitz, M., Said, S.I. *et al.* (1984) Evidence that vasoactive intestinal polypeptide is a dilator transmitter to some cerebral and extracerebral cranial arteries. *Peptides*, 5, 385–8.
49. Kim, N., Azadzoi, K.M., Goldstein, I. *et al.* (1991) A nitric oxide-like factor mediates nonadrenergic, noncholinergic neurogenic relaxation of penile corpus cavernosum smooth muscle. *J. Clin. Invest.*, 88, 112.
50. Bush, P.A., Aronson, W.J., Buga, G.M. *et al.* (1992) Nitric oxide is a potent relaxant of human and rabbit corpus cavernosum. *J. Urol.*, 147, 1650–5.
51. Saenz de Tejada, I., Goldstein, I., Azadzoi, K. *et al.* (1989) Impaired neurogenic and endothelium-mediated relaxation of penile smooth muscle from diabetic men with impotence. *N. Engl. J. Med.*, 320, 1025–30.
52. Lue, T.F. and McAninch, J.W. (1988) Priapism, in *Contemporary Management of Impotence and Infertility* (eds E.A. Tanagho, T.F. Lue and R.D. McClure), Baltimore, MD, Williams and Wilkins, ch. 19, pp. 201–10.
53. Walther, P.J., Meyer, A.F. and Woodworth, P.E. (1987) Intraoperative management of penile erection with intracorporeal phenylephrine during endoscopic surgery. *J. Urol.*, 137, 738–9.
54. Cocchia, D., Rende, M., Toesca, A. *et al.* (1990) Immunohistochemical study of neuropeptide Y-containing nerve fibers in the human clitoris and penis. *Cell Biol. Int. Rep.*, 14, 865.
55. Diederichs, W., Lue, T. and Tanagho, E.A. (1991) Clitoral response to cavernous nerve stimulation in dogs. *Int. J. Impotence Res.*, 3, 7.
56. Pescatori, E.S., Engelman, J.C., Davis, G. *et al.* (1993) Priapism of the clitoris: a case report following trazodone use. *J. Urol.*, 149, 1557–9.
57. Valleroy, M.L. and Kraft, G.H. (1984) Sexual dysfunction in multiple sclerosis. *Arch. Phys. Med. Rehab.*, 65, 125–8.
58. Krane, R.J. and Siroky, M.D. (1980) Studies of sacral evoked potentials. *J. Urol.*, 124, 872–6.
59. Halderman, S., Bradley, W.E., Bhatia, N.N. *et al.* (1982) Pudendal evoked responses. *Arch. Neurol.*, 39, 280–3.
60. Gerstenberger, T.C. and Bradley, W.E. (1983) Nerve conduction velocity measurement of dorsal nerve of penis in normal and impotent males. *Urology*, 21, 90–2.
61. Bennett, A.H., Carpenter, A.J. and Barada, J.H. (1991) An improved vasoactive drug combination for a pharmacological erection program. *J. Urol.*, 146, 1564–5.
62. Lue, T.F. (1990) Intracavernous drug administration: its role in diagnosis and treatment of impotence. *Semin. Urol.*, 8, 100–6.
63. Lue, T.F., Hricak, H., Marich, K.W. *et al.* (1985) Evaluation of arteriogenic impotence with intracorporal injection of papaverine and the duplex ultrasound scanner. *Semin. Urol.*, 3, 43–8.
64. Bookstein, J.J., Valji, K. and Parsons, L. (1987) Pharmacoarteriography in the evaluation of impotence. *J. Urol.*, 137, 333–7.
65. Sharlip, I.D. (1991) The incredible results of penile vascular surgery. *Int. J. Impotence Res.*, 3, 1–6.
66. Padma-Nathan, H. and Goldstein, I. (1988) Arterial reconstruction, in *Contemporary Management of Impotence and Infertility* (eds E.A. Tanagho, T.F. Lue and R.D. McClure), Baltimore, MD, Williams and Wilkins, pp. 163–74.
67. Goldstein, I. (1987) Penile revascularization. *Urol. Clin. North Am.*, 14, 805–13.
68. Lewis, R.W. (1988) Venous surgery for impotence. *Urol. Clin. North Am.*, 15, 115–21.
69. Fisher, C., Gross, J. and Zuch, J. (1965) Cycle of penile erection synchronous with dreaming (REM) sleep. *Arch. Gen. Psychiatry*, 12, 29–45.
70. Karacan, I., Scott, F.B., Solis, P.J. *et al.* (1977) Nocturnal erections, differential diagnosis of impotence, and diabetes. *Biol. Psychiatry*, 12, 373–80.
71. Seagraves, R.T., Schoenberg, H.W. and Seagraves, K.A.B. (1985) Evaluation of the etiology of erectile failure, in *Diagnosis and Treatment of Erectile Disturbances* (eds R.T. Seagraves and R.T. Schoenberg), New York, Plenum Press, p. 177.
72. Karacan, I., Goodenough, D.R., Shapiro, A. *et al.* (1966) Erection cycle during sleep in relation to dream anxiety. *Arch. Gen. Psychiatry*, 15, 183–9.
73. Benkert, O., Witt, W., Adam, W. *et al.* (1979) Effects of testosterone undecanoate on sexual potency and the hypothalamic pituitary-gonadal axis of impotent males. *Arch. Sex. Behav.*, 8, 471–9.
74. Benson, G.S. (1994) Endocrine factors related to impotence, in *Impotence. Diagnosis and Management of Erectile Dysfunction* (ed. A.H. Bennett), Philadelphia, W.B. Saunders, ch. 3, pp. 31–41.
75. Morales, A., Surridge, D.H.C., Marshall, P.G. *et al.* (1982) Nonhormonal pharmacological treatment of organic impotence. *J. Urol.*, 128, 45–47.
76. Morales, A., Condre, M., Owen, J.A. *et al.* (1987) Is yohimbine effective in the treatment of organic impotence? Results of a controlled trial. *J. Urol.*, 137, 1168–72.

77. Corriere, J.N., Fishman, I.J., Benson, G.S. *et al.* (1988) Development of fibrotic penile lesions secondary to the intracorporal injection of vasoactive agents. *J. Urol.*, **140**, 615–17.

78. Levine, S.B., Althof, S.E., Turner, L.A. *et al.* (1989) Side effects of self administration of intracavernous papaverine and phentolamine for the treatment of impotence. *J. Urol.*, **141**, 54–7.

79. Abozeid, M., Juenemann, K.P., Luo, J.A. *et al.* (1987) Chronic papaverine treatment: the effect of repeated injections on the simian erectile response and penile tissue. *J. Urol.*, **138**, 1263–6.

80. Lue, T.F., Hellstrom, W.J.G., McAninch, J.W. *et al.* (1986) Priapism: a refined approach to diagnosis and treatment. *J. Urol.*, **136**, 104–8.

81. Dittrich, A., Albrecht, K., Bar-Moshe, O. *et al.* (1991) Treatment of pharmacological priapism with phenylephrine. *J. Urol.*, **146**, 323–4.

82. Roy, A.C., Tan, S.M., Kottegoda, S.R. *et al.* (1984) Ability of human corpora cavernosa muscle to generate prostaglandins and thromboxanes in vitro. *IRCS Med. Sci.*, **12**, 608–9.

83. Ishii, N., Watanabe, H., Irisawa, C. *et al.* (1989) Intracavernous injection of prostaglandin E_1 for the treatment of erectile impotence. *J. Urol.*, **141**, 323–5.

84. Nadig, P.W., Ware, J.C. and Blumoff, R. (1986) Noninvasive device to produce and maintain an erection-like state. *Urology*, **27**, 126–31.

85. Witherington, R. (1989) Vacuum constriction device for management of erectile impotence. *J. Urol.*, **141**, 320–2.

86. Meinhardt, W., Kropman, R.F., Lycklama, A.A.B. *et al.* (1990) Skin necrosis caused by use of negative pressure device for erectile impotence. *J. Urol.*, **144**, 983.

87. Montague, D.K. (1989) Penile prostheses. *Urol. Clin. North Am.*, **16**, 7–12.

88. Barry, J.M., Giesy, J.D. and McDuffie, R. (1982) Actuarial survivals of inflatable and flexible hinged prostheses. *Urology*, **20**, 605–7.

89. Malloy, T.R. and von Eschenbach, A.C. (1977) Surgical treatment of erectile impotence with inflatable penile prosthesis. *J. Urol.*, **118**, 49–51.

90. Furlow, W.L. and Barrett, D.M. (1984) Inflatable penile prosthesis. New device design and patient–partner satisfaction. *Urology*, **24**, 559–63.

23 MULTIPLE SCLEROSIS: A CLINICAL VIEWPOINT TO MANAGEMENT

Randall T. Schapiro, Robert W. Baumhefner and Wallace W. Tourtellotte

23.1 Introduction

Multiple sclerosis (MS) is a unique disease process which can be devastating, not only because it affects the myelin of the central nervous system but also because it affects the lives of the people with MS, their families and their friends. It is particularly devastating because it causes disability in young adults when meaningful relationships are beginning, families are developing, personalities are maturing and careers are starting. An estimated one and a half million people in the world suffer with MS, of whom 350 000 are in the United States alone [1], and the disease clearly affects two to three times that number psychologically and fundamentally by its effect on families. The specific cause of MS remains unknown, and any hope for its eradication will require an understanding of its etiology and pathogenesis [2, 3]. Effective management, however, requires a comprehensive understanding of its symptoms, signs and problems, and appropriate methods of dealing with them. Much progress has been made in this area, and what follows is intended to be a critical anthology.

MS has a variety of presentations, a highly variable rate of progression and a multiplicity of symptoms and abnormalities. Patients may exhibit significant disabilities in many spheres. It is impossible for the average primary care physician to have the knowledge to handle almost any one of the symptom complexes. Thus while all patients should have a primary care physician, they all require a specialist who understands MS problems and management and can provide principal care for their MS. This is usually a neurologist but any physician with special knowledge of MS may function as the main physician for these patients. Physician assistants, nurse clinicians and clinical nurse specialists may, if appropriately trained, serve as an interface allowing the specialist to serve more patients efficiently. Being a neurologist or physiatrist does not, in itself, make for an appropriate manager of MS. The physician must have a therapeutic bent to be successful in this arena. Specialists who emphasize diagnosis without treatment will not succeed with the complex symptoms of MS. The practice of 'diagnose and adios' was very popular among neurologists before there was a greater understanding of neurorehabilitation and symptom management.

The entire handicap associated with the MS patient must be assessed and managed. Physicians must recognize that there are many non-medical problems which are common in MS. These include the psychosocial difficulties of families, the workplace, friends and life in general. Thus the management of MS encompasses the totality of a person's life. It takes kindness, maturity, understanding and science.

With the multiplicity of symptoms and functional disturbances found in MS, the physician rendering the care of MS must understand how to obtain services for the patient. A 'case manager', usually a nurse clinician, clinical nurse specialist, physician's assistant or a social worker, may ensure that the plan of management is performed efficiently.

The MS care specialist 'quarterbacks' the decision-making process. This may include the input of nurses, physical therapists, occupational therapists, speech pathologists, social workers, psychologists and other health professionals. Sometimes this is done with independent collaboration, written or oral, in what is called a 'multi-disciplinary approach'. Other times the collaboration is more direct, with each discipline actually influencing the patterns of treatment of the others – an 'inter-disciplinary approach'.

An important member of whatever team is the person with MS. Education must be emphasized and done well to insure compliance with the treatment program. This can only occur through an emphasis on communication and understanding. Patients must be 'MS smart'. The

Multiple Sclerosis: Clinical and pathogenetic basis. Edited by Cedric S. Raine, Henry F. McFarland and Wallace W. Tourtellotte. Published in 1997 by Chapman & Hall, London. ISBN 0 412 30890 8.

patient's support system must be identified and brought into the decision-making. Support with an aim of motivation makes the difference between success and failure with life management.

It is important to understand that the management plan should not only be directed toward the disease, MS, but also to the person with the disease. Disease management includes medication and exercise; 'person management' includes the psychological, spiritual, social, vocational aspects of life. These need to be consciously approached and directed.

23.2 Diagnosis (see also Chapter 1)

The diagnosis should be made by an experienced neurologist with the patient understanding how the diagnosis was made. Because there is no specific laboratory test for MS, one must rely on the history and physical examination for diagnostic clues. Serial observations of the patient, sometimes over extended periods of time, may be necessary. Certain characteristics of the disease are helpful. MS symptoms and signs initiate predominantly in young adults (age 15–50). While older and younger cases are diagnosed more commonly than in the past, they remain unusual. MS disease activity characteristically fluctuates, with exacerbations and remissions. As its name implies, the neurological exam is characterized by multiple abnormalities within the central nervous system (dissociated in time and space). When these characteristics are evident the vast majority of MS cases can be diagnosed without expensive diagnostic studies.

In clinical practice it is important to adhere to established criteria for the definition of clinically possible, probable and definite MS in order to standardize the diagnostic process and aid in communication between clinicians [4–6]. Poser et al. [7] defined the term 'laboratory supported' definite MS to characterize a patient that satisfied the classical criteria for 'probable MS' and also had evidence for abnormal intrathecal IgG synthesis by cerebrospinal fluid (CSF) and blood examination. To satisfy this classification patients with only one clinical attack of signs and symptoms of MS must also have evidence of at least two lesions in the CNS separated in onset by at least one month, with clinical evidence of at least one of these lesions [7, 8]. This term should not be confused with clinically definite MS, because it defines patients in whom the diagnosis of MS is much less certain. In one study less than half of these patients developed clinically definite MS in 2 years and 7.5% were eventually found to have another diagnosis [8].

Examination of CSF and blood, however, is still an important tool in the diagnosis of MS. Not only is evidence for intrathecal IgG synthesis rate and/or the presence of unique oligoclonal banding a strong confirmation of the diagnosis and observed in greater than

95% of patients with clinically definite MS, identification of CSF patterns inconsistent with MS and thus broadening the differential diagnosis is also important (Chapter 5).

The MRI has been one of the most important advances in the diagnosis of MS and clearly has promoted an earlier diagnosis in many patients (Chapter 3). However, it is not a definitive laboratory test for MS, because MRI findings are not specific for the disease [9, 10]. Between 4 and 20% of patients with an MRI compatible with MS have another diagnosis [8]. In addition, a significant number of patients have asymptomatic white matter hyperintensities accompanying aging and these give an MRI picture consistent with demyelination [11]. MRI is becoming more sensitive with newer techniques. These are discussed elsewhere in this book (Chapter 3). What is clear is that the clinical implication of a positive MRI in a patient with the initial symptoms consistent with MS is not necessarily pessimistic. The majority of these patients do well over the ensuing years: many remain asymptomatic for much of their lifetimes. Autopsy studies demonstrate a frequency of unsuspected MS twice that of the actual clinical incidence [12]. However, as more is learned about MRI, it has become easier to use this tool as a marker for the progress of MS and it is becoming more appropriate to utilize this marker as a predictor of disability. Further, its use as a secondary outcome assessment in clinical trials is accepted (Chapters 3 and 19).

Evoked potentials provide a physiological way of measuring disturbance in conduction within the central nervous system (CNS). Visual, brain stem and somatosensory testing may provide the evidence of a separate lesion, complementing the clinical criteria to diagnose MS with no morbidity to the testing, and it is objective (Chapter 4) [13].

All of these diagnostic tools add to the ease of approaching MS with an understanding of anatomy, physiology and immunology. They allow for earlier diagnosis and potentially for earlier management strategies

23.3 Informing the patient

The diagnosis has profound sociological, psychological and possibly economic implications for the patient, thus making the diagnosis should not be considered inconsequential. With the advent of FDA-approved treatments that slow down the progression of the disease, and that are most beneficial the earlier in the course they are administered, the diagnosis should be made as expeditiously as possible.

Discussing the diagnosis with the patient takes understanding of human nature, knowledge of accurate facts about the epidemiology of MS (Chapters 6, 7 and 8), patience and time. Ideally the patient should be accompanied by a family member or other support person. Honesty is important in the discussions with the patient, who will need to be as informed as soon as possible in order to make important decisions about his/ her life goals. With an element of kindness the discussion should center on what is known about the nervous system in health and disease. An understanding of the unpredictable nature of the condition is necessary but the emphasis should be on the positive aspects of the statistics. It is helpful to start the discussion, let it settle for a day or two, and then finish it after the initial emotional upheaval has resolved to some degree. This will also allow time for the patient to generate questions. The handing out of written material emphasizing the points made in the verbal discussion decreases misunderstanding [14]. If there is some question mark against the diagnosis it is reasonable to explain this, and stress that time will allow for a more complete understanding of the process. If the term 'MS' is used, nothing short of a full explanation will suffice. Substituting the words 'demyelinating disease', or 'myelitis' will not fool today's patients. They will look up these processes and then will have to explain the problems to themselves. It is appropriate to explain that not all demyelinating or inflammatory problems of the nervous system are MS and that other possibilities are being considered. Discussion of viruses, allergic reactions, vasculitis and other agents may be of value.

The discussion may include the fact that sometimes MS is easily diagnosed and that a definite diagnosis can then be made. But occasionally, especially at the initial presentation, an absolute conclusion is not possible and that more appropriately the process is classified as possible or probable MS. Obviously sometimes MS is not the problem and should be disposed of as 'not MS'.

The messenger of the diagnosis is often intertwined with the message. Often the purveyor of bad news in any chronic disease is looked upon by the patient with negative views. Care must be taken to separate the message from the messenger by discussing the topic with understanding and appropriate facts. Time for questions and knowledge of answers will usually defuse anxiety greatly.

Follow-up visits are also important for detecting and treating new symptoms of MS and managing complications before they become severe, the continued counseling of the patient and the family, and for discussing new treatments and research. We instruct patients to report by telephone any significant change in their neurological function and new physical problems as they arise, since symptomatic treatments are available for some MS-related difficulties.

We emphasize that benign and even subclinical cases of MS are well known and constitute a substantial percentage of all MS patients. In most series this is about 30–40% of all cases with a duration of disease of 10–15 years (Chapters 6 and 7; [15–17]). MS is commonly associated with patients in wheelchairs since these are the easily recognizable cases. Systematic studies reveal that most MS patients do not require wheelchairs, and that many are only mildly incapacitated. Others have no physically disabling symptoms. Fifteen years after onset, about 50% of patients will require a cane to walk half a block and only 15% will be confined to a wheelchair (Chapter 6 and 7; [18]). Clinical studies of the progress of MS point to the fact that no two cases are exactly alike. MS can be classified according to the majority of clinical symptoms anatomically: cerebral, brain stem, spinal cord, cerebellar and multi-focal. More often it is classified according to the clinical progression into:

1. benign;
2. relapsing-remitting;
3. secondary-progressive;
4. primary-progressive;
5. progressive-relapsing.

The benign form of relapsing-remitting MS is more common than is universally understood. Significant numbers of diagnosed cases have mild, usually sensory, symptoms with little obvious activity to the disease. Relapsing-remitting disease (66–79%) is a common presentation with attacks of symptoms followed by stabilization or improvement. This can go on for many years with relatively little permanent disability. Secondary-progressive (3–15%) is characterized by attacks with periods of less activity, but with each attack disability mounts allowing for the progressive nature of the process. Primary-progressive MS (about 10%) is progressive from onset, eventually causing significant disability. A small percentage of MS is progressive from onset, but may have superimposed relapses. Finally there is acute progressive (progressive-relapsing) MS (< 5%) which leads to severe disability over months with rapid progression. This diversity in the course of disease leads to difficulties in the planning of clinical studies with certain drugs being reserved for certain kinds of MS, and makes it harder to capture a uniform group of study patients while expanding the potential therapeutic options according to type [4].

Since heat can exacerbate symptoms, patients should be told to avoid excessive heat exposure, including excessive exercise, and be taught how to take care of infections, such as urinary tract infections, which may cause fever. Patients should be instructed on methods to reduce fever quickly.

Patients must prepare to deal with MS usually for their entire lifetimes. One way to prepare is to become as knowledgeable as possible about the disease. The physician should be open to discussion of news releases about MS and neurorehabilitation which the patient may find vitally important.

23.4   Responding to common inquiries

Certain questions arise from both patients and their physicians in the course of the disease that the managing physician should specifically answer.

1. Diagnostic procedures such as lumbar puncture, angiography and myelography can be performed safely in people with MS[19].
2. Heredity is important to discuss with each patient. This is discussed in detail elsewhere in this book (Chapter 13) but it should be emphasized that while there is an increased risk of MS appearing in the family, it is usually not great enough to warrant genetic counseling.
3. The question of infectiousness is high in the newly diagnosed. The role of infectious agents in MS is discussed elsewhere in this book (Chapter 16) but it can be said here that a specific exogenous agent causing MS has not been identified and MS is not a contagious disease.
4. Because studies indicate a higher prevalence of MS away from the Equator, the question is often raised as to whether one can 'move away from acquiring it'. While migration studies are discussed fully elsewhere (Chapter 7), one can state that movement after the fact appears to have no effect on the disease process and that the likelihood of acquiring MS is small enough that migrating to an area of lower incidence will not lower its incidence in children of MS patients.
5. Temperature sensitivity is common among people with MS. There are physiological reasons for this. If a patient is temperature-sensitive, undue heat exposure is not advisable; cooling techniques are recommended which will be discussed later in this chapter.
6. Immunization remain controversial. It is better to avoid vaccinations except where benefits are likely to be substantial, such as in old, disabled or respiratorily impaired patients where pneumonia or influenza could be fatal.
7. Pregnancy is discussed fully elsewhere in this volume (Chapter 8) but it is important to emphasize that pregnancy, breast feeding or child rearing do not appear to influence the long-term prognosis of MS. Nor does MS affect fetal development or childbirth.
8. Physical trauma does not cause MS exacerbations, but prolonged bedrest should be avoided (Chapter 8). If bedrest cannot be avoided, a daily range of motion exercises and low dose heparin are indicated to avoid pulmonary emobli.
9. Emotional stress makes the symptoms of all neurological diseases worse and MS is no exception. Dealing with stress and its influences in MS is discussed elsewhere in this book (Chapter 8).
10. If diet and vitamins were the answer, MS would no longer exist. Virtually every combination of diet and vitamins has been tried with no systematic success. Limited data indicate that low animal fat and supplemental polyunsaturates may be beneficial, thus, we recommend adding 2 tablespoons of canola oil to a 10% saturated lipid high fiber diet[20, 21].

23.5   Planning an exercise program for the MS patient

Exercise for MS patients has gone from controversial to routinely accepted in the past decade[22–25]. An appropriate program of exercise is of primary importance and one the most important treatments for the MS patient. It is often difficult to determine whether functional impairment in MS is due to disease of the nervous system, disuse or despair. The 'anticipation of disability' is a principle that is operative in most patients with MS, stemming from a universal principle that people do not work up to their full capacity and reinforced by the physician and family, who assume that rest is part of the treatment of MS. Thus the MS patient functions below his/her ability and often discontinues ambulation and other activities too early, making disuse the most important factor. If patients are active and exercise regularly they are better able to maintain their functional level, and future impairment can be more reliably assessed. Patients are told that research will eventually find the cure, but it will be of most value to those patients who have prevented disuse by regular active and passive exercises.

Certain principles should be kept in mind in an MS exercise program. There are different kinds of exercise, each with a different goal. The goal determines the type of exercise. MS affects each patient differently, so the program needs to be tailored to the individual patient[26]. MS has an unpredictable course and a patient's impairments may change, requiring periodic reassessment and possible alteration in the exercise program. Fatigue, while common in MS, should not be a major limiting factor for exercise if frequent rest periods during an exercise session are planned. Exertion should never be excessive, causing prolonged fatigue or exhaustion, for this can be detrimental. Exercises should be aerobic and should be done at a level that allows the patient to carry on a conversation throughout the exercise period[26]. Spasticity can impair efficient exercise by increasing the energy cost of movement. Stretching exercises at the beginning of a session and antispasmodic drugs can be useful in combating this problem. The value of an exercise program for MS patients with rapidly progressive disease can only be determined by a trial of such a program. If progression is slow enough, exercise may delay or alleviate disuse and its complications, and even increase function.

Vigorous water activities have multiple benefits. With the body submerged, water pressure automatically increases blood circulation to some extent. Patients having trouble with land exercise can often easily complete exercises in the pool. Buoyancy lessens gravitational pull: a person immersed to the neck in water experiences an apparent loss of 90% of his/her weight. Thus, even with painful joints or weak leg muscles, patients will usually find it possible to move comfortably in the water. The temperature of the water can be varied easily according to the patient's preference. Some patients prefer a cooler water temperature of about 80 °F, most prefer 85 °F. During exercise, an individual's body temperature rises, which in MS can result in restriction in movement, decreased muscular function, fatigue, temporary blindness (Uhthoff's symptom), or dizziness. With hydrotherapy the water removes the excess heat built up during exercise, permitting the patient to exercise without suffering severe discomfort. The benefits derived from a particular water exercise can be changed depending on the way it is done. An exercise done with stretching movements can increase flexibility and improve posture, while a similar one done with 'water resistance' movements can build muscle tone and coordination. Water provides more resistance for muscles, making them work harder and toning them more efficiently. The buoyancy of the water eliminates shock and trauma to the joints and bones, which can occur with other forms of exercise, such as jogging. Hydrotherapy is an exercise form for both the wheelchair patient and the patient with less severe impairment whose goal is to remain ambulatory.

Reminder: After hydrotherapy we recommend cooling in the pool or cool shower for about 30 minutes. During this time the heat of exercise should be dissipated, and the patient will not suffer worsening of function due to hyperthermia.

We recommend that patients continue vigorous active exercise and an active physical therapy program to the best of their ability without over-exertion during a relapse. We have found that having the patient exercise regularly can also enhance the benefit of corticosteroid therapy and decrease adverse effects. Exercise should of course continue during recovery from the exacerbation, which is more widely practiced [22].

Exercise is good for the spirit as well as the body. It should be enjoyable and appropriate for the circumstance. It is part of a general wellness program which includes good nutrition, socialization, spiritual understanding and education. A positive attitude means more to good living than almost any other aspect of treatment. Patients say they feel better and we find they do maintain a better functional level. We must emphasize that MS patients have a remarkable inability to attain a maintenance level of physical fitness. We recommend that the neurologist-in-charge plan the patient's day to include exercise as described above on top of the usual activities of living, to encourage the patient to be persistent, because if he/she gets physically conditioned, enjoyment and 'addiction to exercise' will be the result. Only a motivated and persistent patient can become physically conditioned.

23.6 Treating neurological symptoms and signs

Despite the lack of definitive knowledge about the cause of MS and the inability to absolutely affect the pathology of MS, management of the disease has improved dramatically in the past decade. This has come about primarily by improved understanding and development of new techniques to alter the symptoms caused by the demyelinating process. Symptoms of MS can be divided into three general categories: those that stem from actual demyelination within the CNS are called primary and include spasticity, weakness, tremor, ataxia, numbness, cognitive difficulties, bladder and bowel dysfunction, blurred and double vision, and occasionally apraxia. Symptoms that originate because of the presence of primary demyelination are called 'secondary' symptoms and include contractures, decubiti, osteoporosis, urinary tract infections and obesity. The symptoms which emanate from the psychological, vocational or marital stress of a chronic disease are labeled 'tertiary' symptoms. The complete management of MS involves the medical, surgical, rehabilitative, psychological and social treatments of these areas.

In Table 23.A.1, which is presented as an Appendix to this chapter, symptoms of MS have been alphabetized and non-medical and medical treatments are listed [27]. In addition, a detailed discussion of major symptoms/signs follows.

23.6.1 WEAKNESS

Weakness is common in MS. This is especially true of the lower extremities. It is almost always of the upper motor neuron type, and hence is associated with spasticity, clonus and involuntary spasms [19, 28]. The physician should look for certain aggravating factors that may be present: excessive exertion, overuse of muscle relaxants, intercurrent infections, fever, environmental increase in temperature, calcium and electrolyte imbalances and malnutrition. Weakness caused by chronic MS lesions cannot be reversed. However, weakness from disuse and despair is common, and a structured program of physical therapy is recommended to determine whether the patient is performing below capacity. Activity to the onset of mild fatigue is encouraged. Moderately to severely weak patients, requiring aids for ambulation or limited to transferring to and from the wheelchair, and bed patients should be referred to a physical therapist or occupational therapist for programmed active (upper extremity) and passive exercises. Devices can be installed in the patient's home to encourage activity and independence, such as grab bars and hand rails, a walker, parallel bars, a stationary bicycle, and a bed trapeze.

A wide range of bathroom safety equipment is available, none of which interferes with the use of the bathroom by others. Such items include elevated toilet seats, grab bars and shower chairs. There are also numerous devices which make everyday tasks easier: built-up silverware, reachers, page turners, telephone holders and utility carts [29]. An experienced occupational therapist can make suggestions. Self-help aid catalogues and magazines for the disabled can also be consulted.

Increasing the efficiency of nerve conduction within demyelinated nerves with 4-aminopyridine and 3,4-diaminopyridine – potassium channel blockers – also combats weakness but these have not as yet been approved for this use in North America [30, 31]. They are stimulatory agents and the excitation appears to lower seizure thresholds. Understanding their use will allow for a chemical strength mediator in the future. For the present physiological cooling appears to be a safer route to a temporary, short duration increase in strength. Cooling may be done with a cooling vest or other means of lowering core body temperature. Ingestion of shaved ice drinks is reasonably efficient at cooling [32].

Frequently patients with severe paraparesis or plegia develop significant edema. This can be relieved by elevation of the extremity together with alternate pressure stockings administered especially during sleep. With these fluid mobilizing stockings the judicious use of diuretics can be successful.

23.6.2 SPASTICITY

Spasticity is one of the most common signs of MS [19]. There may be difficulty in walking or in using the hands despite adequate muscle strength. At times spasticity is necessary to maintain mobility, described as walking with the stiffness of spasticity. Stiff legs may be used to pivot the patient from one location to another. Loss of this function may complicate any treatment for spasticity. Patients learn that inactivity causes increased stiffness, and arising several times at night (as with nocturia) and several times during the day (doing 'stand ups') is helpful. Standing for a few seconds after arising before taking a step achieves balance and the legs limber up somewhat after the first few steps. Spasticity in MS can be aggravated by conditions for which the patient should be screened, such as urinary tract infections, decubiti, fever and rectal or bladder distension.

Non-drug treatments include splints, braces or bivalved casts to maintain a neutral or slightly stretched position [33], massage, hydrotherapy and the application of external cold [22]. Physical therapy can decrease spasticity. A daily program of active and passive exercises is most useful for forestalling progressive shortening of muscles [22, 34]. The patient or a significant other can be trained to administer this program. Stretching the muscles of the calf by standing on a tilt board can lead to generalized relaxation of all muscles of the leg, allowing passive stretching exercises of the other muscles of the legs. Other aids useful in these exercises are a towel or long belt used to pull up on the distal foot to stretch the calf muscles and a beach ball over which a patient can lie, rocking forward and backward to stretch the trunk muscles [34]. Performing exercises in a swimming pool is beneficial, the water allowing vigorous stretching and a range of motion calisthenics with the water temperature kept lukewarm at 85 °F. Stretching, range of motion and aerobic exercises can relieve mild to moderate spasticity and have the advantage of being low cost and without side-effects. They must be performed regularly, however, and the effect is of short duration.

Antispasmodic drugs can then be of significant help and have a longer duration of effect. Four have been demonstrated superior to placebo for MS spasticity: baclofen (Lioresal), diazepam (Valium) and dantrolene sodium (Dantrium) and tizanidine (Zanaflex) [35].

Baclofen (Lioresal)

A blocker of release of excitatory amino acids and possibly of inhibitory GABA receptors in the central nervous system, baclofen is the drug of choice for MS and is well tolerated. It may also improve bladder and bowel function in patients with spinal cord lesions [36]. The starting dose is 5 mg (half a tablet) three times a day, increased by half a tablet every three days until benefit is achieved. A common error is to stop short of finding the optimal dose. Much higher doses than the usual maximum of 20 mg four times a day may be required, occasional patients tolerating 150–350 mg a day with increased benefit [35a]. Side-effects include confusion, sedation and somnolence at higher doses, but much less than with diazepam and usually dissipating in a few days. Muscle weakness, occasionally experienced, especially by those barely ambulating due to severe leg paresis, is amenable to dosage reduction [36]. Abrupt withdrawal of the drug can cause seizures or a period of hallucinations.

Benzodiazepines

The benzodiazapines diazepam (Valium) and clonazepam (Klonopin) enhance presynaptic inhibition by increasing the affinity of GABA receptors and enhancing the endogenous release of GABA in the central nervous system [35]. Studies comparing the effect of diazepam with baclofen found comparable efficacy but more side-effects with diazepam, such as somnolence, dizziness and increased muscle weakness [35, 37, 38]. Because of sedation, these drugs are most useful for nocturnal spasms. Calming side-effects may be beneficial in some agitated patients, but exacerbation of underlying depression is possible. Sedation and confusion is more of a problem in the elderly, thus the starting dose should be lower. Addiction or physical dependence can occur, and diazepam should not be prescribed for patients known to abuse other drugs, including alcohol, and with caution where there is evidence of depression because of the possibility of suicide. Abrupt withdrawal of diazepam may produce seizures or even fatal withdrawal symptoms. Starting dose is 2 mg twice a day, increased by 2 mg every three days until unwanted side-effects develop, adequate benefit is obtained, or a level of 20 mg three times a day is reached. Large doses produce sedation if given initially, but when reached slowly as recommended, they are often well tolerated.

Dantrolene (Dantrium)

Dantrolene reduces depolarization-induced calcium efflux into the muscle sarcoplasm. Muscle contraction is weakened, which is the basis for its antispastic effect. While effective for spasticity in MS patients [39], and causing less drowsiness, it has not been found superior to diazepam [40]. The induced weakness frequently increases the disability of MS patients, often making it useless for ambulatory patients. Some ambulatory patients may benefit if their walking is impaired by tonic spasms of the back or proximal muscles. It is difficult to predict which patients will benefit prior to an actual trial of therapy [35]. Wheelchair-bound patients whose nursing care is impaired by severe muscle contractures and scissoring of the legs are often benefited. Side-effects include drowsiness, light-headedness, diarrhea and occasionally pleuritis or pericarditis as part of a hypersensitivity reaction. The most important side-effect is hepatic damage [41]. Starting dose is 25 mg daily. Benefit may be delayed for a week or more, so dosage increases should not be more frequent than once a week. Maximum doses greater than 100 mg four times a day are rarely indicated, as higher dosages often lead to weakness and/or diarrhea. If no benefit occurs within six weeks, or within two weeks of the maximum dose, the dose should be gradually discontinued, because of the risk of hepatotoxicity and also pleuropericardial reactions [42]. Liver function tests should be obtained before dantrolene is given, and repeated during therapy.

Combinations of the above agents, usually baclofen and diazepam, have been beneficial, because of a synergistic effect, but the sedative effects of both drugs may also be potentiated. The excessive soporific effect of diazepam can sometimes be avoided if it is added in very small doses (0.5–1 mg twice daily) to an optimal baclofen dose. However, baclofen at higher than usual doses should be tried before a combination with a moderate dose with diazepam.

Tizanidine (Sirdalud, Zanaflex)

Tizanidine has been found to be superior to placebo for treating MS spasticity [43, 44]. This drug is an alpha-2-adrenergic agonist at the locus ceruleus and spinal cord interneurons, impairing excitatory amino acid release and inhibiting facilitatory ceruleospinal pathways [45]. Individual comparative studies of baclofen and tizanidine in the treatment of MS spasticity have shown equivalent efficacy [46, 47]. A meta-analysis of more than 20 double-blind comparative studies in MS and cerebrovascular disease indicated no significant difference in efficacy when tizanidine was compared to baclofen and diazepam. The side-effect of muscle weakness was more common with baclofen. While somnolence was more evident with tizanidine, it was less than that experienced with diazepam [48]. Tizanidine is well tolerated by MS patients in large multicenter studies, the main side-effects being drowsiness, dry mouth, dizziness, tiredness and hypotension. A small percentage of patients have an elevation of liver enzymes, which return to normal after reduction or withdrawal of the drug. Single instances of drug-induced hepatitis and hallucinations are reported, both reversed with drug withdrawal [44, 49]. Starting dose of this drug is 2 mg b.i.d., increasing by 4 mg every 4–7 days to a maximum of 36 mg t.i.d. to q.i.d.

Intrathecal baclofen

Baclofen administered using a subcutaneously implanted, programmable infusion pump and an intrathecal catheter is often dramatic in the treatment of spasticity intractable to oral agents [50]. Marked improvement of spasticity occurred in all 35 patients in the original report. Several bedridden patients returned to active rehabilitation, some returned to work or schooling. Bladder function improved in many with a marked reduction of incontinence in some. Some patients have now been followed for 5 years with continued benefit. Slight fatigue and drowsiness can be averted by a slow stepwise increase in the infused dose. This procedure appears to be an important advance and may obviate the need for ablative procedures outlined below.

Botulinum toxin

Another new approach in spasticity treatment has been the injection of botulinum toxin (Botox) into overactive muscles. Good results have been reported from open-label trials of patients with spasticity from a number of conditions including MS [51–54]. Advantages over procedures listed below are ability to target specific muscle groups, weaken muscles in a graded fashion and absence of chemicals causing irreversible neurotoxicity [51]. The amount of toxin necessary for the large muscle spasticity so often seen in MS can, however, militate against its use.

When spasticity is extremely severe and unresponsive to oral medication or physical therapy, when drugs are not tolerated, or deforming contractures begin, other modalities must be considered [55]. Our next recommendation is to place an intrathecal pump to administer baclofen. If intrathecal baclofen does not give relief we use phenol motor point or peripheral nerve blocks. Obturator, perineal, adductor or pudendal, and even sciatic and femoral nerve blocks can be performed with considerable safety. Phenol blocks are time-consuming, requiring several hours to administer properly. The effects are also transient, lasting anywhere from several weeks to 2 years, but usually at least 6 months. Phenol is caustic and irreversibly neurotoxic, which limits the amount that can be injected safely and the number of repeat procedures.

In patients who are wheelchair-bound and cannot stand, a selective nerve root neurolysis or block, usually from L1 to L4, can be done using a paravertebral approach [55]. Phenol is injected or radiofrequency heat lesions can be made using a radiofrequency heat generator [56]. This can abolish hip flexor and adductor spasticity in selected areas of the lower extremities. Cervical blocks have not been as effective for the upper extremities. Sensory loss is variable. Repetition of the process has occasionally been required for recurrences of spasticity. A temporary loss of bladder or bowel function may occur, but it usually returns with time [56].

A chemical rhizotomy can be done as a last resort when all else fails. Phenol in glycerin is injected intrathecally. The dorsal roots will be affected if the patient is in the supine position and the ventral roots if the patient is prone. The risk is too high for patients who have any prospect of ambulation, and it is usually done in cases of fixed paraplegia, impotence and urinary and/or bowel incontinence with an indwelling catheter. It has been quite effective in MS patients, 50% of patients with extreme spasticity gaining some improvement [57]. The success of the baclofen pump has made most of these destructive procedures obsolete.

23.6.3 CONTRACTURES

Spasticity can cause shortening and contractures of muscles leading to fixation of joints. In patients who have severe to total loss of function and are confined to wheelchair or bed, contractures may interfere with nursing care and lead to decubitus ulcer formation. Control of spasticity (section 2.6.2), prophylactic use of physical therapy, and exercises to stretch muscles and maintain range of motion, can forestall contracture formation. Passive range of motion exercises can reduce mild contractures by stretching tight or fibrotic muscles and breaking up adhesions around periarthritic joints. Joints are slowly mobilized, sometimes using a tilt board, and heat or ice prior to stretching to ease pain and increase relaxation. Spasmolytic drugs to decrease muscle tone and occasionally cortisone injected directly into the joint to decrease inflammation and increase mobility have also been found useful [34]. In moderate to severe cases night splints, bivalved casts, arthrodeses, or the neural destructive operations outlined above [55] can be employed. A tenotomy can be used in cases of severe contracture not reversible through nerve blocks [55]. Commonly the adductors of the thigh, the heel cord and the hamstring tendons are severed. Spinal anesthesia and passive stretching should be done first to determine how much of the deformity is due to contracture. Occasionally procedures such as an Achilles tendonotomy may cure an equinous deformity and allow more effective ambulation, but usually these procedures only facilitate nursing care [33]. Tenotomies require an overcorrected position be maintained in a cast to allow the cut ends of the tendon to heal with the longest possible length. The inactivity promoted by the casting can cause increased disability in an MS patient but this can be reversed with physical therapy once the cast is off.

23.6.4 BALANCE SENSE DYSFUNCTION

Cerebellar dysfunction may cause truncal titubation, difficulty in maintaining an upright posture and propensity for falls. No medication or operation can alleviate this difficulty. Frankel exercises have only limited value. Vestibular stimulation by rocking, swinging or spinning may improve a patient's balance sense. Stabilization of ambulation can be effected by the proper use of aids, such as a weighted cane with a tripod base, Lofstrand crutches, full crutches or a weighted walker. Both the selection and adjustment of aids should be done by an experienced physical therapist. Bracing a limb to limit excursion to a single plane of movement may also help [22, 26, 33].

Techniques to compensate for impaired balance are useful for patients, such as pausing after rising for balance before taking a step; purposely broadening the walking base; watching steps; touching or using stair handrails; stepping up first with the strong leg when climbing stairs and stepping down first with the weak leg in descending; taking short rest periods after fatigue sets in; and avoiding walking on bumpy surfaces, slippery floors, in crowds, or in the dark. They should carry on with vigor, but the gait must be slow and cautious to prevent accidental falls. Exercising in a bath tub or swimming pool is much easier because the balance sense is improved in water.

23.6.5 INCOORDINATION AND TREMOR

Frustration in the management of these symptoms is high. Tremor often lessens as the day progresses and is provoked by excitement, fatigue and elevation of body temperature. If seen during a relapse, it may be relieved during remission. Compensation techniques are of benefit when the condition is mild [58]. The patient can stabilize movements by reaching with both hands or by bracing the affected hand. Training for basic movement patterns by repetition, first guided and assisted by physical and occupational therapists and then independently, makes the movements more or less automatic and the patient gains more control when the patterns are used in accomplishing functional tasks. Joints can be immobilized by bracing them in one position to reduce tremor. While most useful for the lower extremity, the upper extremity can be fixed in a position of function for tasks such as writing or eating. Weighting a limb causes more muscles to be used to stabilize it, which reduces tremor and provides more sensory feedback to the central nervous system. Weighted bracelets and weighted utensils can reduce tremor in a minority of patients, but provocation of weakness limits their usefulness [59]. Occupational therapy can reorganize daily tasks and incorporate adaptive devices that are non-skid, easy to grasp and stable to accomplish tasks requiring dexterity [58]. A head rest or a soft neck collar may minimize head tremor. Ataxic speech is aided by speech therapy.

Drug treatment of cerebellar tremor has proved difficult. Alleviating associated stress with agents such as diazepam or hydroxyzine (Atarax or Vistaril), is sometimes effective, although these agents can cause too much sedation. Phenothiazines such as chlorpromazine (Thorazine) can be useful, but in some patients may cause the tremor to worsen and produce a resting tremor. Spasticity may contribute to action tremors of MS, and baclofen may be beneficial when this occurs [58]. Clonazepam can be of some use in MS tremor, starting at 0.5 mg twice daily and gradually increased to 2–5 mg daily in divided doses to minimize sedation. Rarely a tremor resembling essential tremor will respond to propranolol [36]. Another drug that may be of help in some patients is primadone (Mysoline). Acetazolamide (Diamox) also has some anti-tremor properties [60]. Several reports have indicated that high doses of isoniazid (INH) at 600–1200 mg/day given with pyridoxine can reduce action tremor and have some effect on postural tremor. Other evidence of cerebellar disease was not affected, however, and there was no improvement in overall function. Adverse side-effects, especially hepatotoxicity with high doses, may occur. Monitoring patients and their liver function tests and discontinuing the drug after several weeks if no significant benefit ensues is prudent [19, 58]. Glutethimide (Doriden) has been of some benefit, but sedation limits its usefulness [61]. After all has been tried, a course of corticosteroids can sometimes be of value. Thalamotomy should be considered in selected patients [19].

23.6.6 BLADDER DYSFUNCTION

Bladder dysfunction is discussed extensively in Chapter 21. Suffice it to note that the MS bladder is not one type: it may be small and muscular – a failure to store, hyperactive bladder; it may be a large, boggy structure – a failure to empty, hypotonic bladder; the bladder may conflict with its sphincter – a dyssynergic bladder. There are rehabilitation strategies involving bladder reflexes and catheterization techniques as well as the use of anticholinergic medications for management. The key to successful management of bladder dysfunction is to make the proper diagnosis of the kind of bladder and follow it with treatment appropriate to that type.

23.6.7 BOWEL DYSFUNCTION

This can take the form of constipation, incontinence or frequency and urgency. Constipation is most common in MS and can be due to a number of causes. Demyelination in the spinal cord causes slowed passage of stool through the bowel, more water absorption and a desiccated hard stool which is difficult to pass. Patients limit their fluid intake because of bladder problems, causing more water absorption from the stool. Decreased activity due to weakness and fatigue and weakness of the abdominal muscles produces slowed bowel activity. Improper diet, lack of exercise, stress, insufficient rest, irregular habits, and drugs, especially anticholinergic agents, can also contribute to constipation [62]. Patients must understand it is not necessary to have a daily bowel movement. Once every other day is adequate, but a frequency of twice a week should be treated. A distended bowel can cause increasing bladder dysfunction and walking disability due to increased spasticity [63].

Treatment in mild to moderate cases includes initiating a good diet with balanced meals taken in a relaxed atmosphere with an adequate consumption of fiber, 23 g per day. However, too rapid an increase in fiber in the diet can lead to gas, distension and occasionally diarrhea. The patient's activity through an exercise program may give improvement. An adequate daily fluid intake, at least 2000 ml/day, and a bowel program stressing regular evacuations is instituted. A convenient time for bowel movements is selected, usually 30 minutes after a meal when the gastrocolic reflex occurs. Patients should adhere to the program even when there is no urge to defecate.

Medications, used when the above methods are unsuccessful, should be geared to the cause of constipation [62]. Inadequate bulk requires bulk formers, such as psyllium hydrophilic mucilloid (Metamusil), Perdiem Plain, or Naturacil. Hard stool requires stool softeners to draw water into the bowel, such as sodium sulphosuccinate (Colace), docusate calcium (Surfak), or lactulose (Chronulac syrup). When the difficulty is expelling stool, laxatives can be used. Initially it is best to avoid the harsh laxatives, such as Exlax, Fenamint, Correctol, Dulcolax tablets or caster oil, on which the bowel can become dependent. Milder laxatives, less harmful to the bowel when used repeatedly, should be used first, such as Doxidan, Pericolace, danthron (Modane) senna concentrate (Senokot), psyllium with senna (Perdiem), or milk of magnesia with or without cascara.

Rectal suppositories, used when the above agents are ineffective, generally work within 15 minutes to an hour. Usually given in the morning after a dose of oral laxative the previous night, glycerin suppositories provide lubrication only while bisacodyl (Dulcolax) contains a medication that stimulates the bowel locally. Enemas, either Fleets or tap water, can be used when the previous methods fail. Routine use of enemas may give the only relief. Digital stimulation of the bowel may help some patients eliminate. Periodic manual removal of stool or disimpaction may be necessary in severely debilitated patients. Establishing a regular routine for elimination with a combination of a number of methods if necessary is the key to controlling constipation. Once established the regimen can often be simplified in time and some medications discontinued [62].

Bowel incontinence is rare in MS and is usually due to some secondary cause [63]. If the condition persists, the patient should be evaluated in the hospital. Dietary irritants, spicy foods, coffee, alcohol, cigarettes, diarrhea due to gastrointestinal flu, drugs, antacids or laxatives may contribute to the problem. Incontinence may be caused by impaction, with loose stool passing around hardened feces. MS can cause incontinence when there is a loss of rectal sensation. The rectum can then become filled and stretched beyond its usual capacity, leading to involuntary relaxation of the anal sphincter.

Incontinence and urgency are difficult problems to treat. However, they can often be managed by a bowel program using laxatives, suppositories or enemas to empty the bowel at fixed times [63]. The patient should be aware of the gastrocolic reflex 30 minutes after meals when incontinence is most likely, and also the stimulatory effects of coffee and hot liquids. Anticholinergics and bulk formers such as Metamucil, taken without the extra fluid and no more than once a day, may be helpful [62]. In extreme cases Kaopectate or diphenoxylate hydrochloride with atropine sulphate (Lomotil), 5 ml four times a day, can relieve acute symptoms. Frequent incontinence often requires protective underpants with absorbent linings and plastic outer shields, such as Attends. Biofeedback is an experimental technique that may have some use in incontinent patients. In the rare patient whose bowel urgency cannot be managed, colostomy might be indicated for hygienic reasons, especially if sacral pressure ulcers exist [62].

23.6.8 SEXUAL PROBLEMS

Sexual dysfunction in both the male and female patient with MS is common [64, 64a, 65]; it is discussed fully in Chapter 22. It should be understood that to manage sexual difficulties effectively it is essential to be able to speak about them without embarrassment and with an ability to develop potential solutions. There are many solutions now available; optimism for a happier sexual life for those with neurologic disabilities should be high and understanding the alternatives is essential.

23.6.9 FATIGUE

Fatigue is very frequently experienced in MS, being present in 78–85% of patients [66, 67]. It is often the presenting symptom of MS when patients have normal neurological examinations and are thus sent for psychiatric evaluations. When evaluating fatigue in MS it is important to determine what type of fatigue is present [68]. One type is the normal tired feeling at the end of the day after working hard, which is relieved with a night's rest. Another is the worn-out feeling, associated not with activity but with depression, accompanied by poor appetite, sleep disturbances and feelings of decreased self-worth. It is relieved when the depression is treated. Another fatigue is that associated with a paretic limb subjected to repeated activity, such as a slight limp which becomes more prominent with continued walking and finally requires rest, during which the strength in the limb returns.

Finally there is the sense of overwhelming tiredness or lassitude, which has been termed MS fatigue [66]. Not related to depression or activity *per se*, it may be present even after a good night's sleep. It is often inexplicable on the basis of the neurological findings, occurring in the face of normal or only minimally abnormal neurological examinations. It occurs on a daily basis, gets worse in the afternoon and evening, may resolve after a few hours. There is usually an overpowering need to rest. The majority of patients find it gets worse with vigorous or moderate exercise, but many – greater than half – will also report it seems to improve with moderate exercise done routinely. Warmer temperatures will exacerbate the fatigue; some relief results from cooling the skin with water. Naps or periods of rest are also helpful in most patients.

Treatment of this type of fatigue includes encouragement and support. Patients should be told they are not fragile and should try to carry on as usual. They will often find that the more they attempt the easier it becomes, improving their morale and gaining a sense of control over their condition. However, over-exhaustion may lead to a temporary increase in symptoms and should be avoided. Patients should be active and busy during the day as long as possible, not nap excessively, but plan for periods of rest during the day, especially during work hours. When rest is required, chair rest rather than bed rest is recommended.

To enable patients to overcome fatigue, maximize energy and minimize over-exertion we suggest:

- sleep regular hours and avoid unnecessary late nights;
- plan ahead and make daily or weekly schedules of activities;
- recognize a limit, which may vary from day to day;
- pace activity, taking short rest periods during prolonged activity.

A particularly difficult activity should be broken down into a series of steps or the help of other people should be sought. Priorities should be set, focusing on tasks that must be done, while others are postponed. Plan most activities for early in the day, when the energy level is the highest. Occupational therapists can organize the home and the workplace to conserve energy by doing work simplification of everyday tasks, such as cooking, cleaning, yard work, desk work, dressing and bathing.

A few medications have been found useful in combating MS fatigue. A randomized study, using retrospective patient reporting, showed that amantadine can be effective in as many as 66% of patients, although the effect was small and was not accompanied by changes in overall disability[69]. Further prospective double-blind placebo-controlled studies have confirmed the effect[70–72]. The starting dose is 100 mg twice a day, increasing to three times a day if necessary and discontinued if there is no effect at the higher dose. Side-effects are mild, usually dry mouth, insomnia, increased constipation and sometimes urinary retention.

Another drug that has been found useful is pemoline (Cylert)[68], a stimulant. Two preliminary clinical trials, one double-blind and placebo-controlled, have shown this drug to be effective in reducing patient rated severity of fatigue[67, 73]. The starting dose is one 18.75 mg tablet daily. Because of a delayed effect, it should only be increased by one tablet every 3 weeks to as much as 10 tablets per day. Side-effects are irritability, insomnia, nausea, transient weight loss, anorexia and hypersensitivity reactions (blotching of the legs, i.e. livedo reticularis, edema) which are reversible with discontinuing the drug. Methylphenidate (Ritalin) and dextroamphedamine are also used for MS fatigue, but these are controlled drugs; they are habit forming, cause weight loss and anorexia and have not been found to be any more effective. More recently the newer activating antidepressants such as fluoxitene (Prozac) seem to have antifatigue properties without significant side-effects[60].

23.6.10 VISUAL DISTURBANCES

The neuro-ophthalmological aspects of MS are presented in Chapter 2. Visual disturbances include oscillopsia, diplopia, reduced visual acuity, uveitis, cataracts, central scotoma, field defects and difficulty tracking associated with internuclear ophthalmoparesis.

The non-infectious uveitis is treated with mydriatics and local corticosteroids. High-powered magnifiers aid patients with central scotomas or decreased vision secondary to optic atrophy. This visual disability is accentuated when light is dim and patients should always optimize their lighting conditions, leaving a light on at night for emergencies[26]. Patients with field defects and/or difficulty in tracking can improve reading by using an engineer's triangular ruler. Visually impaired patients should be made aware of the talking book programs available through city library systems and local MS groups[74].

Many patients compensate for diplopia by suppression of one of the images after several months[26, 33]. When it continues to be a problem, a plastic eye shield over one eye, alternated between eyes, is recommended for reading and driving, but it should not be worn constantly, so that the brain can eventually compensate for the diplopia. Patients complain of oscillopsia usually when nystagmus is present in primary or downward gaze. Visual acuity can be affected, because of slippage of the retinal image induced by the nystagmus. If nystagmus and oscillopsia can be suppressed by convergence, glasses with converging (base-out) prisms may be helpful[75]. Patching may aid patients in whom oscillopsia is dissociated. Certain drugs may suppress pendular nystagmus with resultant improvement in oscillopsia and visual acuity: isoniazid in doses of 800–1000 mg/day[75], clonazepam[76] and, in a few cases, baclofen. Other beneficial drugs have been valproic acid and trihexyphenidyl[77, 78]. In patients with severe oscillopsia and impaired visual acuity, the acuity should be retested after 1–2 mg of oral clonazepam.

Acute optic neuritis, occurring at the onset of clinical manifestations of MS in 20–30% and sometime in the course of the disease in about half of patients, gives rise to ocular pain, impaired visual acuity and field defects. Its treatment is discussed in Chapter 2.

23.6.11 DYSARTHRIA

As an initial symptom of MS this is uncommon, but the speech pathways are frequently involved later in the course of MS [19, 28, 79]. Brain stem lesions cause the speech to be slurred and have a low volume. Shallow breathing and low breath pressure due to bulbar paresis may also affect speech. Cerebellar disturbances can cause a dysmetria of speech, and an inability to talk rapidly. Cerebral lesions leave a halting combined with a fast, unintelligible speech pattern. Dysarthria may be more severe when the patient is excited, or overheated due to weather or fever. Instruction by a professional speech therapist in articulation and breathing can be beneficial, as may progressive resistive exercises given to the muscles of phonation [33]. A pacing board is often used in treatment which the patient touches while speaking each syllable to slow the speech pattern down. Cerebellar speech disturbances have been less responsive to treatment. Continuous encouragement to speak and read aloud slowly, distinctly and frequently is important, because the effort to speak can be especially tiring and depressing to some patients with moderate to severe dysarthria. In some cases tremor of the lips, tongue or jaw may make it impossible to speak and alternative communication devices are then indicated [26]. Computer-driven communication aids or voice synthesizers are coming into much wider use, allowing greater efficiency and a higher rate of output than older devices.

Paroxysmal dysarthria when present is highly characteristic of MS and occurs in 2–4% of patients in large series [19]. It is characterized by frequent (every half hour or more often) brief (20 seconds or less) episodes, usually accompanied by other symptoms, such as paroxysmal ataxia or paresthesias of one or more limbs, and sometimes precipitated by talking, movement or hyperventilation. Carbamazepine (Tegretol) has been found to be efficacious, usually in less than therapeutic anticonvulsant doses. If not tolerated, acetazolamide [80] can be used, whereas phenytoin and baclofen have not been found to be particularly useful [37].

23.6.12 DYSPHAGIA

Severe dysphagia is relatively uncommon in ambulatory MS patients, although many have a mild dysphagia, especially when they drink liquids [19, 28]. Choking intermittently on saliva is also common. Dysphagia can be increased by excitement, tiredness or being overheated. Teaching patients to take a deep breath before swallowing has been beneficial. Other helpful techniques have been: modifying food texture by commercially available thickening agents; moisturizing food with broth, juice, or gravy; warming or cooling food to stimulate the swallowing reflex; changing the position of the head; alternating liquid with solids; reducing the size of bites and meals, and eating less more frequently. The speech pathologist, occupational therapist, clinical dietitian, radiologist, neurologist, otolaryngologist, and specialist in rehabilitation medicine (physiatrist) all may be involved with dysphagia management. The cineesophagram and videofluoroscopy can be very useful for diagnosing the problem, planning rehabilitative measures and to test improvement. It can also indicate aspiration is occurring, which may be missed by clinical evaluation in up to 40% of patients. A feeding strategy based on the consistency, amount and order of oral intake may then be developed. Food thickeners (such as Diafoods Thick-It, Milani Foods, 2525 Armatage Avenue, Melrose Park, Illinois 60160, USA) may be a part of this strategy.

Dysphagia made worse by an elevation of body temperature, such as a fever, is one of the most distressing symptoms of MS. It should be considered an emergency because of possible pulmonary aspiration. In cases of severe ongoing dysphagia percutaneous endoscopic gastrostomy is recommended for long-term enteral feeding [81] and prevention of aspiration pneumonia.

23.6.13 DIZZINESS

Nonspecific dizziness, termed light-headedness, dizziness, giddiness, or vertigo by various authors, occurs as an initial symptom in 5–9% of MS patients in large series [19, 28]. However, electronystagmography and caloric vestibular measurements reveal vestibular abnormalities in as many as 40–48% of nonselected patients. Equilibrium is complex with input from the cerebrum, eyes, ears, brain stem, posterior columns, cerebellum and peripheral nervous system. Treatment begins with diagnosing the region of demyelination. Following appropriate diagnosis an exercise program may be developed based specifically on appropriate anatomical rehabilitation techniques. This may vary from vestibular rehabilitation with techniques designed to fatigue the abnormal impulses to simply giving an assistive device (cane, crutch) to allow for stabilization of the body. Postural dizziness is usually exacerbated by a sudden change of position, and is not a bothersome symptom. Problematic dizziness can usually be controlled with administration of dimenhydrinate (Dramamine), meclizine HCl (Antivert or Bonine), oxazepam, chlorpromazine (Thorazine), fentanyl plus droperidol (Innovar), or diphenhydramine (Benadryl) [26, 82]. Attacks of true vertigo resembling acute labyrinthitis, exhibiting nausea, vomiting and prostration, do occur and may be the initial manifestation of MS or occur as part of a relapse. They last a few days to several weeks, and usually do not recur. Bed rest with restriction of head movement and administration of the above named agents usually gives relief. If vomiting is severe, preventing oral medication, intravenous fluids to maintain hydration should be given, and pulse high-dose intravenous methylprednisolone to reduce brain stem inflammation may be warranted.

23.6.14 PARESTHESIAS

Sensory symptoms are very common in MS and part of the initial symptomatology in 21–23% of cases [19, 28]. Pure sensory relapses are frequent in early clinical MS. They occur most commonly in one leg, and spread to both legs and the lower part of the trunk. Other attacks may involve the arms or the face. The perineum may be involved, impairing sensation of urination, defecation and the vagina, but control is preserved. Light touch and pinprick sensations are preserved but dysesthetic. The relapses may last 10 days to 6–8 weeks. In another distinctive relapse, proprioception is lost in one or both upper extremities giving the complaint of useless hands. Cutaneous sensation is preserved and the lesion has been localized to the posterior columns of the spinal cord. Remission usually occurs but may not be complete.

Persistent paresthesias are very common, present in as many as 84% of patients [83]. They are diffuse or segmental, involving one dermatome, and described variously as: 'tingling-pricking', 'numbness', 'like after Novocain', 'tightness around knees', 'fingers too big', 'can't identify by touching', 'girdle sensation', 'swelling', 'like a bandage or plaster cast'. They should be regarded as an annoyance rather than truly disabling symptom. Patients should be dissuaded from focusing on the symptoms, as this only makes the problem worse [26]. Corticosteroids may alleviate the symptoms, but should be reserved for more disabling exacerbations. In our experience amitriptyline (Elavil) or carbamazepine may be of help when bothersome symptoms cannot be ignored.

Lhermitte's sign is a particular type of intermittent paresthesia, most commonly caused by MS, and is present in 33–38% of patients at some time in their clinical course [19]. Precipitated by neck flexion, its probable cause is a demyelinating lesion in the posterior columns of the cervical spinal cord. Only rarely does it require treatment with analgesics and tranquilizers. In one study it was abolished by carbamazepine [84]. Treatment can often be discontinued in a few months, as this condition usually does not persist longer than this.

23.6.15 TRIGEMINAL NEURALGIA

This is a specific type of brief, severe, recurrent, radicular pain in the trigeminal nerve distribution occurring in approximately 1–2% of MS patients. When series of patients with trigeminal neuralgia are studied, the incidence of multiple sclerosis is between 2 and 3% [19, 24]. The pain is more likely to be bilateral in MS than in idiopathic cases [85].

The first treatment of choice is carbamazepine [26, 86]. Low doses are given initially to avoid sedation, starting at 100 mg three times a day and increased over 3 or 4 days to 200 mg three times per day. Further increases are made every 7 days as tolerated to obtain pain relief, up to 2000 mg per day. Dosage should be kept as low as possible, consistent with adequate pain relief and adverse side-effects. A blood level of 6–8 µg/ml is usually necessary to achieve a response [36]. The drug aggravates many symptoms of MS, most notably weakness in the legs, and may not be tolerated in the higher doses [19]. If patients cannot tolerate carbamazepine, phenytoin (Dilantin, 300–600 mg/day) may be used, but it is less effective. Clonazepam has also been shown to be effective. An initial dose of 0.5 mg twice a day may be increased at intervals of 5 days. Baclofen (30–80 mg/day) also has been reported to be effective [87]. Amitriptyline (50–150 mg/day) has been shown to be effective in as many as half of affected patients [36]. Other patients respond to a combination of perphenazine (2–12 mg/day) and 50 mg/day amitriptyline, started twice daily and gradually increased weekly to a maximum of 12 mg perphenazine and 150 mg amitriptyline. Misoprostol, a long-acting PGE$_1$ analogue, has also been beneficial [88]. If the pain is controlled with drug therapy it should be tapered after 3 months to determine whether a remission has occurred. If the pain proves refractory to drug treatment, percutaneous stereotactic thermal rhizotomy of the appropriate trigeminal nerve branch using radiofrequency or a laser has given excellent results [60, 89, 90]. Good results have also been obtained using glycerol rhizotomy [91].

23.6.16 PAIN

Traditionally pain was not thought to be a common feature of MS [28]. However, more recent studies report pain due to the disease of MS in 29–65% of patients, with 20–32% having significant pain and 20% having pain at the onset of MS. Pain may be due to optic neuritis, trigeminal neuralgia, painful tonic seizures, headache, low back ache, neck ache, painful reflex spasms, paroxysmal burning extremity pain, or dysalgesia [19, 92–95]. Many MS patients have a chronic back or neck ache, probably secondary to spasticity or low back strain produced by an abnormal gait or posture. Localized spinal root pain due to MS is rare, and should lead to a search for another cause. Poor walking posture should be corrected through rehabilitation. Mild analgesics and anti-inflammatory agents – aspirin, acetaminophen or non-steroidal anti-inflammatories – muscle relaxants – baclofen, diazepam, methocarbamol (Lobaxin) or carisoprodol (Soma) – cyclobenzaprine (Flexeril), physical therapy, exercise, a firmer mattress or a bed board, local heat, massage, ultrasound and hydrotherapy may all be helpful. Spinal manipulation, however, may irritate the spinal cord and increase neurologic dysfunction problems [26]. An acute flare-up of backache may necessitate bed rest on a firm mattress with leg elevation.

Leg weakness, which can lead to knee hyperextension, ligament damage and a swollen and painful knee can occur. A load-relieving cane or crutch and a knee brace can give relief [60].

Muscle cramps trouble certain patients, and baclofen and diazepam can give significant relief.

Dysesthetic limb pain or pseudoradicular pain, possibly due to involvement of the sensory root zone or spinothalamic tracts of the spinal cord, can be refractory to milder analgesics. It is manifested by a persistent burning sensation, predominantly in the lower extremities, worse at night and aggravated by heat and walking [19]. Opiates or codeine, except acutely, should be avoided to prevent dependency. Phenytoin, carbamazepine and amitriptyline in doses used for trigeminal neuralgia have been effective for this pain in some cases. Desipramine (Norpramin) or nortriptyline (Pamelor) can be used if amitriptyline causes too much sedation. Occasionally transcutaneous nerve stimulation may help, but it may have the opposite effect in some cases. Biofeedback techniques, meditation and acupuncture may also be helpful in some cases [26]. Capsaic acid cream (Axsain, Zostrix HP), topically at least three times a day to areas of pain, has become available, and has been reasonably effective for this paresthetic pain with few side-effects. Phenol nerve root blocks, posterior root section or cordectomy may be considered in rare cases refractory to other therapy.

23.6.17 EPILEPTIC SEIZURES

After excluding coincidental occurrence of epilepsy and MS and unilateral 'tonic seizures' in earlier case studies, a higher prevalence of seizures in MS patients versus the general populace remains. Studies indicate 1–5% of clinically definite MS patients had seizures during the course of the disease [96–99]. On the other hand, Ritter and Poser [100] found only 5 cases out of 812 patients, a frequency equal to the general population. Therefore, a search for other causes of seizures must be made. A few autopsied cases demonstrated plaques immediately beneath the cortex or massive demyelination of the cerebral white matter. Edema, inflammation or gliosis of a plaque immediately adjacent to the cortex may initiate epileptiform spike discharges in cortical neurons [19]. All types of seizures can be seen, except for petit mal epilepsy. Most common are generalized motor seizures with or without a focal onset. Temporal lobe seizures, epilepsia partialis continua, and status epilepticus can also occur. In many instances different seizure types may occur in the same patient [97]. Rarely epilepsy can

precede the onset of other manifestations of MS. In most cases seizures are benign, infrequent and easily controlled with anticonvulsants, and actually remitted in half the patients in one study [98]. Seizures may also occur during an acute relapse and not be followed by recurrent epilepsy. A small number of patients have seizures in association with rapidly increasing disability that are difficult or impossible to control [19], but usually efficacy is high with standard anticonvulsant doses of phenytoin (Dilantin) or carbamazepine (Tegretol). After a 6-month seizure-free period, anticonvulsants can also be tapered and finally discontinued over 3 months. Treatment may be restarted if seizures return, which is unlikely. Failure of treatment in the absence of rapid progression of MS should lead to a reassessment for another etiology.

23.6.18 TONIC SEIZURES

These and other forms of paroxysmal symptoms are a characteristic feature of MS [101–103]. In fact, when paroxysms of brain stem or spinal cord origin occur in young adults, the most likely etiology is MS. The incidence varies from 4 to 9% of MS patients in Western studies [19] to as high as 17% in the Japanese literature [99], and were the first symptom of MS in 8–10% of the reported cases. About half of the patients note precipitating factors, most commonly truncal movement or tactile stimulation, but also hyperventilation. The duration of the episodes is usually less than two minutes (usually 15–90 seconds), and their frequency up to 30 times a day, but less frequent than paroxysmal dysarthria. They usually occur in a hemiparetic distribution and are very similar to dystonic seizures. One or both limbs on the same side and often the face go into tonic contraction without loss of consciousness or involuntary micturition. Bilateral attacks, sometimes involving all four limbs, have been reported, especially in Japan. The upper extremity is most commonly involved, but rapid spread to other areas may occur. Sensory symptoms on the same or opposite side, usually unpleasant burning or tingling, may precede the tonic spasm. The spasms are painful in about half of the cases. They may be associated with other paroxysmal symptoms, such as dysarthria and ataxia. The pathophysiology remains conjectural. Possibly impulses, especially afferent ones, reach an area of demyelination and spread laterally to neighboring afferent and efferent axons within the plaque. Fluxes of ionized calcium at the site of the plaque may also be involved, hence the resemblance of tonic seizures to hemitetany of metabolic origin and their precipitation by hyperventilation.

Tonic seizures are just one of a number of paroxysmal symptoms that can be the first clinical manifestation of MS, such as dysarthria and ataxia, diplopia, paresthesias, pain, itching and akinesia. Carbamazepine (Tegretol) has been an effective agent for all of these [36, 103]. Low doses (200 mg twice a day) with blood levels below the anticonvulsant therapeutic range are often adequate, and can be tolerated by even ataxic patients. Acetazolamide (Diamox), 125–250 mg three times a day, has also been reported to be effective [80], while phenytoin or phenobarbital have been less so, and baclofen has been ineffective. Drug therapy should be discontinued in a few months, as symptoms often spontaneously remit in patients within this time period [102].

23.6.19 NEUROBEHAVIORAL DISORDERS

Those that occur in MS include depression, euphoria, cognitive impairment, and less frequently bipolar disease, psychosis and emotional incontinence [36].

Rather than euphoria, MS patients have evidence of concealed and overt depression more frequently than other patients with neuromuscular disease of comparable severity [19]. With progression of the disease, overt depression increases, while denial decreases [104]. Helping the MS patient cope with depression should be a major therapeutic goal. Studies have not shown depression to be related to functional disability or the extent of disease on MRI. Depression in MS is more a reaction to the prospect of chronic progressive disability and isolation than a direct result of the disease [19]. If euphoria exists at all, it is part of a coping strategy in some patients [105] or it may be seen with moderate to severe cognitive impairment [19].

Psychiatric counseling should be available not only to the patient but also to the family, which is also coping with the changes in lifestyle and member relationships. The potential for suicide should be considered in all patients. More frequent doctor visits to foster support and reassurance, discussions with family members with regard to altering the patient environment to help deter suicide, and limiting the amount of certain medications prescribed at one time may be appropriate in some cases. Good trials assessing drugs for depression in MS are limited. Only occasionally are drugs, such as imipramine (Tofranil), amitriptyline (Elavil), doxepin, trazodone, or rarely CNS stimulants such as pemoline (Cylert) indicated. Desipramine has also been found to be useful for MS patients, due to a lower anticholinergic profile than amitriptyline [36]. The dose is started at 25 mg each night and slowly brought up to 75–100 mg, usually the minimum effective level. An adequate period of assessment at each dose level is necessary, as patient response may be delayed by 2–4 weeks. Fluoxetine (Prozac) has been shown recently to be effective in treating depression in MS. It should be kept in mind that drugs are never a substitute for verbalizing interpersonal relationships.

Cognitive impairment, in the past reported in 20 and 30% of patients at some time in their course of MS [19, 106], was often underestimated because of the insensitivity of bedside mental status testing [107]. More recently formal neuropsychological studies have indicated that cognitive dysfunction is present in 48–65% of MS patients [108]. However, less than 10% of patients have moderate to severe dementia that is associated with severe disability [109]. Rather than duration of disease or disability, the strongest correlate with cognitive impairment has turned out to be total lesion area in the cerebral hemispheres on MRI or by neuropathological examination [19, 110–112]. Cognitive dysfunction is discussed in more detail in Chapter 20. We will emphasize here that its pattern in MS is consistent with a subcortical dementia or a frontal lobe disconnection syndrome, distinctly different from the pattern present in Alzheimer's disease [108, 113, 114], and it can be a major cause of employment disability in MS patients [115]. Neuropsychological testing should be performed at the first sign of difficulties at work or alterations in social behaviour, formerly often attributed to depression or fatigue. Early initiation of adaptations in the workplace and treatment modalities aimed at keeping the MS patient employed can then be made. Such testing should also play a greater role in the determination of MS disability for social security and employment compensation benefits [115].

Treatment of cognitive dysfunction in MS is still in its infancy. A thorough assessment of the patient should be made to distinguish the problem from depression or fatigue. Individual psychotherapy may help some patients who have more difficulty dealing with the emotional impact of the problem. Drug treatment of cognitive impairment in MS is still experimental. Compensatory measures, such as notebooks and pocket electronic databanks, and cognitive strategies (enhancing memory by association) are helpful for many patients. More promising are formalized cognitive retraining programs, used with success for other types of cognitive dysfunction such as that following head injury [116]. Moderate to severe dementia, while rare, currently has no treatment, often interferes with rehabilitation, and may require custodial care.

The syndrome of emotional incontinence or pathologic laughing and crying is common in MS and is part of pseudobulbar palsy [36]. It can be very distressing for patients, lead to serious impairment of interpersonal relationships and mask a severe underlying depression. Clinicians should be aware of this condition, because it is usually amenable to treatment with amitriptyline (25 mg two to three times a day). The drug can periodically be tapered to assess the continued need for treatment. Other tricyclic antidepressants as well as levodopa or bromocriptine may also be effective.

23.7 Preventing and treating secondary complications

Better medical care and a more aggressive approach toward the containment of preventable secondary complications has resulted in lower mortality, morbidity and disability rates in MS in the past four decades [92, 117]. More efficient antibiotics and symptomatic management of movement disorders have been important elements in producing this favourable trend. The most common complications of MS are infections of the urinary tract, skin or respiratory tract, septicemia, respiratory failure, pulmonary embolism, bladder and renal calculi, and pressure ulcers of the skin. Most of these do not become evident until the patient is severely disabled, confined to a wheelchair or bed. Infection or fever sufficient to cause symptomatic worsening in MS should always be considered a neurological emergency. Patients should always call their physicians when this occurs. Immediate treatment with antipyretics is necessary if worsening is associated with fever to prevent possible dysphagia and aspiration.

23.7.1 PULMONARY INFECTIONS

The most life-threatening of all complications is pneumonia, usually of the aspiration type. Proper assessment of dysphagia severity is required to prevent aspiration, and the diet altered to ease swallowing if necessary. A transesophageal feeding or a gastrostomy tube should be considered in severe cases. In bedridden patients progressive range of motion of the extremities, turning the body from side to side, and propping the patient up in a chair during the day is important for preventing fluid collection in the lungs which may result in lung congestion and pneumonia [118]. Pneumonia is managed in the usual way, but aggressive means of fever control are employed, such as a hypothermia mattress and/or alcohol sponges to prevent further decompensation of brain stem function caused by the fever, leading to impaired cough and clearing of secretions, or dysphagia and aspiration [119].

23.7.2 PRESSURE SORES

Pressure sores or decubitus ulcers are particularly prone to occur in severely disabled wheelchair- or bed-bound MS patients who have impaired skin sensation. The ulcers frequently appear quietly with little or no pain. Areas of the skin under constant pressure for even one hour, such as those in contact with a bed or wheelchair, can experience obstructed blood flow leading to tissue necrosis and breakdown. The thorough, precise report by Reuler is still recommended for all who care for MS patients with pressure sores [120].

Once an ulcer is established it can be difficult to cure. The key to the management of decubitus ulcers is prevention, which can be done in the majority of cases if the causative factors are understood [121]. The causative factors include: (a) configuration of the bony skeleton where bony prominences occur (especially shoulders, ischial tuberosity, sacrum, ankles and heels); (b) immobility; (c) rubbing movements; (d) moisture and bacterial contamination of bedclothes and skin of the pelvis and adjoining areas due to urinary and fecal incontinence; (e) inadequate nutrition; (f) lack of education regarding prevention. Braces and splints should be carefully adjusted to avoid pressure points and padded if necessary. A wheelchair patient should have a change in position every 30 minutes to an hour (doing push-ups on the arms of the chair or being lifted in the wheelchair or standing up for 4 or 5 minutes if that is possible) [118]. A foam rubber wheelchair cushion at least 6 inches thick or a silastic cushion should be used, covered with clean sheepskin. A columnar air cushion such as the Roho is also excellent as long as it is kept inflated. The seat and cushion should be dry and free of wrinkles. If there is dependent edema and/or discoloration of the ankles and feet, the legs should be elevated periodically on wheelchair foot rests, a chair or sofa. Active or passive range of motion exercises of the legs should be done daily, and support stockings worn during the day.

The bedridden patient with ulcers should have a rotating-pressure, air or water mattress covered with a clean sheepskin, and should also undergo a change of posture (turning from side to side or on the abdomen) every 1–2 hours, facilitated by an electric bed with side rails and an overhead trapeze. However, the traditional sidelying position with the upper leg flexed at the hip and knee over the body should not be used, as this puts too much pressure on the trochanteric areas, actually promoting pressure ulcers over these areas, and also conductive to flexion contracture development in the legs. A modified dorsilateral position with the top leg behind the body and the arms and legs extended is preferred. Bony prominences should be checked daily for areas of redness or irritation, and if found massaged with a skin lotion. Sun lamps and heating pads should be used with caution. Foam rubber rings or bootees under the feet can prevent heel ulceration. Rubbing movements of pressure points over bedclothes during change of position and direct trauma that might cause a break in the skin must be avoided. Friction of the skin caused by spastic movements, such as legs held together by abductor spasm should be controlled by the procedures mentioned here. Spastic legs can be separated by a foam rubber insert or pillow. The skin must be kept as clean and dry as possible, facilitated by the use of an indwelling bladder catheter and a change of diapers soon after a bowel movement in incontinent patients. A daily bath (bed or tub) is recommended. Wet areas should be cleansed, dried and powdered. Tincture of benzoin can be applied several times a week to toughen the skin. The nails should be kept short to prevent scratching and adequate nutrition should be ensured [118].

23.7.3 URINARY TRACT INFECTIONS AND CALCULI

The key to managing urinary tract infections is to prevent them from occurring. Residual urine in the bladder should be kept as low as possible by frequent and complete voiding using the Credé method of bladder pressure if necessary (pressure applied with both hands over the lower abdomen during Valsalva in the sitting position on a toilet or commode) [122]. If residual urine is still above 150 ml, a program of intermittent self-catheterization should be employed. Adequate amounts of fluid (6–8 glasses/day) should be consumed to promote flushing of the bladder contents. Women should be careful to wipe from front to back, especially after a bowel movement, avoid undergarments made of synthetic fabrics which trap moisture, and empty the bladder before and after intercourse. All patients should keep their urine acidic with vitamin C, 1000 mg four times a day and by drinking cranberry juice twice a day as part of fluid intake [118]. Prophylactic antibiotics, such as methenamine mandelate (Mandelamine) 1 g four times a day, methenamine hippurate 500 mg four times a day or trimethoprim-sulphamethoxazole (Bactrim or Septra) one tablet daily, should be reserved for patients with repeated infections, indwelling catheters or significant post-void residual urines [123]. Indwelling Foley catheters should be avoided if possible in favor of intermittent daily catheterization. If they become necessary, one should keep the catheter and drainage apparatus as clean as possible, and a closed drainage system should be employed at all times. When infection occurs, identification of the organism and its antibiotic sensitivities, forced fluids and appropriate antibiotic therapy are indicated, as well as quick reduction of fever and the maintenance of adequate bladder drainage, which may be a predisposing factor to these infections. Repeated infections require further investigation by a urologist.

Bladder and renal calculi usually do not become a problem until an indwelling bladder catheter is used. Calculi can usually be prevented by encouraging a large fluid intake (approx. 3500 ml) and an upright posture to assist bladder drainage. Regular urinalysis and periodic urological evaluations with residual urine determinations are recommended. If bladder and renal calculi are suspected, urological consultation for evaluation and surgical removal is indicated.

23.8 Treating relapses with ACTH and corticosteroids – putative treatments

The etiology and pathogenesis of MS are unknown, thus any rational therapeutic approach aimed at proposed specific disease processes must remain putative. Immunosuppressive and immunomodulatory treatments of MS are discussed in Chapter 17. We will confine our discussion to some general comments about these treatments, a more detailed presentation of treatments that do not fall into these two categories, and our method of treating the acute exacerbation with corticosteroids.

23.8.1 ACTH AND/OR CORTICOSTEROIDS

These agents can have a strong anti-inflammatory effect on the central nervous system of MS patients, as manifested by the marked suppression of intrathecal IgG synthesis rate [124, 125] and the ability of high-dose intravenous methylprednisolone to reduce the number of enhancing lesions demonstrated by serial double-dose delayed contrast enhanced CT scans [126] and gadolinium enhanced lesions appearing on the MRI [127, 128]. In a study of 143 MS brains, a reduction in perivascular infiltrates was found in patients treated with corticosteroids or immunosuppressive drugs [129].

In one of the first studies of its kind in MS, the USA National Cooperative ACTH Study found that ACTH gel, 40 units intramuscularly twice a day for 1 week followed by a 1-week taper, was superior to placebo at the 4 week follow-up period for 197 patients in exacerbation. However, the statistical significance between the two patient groups was marginal. Despite a number of criticisms of this trial, subsequent studies supported the use of ACTH and corticosteroids for acute relapse [86, 130–133], and the US Food and Drug Administration approved the use of ACTH for the treatment of acute relapses of MS.

If ACTH is to be used for clinical relapse of MS, from our clinical experience we suggest the patient be hospitalized and a dose of 100 units be given intramuscularly twice a day for 2–3 weeks depending on the side-effects encountered. The dose should then be tapered to zero at a rate of 20 mg every day. To prevent a possible rebound of symptoms and minimize withdrawal effects, 100 mg of oral prednisone on alternate days should follow ACTH with a tapering of the dose to zero over 2 months.

If a worsening occurs, the dose is returned to minimum necessary to suppress symptoms and signs, and tapering is prolonged. Improvement in neurological function rarely begins before the third day and may continue after therapy is stopped. During treatment the patient is on a 1 g sodium 1800 calorie diet. Potassium supplementation (25 mEq) is given twice a day along with an antacid such as Tums (calcium carbonate, 200 mg of calcium) between meals and at bedtime, or ranitidine [133]. Full activity as tolerated should be encouraged during treatment and the patient should be given physical therapy at least once a day.

Side-effects of ACTH therapy occur quite commonly and can be severe [133a]. The most frequent of these include acne, Cushingoid facies, hirsutism, water retention, increased appetite and weight gain, glucose intolerance, hypertension, purpura, edema, heartburn, euphoria, irritability, insomnia, lassitude, severe depression and anxiety. More serious psychological effects including confusion, flight of ideas, hallucinations, delusions, marked depression, suicidal ideation, mood swings, manic episodes and psychosis are possible. Peptic ulcer and gastrointestinal bleeding, severe hypertension, uncontrollable diabetes and precipitation of seizures in MS patients occur rarely. Symptoms suggestive of hypothalamic pituitary suppression can be seen if ACTH is withdrawn too quickly. Osteoporosis with vertebral compression fractures and cataracts has occurred after repeated courses of ACTH. In MS patients one must watch for new infections, such as pneumonitis and urinary tract infections, as ACTH will suppress the usual systemic manifestations of infection and cause an elevated white cell count in the blood, interfering with the use of this test in the assessment of infection.

No adequate controlled trials have compared prednisone with ACTH for treating acute relapses of MS, and it should not be assumed that these two agents can be used interchangeably [134]. However, we have had a favourable experience using this agent and dexamethasone (Decadron), 16 mg per day (four divided doses) in reducing MS intrathecal IgG synthesis rate [125]. After acute treatment, a tapering regimen should be used to prevent rebound of symptoms.

Our regimen to treat exacerbations is oral prednisone in a dose of 160 mg per day (four divided doses) for 1 week followed by 160 mg every other day tapering by 20 mg per week [27]. We also use supplemental treatments mentioned above. If our oral regimen is not effective we recommend intravenous prednisolone.

Within the past decade a new mode of corticosteroid treatment for MS relapses has been gaining popularity – intravenous (IV) bolus or 'pulse' methylprednisolone (MP). Two double-blind studies have reported the superiority of high-dose IV MP over placebo for accelerating the recovery from MS relapse [135, 136]. Three studies have shown either no significant differences in outcome or an advantage for IV MP when it was compared to ACTH for the treatment of MS exacerbations [137–139]. Pulse high-dose MP therapy has also been well tolerated in MS patients, with few significant adversities experienced [124, 140], the common ones being the same as ACTH described above. A corticosteroid 'let down' also occurs in some patients by the abrupt withdrawal of treatment, manifested by generalized weakness, but no Addisonian crises are precipitated. Avascular necrosis of the femoral or humoral head has occurred. Sudden deaths, fatal arrhythmia and nearly fatal anaphylactic reactions have been reported [141], but have not occurred in a retrospective review of 240 treated patients [140]. From the literature, little support can be found for long-term treatment with ACTH and corticosteroids. Several researchers have concluded that pulse high-dose intravenous methylprednisolone is the best treatment of acute relapses of MS [19, 141–143]. We tend to support this view. While studies comparing this treatment with ACTH therapy have been flawed for various reasons, no significant differences in outcome have been found. Yet pulse MP treatment is safer, with fewer significant side-effects. If required, patients can tolerate repeated courses of treatment over a shorter time span than with ACTH. The treatment with pulse MP is also shorter, requiring less hospitalization. The optimum dose of MP has not been determined; however, we are in agreement with Myers [141] in recommending 1 g of MP in 50 ml of 5% dextrose given over 30 minutes daily for 5 days. The patient should be hospitalized for the infusions, but the treatment is safe enough to allow home treatment by a visiting nurse. We recommend the first IV dose be given under observation in the outpatient clinic or office. Antacids, in the form of calcium carbonate or ranitidine between meals and at bedtime, will decrease indigestion. Low sodium diet will decrease the likelihood of extremity edema. To counteract withdrawal symptoms and prolong treatment effects we also recommend a tapering course of alternate day oral prednisone as outlined above for ACTH. If no improvement occurs after the first 5 days of MP infusion, extending intravenous MP treatment for an additional 3–5 days may be beneficial [141a]. If response is poor while on alternate day prednisone over the course of the next month, we would recommend treatment with ACTH as defined above.

23.9   Drugs affecting demyelinated axonal conduction

4-Aminopyridine (4-AP) is a potassium channel blocker that prolongs the repolarization phase of nerve action potentials and thus the total duration and current of the action potential, restoring conduction in blocked demyelinated nerves in animals [31]. Early pilot trials of oral or intravenous 4-AP improved motor, oculomotor and visual defects in the majority of MS patients, but with limiting side-effects of dysesthesias, dizziness and gait imbalance [144, 145]. Side-effects were minimal – transient mild paresthesias or dizziness – in 10 of 15 patients without seizures [31]. There was no correlation between 4-AP serum level or half-life and the magnitude or pattern of clinical improvement [146]. Seizures have been reported by others with 4-AP treatment of MS and other neurologic conditions, which was often related to serum levels above 100 μg/ml. A phase II randomized, double-blind, placebo-controlled, crossover study was able to show a significant change in the Kurtzke EDSS with 4-AP treatment [147].

A sustained release preparation of 4-AP may increase the ratio between efficacy and safety [147]. About 30% of patients report a beneficial clinical response to 4-AP: in 14% this response was significant, and 80–90% of responders will benefit from long-term treatment [148]. 4-AP is a promising drug for the symptomatic treatment of MS, although serum levels may have to be monitored to control side-effects and limit the potential for seizures. Further studies of this agent are warranted.

Digitalis can inhibit the neuronal electrogenic sodium/potassium pump, responsible for part of the resting membrane potential and the activity-related membrane hyperpolarization following high-frequency impulses, thus possibly reversing demyelinative conduction blocks. A short acting digitalis-like agent, ouabain, was found to reverse slowed conduction velocity in rats with spinal cord demyelination [149], and intravenous digoxin (0.02 mg/kg) given to seven MS patients with temperature-dependent symptoms caused improvement in clinical effects and evoked potentials in three of them [150].

23.10 Cooling

Cooling suits are being marketed for MS. In a pilot trial, nine heat-sensitive MS patients were each cooled for 90 minutes with a garment using circulating coolant cooled by frozen cartridges (Life Support Systems Inc., Mountain View, CA), or a vest holding pre-frozen gel packets (Steele Inc., Kingston, WA). Patients were tested before and 90 minutes after cooling: no significant changes in neuroperformance testing or neuropsychological tests occurred immediately post cooling. A prospective study of 20 patients undergoing cooling twice a day for 3 weeks, sham cooling or no cooling failed to show a cumulative effect of cooling on disability, neuroperformance or neuropsychological testing [32]. Even though we are unable to show significant improvement in neuroperformance tests, patients report lowering body temperature permits them to exercise for longer periods of time, to tolerate hot environments better and lessens fatigue. Accordingly, we recommend the cooling vest.

23.11 Conclusion: modern management of MS

In the past several decades MS management has changed dramatically. In the 1950s fever therapy along with histamine desensitization were considered mainstream medical treatments. In relatively rapid succession steroids, aggressive immunosuppression and now interferon have been introduced. In a disease as unpredictable as MS, it is essential to follow individual patients' neurological function and behavior and administer treatments based on clinical judgment. In our experience the backbone of MS management, now and into the foreseeable future, will remain symptom management. (See Table 23.1.1 in the Appendix for a tabulation of non-medical and medical treatment of MS symptoms listed alphabetically.) This includes not only the symptoms of demyelination but also the psychological, social and vocational stresses of living with MS. As the future becomes the present, hopefully newer management techniques will alleviate the stresses and pain of living with the problems of MS. As we wait for the final solution, there is much to do now to allow persons with MS to live independently with satisfaction.

In summary, to assist in managing MS patients we have formulated four algorithms based on our experience, the course of the disease and the level of disability. They are shown in the Appendix as Figures 23.A.1–23.A.4.

Addendum

Since this chapter was completed, two publications on value of exercise to the wellbeing of multiple sclerosis patients have been reported. Petajan et al. [151] have reported a controlled clinical trial which recruited patients with multiple sclerosis Kurtzke 2–5 ratings; they then randomized to a non-exercise or exercise or an exercise group. Utilizing various measuring devices, they presented evidence that multiple sclerosis patients can and should be involved in an aerobic exercise program. This resulted in significant improvement of fitness and had a positive impact on factors related to quality of life, which they measured by accepted questionnaires

Additionally, a controlled randomized two-treatment double-blind microclimate cooling trial in multiple sclerosis patients (Kurtzke 4–6) was carried out to determine the effect of lowering body temperature on a non-exercise and an exercise group (Kraft, personal communication). Patients were subjected to low and high cooling. Heat loss in the low cooling group was on the average 9 watt hours and the high cooling averaged 87. Leg cycling was improved 11% at low cooling and 24% at high cooling, and tandem gait 4 and 13%, respectively. Other significant differences between the two cooling regimens were single leg standing balance, self-select ambulation velocity and quadriceps peak strength.

Accordingly, we recommend that patients should have an aerobic exercise program for 40 minutes three times a week [151] and should cool for about an hour before and during the exercise program. Both the microclimate vest and the Steele vest will lower body temperature about 0.6°C in an hour and maintain it for 2 more [152, 153].

Appendix: treatment of symptoms and algorithms for management

Table 23.A.1 Treating multiple sclerosis neurological symptoms

Symptoms	Non-medical treatments and comments	Medical procedures and medications
Balance sense dysfunction (incoordination of lower and/or upper extremities and/or truncal ataxia)	Balance/coordination exercises; hydrotherapy; strengthening exercises; cooling; weighted aids of ambulation; bracing; compensation techniques. Education on safe walking	Corticosteroids
Bladder impairment 1. Failure to store (small capacity, spastic urgency, frequency, dribbling)	Classification of the type of impairment by measuring the residual urinary volume is necessary for proper diagnosis: get 2-day voiding history and check post-void residual urine, urinalysis, culture, BUN, creatinine. Refer to urologist for refractory problems, recurrent infections or hematuria	1. *Failure to store*: baclofen (Lioresal), oxybutynin chloride (Ditropan), propantheline bromide (Probanthine), flavoxate HCl (Urispas), hyoscyamine (Cystospaz), imipramine (Tofranil). Try more than one drug of the same class; combine imipramine with another drug. Use high doses to medically paralyze the bladder and use intermittent catheterization
2. Failure to empty (large capacity, infrequency, and hesitancy; frequency and urgency, when bladder stretched)	*Prevent infection*: reduce residual urine by frequent complete voiding, Credé maneuver, intermittent catheterization if residual > 150 ml. Adequate fluid intake (6–8 glasses/day); proper perineal hygiene for women. Avoid indwelling catheters, if used keep a closed system, do asepsis of the catheter meatal junction and drainage apparatus, and change catheter monthly, and bag and drainage apparatus every 2 weeks. Cranberry juice, two glasses a day. Do regular urinalysis and culture with serum creatinine	2. *Failure to empty*: bethanechol (Urecholine), phenoxybenzamine (Dibenzyline), baclofen, imipramine. Medically paralyze bladder (see 1) and use intermittent catheterization. Surgical dilatation of bladder neck: total urethral sphincterotomy with condom catheter in males; suprapubic cystostomy for both sexes
3. Combination of 1 and 2	*For cystitis*: maintain adequate bladder drainage; force fluids; reduce fever; urinalysis and culture to determine antibiotic sensitivities; use appropriate antibiotic with broad spectrum coverage prior to culture results. Intravenous pyelography or sonography and bladder dynamic studies if infections are frequent	3. *Combination of 1 and 2*: anticholinergic drug with intermittent catheterization
4. Detrusor–sphincter dyssynergia (combination of 1 and 2)	*Failure to store*: bladder training program; fluid restriction at certain hours; for nocturia fluid restriction 5 hours before sleep; regular scheduled voiding using Credé or rectal stimulation; condom catheter with leg bag for men; protective underpants with adult diapers for women	4. *Detrusor–sphincter dyssynergia*: imipramine, baclofen, terazosin HCl (Hytrin); intermittent catheterization with or without medically paralyzing bladder; external sphincterotomy
5. Antisepsis	*Failure to empty*: regular voiding using Credé or rectal stimulation. Intermittent catheterization; indwelling catheter if this is not practical	5. *Antisepsis*: ascorbic acid (4 g/day), methenamine mandelate (Mandelamine), co-trimoxazole (Bactrim or Septra) once a day
6. Cystitis		6. *Cystitis*: co-trimoxazole, norfloxacin (Noroxin), ofloxacin (Aoxin), antibiotic appropriate to sensitivities of the bacteria involved
7. Nocturia	*Detrusor–sphincter dyssynergia*: see Failure to empty	7. *Nocturia*: intranasal vasopressin

Problem	Management	Medications
Constipation	Exercise. High fiber diet (23 g per day) with adequate fluid intake (6–8 glasses per day). Bowel program stressing regular evacuations, enemas and digital stimulation or removal, especially if urgency results in incontinence. Disimpaction. Protective underpants and adult diapers	Metamucil or another bulk former. Stool softeners, such as dulcosate sodium (Colace or Surfak). Mild laxatives such as Doxidan, Pericolace, Senokot or Milk of Magnesia with or without cascara. Bisacodyl (Dulcolax), suppositories initially and then the tablets orally the night before and suppositories at the time of defecation. Sodium phosphate (Fleet) enemas. Rarely colostomy for uncontrollable constipation
Contractures	Range of motion and stretching exercise. Cooling. Night splints, bivalved casts	Spasmolytic drugs (see **Spasticity**). Surgery: motor nerve blocks, rhizotomies, tendonotomies, myelotomy, arthrodesis
Convulsive seizures	Search for other causes of seizures since they are only about 10 times more frequent in MS	Carbamazepine (Tegretol), valproic acid (Depakene or Depakote), phenytoin (Dilantin). After 6 months without seizures, taper anticonvulsants over 3 months if no other etiology present
Depression and behavioral problems	Education of patient, family and all social contacts. Guide patient toward acceptance of disease. Fostering a good doctor–patient relationship. Psychotherapy. Suicide preventive measures. Group therapy for patients and families	Amitriptyline (Elavil), desipramine (Norpramin), fluoxetine (Prozac), imipramine (Tofranil), doxepin, trazodone (Desyrel), lithium (Eskalith), carbamazepine (Tegretol)
Diarrhea/bowel incontinence	Unusual in MS; check for secondary causes, e.g. impaction, infection. Avoid dietary irritants. Bowel program stressing regular evacuations, enemas, suppositories. Protective underpants and adult diapers	Anticholinergics (see **Bladder, Failure to Store**), metamucil, attapulgite (Kaopectate), diphenoxylate HCl with atropine sulfate (Lomotil), loperimide (Imodium). In extreme cases, colostomy
Decubitus ulcer	See **Pressure ulcer**	
Diplopia	Use alternating patch, but not constantly. Teach to gaze in the direction least affected. Cooling	Corticosteroids
Dysarthria	Read aloud and speak often, slowly and distinctly. Pacing board. Speech therapist. Chew gum. Cooling. Alternative communication devices. Computer-driven communication aids or voice synthesizers	
Dysarthria, paroxysmal	Cooling	Carbamazepine (Tegretol), valproic acid (Depakene), acetazolamide (Diamox), phenytoin (Dilantin)
Dysphagia	Change position of head; alternate liquids with solids; reduce size of bites and meals, chew well, deep breath before swallowing. Chew gum. Food thickeners (Thick-It). Cooling. Stand-by aspirator. Evaluation with cine-esophagram and videofluoroscopy. Speech pathology/dietitian referral. With fever, dysphagia can worsen and result in aspiration: cool immediately. See **Pulmonary infections**	Anticholinergics to dry salivary secretions with or without gastrostomy. For severe ongoing dysphagia, percutaneous endoscopic gastrostomy for long-term enteral feeding

(Continued)

Table 23.A.1 (Continued)

Symptoms	Non-medical treatments and comments	Medical procedures and medications
Edema	Extremity elevation; compressive stockings; physical therapy (range of motion); Jobst pump stocking	Hydrochlorothiazide (Hydrodiuril)
Fatigue	Positive attitude to 'fight' fatigue; remain active, fatigue begets fatigue. Rest in chair rather than bed. Plan day in detail and do it. Pace activities. Sleep regular hours; avoid late nights. Progressive exercise program. Occupational therapy to maximize efficiency in home. Aids of ambulation to conserve energy. Cooling	Treat depression if present. Pemoline (Cylert), amantadine HCl (Symmetrel), fluoxetine (Prozac), methylphenidate HCl (Ritalin), dextroamphedamine, selegiline HCl (Eldepryl), isoniazid (INH) with pyridoxine 2 mg
Flexor spasms	Frequently occur on falling asleep. Cooling	Baclofen (Lioresal), diazepam (Valium), clonazepam (Klonopin). Dantrolene (Dantrium), cyclobenzaprine HCl (Flexeril). Timing: extra medication 30 minutes prior to sleep if nocturnal spasms
Hypoventilation	This is an emergency. Usually with fever. Respiratory assistance with or without intubation. Cooling	Oxygen
Insomnia (see Bladder, nocturia; Flexor spasms)	No caffeinated drinks or food (chocolate) 5 hours before sleep. No vigorous exercise. Quiet and dark room with comfortable bed. Minimal naps taken throughout the day.	Zolpidom (Ambien), temazepam (Restoril), flurazepam (Dalmane), triazolam (Halicion), amitriptyline (Elavil), diazepam (Valium), ethchlorvynol (Placidyl)
Intellectual impairment	Impairment of recent memory, sustained attention, conceptual reasoning, verbal fluency, speed of informational processing while IQ and language functions are relatively spared. Sometimes difficult to distinguish depression and fatigue as the main factors. Assess with neuropsychological testing; may be important for disability benefits and early adaptation in workplace Education: read and recite; read aloud. Social stimulation and frequent speaking. Adaptive computers. Cognitive retraining. Use notebooks, pocket electronic databanks. Cooling. Severe cases: confinement with full-time caregivers	Amitriptyline (Elavil) and fluoxetine (Prozac) if depression present. Pemoline (Cylert), amantadine HCl (Symmetrel), methylphenidate HCl (Ritalin), physostigmine
Intention tremor	Made worse with stress. Physical and occupational therapy. Compensation techniques; bracing. Weighted bracelets and utensils. Cooling. Headrest, soft collar	Diazepam (Valium), lorazepam (Ativan), chlordiazepoxide HCl (Librium), hydroxyzine HCl (Atarax), propranolol (Inderal), primidone (Mysoline), hydroxyzine pamoate (Vistaril), clonazepam (Klonopin), buspirone (Buspar), chlorpromazine (Thorazine), baclofen (Lioresal), isoniazid (INH) with pyridoxine 2 mg, haloperidol (Haldol), 5-hydroxy-tryptophan, glutethamide (Doriden). Ondansetrone thalamotomy in extreme cases with good strength and mild dementia

Labile emotions or emotional incontinence	Stress can enhance. Cooling	Amitriptyline (Elavil), diazepam (Valium), carbidopa-levodopa (Sinemet), bromocriptine mesylate (Parlodel)
Oscillopsia	Can produce low vision, so use refraction. Can be dissociated, so use patching. Cooling. Low vision clinic. Glasses with converging prisms	Isoniazid (INH) with pyridoxine 2 mg, clonazepam (Klonopin), baclofen (Lioresal), valproate (Depakote), trihexyphenidyl (Artane). Corticosteroids
Pulmonary infections	This is the most common cause of death and an emergency. Usually secondary to aspiration. Proper assessment of dysphagia is needed to prevent this. Cool aggressively (hypothermia mattress or alcohol sponges)	Oxygen. Broad spectrum antibiotics. IV fluids. Respiratory assistance with or without intubation
Pain		
● Neckache	Rule out surgically treatable spondylosis. Neck brace. Physical therapy. Exercises. Local heat. Massage. Ultrasound. Hydrotherapy	Mild analgesics, non-steroidal anti-inflammatory drugs, and muscle relaxants
● Backache	See Neckache. Rule out surgically treatable spondylosis. Firm mattress or bed board. Correct walking posture. Avoid chiropractic manipulation. Bedrest with leg elevation for flare-ups. Cane, crutch, or knee brace. Rockport prowalker shoes, airpillow in soles.	Mild analgesics, non-steroidal anti-inflammatory drugs, and muscle relaxants
● Headache	Rule out migraine	If migraine, treat with anti-migraine medication(s). If not migraine, use headache analgesics and anti-depressants
● Muscle cramps	Physical therapy. Range of motion. Oral fluids	Baclofen (Lioresal), diazepam (Valium), quinine sulfate (Quinamm), calcium carbonate (Tums)
● Paroxysmal extremity burning pain and dysalgesia	Persistent burning predominantly in lower extremities, worse at night, aggravated by heat and walking. Cooling. Transcutaneous nerve stimulation, biofeedback, meditation, acupuncture	Amitriptyline (Elavil), trazodone (Desyrel), carbamazepine (Tegretol), valproic acid (Depakene), phenytoin (Dilantin), desipramine (Norpramin), nortriptyline (Pamelor), haloperidol (Haldol), chlorpromazine (Thorazine), capsaicin (Zostrix topical analgesic cream, rub in lidocaine ointment first). Gabapentin. Phenol nerve root blocks, posterior nerve root section, or cordectomy in rare refractory cases
Paresthesias	Medically treat only if painful. Cooling	Amitriptyline (Elavil), desipramine (Norpramin), carbamazepine (Tegretol), gabapentin (Neurontin)
Pressure ulcer	Prevention and vigilance: cushions, pads, special mattresses. Change position every 30 minutes to an hour in wheelchair. Prevent wetness. Turn a bed patient every 1–2 hours on a rotating pressure air or water mattress. Use modified dorsolateral position. Prevent rubbing movements and adductor spasm. Daily bed or tub bath, drying and powdering all wet areas. Good nutrition. Debride. Expose to air. Heat lamps or blow dryer. DuoDERM covering. Wet to dry dressing	Tincture of benzoin, povidone-iodine (Betadine), hydrogen peroxide 3%, thymol iodine powder, cornstarch, Aeroplast dressing. Hospitalize; use of Clinitron, Egerton, sand, or water bed; surgical debridement; ulcer resection with full-thickness skin grafting

(Continued)

Table 23.A.1 (*Continued*)

Symptoms	Non-medical treatments and comments	Medical procedures and medications
Sexual dysfunction	Appropriate evaluation: detailed interview with patient and significant other; musculoskeletal survey; assessment for bladder and bowel dysfunction. Sex therapy and psychotherapy. Treat spasticity, bladder and bowel dysfunction, fatigue	Treat spasticity, bladder and bowel dysfunction, fatigue. See appropriate sections in this Table
● Libido	Check testosterone level. Sex therapy and psychotherapy	Testosterone, yohimbine
● Erection dysfunction	Tactile or oral/manual stimulation of penis by partner or patient. Vacuum pump with elastic constricting band	Inject penis with papaverine hydrochloride or prostaglandins; Cavar Jet kit; consult urologist. Penile prosthetic devices surgically implanted
● Ejaculation dysfunction	Treat spasticity, bowel and bladder dysfunction, fatigue. Prostatic stimulation	Treat spasticity; bowel and bladder dysfunction: See appropriate sections in this Table.
● Female sexual dysfunction	Stimulation: manual, vibrator. Water soluble lubrication. Treat spasticity, bladder, and bowel dysfunction, fatigue	K–Y jelly. Treat spasticity, bowel and bladder: See appropriate sections in this Table. Painful genital sensations: see pain treatment in this Table
Spasticity	Check for fever, infection, rectal or bladder distension. Physical therapy: stretching, range of motion, active and passive exercise. Cooling. Aids of ambulation, braces. Daily exercises. Hydrotherapy. Prevent contractures	Baclofen (Lioresal), diazepam (Valium), lorazepam (Ativan), clonazepam (Klonopin), dantrolene (Dantrium), tizanidine, clonidine. Combinations of above. Botulinum (Botox) injections. In extreme cases intrathecal baclofen, lidocaine or (Xylocaine) nerve or motor point blocks; if there is improvement follow with phenol blocks. Selective nerve root neurolysis or block; chemical rhizotomy; surgical neurectomy or rhizotomy; myelotomy
Thermoregulation (heat sensitivity)	Air condition one room in home and car. Take care with dress; drink iced drinks, ice pops and eat cool. Spray skin. Alcohol sponging. Cool showers. Cool swimming pool. Cool mattress. SteeleVest (body cooling system)	
Tonic seizures	Avoid the movement or touch which precipitates them. Avoid hyperventilation	Carbamazepine (Tegretol), acetazolamide (Diamox), phenytoin (Dilantin), phenobarbitol, valproic acid (Depakene). Can usually be discontinued after 2 months

Trigeminal neuralgia	Carbamazepine (Tegretol) with gradual increase, phenytoin (Dilantin), valproic acid (Depakene), clonazepam (Klonopin), baclofen (Lioresal), amitriptyline HCl (Elavil), nortriptyline HCl (Pamelor), perphenazine (Trilifon, Etrafon) and amitriptyline in combination, misoprostol. Avoid narcotic analgesics. Percutaneous stereotactic thermal rhizotomy; glycerol rhizotomy	Avoid the trigger point
Vertigo	Dimenhydrinate (Dramamine), meclizine HCl (Antivert), chlorpromazine (Thorazine), fentanyl plus droperidol (Innovar), diphenhydramine (Benedryl), oxazepam, corticosteroids. Decongestants if due to eustachian tube dysfunction and/or otitis media. Intravenous fluids if vomiting is severe	Avoid sudden changes in posture, or find lying head position that dampens spin sensation. Ear exam is essential to distinguish peripheral (non-CNS) causes. Vestibular desensitization
Visual loss		
● Acute optic neuritis	High dose IV methylprednisolone (Solu-Medrol)	
● Loss of acuity	Uveitis: mydriatics and local corticosteroids. Cataract surgery	Check for cataracts, uveitis and diabetes. Ophthalmologic and occupational therapy referral. After best refraction, use magnifiers with optimal lighting. Cooling. Low vision books, computers, talking books. Low vision clinics
● Fixed defects		See **Loss of acuity**. Engineer's triangular ruler for reading with visual field defect or eye tracking problems. Cooling. Braille system of reading. Referral to Federal Commission for the Blind and Visually Handicapped or appropriate national institution
Weakness	Corticosteroids. 4-aminopyridine (experimental)	Check for infection, fever, heat exposure, dehydration, calcium and electrolyte disturbances, malnutrition, overuse of muscle relaxants, over-exercise, over-exertion. Physical therapy. Home exercise program. Hydrotherapy (walking, deep knee bends). Aids for ambulation and mobility. Occupational therapy aids. Braces. Cooling. Energy conservation techniques

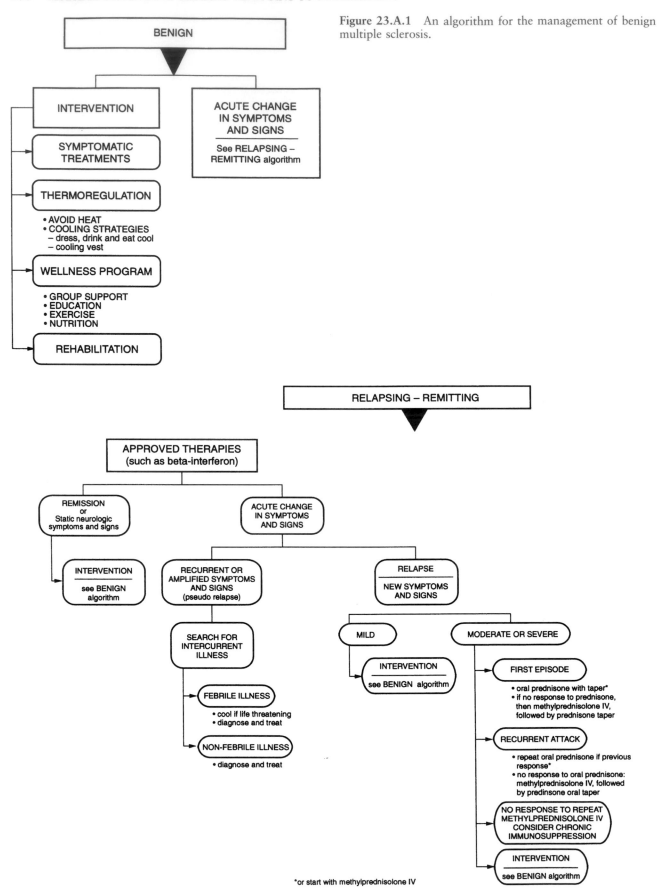

Figure 23.A.1 An algorithm for the management of benign multiple sclerosis.

Figure 23.A.1 An algorithm for the management of relapsing-remitting multiple sclerosis.

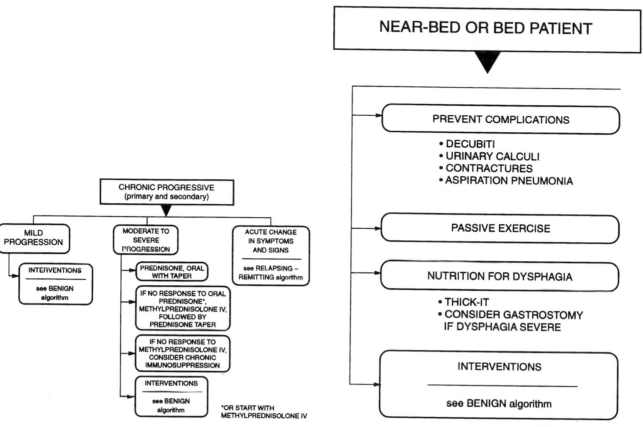

Figure 23.A.2   An algorithm for the management of chronic progressive (primary and secondary) multiple sclerosis.

Figure 23.A.3   An algorithm for the management of the near-bed or bed patient with multiple sclerosis.

References

1. Anderson, D.W., Ellenberg, J.H., Leventhal, C.M. *et al.* (1992) Revised estimate of the prevalence of multiple sclerosis in the United States. *Ann. Neurol.*, **31**, 333–6.
2. Lisak, R.P. (1988) Overview of the rationale for immunomodulating therapies in multiple sclerosis. *Neurology*, **38**, (Suppl. 2), 5–8.
3. Waksman, B.H. (1983) Rationales of current therapies for multiple sclerosis. *Arch. Neurol.*, **40**, (11), 671–2.
4. McDonald, W.I. and Halliday, A.M. (1977) Diagnosis and classification of multiple sclerosis. *Br. Med Bull.*, **33**, 4–8.
5. Rose, A.S., Ellison, G.W., Myers, L.W. and Tourtellotte, W.W. (1976) Criteria for the clinical diagnosis of multiple sclerosis. *Neurology*, **26** (6), 20–2.
6. Schumacher, G.A., Beebe, G., Kibler, R.F. *et al.* (1965) Problems of experimental trials of therapy in multiple sclerosis. Report by the panel on the evaluation of experimental trials of therapy in multiple sclerosis. *Ann. NY Acad. Sci.*, **122**, 552–68.
7. Poser, C.M., Paty, D.W., Scheinberg, L. *et al.* (1983) New diagnostic criteria for multiple sclerosis: guidelines for research protocols. *Ann. Neurol.*, **13** (3), 227–31.
8. Lee, K.H., Hashimoto, S.A., Hooge, J.P. *et al.* (1991) Magnetic resonance imaging of the head in the diagnosis of multiple sclerosis: a prospective 2-year follow-up with comparison of clinical evaluation, evoked potentials, oligoclonal banding, and CT. *Neurology*, **41**, 657–60.
9. Gebarski, S.S., Gabrielson, T.O., Gilman, S. *et al.* (1985) The initial diagnosis of multiple sclerosis: clinical impact of magnetic resonance imaging. *Ann. Neurol.*, **17**, 469–74.
10. Ormerod, I.E.C., Miller, D.H., McDonald, W.I. *et al.* (1987) The role of MRI imaging in the assessment of multiple sclerosis and isolated neurological lesions. *Brain*, **110**, 1579–616.
11. Kozachuk, W.E., DeCarli, C., Schapiro, M.B. *et al.* (1990) White matter hyperintensities in dementia of Alzheimer's type and in healthy subjects without cerebrovascular risk factors. *Arch. Neurol.*, **47**, 1306–10.
12. Gilbert, J.J. and Salder, M. (1983) Unsuspected multiple sclerosis. *Arch. Neurol.*, **40**, 533–6.
13. Cutler, J.R., Aminoff, M.J. and Brant-Zawadzki, M. (1986) Evaluation of patients with multiple sclerosis by evoked potentials and magnetic resonance imaging: a comparative study. *Ann. Neurol.*, **20**, 645–8.
14. Schapiro, R.T. (1991) Multiple Sclerosis, An Explanation. Handout sheet, Fairview MS Center at the Riverside Medical Center, 701 25th Avenue South, Minneapolis, Minnesota, 55454,
15. McAlpine, D. (1961) The benign form of multiple sclerosis. A study based on 241 cases seen within three years of onset and followed up until the tenth year or more of the disease. *Brain* **84**, 186–203.
16. Phadke, J.G. (1990) Clinical aspects of multiple sclerosis in north-east Scotland with particular reference to its course and prognosis. *Brain*, **113**, 1597–628.
17. Thompson, D.S., Nelson, L.M., Burns, A., Burks, J.S. and Franklin, G.M. (1986) The effects of pregnancy in multiple sclerosis: a retrospective study. *Neurology*, **36**, 1097–9.
18. Runmarker, B. and Anderson, O. (1993) Prognostic factors in a multiple sclerosis incidence cohort with twenty-five years of follow-up. *Brain*, **116**, 117–34.
19. Matthews, W.B., Compston, A., Allen, I.V. and Martyn, C.N. (1991) *Multiple Sclerosis*, Edinburgh, Churchill Livingstone.
20. Dworkin, R.H., Bates, D., Millar, J.H.D. and Paty, D.W. (1984) Linoleic acid and multiple sclerosis: a reanalysis of three double-blind trials. *Neurology*, **34**, 1441–5.
21. Swank, R.L. (1970) Multiple sclerosis: twenty years on a low fat diet. *Arch. Neurol.*, **23**, 460–74.
22. Alexander, J. and Abramson, A.S. (1983) Physical and surgical therapy, in *Multiple Sclerosis. A Guide for Patients and Their Families* (eds L.C. Scheinberg *et al.*), New York, Raven Press, pp. 71–90.
23. Cailliet, R. (1968) Rehabilitation in multiple sclerosis in *Rehabilitation and Medicine* (eds S.H. Licht *et al.*), Baltimore, MD, Waverly Press, pp. 446–59.
24. Cailliet, R. (1978) *Exercise in Multiple Sclerosis*, Baltimore, MD, Williams and Wilkins,
25. Schapiro, R. (1993) *Multiple Sclerosis: a Rehabilitation Approach*, New York, Demos Vermande.
26. Schapiro, R.T. (1987) *Symptom Management in Multiple Sclerosis*, New York, Demos Publications.
27. Tourtellotte, W.W. and Baumhefner, R.W. (1994) Multiple sclerosis, in *Conn's Current Therapy, 1994* (ed. R.E. Rakel), W.B. Saunders, Philadelphia, 883–905.
28. McAlpine, D., Lumsden, C.E. and Acheson, E.G. (1972) *Multiple Sclerosis: a Reappraisal* 2nd edn, Baltimore, MD, Williams and Wilkins.
29. Robbins, K. and Abramson, A.S. (1983) Aids to ease the activities of daily living, in *Multiple Sclerosis: a Guide for Patients and Their Families* (eds. L.C. Scheinberg *et al.*), New York, Raven Press, pp. 91–110.
30. Bever, C.T., Leslie, J., Camenga, D.L., Panitch, H.S. and Johnson, K.P. (1990) Preliminary trial of 3,4-diaminopyridine in patients with multiple sclerosis. *Ann. Neurol.*, **27**, 421–7.
31. Davis, F.A., Stefoski, D. and Rush, J. (1990) Orally administered 4-aminopyridine improves clinical signs in multiple sclerosis. *Ann. Neurol.*, **27**, 186–92.
32. Syndulko, K., Woldanski, A., Baumhefner, R.W. and Tourtellotte, W.W. (1995) Preliminary evaluation of lowering tympanic temperature for the symptomatic treatment of multiple sclerosis. *J. Neurol. Rehabil.*, **9** (4), 205–14.
33. Schneitzer, L. (1978) Rehabilitation of patients with multiple sclerosis. *Arch. Phys. Med. Rehabil.* **59** (9), 430–7.
34. Deloya, A., Arndt, J. and Schapiro, R.T. (1987) Spasticity, in *Symptom Management in Multiple Sclerosis* (eds R.T. Schapiro *et al.*), New York, Demos Publications, pp. 11–16.
35. Young, R.R. and Delwaide, P.J. (1981) Drug therapy, spasticity. *N. Engl. J. Med.*, **304**, 28–33, 96–9.
35a.Scheinberg, L. and Giesser, B.S. (1983) Drug therapy, in *Multiple Sclerosis. A Guide for Patients and Their Families* (eds L.C. Scheinberg), New York, Raven Press, pp. 45–55.
36. Rudick, R., Schiffer, R.B. and Herndon, R.M. (1987) Drug treatment of multiple sclerosis. *Sem. Neurol.*, **7**, 150–9.
37. Cartlidge, N.E.F., Hudgson, P. and Weightman, D. (1974) Comparison of baclofen and diazepam in the treatment of spasticity. *J. Neurol. Sci.*, **23**, 17–24.
38. From, A. and Heltberg, A. (1975) A double-blind trial with baclofen (Lioresal) and diazepam in spasticity due to multiple sclerosis. *Acta Neurol. Scand.*, **51**, 158–66.
39. Ladd, H., Oist, C. and Jonsson, B. (1974) The effect of Dantrium on spasticity in multiple sclerosis. *Acta Neurol. Scand.*, **50**, 397–408.
40. Schmidt, R.T., Lee, R.H. and Spehlemann, R. (1976) Comparison of dantrolene sodium and diazepam in the treatment of spasticity. *J. Neurol. Neurosurg. Psychiatry*, **39**, 350–6.
41. Wilkinson, S.P., Portmann, B. and Williams, R. (1979) Hepatitis from dantrolene sodium. *Gut*, **20**(1), 33–6.
42. Petusevsky, M.L., Faling, L.J., Rocklin, R.E. *et al.* (1979) Pleuropericardial reaction to treatment with dantrolene. *J. Am. Med. Assoc.*, **242**(25), 2772–4.
43. Lapierre, Y., Bouchard, S., Tansey, C. *et al.* (1987) Treatment of spasticity with tizanidine in multiple sclerosis. *Can. J. Neurol. Sci.*, **14**, 513–17.
44. United Kingdom Tizanine Trial Group (1994) A double-blind, placebo-controlled trial of tizanidine in the treatment of spasticity caused by multiple sclerosis. *Neurology*, **44** (Suppl. 9), S70–S78.
45. Coward, D. (1994) Tizanidine: neuropharmacology and mechanisms of action. *Neurology*, **44** (Suppl. 1), S6–S11.
46. Bass, B., Weinshenker, B., Rice, G.P.A. *et al.* (1988) Tizanidine versus baclofen in the treatment of spasticity in patients with multiple sclerosis. *Can. J. Neurol. Sci.*, **15**, 15–19.
47. Stein, R., Nordal, H.J., Offedal, S.I. and Slettebo, M. (1987) The treatment of spasticity in multiple sclerosis: a double-blind clinical trial of a new anti-spastic drug tizanidine compared with baclofen. *Acta Neurol. Scand.*, **75**, 190–4.
48. Lataste, X., Emre, M., Davis, C. and Groves, L. (1994) Comparative profile of tizanidine in the management of spasticity. *Neurology*, **44**(Suppl. 9), S53–S59.
49. Smith, C., Birnbaum, G., Carter, J.L. *et al.* and US Tizanidine Study Group (1994) Tizanidine treatment of spasticity caused by multiple sclerosis: results of a double-blind, placebo-controlled trial. *Neurology*, **44**(Suppl. 9), S34–S43.
50. Penn, R.D., Savoy, S.M., Corcos, D. *et al.* (1989) Intrathecal baclofen for severe spinal spasticity. *N. Engl. J. Med.*, **320**, 1517–21.
51. Borg-Stein, J., Fine, Z., Mille, R.J. and Brin, M. (1993) Botulinum toxin for the treatment of spasticity in multiple sclerosis. *Am. J. Phys. Med. Rehabil.*, **72**(6), 364–468.
52. Dunne, J. and Dunne, S. (1995) Treatment of chronic limb spasticity with botulinum toxin A. *J. Neurol. Neurosurg. Psychiatry*, **58**, 232–5.
53. Hesse, S., Lucke, D., Malezic, M. *et al.* (1994) Botulinum toxin treatment for lower limb extensor spasticity in chronic hemiparetic patients. *J. Neurol. Neurosurg. Psychiatry*, **57**, 1321–4.
54. Selzer, M. (1994) Clinical experience with BTX in spasticity encourages additional double-blind investigations. *Neurorehabilitation News*, September, pp. 1–7.
55. DeLisa, J. and Little, J.W. (1982) Managing spasticity. *Am. Fam. Phys.*, **26**, 117–22.
56. Kasdon, D.L. and Lathi, E.S. (1984) A prospective study of radiofrequency rhizotomy in the treatment of posttraumatic spasticity. *Neurosurg.*, **15**, 526–9.
57. Dimitrijevic, M.R. and Sherwood, A.M. (1980) Spasticity: medical and surgical treatment. *Neurology*, **30**, 19–27.
58. Schapiro, R.T., Harris, L. and Lenling, M. (1987) Tremor, in *Symptom Management in Multiple Sclerosis* (eds R.T. Schapiro *et al.*), New York, Demos Publications, pp. 17–20.
59. Hewer, R.L., Cooper, R. and Morgan, M.H. (1972) An investigation into the value of treating intention tremor by weighting the affected limb. *Brain*, **95**, 579–90.
60. Schapiro, R. (1994) *Symptom Management in Multiple Sclerosis*, New York, Demos Vermande.

61. Aisen, M., Holzer, M., Rosen, M., Dietz, M. and McDowell, F. (1991) Glutethimide treatment of disabling action tremor in patients with multiple sclerosis and traumatic brain injury. *Arch. Neurol.*, **48**, 513–15.

62. Brelje, B., Phair, C. and Schapiro, R.T. (1987) Bowel, in *Symptom Management in Multiple Sclerosis* (eds R.T. Schapiro *et al.*), New York, Demos Publications, pp. 61–8.

63. Holland, N.J. and Abramson, A.S. (1983) Bladder and bowel management, in *Multiple Sclerosis. A Guide for Patients and their Families* (eds L.C. Scheinberg *et al.*), New York, Raven Press, pp. 129–53.

64. Kirkeby, H.J., Poulsen, E.U., Petersen, T. and Dorup, J. (1988) Erectile impotence in multiple sclerosis. *Neurology*, **38**, 1366–71.

64a. Kalb, R., LaRocca, N. and Kaplan, S.R. (1983) Sexuality, in *Multiple Sclerosis. A Guide for Patients and Their Families* (eds L.C. Scheinberg), New York, Raven Press, pp. 155–73.

65. Miller, A. (1994) Sexual dysfunction in multiple sclerosis, in *Sexual Dysfunction: a Neuro-Medical Approach* (eds C. Singer and W.J. Weinger), New York, Futura.

66. Freal, J.E., Kraft, G.H. and Coryell, J.K. (1984) Symptomatic fatigue in multiple sclerosis. *Arch. Phys. Rehabil.*, **65**, 135–8.

67. Krupp, L.B., Alvarez, L.A., LaRocca, N.G. and Scheinberg. L.C. (1988) Fatigue in multiple sclerosis. *Arch. Neurol.* **45**, 435–7.

68. Schapiro, R.T., Harris, L., Lenling, M. and Metelak, J. (1987) Fatigue, in *Symptom Management in Multiple Sclerosis* (eds R.T. Schapiro *et al.*), New York, Demos Publications, pp. 23–8.

69. Murray, T.J. (1985) Amantadine therapy for fatigue in multiple sclerosis. *Can. J. Neurol. Sci.*, **12**, 251–4.

70. Cohen, R.A. and Fisher, M. (1989) Amantadine treatment of fatigue associated with multiple sclerosis. *Arch. Neurol.*, **46**, 676–80.

71. Rosenberg, G.A. and Appenzeller, O. (1988) Amantadine, fatigue, and multiple sclerosis. *Arch. Neurol.*, **45**, 1104–6.

72. Canadian MS Research Group (1987) A randomized controlled trial of amantadine in fatigue associated with multiple sclerosis. *Can. J. Neurol. Sci.*, **14**, 273–8.

73. Bass, B., Weinshenker, B.G., Penman, M., Ebers, G.C. and Rice, G.P.A. (1990) A double-blind, placebo-controlled, randomized trial to compare the efficacy of cylert (pemoline) and placebo in the control of fatigue in multiple sclerosis. *Neurology*, **40** (Suppl. 1), 261.

74. Stetten, D. (1981) Coping with blindness. *N. Engl. J. Med.*, **305**, 458–60.

75. Traccis, S., Rosati, G., Monaco, M.F., Aiello, I. and Agnetti, V. (1990) Successful treatment of acquired pendular elliptical nystagmus in multiple sclerosis with isoniazid and base-out prisms. *Neurology*, **40**, 492–4.

76. Currie, J.N. and Matsuo, V. (1986) The use of clonazepam in the treatment of nystagmus-induced oscillopsia. *Ophthalmology*, **93**, 924–32.

77. Herishanu, Y. and Louzoun, Z. (1986) Trihexyphenidyl treatment of vertical pendular nystagmus. *Neurology*, **36**, 82–4.

78. Lefkowitz, D. and Harpold, G. (1985) Treatment of ocular myoclonus with valproic acid. *Ann. Neurol.*, **17**, 103–4.

79. Beukelman, D.R., Kraft, G.H. and Freal, J. (1985) Expressive communication disorders in persons with multiple sclerosis: a survey. *Arch. Phys. Med. Rehabil.*, **66**, 675–7.

80. Voiculescu, V., Pruskauer-Apostol, B. and Alecu, C. (1975) Treatment with acetozolamide of brain-stem and spinal paroxysmal disturbances in multiple sclerosis. *J. Neurol. Neurosurg. Psychiatry*, **38**, 191–3.

81. Eisdorfer, R.M. and Weg, A. (1990) Percutaneous endoscopic gastrostomy: a retrospective. *J. Neurol. Rehabil.*, **4**, 75–7.

82. Johnson, W.H., Fenton, R.S. and Evans, A. (1976) Effects of droperidol in management of vestibular disorders. *Laryngoscope*, **86**, (7), 946–54.

83. Sanders, E.A.C.M. and Arts, R.J.H.M. (1986) Paresthesiae in multiple sclerosis. *J. Neurol. Sci.*, **74**, 297–305.

84. Ekbom, K. (1971) Carbamazepine: a new symptomatic treatment for the paresthesiae associated with Lhermitte's sign. *Zeitschr. Neurol.*, **200**, 341–4.

85. Hooge, J. and Redekop, W. (1995) Trigeminal neuralgia in multiple sclerosis. *Neurology*, **45**, 1294–6.

86. Eadie, M.J. and Tyrer, J.H. (1980) *Neurological Clinical Pharmacology*, Lancaster, MTP Press.

87. Fromm, G.H., Terrence, C.F. and Chattha, A.S. (1980) Treatment of face pain with baclofen. *Trans. Am. Neurol. Assoc.*, **105**, 486–8.

88. Reder, A. and Arnason, B. (1995) Trigeminal neuralgia in multiple sclerosis relieved by a prostaglandin E analogue. *Neurology*, **45**, 1097–100.

89. Brett, D.C., Ferguson, G.G., Ebers, G.C. and Paty, D.W. (1982) Percutaneous trigeminal rhizotomy. Treatment of trigeminal neuralgia secondary to multiple sclerosis. *Arch. Neurol.*, **39**, 219–21.

90. Brisman, R. (1987) Trigeminal neuralgia and multiple sclerosis. *Arch. Neurol.*, **44**, 379–81.

91. Kondzioka, D., Lunsford, L. and Bissonette, D. (1994) Long term results after glycerol rhizotomy for multiple sclerosis-related trigeminal neuralgia. *Can. J. Neurol. Sci.*, **21**, 137–40.

92. Bauer, H.J. (1977) *A Manual of Multiple Sclerosis*, National Multiple Sclerosis Society, 205 East 42nd Street, New York, NY, 10017–5706, New York.

93. Clifford, D.B. and Trotter, J.L. (1984) Pain in multiple sclerosis. *Arch. Neurol.*, **41**, 1270–2.

94. Moulin, D.E., Foley, K.M. and Ebers, G.C. (1988) Pain syndromes in multiple sclerosis. *Neurology*, **38**, 1830–4.

95. Stenager, E., Knudsen, L. and Jensen, K. (1991) Acute and chronic pain syndromes in multiple sclerosis. *Acta Neurol. Scand.*, **84**, 197–200.

96. Elian, M. and Dean, G. (1977) Multiple sclerosis and epilepsy, in *Epilepsy, the 8th International Symposium* (eds J.K. Perry *et al.*), New York, Raven Press, pp. 341–4.

97. Gozzoli, L., Faggi, L. and Costi, V. (1979) Epilepsy and multiple sclerosis. Report of 5 cases. *Acta Neurol. (Napoli)*, **34**(5), 396–404.

98. Kinnunen, E. and Wilström, J. (1986) Prevalence and prognosis of epilepsy in patients with multiple sclerosis. *Epilepsia*, **27**, 729–33.

99. Shibasaki, H. and Kuroiwa, Y. (1974) Painful tonic seizure in multiple sclerosis. *Arch. Neurol.*, **30**, 47–51.

100. Ritter, G. and Poser, S. (1974) Epilepsie und multiple sklerose. *Münch. Med. Wochenschr.*, **116**, 1983–6.

101. Heath, P.D. and Nightingale, S. (1982) Clusters of tonic seizures as an initial manifestation of multiple sclerosis. *Ann. Neurol.*, **12**, 494–5.

102. Matthews, W.B. (1975) Paroxysmal symptoms in multiple sclerosis. *J. Neurol. Neurosurg. Psychiatry*, **38**(6), 617–23.

103. Twomey, J.A. and Espir, M.L. (1980) Paroxymal symptoms as the first manifestation of multiple sclerosis. *J. Neurol. Neurosurg. Psychiatry*, **43**(4), 296–304.

104. Baretz, R.M. and Stephenson, G.P. (1981) Emotional responses to multiple sclerosis. *Psychosomatics*, **22**, 117–27.

105. LaRocca, N.G. (1984) Psychosocial factors in multiple sclerosis and the role of stress, in *Multiple Sclerosis: Experimental and Clinical Aspects* (eds L. Scheinberg and C.S. Raine) The New York Academy of Sciences, New York, *Annals of the New York Academy of Sciences*, **436**, pp. 435–42.

106. Kahana, E., Leibowitz, V. and Alter, M. (1971) Cerebral multiple sclerosis. *Neurology*, **21**, 1179–85.

107. Peyser, J.M., Edwards, K.R., Poser, C.M. and Filskov, S.B. (1980) Cognitive function in patients with multiple sclerosis. *Arch. Neurol.*, **37**, 577 9.

108. Rao, S.M., Leo, G.J., Bernardin, L. and Unverzagt, F. (1991) Cognitive dysfunction in multiple sclerosis. I. Frequency, patterns and prediction. *Neurology*, **41**, 685–91.

109. Staples, D. and Lincoln, N.B. (1979) Intellectual impairment in multiple sclerosis and its relation to functional abilities. *Rheum. Rehabil.*, **18**, 153–60.

110. Baumhefner, R.W., Tourtellotte, W.W., Syndulko, K. *et al.* (1990) Quantitative multiple sclerosis plaque assessment with magnetic resonance imaging. Its correlation with clinical parameters, evoked potentials and intra-blood–brain-barrier IgG synthesis. *Arch. Neurol.*, **47**, 19–26.

111. Franklin, G.M., Heaton, R.K., Nelson, L.M., Filley, C.M. and Seibert, C. (1988) Correlation of neuropsychological and MRI findings in chronic progressive multiple sclerosis. *Neurology*, **38**, 126–9.

112. Rao, S.M., Leo, G.J., Haughton, V.M., St Aubin-Faubert, P. and Bernardin, L. (1989) Correlation of magnetic resonance imaging with neuropsychological testing in multiple sclerosis. **39**, 161–6.

113. Cummings, J.L. and Benson, F. (1984) Subcortical dementia: review of an emerging concept. *Arch. Neurol.*, **41**, 874–9.

114. Filley, C.M., Heaton, R.K., Nelson, L.M., Burks, J.S. and Franklin, G.M. (1989) A comparison of dementia in Alzheimer's disease and multiple sclerosis. *Arch. Neurol.*, **46**, 157–61.

115. Rao, S.M., Leo, G.J., Ellington, L. *et al.* (1991) Cognitive dysfunction in multiple sclerosis. II. Impact on employment and social functioning. *Neurology*, **41**, 692–6.

116. Ben-Yishay, Y. and Dillar, L. (1983) Cognitive rehabilitation, in *Rehabilitation of the Head Injured Adult* (eds M. Rosenthal, E.R. Griffith, M.R. Bond and J.D. Millar), Philadelphia, F.A. Davis, pp. 367–80.

117. Bauer, H. (1978) Problems of symptomatic therapy in multiple sclerosis. *Neurology*, **28**, 8–20.

118. Holland, N.J., Weisel-Levison, P. and McDonnell, M. (1983) Nursing care, in *Multiple Sclerosis. A Guide for Patients and Their Families* (eds L.C. Scheinberg *et al.*), New York, Raven Press, pp. 111–28.

119. Stefoski, D. and Davis, F.A. (1980) Central disturbances of respiration in multiple sclerosis, in *Respiratory Dysfunction in Neurologic Disease* (eds W.J. Weiner *et al.*), Mount Kisco, NY, Futura.

120. Reuler, T.W. and Cooney, T.G. (1981) The pressure sore: pathophysiology and principles of management. *Ann. Intern. Med.*, **94**, 661–6.

121. Werner, R. and Schapiro, R.T. (1987) Pressure sores (decubiti), in *Symptom Management in Multiple Sclerosis* (eds R.T. Schapiro *et al.*), New York, Demos Publications, pp. 79–82.

122. Phair, C., Brelje, B. and Schapiro, R.T. (1987) Bladder, in *Symptom Management in Multiple Sclerosis* (eds R.T. Schapiro *et al.*), New York, Demos Publications, pp. 49–59.

123. Blaivas, J.G., Holland, N.J., Geisser, B. *et al.* (1984) Multiple sclerosis bladder, in *Multiple Sclerosis: Experimental and Clinical Aspects* (eds L. Scheinberg and C.S. Raine), The New York Academy of Sciences, New York, *Annals of the New York Academy of Sciences*, **436**, pp. 328–43.

124. Baumhefner, R.W., Tourtellotte, W.W., Syndulko, K. and Shapshak, P.

(1986) Neuroimmunologic pharmacology of multiple sclerosis. II. Evaluation of immunosuppressive agents, in *Immunotherapies in Multiple Sclerosis* (eds O.R. Hommes, J. Mertin and W.W. Tourtellotte), Suffolk, Stuart Phillips, pp. 226–36.

125. Tourtellotte, W.W., Baumhefner, R.W., Potvin, A.R. *et al.* (1980) Multiple sclerosis de novo CNS IgG synthesis: effect of ACTH and corticosteroids. *Neurology*, **30**, 1155–62.

126. Troiano, R., Hafstein, M., Ruderman, M. *et al.* (1984) Effect of high-dose intravenous steroid administration on contrast-enhancing computed tomographic scan lesions in multiple sclerosis. *Ann. Neurol.*, **15**, 257–63.

127. Barkhof, F., Hommes, O.R., Scheltens, P. and Valk, J. (1991) Quantitative MRI changes in gadolinium-DTPA enhancement after high-dose intravenous methylprednisolone in multiple sclerosis. *Neurology*, **41**, 1219–22.

128. Burnham, J.A., Wright, R.R., Dreisbach, J. and Murray, R.S. (1991) The effect of high-dose steroids on MRI gadolinium enhancement in acute demyelinating lesions. *Neurology*, **41**, 1349–54.

129. Guseo, A. and Jellinger, K. (1975) The significance of perivascular infiltrations in multiple sclerosis. *J. Neurol.*, **211**, 51–60.

130. Kibler, R.F., Daty, D.W., Re, P.K., McPhedran, A.M. and Karp, H.R. (1972) Effects of large doses of adrenocorticosteroids on the course of EAE and multiple sclerosis, in *Multiple Sclerosis: Immunology, Virology and Ultrastructure* (eds F. Wolfgram, G.W. Ellison, J.G. Stevens and N.M. Andrews), New York, Academic Press, pp. 511–38.

131. Liversedge, L.A. (1977) Treatment and management of multiple sclerosis. *Br. Med. Bull.*, **33** (1), 78–83.

132. Poser, C.M. (1978) Diseases of the myelin sheath, in *Clinical Neurology* (eds A.B. Baker and L.H. Baker), Hagerstown, MD, Harper and Row, vol. 2, ch. 25, pp. 1–188.

133. Zinner, M.J., Zuidema, G.D., Smith, P.L. and Mignosa, M. (1981) The prevention of upper gastrointestinal tract bleeding in patients in an intensive care unit. *Gynaecol. Obstet.*, **143**, 214–20.

133a. Baumhefner, R.W. and Tourtellotte, W.W. (1986) Neuroimmunologic pharmacology of multiple sclerosis. III. Adversities to immunosuppression, in *Immunotherapies in Multiple Sclerosis* (eds O.R. Hommes, J. Mertin and W.W. Torutellotte), Stuart Phillips Publications, St Edmundsbury Press, Suffolk, pp. 237–60.

134. Goodkin, D.S. (1991) The use of immunosuppressive agents in the treatment of multiple sclerosis: a critical review. *Neurology*, **41**, 980–5.

135. Durelli, L., Cocito, D., Riccio, A. *et al.* (1986) High-dose intravenous methylpredisolone in the treatment of multiple sclerosis. *Neurology*, **36**, 238–43.

136. Milligan, N.M., Newcombe, R. and Compston, D.A.S. (1987) A double-blind controlled trial of high dose methylprednisolone in patients with multiple sclerosis. *J. Neurol. Neurosurg. Psychiatry*, **50**, 511–16.

137. Abbruzzese, G., Gandolfo, C. and Loeb, C. (1983) 'Bolus' methylpredniso-lone versus ACTH in the treatment of multiple sclerosis. *Ital. J. Neurol. Sci.*, **2**, 169–72.

138. Barnes, M.P., Bateman, D.E., Cleland, P.G. *et al.* (1985) Intravenous methylprednisolone for multiple sclerosis in relapse. *J. Neurol. Neurosurg. Psych.*, **48**, 157–9.

139. Thompson, A.J., Kennard, C., Swash, M. *et al.* (1989) Intravenous methylprednisolone and ACTH in the treatment of acute relapse in MS. *Neurology*, **39**, 969–71.

140. Lyons, P.R., Newman, P.K. and Saunders, M. (1988) Methylprednisolone therapy in multiple sclerosis: a profile of adverse effects. *J. Neurol. Neurosurg. Psychiatry*, **51**, 285–7.

141. Myers, L.W. and Ellison, G.W. (1990) The peculiar difficulties of therapeutic trials for multiple sclerosis. *Neurol. Clin.*, **8** (1), 119–41.

141a. Myers, L.W. (1990) Management of multiple sclerosis. *Autoimmun. Forum-Neurol.*, **2** (1), 3–5, 11.

142. Compston, A. (1988) Methylprednisolone and multiple sclerosis. *Arch. Neurol.*, **45**, 669.

143. Troiano, R., Cook, S.D. and Dowling, P.C. (1987) Steroid therapy in multiple sclerosis: point of view. *Arch. Neurol.*, **44**, 803–7.

144. Jones, R.E., Heron, J.R., Foster, D.H. *et al.* (1983) Effects of 4-aminopyr-idine in patients with multiple sclerosis. *J. Neurol. Sci.*, **60**, 353–62.

145. Stefoski, D., Davis, F.A., Faut, M. and Schauf, C.L. (1987) 4-aminopyr-idine improves clinical signs in multiple sclerosis. *Ann. Neurol.*, **21**, 71–7.

146. Stefoski, D., Davis, F.A., Fitzsimmons, W.E. *et al.* (1991) 4-aminopyridine in multiple sclerosis: prolonged administration. *Neurology*, **41**, 1344–8.

147. Van Diemen, H.A., Polman, C.H., Koetsier, J.C. *et al.* (1993) 4-Aminopyr-idine in patients with multiple sclerosis: dosage and serum level related to efficacy and safety. *Clin. Neuropharmacol.*, **16** (3), 195–204.

148. Polman, C.H., Bertelsmann, F.W., van Loenen, A.C. and Koetsier, J.C. (1994) 4-aminopyridine in the treatment of patients with multiple sclerosis. Long-term efficacy and safety. *Arch. Neurol.*, **51** (3), 292–6.

149. Kaji, R. and Summer, A.J. (1989) Effect of digitalis on central demyelinative conduction block *in vivo*. *Ann. Neurol.*, **25**, 159–65.

150. Kaji, R., Happel, L. and Summer, A.J. (1990) Effect of digitalis on clinical symptoms and conduction variables in patients with multiple sclerosis. *Ann. Neurol.*, **28**, 582–4.

151. Petajan, J.H., Gappmaier, E., White, A.T. *et al.* (1996) Impact of aerobic training on fitness and quality of life in multiple sclerosis. *Ann. Neurol.*, **39**, 432–41.

152. Sundulko, K., Woldanski, A., Baumhefner, R. W. and Tourtellotte, W.W. (1995) Preliminary evaluation of lowering tympanic temperature for the symptomatic treatment of multiple sclerosis. *J. Neurol. Rehab.*, **91**, 205–15.

150. Syndulko, K., Jafari, M., Woldanski, A., Baumhefner, R. and Tourtellotte, W.W. (1995) Effects of temperature in multiple sclerosis: a review of the literature. *J. Neurol. Rehab.*, **10**, 23–34.

INDEX